D0825629

Wellness

Choices for Health and Fitness

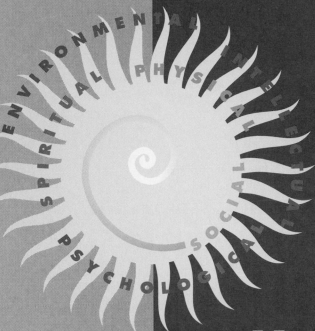

ENVIRONMENTAL
SPIRITUAL PHYSICAL INTELLECTUAL
PSYCHOLOGICAL SOCIAL

Second Edition

Wellness
Choices for Health and Fitness

Rebecca Donatelle
Christine Snow
Anthony Wilcox
Oregon State University

Wadsworth Publishing Company

 An International Thomson Publishing Company

Belmont • Albany • Bonn • Boston • Cincinnati • Detroit • Johannesburg • London • Madrid
Melbourne • Mexico City • New York • Pacific Grove • Paris • Singapore • Tokyo • Toronto • Washington

Sponsoring Editor: *Marianne Taflinger*
Project Development Editor: *James Strandberg*
Marketing Team: *Alicia Barelli/Aaron Eden/Jean Thompson*
Editorial Assistants: *Scott Brearton/Rachael Bruckman*
Production Editor: *Tessa A. McGlasson*
Manuscript Editor: *Patterson Lamb*
Permissions Editor: *The Permissions Group*
Design Editor: *Vernon T. Boes*

Interior and Cover Design: *Delgado Design Inc.*
Interior Illustration: *Delgado Design Inc./Precision Graphics*
Art Editor: *Lisa Torri*
Photo Editor: *Robert J. Western*
Indexer: *Meg McDonnell*
Typesetting: *GTS Graphics*
Cover Printing: *Phoenix Color Corp.*
Printing and Binding: *World Color Corp.*

COPYRIGHT © 1999 by Wadsworth Publishing Company
A division of International Thomson Publishing Inc.

I⊤P The ITP logo is a registered trademark used herein under license.

For more information, contact:

WADSWORTH PUBLISHING COMPANY
10 Davis Drive
Belmont, CA 94002
USA

International Thomson Publishing Europe
Berkshire House 168-173
High Holborn
London WC1V 7AA
England

Thomas Nelson Australia
102 Dodds Street
South Melbourne, 3205
Victoria, Australia

Nelson Canada
1120 Birchmount Road
Scarborough, Ontario
Canada M1K 5G4

International Thomson Editores
Seneca 53
Col. Polanco
México, D. F., México
C. P. 11560

International Thomson Publishing GmbH
Königswinterer Strasse 418
53227 Bonn
Germany

International Thomson Publishing Asia
60 Albert Street #15-01
Albert Complex
Singapore 189969

International Thomson Publishing Japan
Hirakawacho Kyowa Building, 3F
2-2-1 Hirakawacho
Chiyoda-ku, Tokyo 102
Japan

All rights reserved. No part of this work may be reproduced, stored in a retrieval system, or transcribed, in any form or by any means—electronic, mechanical, photocopying, recording, or otherwise—without the prior written permission of the publisher, Wadsworth Publishing Company, Belmont, California, 94002.

Printed in the United States of America

10 9 8 7 6 5 4 3 2 1

Library of Congress Cataloging-in-Publication Data
Donatelle, Rebecca J., [date]
    Wellness : choices for health and fitness / Rebecca Donatelle,
Christine Snow, Anthony Wilcox. — 2nd ed.
      p. cm.
    Includes bibliographical references and index.
    ISBN 0-534-34836-X
    1. Health. 2. Physical fitness. I. Snow, Christine,
[date] II. Wilcox, Anthony Robert, [date] . III. Title.
613--dc21

98-26394
CIP
AC

Brief Contents

Contents

Features

Preface

To The Student

Wellness: Choices for Health & Fitness may be your required class text-book, but it is intended to be more than that. This book has been written to provide you with the knowledge and skills that will enable you to achieve optimal health.

Wellness is a condition of positive health and fitness, and it is the product of the many choices you make every day. Your wellness is determined by such factors as your level of physical activity, your selection of foods to eat, your ability to manage stress, your capacity to build and maintain satisfying relationships, your ability to avoid abusing substances, and your adoption of safer sex practices. Wellness is achieved by making the right choices, which you can do only if you are aware of different options and strategies and understand all the issues and implications surrounding your decisions.

In this text we offer a comprehensive discussion of the various dimensions of wellness, including such topics as physical fitness, nutrition, psychological well-being, stress management, preventing AIDS and STDs, substance abuse and addictive behaviors, and chronic diseases. Throughout each chapter we offer practical advice for adopting a wellness lifestyle that takes into account individual interests, goals, and life situations. Our goal: to encourage you to make healthy choices which will lead to a lifetime of wellness!

To the Instructor

Wellness is intended for use in courses in which equal weight is given to the physical fitness and health components of wellness. This book may also be used in fitness courses since there is thorough treatment of the components of physical fitness, and extensive laboratory activities in the fitness chapters of the book. The authors—Rebecca Donatelle, Ph.D., Christine Snow, Ph.D., and Anthony Wilcox, Ph.D.—have combined their teaching, writing, and subject area expertise to bring you a balanced approach to wellness. Snow and Wilcox are trained in the exercise and sport sciences, while Donatelle specializes in public health. All three are scientists who have developed and team-taught the wellness course to thousands of students at Oregon State University.

Our key goals in this text are to:

- Provide balanced, in-depth coverage of the dimensions of wellness.

- Offer a range of choices that can be adapted readily to students' lifestyles and that are appropriate for a lifetime of wellness.

- Engage students with a multitude of examples and up-to-date information to make the material both interesting and relevant.

- Provide laboratory experiences that promote application of knowledge for all topic areas and self-assessments in the dimensions of wellness.

- Offer a comprehensive wellness questionnaire for students to evaluate their current status. Specific questions from this tool are woven into the appropriate topic areas so that students can refer to their answers and make choices based upon their responses.

New in the Second Edition

In this second edition of *Wellness,* we have retained the overall chapter organization and the breadth of coverage that have made this book a success. We have **updated every chapter** to reflect newly available information and research, and revised a considerable number of areas to reflect suggestions from colleagues and reviewers. Beyond this updating, we have also worked to strengthen the book's applicability in promoting healthy choices, to build on the well-received pedagogical features, to introduce ways in which aspects of wellness can be enhanced using the Internet, and to improve the overall design of the text to make it more visually vibrant and appealing.

NEW! Sound Decision Making.

A new feature to this edition is an applied feature box, appearing in every chapter, which takes a look at how an individual can change behavior by making the right choices. Building on the Prochaska model of stages of behavior change (this model is discussed in the Sound Decision Making box in Chapter 1), these boxes focus on specific examples germane to the lives of college students—making time in one's schedule to exercise, finding alternatives to a constantly poor diet, dealing with a drinking problem, adopting strategies for reducing stress, and similar scenarios. The first edition of *Wellness* had a strong applications focus, and the Sound Decision Making feature builds on that focus to show models of constructive change appropriate for the topic of every chapter.

Sound Decision Making

STAGES OF BEHAVIOR CHANGE

You have probably noticed that making lasting changes in your habits and behaviors is sometimes difficult. Why is it that some people are successful in maintaining an exercise program or stopping smoking while others struggle less successfully? One possible explanation for success relates to your "readiness" to make a change. Psychologists James Prochaska, John Norcross, and Carlo DiClemente studied individuals who had successfully changed health-related behaviors on their own to see what strategies were most helpful. They found that individuals progressed through distinct *stages of change* on their way to increased health wellness, and that different strategies are effective at different stages.

- At the *precontemplation* stage, you either don't realize that you have a problem, or you deny it. Although you may have heard that a certain behavior is risky, you fail to really acknowledge your own problems and have no intention of changing your habits. In order to move to the next stage, you need to become convinced that there would be benefits to making behavior changes.

- At the *contemplation* stage, you acknowledge that you have a problem and begin to think about doing something about it. You may struggle to understand your problem, what caused it, and why changing your behavior might be worthwhile. To move to the preparation stage, you can think about successful changes you've made in the past and list the short- and long-term benefits of making the change you're contemplating.

- At the *preparation* stage, you are planning to make a behavior change within the next month and are putting together strategies and mobilizing your resources to put your plan into action. To move into the next stage, it may be helpful to make a written plan or contract and to talk with friends and relatives about your plan.

- The *action* stage is the busiest stage and the one that requires the most commitment. You are putting your plan into motion, and changes made at this stage are most likely to be noticed by others. During the action phase, it is important to stick to your plan, use your friends for support, and reward yourself for progress toward your goal.

- After the intense effort of the action stage, you move into the *maintenance* stage. At this point you work to keep up the changes you made and to avoid relapse to old problem behaviors. In some ways, maintenance is a lifelong process.

Although the stages of change represent one popular explanation for behavioral change, it is important to remember that behaviors are extremely complex and have many possible explanations. Your attitudes, beliefs, values, social support, perceived susceptibility for risks, perception of threat, and other factors influence what any of us will do or not do to help ourselves gain in "health" years.

In each chapter of this book the Sound Decision Making feature will focus on how students go through these stages of change in their quest to make decisions that will lead to a lifetime of wellness.

Source: Prochaska, J., J. Norcross, and C. DiClemente. *Changing for Good.* New York: William Morrow, 1994.

NEW! Websites for Wellness. Each chapter now includes a special box called Websites for Wellness. Rather than list several relevant sites appropriate to many chapter topics, each of these new boxes focus instead on one particular site, which the student is encouraged to visit and explore. These have been selected to help promote good decision-making, thus building once again on the applied theme of this text. Topics covered on these sites include improving flexibility, recovering from a sports-related injury, practicing safer sex, and similar health-enhancing strategies. Each of these features ends with a set of critical thinking questions, thus adding another pedagogical element to the text.

Other Significant Changes in the 2nd Edition.

- A new Laboratory 3.3 has been added on YMCA Submaximal Bicycle Ergometer Test for Estimating Maximal Aerobic Capacity.

- Chapter 4 contains a new subsection on Gender Differences in Strength and Response to Training.

- Chapter 5 has been expanded, with additional illustrations of stretching and back-strengthening exercises in Figures 5.3 and 5.8, and the hurdler's stretch now shown as another contraindicated stretch in Figure 5.4.

- Chapter 6 now includes coverage of the new gel ice packs, and new figures have been added to show typical sites of shin splints and plantar fasciitis.

- A new section on The Modern Diet has been added to Chapter 7, with American Eating Habits now a subsection, the three types of vegetarian diets now described, and Food Irradiation discussed.

- New subsections have been added to Chapter 9, including one on Spiritual Health and Wellness.

- Eustress is now discussed and made a key term in Chapter 10, and Road Rage is now covered in expanded material on individual differences in reacting to stressors.

- Chapter 11 now covers substance abuse as well as addictive behaviors and has been reorganized significantly. A new section has been added on Anabolic Steroids, and two new laboratories are included: Laboratory 11.1 on Assessing Your Level of Alcohol Use, and Laboratory 11.3 on Assessing Your Gambling Behavior.

- Chapter 12 on AIDS/STDs has been significantly revised to reflect current information on incidence rates, treatments, and so forth.

- In Chapter 13, new coverage is included on cigar smoking and the health risk this new fad poses, the Prevention of Cancer section has been significantly expanded, and a new section has been added on Advocating for Your Health.

- New Food Composition Tables have been added as Appendix A.

- The Wellness Directory is now Appendix B, and it has been updated to

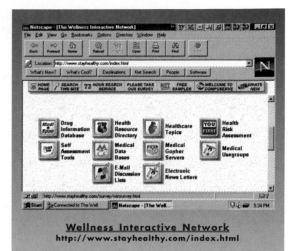

Wellness Interactive Network
http://www.stayhealthy.com/index.html

This wellness megasite includes thousands of Internet resources related to all areas of health and wellness. Users can start by taking a confidential online health risk assessment questionnaire that will pinpoint areas where behavior change can minimize current health risks. Additional assessment tools are available for cardiovascular health, weight control, and nutrition. There is a searchable database of drug information and links to sites on a wide variety of health and wellness topics, including sites on women's health, mental health, fitness, and aging. In addition, users can search medical information databases for additional information on specific diseases, subscribe to electronic newsletters on a variety of topics, or learn about mailing lists and newsgroups related to wellness.

Critical thinking: This Web site contains some advertisements. Do you think the ads change the value of the site? Can you think of any ways that the group that maintains this site might be influenced by its advertisers?
Source: From Avalon Group, Inc. 1998.

provide current information, including Web addresses for those organizations that have their own websites.

Retained Features

Reviewers and colleagues were strongly supportive of the special features included in our first edition, so we have retained them, revised several, and have now included them across all chapters.

Myths and Controversies. This feature addresses common misconceptions and current controversies about wellness. The new Myths and Controversies for Chapter 2 includes the debate over how much exercise is "enough," while the new one in Chapter 12 explores (and debunks) three prevalent myths about HIV and AIDS.

Do's and Don'ts. This feature lists concise, practical tips on what to do—and what not to do—to achieve optimal health. For example, in Chapter 9, this feature looks at

---

MYTHS & CONTROVERSIES

Myth 1 **Behaviors during the college years don't matter.** In fact, the young adult years are a time when habits are formed that will last a lifetime. If you develop healthy habits like eating well, exercising, managing your level of stress, and drinking alcohol responsibly, they are likely to stay with you for years to come. You'll reap the benefits of your healthy behaviors now as a greater sense of well-being, and as you grow older, you'll be rewarded with a reduced risk of heart disease, some form of cancer, and other diseases. On the other hand, if you spend your college years eating poorly, being sedentary, or drinking too much alcohol, you will feel the consequences both now and in the future. The good news is that the college years are a great time to establish healthy habits and change unhealthy ones. Taking this course is a great first step.

Myth 2 **Genetics (or luck) determine who will get a disease.** Actually, lifestyle factors play a major role in all of the five leading causes of death in the United States. It is true that your heredity may put you at higher risk for getting certain diseases, but you may reduce your risk and/or have many more years of health through a healthy lifestyle. For example, if you have a genetic predisposition to diabetes, you may delay its onset for decades through diet and exercise. Likewise, heart disease, the leading killer of Americans, is influenced by diet, activity level, smoking, alcohol consumption, and stress management factors. Even if you have a family history of heart disease, you can tip the balance in favor of good health by eating well, exercising regularly, not smoking, and controlling your stress. Similarly, you can greatly reduce your risk of cancer, stroke, lung disease, and deadly injury by making changes in your behavior.

Source: U.S. Department of Health and Human Services, National Center for Health Statistics, 1997.

A · WELLNESS · LIFESTYLE

Do

▲ Learn all you can about the benefits of a wellness lifestyle.

▲ Ask yourself what you want for yourself now and in the future.

▲ Take responsibility for your own health and happiness in life.

▲ Start with small changes to boost your self-confidence.

▲ Enlist the help of others: friends, relatives, co-workers, and health professionals.

▲ Set specific goals and reward yourself when you reach them.

▲ Visualize yourself achieving your goals and enjoying the benefit.

▲ Think critically about health-related information.

▲ Keep trying if you slip up.

Don't

▼ Try to tackle all your problems at once.

▼ Start a behavior change program at a time of great stress.

▼ Procrastinate—pick a date and stick with it.

▼ Ignore outside sources of help. Friends, teachers, campus resources, and outside organizations can all be tremendous resources.

▼ Get down on yourself if you have difficulty with some aspect of behavior change. Almost everyone struggles to make changes, and many people have to try more than once before they are successful.

▼ Give up—try other strategies if one doesn't seem to work.

concrete ways to improve one's psychological well-being and lists harmful traps to avoid.

Stats-at-a-Glance. Up-to-date and thought-provoking data are summarized in these bulleted lists, reflective of such issues as Muscular Fitness and Aging in Chapter 4, and Current Eating Patterns of Americans in Chapter 7.

Lifestyle Choices: Plan for Action. At the end of every chapter are worksheets to encourage students to translate what they have read into practical goals, and to help them establish their own self-assessment devices to measure progress in meeting their goals.

One Student's View. In each chapter opener, a relevant comment from a real student is included to emphasize the book's real-life orientation and to offer a point of view. Two-thirds of the selections are new to this edition, having been solicited from students at several schools around the country who were taking a wellness course.

Pedagogy

Chapter Objectives. Each chapter opens with a list of learning objectives, focusing on the most important aspects students should master.

Running Glossary. Key terms are boldfaced in the text and defined in the margin on the same page as they appear.

Chapter Summary. Each chapter concludes with a brief prose summary, followed by a bulleted listing of key points.

Laboratories. Twelve chapters include one or more laboratories following the references, and these are meant to be used either in labs accompanying these courses, or for students' own use in assessing themselves and helping them realize individual goals. The pages are perforated so that worksheets can be turned in as assignments.

Topic Coverage

The second edition of this text offers thirteen chapters which provide the reader with thorough coverage of the basic components of wellness, up-to-date information, and a host of strategies for implementing healthy lifestyle changes.

Chapter 1—Lifestyle Choices for Wellness. Provides an overview of key concepts related to individual wellness. Health, wellness, health promotion, and disease prevention are discussed in relation to lifestyle choices. The laboratory following Chapter 1 is a comprehensive wellness inventory.

Chapter 2—Becoming Physically Fit. Explains the principles behind the training effects from exercise and the ways in which muscles generate energy during exercise. These principles are applied to developing a personal exercise program.

Chapter 3—Achieving Aerobic Fitness. Covers the structure of the cardiovascular system, the basic concepts of aerobic fitness, and the principles for designing an aerobic fitness program to meet personal needs. The labs associated with this chapter teach students how to take their heart rate and help them to assess their level of aerobic fitness.

Chapter 4—Building Muscular Strength and Endurance. Discusses the basics of muscular fitness and its benefits and provides the necessary information on how to develop a personal program of muscular fitness. Labs for assessing muscular strength and endurance are included.

Chapter 5—Flexibility and Back Health. Addresses the importance of including flexibility and back health exercises in a fitness program and in daily activities. A comprehensive program for back health and selected stretching exercises to improve range of motion are included.

Chapter 6—Exercise-Related Injuries (by Rod Harter, Ph.D., A.T.C.). Provides a thorough and comprehensive overview of exercise-related problems—information that will help students prevent injuries and accidents.

Chapter 7—The Wellness Diet. Covers the basics of nutrition and presents a strategy for dietary planning to ensure adequate intake of carbohydrates, fats, protein, water, vitamins, and minerals to meet daily needs. Food intake and energy expenditure in relation to weight management are discussed.

Chapter 8—Body Composition and Managing Your Weight. Describes the functions of fat in the body, the methods of measuring body fat, and criteria for evaluating what level of fatness may present a health risk. The chapter also examines the physiological controls of body fat and ways to maintain an appropriate body fat level.

Chapter 9—Being Psychologically Well. Discusses families, social and cultural experiences, genetics, social services, and other factors in relation to psychological well-being. Active thinking about personal psychosocial wellness is emphasized, and suggestions are offered for optimizing emotion, spiritual, and psychological health.

Chapter 10—Stress and Well-Being: Facing Life's Challenges. Introduces students to the complex interaction between psychological perception, physical challenges, and health-damaging physiological responses. Factors that contribute to individual stress are discussed, as well as the actions that individuals can take in avoiding, coping with, and managing the inevitable stresses and strains of living.

Chapter 11—Addictive Behavior: Substance Use and Abuse (by Pat Ketcham, M.A.). Students are provided with information concerning risk factors and warning signs of substance abuse and addictive behaviors. Strategies for making lifestyle choices to prevent or reduce the negative impact of substance abuse and addiction, and to promote enhanced wellness, are highlighted.

Chapter 12—AIDS and STDs. Provides an overview of the major risks from sexually transmitted diseases and outlines ways to prevent their transmission. Risks associated with sexual activities are discussed, and personal responsibility for sexual behavior is emphasized.

Chapter 13—Chronic Diseases. Discusses the major chronic diseases, the risk factors associated with them, and lifestyle modifications that can be made to reduce risk. The accompanying laboratories help students develop a risk factor profile.

A Complete Teaching Package

For your convenience, a complete instructional package featuring high-quality supplements is available to complement *Wellness.*

Instructor's Guide and Testbank. Written by Janet M. Shaw of the University of Utah and Peggy Pedersen of Northern Illinois University, the Instructor's Guide for *Wellness* 2e offers ideas for presenting healthier lifestyle choices to students and for helping students to understand how these choices fit into a comprehensive view of wellness. Included in the Instructor's Guide are lecture outlines with learning objectives, review questions, class discussions and activities, teaching hints, Trigger Video tie-ins, transparency masters, and strategies to promote independent thinking. The written testbank is included as part of the Instructor's Guide, and provides test items in multiple-choice, scenario-based, and true-false formats.

Thomson World Class Testing Tool. A computerized testbank is also available in Macintosh and Windows formats. This fully integrated suite of test creation, delivery, and classroom management tools includes World Class Test, Test Online, and World Class Management software. World Class Testing Tools allows professors to deliver tests via print, floppy, hard drive, LAN, or Internet. With these tools, professors can create cross-platform exam files from publisher files or existing WESTest 3.2 test banks, edit questions, create questions, and provide their own feedback to objective test questions—enabling the system to work as a tutorial or an examination. In addition, professors can generate questions algorithmically and create tests that include multiple-choice, true/false, or matching questions. Professors can also track the progress of an entire class or an individual student. Testing and tutorial results can be integrated into the class management tool which offers scoring, gradebook, and reporting capabilities.

Transparency Acetates. Four-color transparency acetates of over forty figures linked to the text are available in a package for use on traditional overhead projectors. These color transparencies are also available as a CD-ROM of electronic transparencies, for use in the Acrobat presentation format (the CD-ROM includes Acrobat Reader, which requires a one-time download).The CD-ROM features a complete set of four-color transparencies, and instructions for using the numbers Acrobat features—such as how to print your own transparency masters.

Diet Analysis Plus Software (Windows and Macintosh). This user-friendly software program helps simplify the process of diet analysis. It contains comprehensive information on nutrients in foods and energy expenditures from exercise. Diet Analysis Plus calculates the Recommended Dietary Allowances, analyzes daily intakes, identifies diet deficiencies and excesses, calculates comparisons and ratios, helps locate alternative foods, and helps plan an exercise program, as well as a weight-gain or -loss program. The database has been updated to include more foods common to college students as well as a comprehensive list of microwaveable foods.

Dine Healthy Software (Windows and Macintosh). Dine Healthy teaches you to eat sensibly, eliminating the need for crash diets. Clear, concise bar charts show how well you eat, with recommendations for food-choice changes. An exercise section enables you to track caloric expenditures and calculate ideal caloric intakes. A recipe analysis feature suggests how your favorite recipes can be improved nutritionally. An expandable database lets you add new food products as they come into the marketplace. Each adopting department is eligible to receive one copy of this powerful personal trainer for nutrition and fitness.

Nutrition Interactive CD-ROM by Frances Sienkiewicz Sizer, Sharon Rady Rolfes, Linda Kelly Debruyne, and Kathy Beerman. Explore nutritional concepts as never before with this CD-ROM for Windows and Macintosh computers. With *Nutrition Interactive,* you can do more than read about a topic—you can read, watch, listen, and interact with it. It covers everything from heart disease to eating disorders. The CD includes more than 100 fully interactive exercises plus a searchable glossary containing over 650 terms. You'll be able to visualize difficult concepts, manipulate variables, analyze data, and receive immediate feedback as you work through each exercise.

Trigger Video Series. During the first year, adopting departments will receive two video tapes containing a series of short "trigger" videos. These topical videos complement the text and help enliven the lecture presentation.

Trigger Video: Fitness. This 30-minute video is designed to promote— or "trigger"—classroom discussion on a variety of topics related to physical fitness. The segments include: Fitness in the Schools, Activity versus Sports Skills, How Much Exercise is Enough?, The Importance of Variety, and Exercise and Osteoporosis.

Trigger Video: Stress. This 60-minute video contains five 8-10 minute long video clips, followed by questions for discussion. Segments include: Running Out of Time, Post-Traumatic Stress Disorder, Stress and Immunity, the Stress Response, and Coping with Stress: Social Support, Personal Perception and Relaxation. An Instructor's Guide includes a description of the content of each video clip, student objectives, key words defined before watching the video, and possible responses to questions posed to students at the completion of the video. The guide also provides helpful hints on how to use the Stress video segments in class.

Other Videos. We feature over 20 additional videos covering eating and weight management, addiction, fitness, and AIDS/STDs. All videos have been carefully reviewed by a panel of health and fitness specialists to confirm their currency, accuracy, and appeal to today's students.

Wadsworth Health Study Center. The Wadsworth Health Study Center is a dedicated site on the World Wide Web for the use of adopters of *Wellness*. Some areas are password protected and available only to faculty and students using this textbook. Contact your local sales representative or Wadsworth Marketing at 1-800-426-2063. To preview the Web site, point your browser to http://healthstudy.wadsworth.com/ and explore.

Personal Health Interactive CD-ROM by Arthur J. Kohn and Wendy Kohn. This powerful teaching and learning tool on CD-ROM for Macintosh and Windows features a comprehensive "Wellness Clinic" that allows students to monitor and improve their daily health behaviors. Students can also access an interactive mix of activities, including Internet-based projects, animations, study pages, surveys, and video clips. The CD-ROM's "CourseWeaver" program allows professors to prepare professional multimedia lectures quickly and easily, and to export multimedia elements to popular presentation packages, such as PowerPoint, Persuasion, and Astound.

Acknowledgments

Many people contributed to the development of this text. First, we want to single out our two contributing authors: Rod Harter, who again provided the expertise required for a comprehensive chapter on exercise-related accidents and injuries, and Pat Ketcham, who drew on her experience with thousands of college students to revise her chapter on substance abuse and addictive behaviors.

This book was originally developed at Benjamin Cummings, and we wish to thank again Pat Coryell, Grace Wong, Jude Berman, Mary Johnson, Shelley Parlante, Donna Linden, Donna Kalal, and Cecelia Mills, as well as Vicki Ebbeck. At Brooks/Cole, which inherited the book from Benjamin Cummings, we thank Marianne Taflinger, Heather Dutton, Jim Strandberg, Tessa McGlasson, Vernon Boes, May Clark, Alicia Barelli, Jennifer Wilkinson, Megan Rundel, Lisa Torri, and Bob Western, and the many others responsible for making this second edition—and its supplements—a reality. We are particularly proud of the new look of our book: much appreciation to Delgado Design in New York City for creating such an appealing layout.

We are especially grateful to the many reviewers, consultants, and focus group members whose comments are reflected in our chapters.

For the second edition, we thank the following reviewers:

Ronnie D. Carda	University of Wisconsin
Dan Connaughton	University of Florida
Steven M. Haynie	College of William and Mary
Lisa Larkin	Marian College
Linda L. Rankin	Idaho State University
Stephen W. Sansone	Chemeketa Community College
Margaret K. Snooks	University of Houston, Clear Lake
Carl Stockton	Radford University

And, our thanks once again to those who assisted us with the first edition:

Kim Barrett	University of Florida
Don Bergey	Wake Forest University

Craig Broeder   East Tennessee State University
Mitchell Collins   Kennesaw State College
Bob Crooks   Portland Community College
Bob Cross   Salisbury State University
Cindy Hanawalt   University of Iowa
Craig Huddy   University of Georgia
Gary Hunter   University of Alabama-Birmingham
Jimmy Jones   Henderson State University
Patricia Kenney   Pennsylvania State University
Deborah McDonald   New Mexico State University
Robert Moffett   Florida State University
J. Dirk Nelson   Missouri Southern State College
Gary Oden   Sam Houston State University
Jacalyn Robert   Texas Tech University
Marge Robertson   Manatee Community College
Rob Shurrer   Black Hills State University
Michael Teague   University of Iowa
Luke Thomas   Northeast Louisiana University
Paul Todd   Polk Community College

To your wellness!!

Rebecca Donatelle

Christine Snow

Anthony Wilcox

Wellness

Choices for Health and Fitness

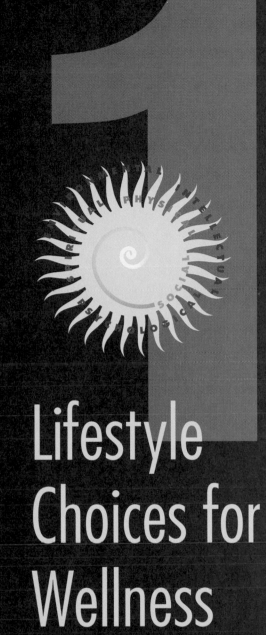

chapter 1

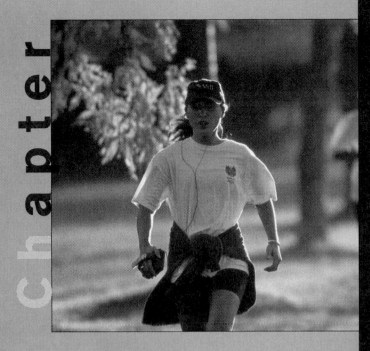

Lifestyle Choices for Wellness

One Student's View

To me, wellness is the key that will enable anyone to utilize all of their given potential in life. Being in a state of wellness allows the body, mind, and soul to be in perfect harmony. By respecting your body and taking care of it properly, life will become easier and more enjoyable.

—Sajjad Nasir

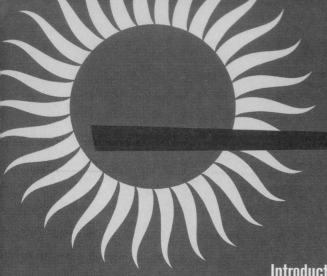

Introduction

"Use it or lose it." "Just do it." "Just say no." "If you have your health, you have everything." Sound familiar? Statements like these have become part of our American vocabulary. Not a day goes by that we don't read, hear, or talk about the latest ways to lose weight, reduce stress, and improve ourselves in some way. We are exhorted to be strong, exercise our willpower and our bodies, avoid harmful substances, fling ourselves into the social arena, and "be all that we can be." Our society seems to have "turned on" to the importance of health and the idea that we can and should make a difference in our personal health and well-being.

Hype aside, there are some very good reasons Americans need to be concerned about the lives they lead. In the United States, the leading causes of death and disability are due, in part, to our unhealthy behaviors (see Table 1.1). We are killing ourselves by what we eat, what we do or don't do, how we interact with others, and how we abuse the environment in which we live. Clearly, our lifestyles and healthstyles have a decided impact on our own health. They can also have an impact on our loved ones, on our health care system, and on the global burden of disease and disability (Murray & Lopez, 1996). Because of this far-reaching effect, we should consider the impact of our choices not only on ourselves as individuals, but also on society at large and on the health/wellness of the planet. Although no one can be sure of the actual extent to which we can prevent illness or prolong our lives by altering our lifestyles, we do know that by acting responsibly to improve selected areas of our health, we can live longer and have healthier, higher quality years of life. In contrast, by making choices that lead away from health/wellness, we contribute to escalating health care

Objectives

After reading this chapter, you should be able to

- **Define health and wellness and explain how they differ**

- **Identify and define the six dimensions of health**

- **Explain how wellness can be viewed on a continuum**

- **Discuss individual and societal influences on wellness**

- **Describe the benefits of a comprehensive wellness lifestyle**

- **Understand the basic elements of successful behavioral change and how your behavior changes may impact your health status, now and in the future**

- **Begin thinking about your own lifestyle choices for wellness and the actions you might take to reduce your risks and improve your health**

costs, reduce the number of our productive years, and contribute to the growing pressures on our health care/treatment systems and the resources that are available to maintain health.

Many Americans have begun to take action to improve their own health, but the majority still remain on the sidelines. For example, the recent Surgeon General's Report on Physical Activity, along with other health-related national documents, shows us to be largely a society of couch potatoes—people who find regular exercise difficult to maintain. It's easy to understand why. The slogans sound good, but putting them into practice is another matter. Many people view problems like heart disease, high blood pressure, and diabetes as things that happen only to someone else or to older people. "What does it have to do with me, and what could I do about it anyway?" they may ask. Often, they view disease as something that somehow won't touch them, or will come many years from where they are now. The immediate risks to them are minimal and they act as if they have their entire lifetimes to practice wellness. Some people are overwhelmed by the barrage of conflicting messages about what is good for them and what is bad. How can we know which "experts" to believe, and where can we obtain accurate and reliable information? Often, people would like to develop healthier habits but just don't know how to start.

You've probably had similar concerns yourself. How healthy are you? What are the greatest threats to your health? What difference might it make if today you began to change your lifestyle in certain ways? These questions are common, but you are a unique individual, and you must find the answers that are right for you. This text is designed to help you understand how the choices you make and the way you live your life can make a difference in the quality of your life—and in how long you live. In an indirect way, what you read in this text and discuss in classes should also help you understand why improving your health is not just good for you, but is good for society as a whole. Before beginning these discussions, it is important for us to explain what being healthy or well really means and to provide a blueprint for making decisions designed to reduce your health risks and improve your overall well-being.

Rather than telling you to "just do it" for the sake of doing it, or because everyone else is doing it, we will explain the scientific basis for asserting that certain lifestyle changes are as important to you today as they will be 20 or 30 or 50 years from now. We hope that once the foundations of health and wellness have been explained, and possible options for your own improvement have been explored, you will be able to make lasting lifestyle choices for optimum health that will become a part of your typical daily routine. Rather than "just doing it," these activities will become an inherent part of "what you do."

TABLE 1.1

Leading Causes of Death in the United States by Age*

RANK	ALL AGES	1–4	5–14	15–24	25–44	45–65	65+
1	Heart diseases (880.0)	Accidents and adverse effects (40.6)	Accidents and adverse effects (22.5)	Accidents and adverse effects (95.3)	Human immuno-deficiency virus (36.9)	Malignant neoplasms (253.0)	Heart diseases (5052.8)
2	Malignant neoplasms (204.9)	Congenital anomalies (4.4)	Malignant neoplasms (2.7)	Homicide and legal intervention (20.3)	Accidents and adverse effects (33.2)	Heart diseases (196.8)	Malignant neoplasms (1136.6)
3	Cerebro-vascular diseases (60.1)	Malignant neoplasms (3.1)	Homicide and legal intervention (1.5)	Suicide (13.3)	Malignant neoplasms (26.4)	Accident and adverse effects (35.5)	Cerebro-vascular diseases (413.8)
4	Chronic obstructive pulmonary disease (39.2)	Homicide and legal intervention (2.9)	Congenital anomalies (1.2)	Malignant neoplasms (4.6)	Heart diseases (20.5)	Cerebro-vascular diseases (29.1)	Chronic obstructive pulmonary disease (263.9)
5	Accidents and adverse effects (35.5)	Heart diseases (1.6)	Suicide (0.9)	Heart diseases (2.9)	Suicide (15.3)	Chronic obstructive pulmonary disease (24.4)	Pneumonia and influenza (221.6)
6	Pneumonia and influenza (31.6)	Human immuno-deficiency virus (1.4)	Heart diseases (0.8)	Human immuno-deficiency virus (1.7)	Homicide and legal intervention (12.3)	Diabetes mellitus (23.3)	Diabetes mellitus (132.6)
7	Diabetes mellitus (22.6)	Pneumonia and influenza (1.0)	Human immuno-deficiency virus (0.5)	Congenital anomalies (1.3)	Chronic liver disease (5.2)	Chronic liver disease (20.3)	Accidents and adverse effects (64.0)
8	Human immuno-deficiency virus (16.4)	Conditions of perinatal period (0.6)	Conditions of perinatal period (0.4)	Conditions of perinatal period (0.7)	Cerebro-vascular disease (4.2)	Human immuno-deficiency virus (20.1)	Alzheimer's disease (60.3)
9	Suicide (11.9)	Septicemia (0.4)	Pneumonia and influenza (0.3)	Pneumonia and influenza (0.6)	Diabetes mellitus (2.9)	Suicide (14.1)	Nephritis-related problems (60.2)
10	Chronic liver disease (9.6)	Cerebro-vascular disease (0.4)	Benign neoplasms and neoplasms of uncertain behavior (0.3)	Cerebro-vascular disease (0.5)	Pneumonia and influenza (2.5)	Pneumonia and influenza (10.6)	Septicemia (50.4)

*Numbers in parentheses are rates per 100,000 population

Source: Anderson, R. N., K. D. Kochenek, and S. L. Murphy. Report of Final Mortality Statistics, 1995. *Monthly Vital Statistics Report,* 45(11), 1997.

Health and Wellness Defined

Today, the terms *health* and *wellness* are often used interchangeably, but their meanings differ in subtle but important ways.

Health

The definition of **health** has evolved over the years, from early notions of health as being synonymous with hygiene and sanitation, to health as the absence of disease, to a more currently accepted definition provided by the World Health Organization in the 1940s—of health as "the state of complete physical, mental, and social well-being; not merely the absence of disease" (WHO, 1947).

Definitions of health have expanded significantly over the years. For example, Shirreffs described health as "a quality of life, involving social, mental, and biological fitness on the part of the individual, which results from adaptations to the environment." Renee Dubois, a noted scientist, has stated, "Measure your health by your sympathy with morning and spring," implying that there is more to health than just the physical or psychological elements. Currently, most people would describe health as being multidimensional, including many different components and encompassing many different aspects of life. Today, health is also ever-changing, implying that you can influence your health status either positively or negatively on an ever-changing basis. Thus, getting there may be only half the struggle. Maintaining good health must be part of an ongoing process involving many different components. These components typically include the following:

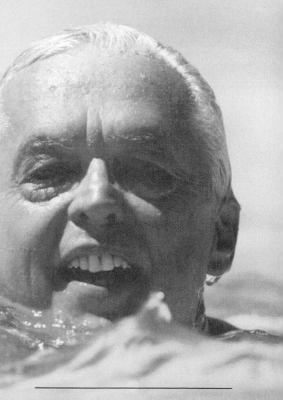

- *Social health.* The process of creating and maintaining healthy relationships through the choices we make. The ability to interact well with people and to have satisfying interpersonal relationships is important to social health.

- *Physical health.* The process of making choices to create a flexible, cardiovascularly fit, energetic, strong body, one that is able to perform daily tasks without undue fatigue. The choices you make regarding exercise, nutrition, rest, stress management, drug use, injury prevention, disease avoidance, and appropriate treatment for illness and disease all influence your physical health.

- *Psychological health.* The process of accepting your worth and the worth of others; creating, recognizing, and expressing your feelings in an appropriate way; and practicing positive "self-talk" designed to keep you "up" rather than focusing on negative aspects of life.

- *Intellectual health.* The process of using your mind to create a greater understanding and appreciation of yourself, others, and your environment. Intellectual health involves the ability to learn and to think rationally.

- *Environmental health.* The process of making choices that will contribute to sustaining or improving the quality of the environment for current and future generations.

- *Spiritual health.* The process of creating and discovering meaning and purpose in life, recognizing one's place in the greater scheme of existence and demonstrating values through behaviors. (See Figure 1.1.)

health quality of life, involving social, physical, psychological, intellectual, environmental, and spiritual well-being

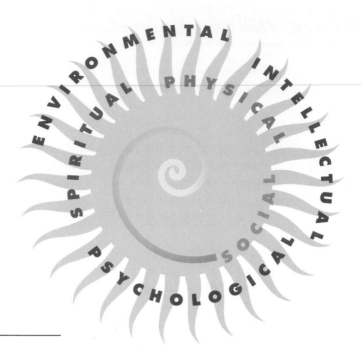

Figure 1.1

Wellness has six key components.

Over the years, people have chosen to focus on one or another component of health, most probably based on their own notions of being "healthy." For example, people who think of health as the absence of disease, illness, or injury will focus their efforts to improve health on the physical aspects of the body: exercising regularly, having regular physical examinations, wearing safety belts, eating healthy foods, and so on. People for whom the intellectual, social, and psychological components of health are most important may aim their health improvement efforts at deriving satisfaction from life rather than improving the physical body. Although each group of people may be making progress toward achieving health, this focus on only one component may actually cause problems. For example, if you quit smoking, take up jogging, and lose weight, these changes would be considered an improvement in your health. However, if the jogging takes time away from your studies or social life, you may find that instead of feeling good about yourself, you feel unhappy or make others unhappy if you shirk your responsibilities. As this example suggests, although physical fitness is an essential component of overall health, social and psychological components should not be ignored. Balance is key to your health planning efforts.

Many health professionals have long understood that health is multifaceted, but getting other people to understand the importance of all of the components has been very difficult. The idea of health as simply a lack of illness has persisted in spite of recent efforts to educate the public otherwise.

Health Promotion. One of two terms that have emerged in our collective efforts to better understand what health means, **health promotion** is defined as any combination of educational, organizational, economic, and environmental supports for behaviors that are conducive to health. It has also been called the art and science of helping people change their lifestyles to move toward a state of optimal health and wellness. Health promotion literature once focused almost entirely on interventions designed to influence individual risk taking directly—behavior such as smoking, drinking, weight con-

health promotion any combination of educational, organizational, economic, and environmental supports for behaviors that are conducive to health

trol, fitness, and so on; now it has begun to acknowledge that individual choices toward positive health change have the best chance to succeed when they are combined with social, environmental, organizational, and policy supports. For example, people will be more likely to choose not to smoke in areas where legislative measures prohibit smoking in public places. Similarly, the decision to not drink and drive is most likely to occur in areas where laws severely penalize offenders.

Disease Prevention. The second term related to our improved understanding of what health means is **disease prevention,** which refers to the process by which we individually and collectively attempt to reduce the occurrence and severity of various diseases. The virtual elimination of some infectious diseases like polio, for example, has been among the greatest public health successes of past years. Major priorities for the nation's current effort to achieve optimal health have been identified as personal responsibility and enlightened behavior by everyone. One such example of an area targeted for disease prevention relates to tobacco usage in the United States. Tobacco alone is estimated to contribute billions of dollars to overall health care costs each year in the form of tobacco-related diseases. When factors such as time lost from work because of tobacco-related respiratory illnesses, reduced productivity due to lung impairment, and other expenses are added to this amount, the costs are staggering.

Based on the efforts of many health organizations, government agencies, policymakers, and individuals, the United States developed a set of guidelines for the nation that described how we might best achieve health and wellness for all. These Objectives for the Nation provided a useful overview of where we needed to be by the year 2000. Unfortunately, we are nearly at the deadline for achieving many of these goals, yet we have a long way to go before reaching a number of them. Highlights from this document are included in Table 1.2.

Wellness

Rather than focusing only on achieving a state of health or on isolated components of health, some health professionals have preferred to focus on "good" or "excellent" health and the challenge of attempting to achieve a high level of physical, intellectual, psychological, environmental, social, and spiritual well-being. In the late 1960s and the 1970s, Dunn first used the term *wellness* in his writings about individual attempts to achieve optimum health. He defined **wellness** as the active process of becoming aware of and making choices to create a healthier life, in all of life's dimensions. Wellness describes a lifestyle in which the physical, social, intellectual, psychological, spiritual, and environmental components of health are integrated. The person committed to wellness is continually striving to achieve the optimum level of health within the framework of his or her own limitations and potential.

Well individuals take an honest look at their own capabilities and limitations and attempt to change those negative factors in life that are within their power to change. Examples of wellness behavior include the following:

■ Exercising aerobically at least three times per week and engaging in other forms of moderate exercise on a daily basis; keeping moving whenever possible

disease prevention process by which we individually and collectively attempt to reduce the occurrence and severity of various diseases

wellness active process of becoming aware of and making choices to create a healthier lifestyle, in all of life's dimensions

- Not smoking
- Limiting the consumption of alcohol to no more than two drinks per day and seven drinks per week
- Taking actions to preserve the environment
- Eating wholesome, nutritious foods
- Reducing caffeine intake
- Practicing safer sex
- Taking time to help others who are less fortunate
- Assessing the stressors in your life and taking action to reduce your stress levels
- Avoiding inappropriately hostile or aggressive behavior or negative situations
- Being an advocate for health-oriented policies and programs
- Balancing work with social and other activities; taking time for yourself

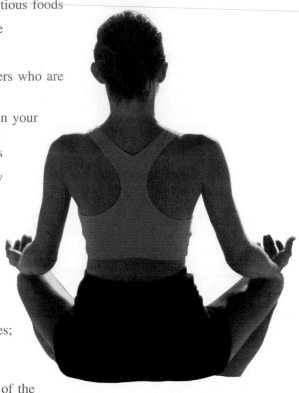

A well person tries to achieve a *balance* in each of the wellness dimensions while also trying to achieve a *positive wellness* position on an imaginary continuum (see Figure 1.2). This person also recognizes that many wellness factors are not totally within the sphere of individual decision making and tries to contribute to overall social policy and community- or system-wide changes. Many people believe that high levels of wellness can best be achieved through adopting a *holistic* approach in which the interaction and positive balance among the mind, body, and spirit are emphasized.

Characteristics of a Wellness Lifestyle

Our outlook on life, our relationships with others, our general appreciation of the world around us, and our respect for the well-being of others are all major elements of a wellness lifestyle. If you are living a wellness lifestyle, you are improving your wellness level, consciously acting to be tolerant of others who are different from you, trying to block negative thoughts and focus on the positive aspects of a situation, and seeking enjoyment in the many things that you do each day. Sometimes these wellness behaviors are small, seemingly incidental steps that you may take to change your thinking or to make an extra effort to do something that brings enjoyment to someone else. Other times, wellness behaviors may involve major shifts in your behaviors, such as cutting fat out of your evening meal or deciding to go for

TABLE 1.2

Health Objectives: Blueprint for the Rest of the Century

The following objectives are where officials from the Office of Disease Prevention and Health Promotion say we should be by the year 2000.

■ No more than one in five adults and less than 15% of teenagers should be overweight.

■ More than 90% of adults should know the risk factors for cardiovascular disease that can be changed (high blood pressure, high blood cholesterol, smoking, and obesity).

■ At least 90% of adults should have had their blood pressure checked in the past 2 years and know what it is.

■ At least one-half of all households should purchase foods low in sodium, prepare foods without salt, and not add salt at the table.

■ More than three-quarters of overweight people age 12 or older should adopt weight loss plans combining diet and exercise.

■ Blood cholesterol of adults over age 20 should be no higher than 200, and more than half of the adults should know that it should be less than 200.

■ Three-quarters of the population should know that saturated fat—the kind found in animal products—raises blood cholesterol. Three-quarters should also know what foods are high in fat, saturated fat, sodium, cholesterol, calories, calcium, and fiber.

■ At least four out of five packaged foods should have nutritional labeling, and two out of five fresh and carry-out foods should have similar labeling.

■ At least 9 out of 10 adults should have had their blood cholesterol checked in the past 5 years. As of 1988, only 59% had ever done so.

■ At least 45% of children in grades 1–12 should participate in daily physical education classes.

■ Nearly two-thirds of those age 6 or older should participate in moderate exercise three or more times per week for 20 minutes or more per session. Nearly one-third of teenagers and adults should participate in vigorous exercise for lungs and heart at least three times per week, 20 minutes per session.

■ One in five adults over age 65 should participate in vigorous heart- and lung-strengthening exercise at least three times per week, 20 minutes or more per session.

■ At least 95% of people age 13 or older should know how AIDS is transmitted, how to prevent it, and how susceptible they are.

■ At least 9 out of every 10 teenagers and adults should know what safer sex is, what the signs and symptoms of sexually transmitted diseases are, and where they can get help.

■ Less than 15% of adults, and not more than 15% of young people, should smoke. About 30% of the adult population still smokes.

■ All tobacco product packages and advertisements should provide information on all major health effects, including addiction, and should name all ingredients and list the potential harm of smoke.

■ At least 85% of teens should link cigarette smoking with great risk to health and with social disapproval.

■ No more than 5% of adults should have more than two alcoholic drinks a day.

Source: Based on U.S. Department of Health and Human Services. Office of Disease Prevention and Health Promotion, *Healthy People 2000: National Health Promotion and Disease Prevention Objectives.* Boston: Jones & Barlett, 1991.

Figure 1.2
Wellness can be viewed on a
continuum from negative (premature
death) to positive (optimal health).

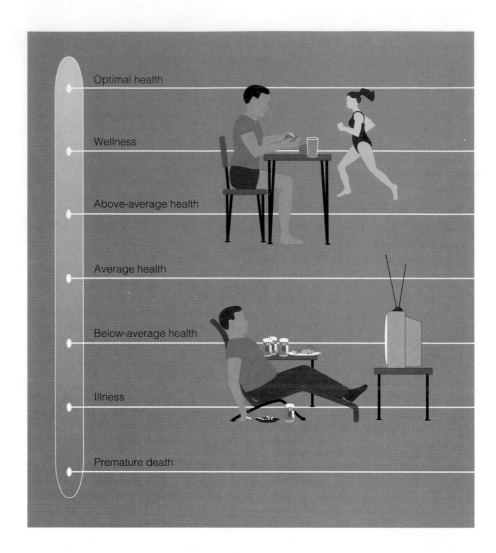

a walk each day. However large or small the action, the sum total of your
daily efforts will add up to an overall improvement in your health actions;
hence, your overall health status may improve. Regardless of age, ability,
intellect, or current physical condition, everyone has something that he or
she can work to improve. Moving in the right direction is more important
than the point at which you may start on the wellness continuum. Today,
health professionals stress the importance of a "mindset for wellness" that
can help you enjoy an enhanced level of well-being. Some of the elements
of this mind-set are described next.

Personal Responsibility

A wellness perspective assumes that rather than adopting a "poor me" attitude and allowing yourself to be consumed by the negative events in your
life, you will take personal responsibility for your actions and the quality
of your own health. You realize, for example, that if your diet is poor, you
don't exercise or get enough rest, and you expose yourself to excessive
stress, you may develop problems. But you also know that if you choose
to take action to improve your lifestyle, your overall wellness will likely
change in a positive direction. For example, suppose you feel that you just
don't have any time for "fun" things in your life. You are resentful because
the weather is great, everyone else seems to be out having fun, and you are

stuck studying for exams. Rather than just feeling sorry for yourself, you need to take a look at your situation. Do you really have *no* time, or could you use your time more effectively? Develop an activity plan for the next day, complete with one hour that is *yours* to do whatever you like. Reward yourself with this *time out* for health/wellness. Take a walk with a friend, read a good book, spend an hour doing something nice for someone else, or just thinking about things that are of concern to you. After you return to work, make note of how you feel. Did the time spent on you help to renew your energy? Were you more productive afterward? Often, such simple time outs from responsibilities may provide the balance that you need to get a good reality check of your priorities. You should always be a key part on your own priority list if you are interested in health and wellness. As a part of personal responsibility, having a positive, optimistic view of life and an interest in taking part in life's pleasures are important elements of wellness. Focusing on being optimistic is much less stressful than continually thinking negative, pessimistic thoughts.

Concern for Others

People who have achieved a high degree of wellness tend to be other-centered rather than self-centered. Well individuals have a strong sense of how "self" fits in the greater environment and act to become more integrated into society at large. They demonstrate a real concern for others by words and actions and through a respectful appreciation for other living things. They are not judgmental and do not impose their own values and attitudes on others. Additionally, although they are tolerant of others' imperfections, they also allow themselves to be less than perfect. They are socially aware, take time to understand health issues, and act in socially responsible ways.

Health Awareness and Sound Decision Making

Achieving a high degree of wellness is not something that just happens. Well individuals are willing to devote a considerable amount of time and energy to developing a sound, factual basis for decision making about wellness. They read, think, and listen, and they choose from various alternatives, based on the best evidence available to them. They value their own health and pay careful attention to signs and signals that something is amiss. When they do have problems, they actively seek the best methods of treatment. Decision making is both a right and a responsibility for these individuals.

Benefits of Wellness

Each dimension of wellness brings its own unique set of benefits that will make the changes it requires worthwhile. Many of the positive choices that you make today will not only yield benefits in the short term, but will contribute to future well-being too. For example, in the physical dimension of wellness, improved cardiovascular fitness may enable you to play a game of volleyball with your friends as well as help you avoid cardiovascular disease later on in your life.

A ◆ WELLNESS ◆ LIFESTYLE

Do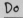

▲ Learn all you can about the benefits of a wellness lifestyle.

▲ Ask yourself what you want for yourself now and in the future.

▲ Take responsibility for your own health and happiness in life.

▲ Start with small changes to boost your self-confidence.

▲ Enlist the help of others: friends, relatives, co-workers, and health professionals.

▲ Set specific goals and reward yourself when you reach them.

▲ Visualize yourself achieving your goals and enjoying the benefit.

▲ Think critically about health-related information.

▲ Keep trying if you slip up.

Don't

▼ Try to tackle all your problems at once.

▼ Start a behavior change program at a time of great stress.

▼ Procrastinate—pick a date and stick with it.

▼ Ignore outside sources of help. Friends, teachers, campus resources, and outside organizations can all be tremendous resources.

▼ Get down on yourself if you have difficulty with some aspect of behavior change. Almost everyone struggles to make changes, and many people have to try more than once before they are successful.

▼ Give up—try other strategies if one doesn't seem to work.

Although a comprehensive listing of benefits derived from a high degree of wellness would fill many pages, the following are among the most important:

■ *Improved cardiovascular efficiency.* Although a stronger heart and circulatory system can benefit you in many ways, the most obvious benefit is your body's improved ability to deliver oxygen-rich blood to all bodily systems with a minimum amount of strain on the cardiovascular system. Improved cardiovascular efficiency also influences cellular response in

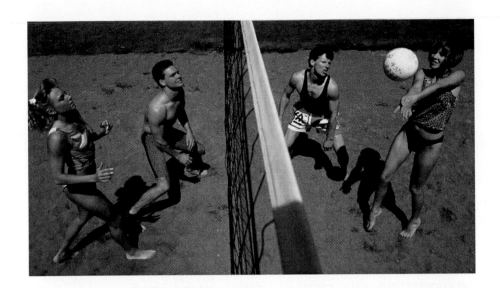

In addition to helping you avoid cardiovascular disease later in life, cardiovascular fitness may enable you to enjoy a spontaneous game of volleyball with your friends.

warding off disease-causing agents and in healing after body systems are damaged, thus resulting in decreased recovery time after injury, illness, or stress.

■ *Increased muscle tone, strength, flexibility, and endurance.* When your muscles are in good shape, you not only function more effectively in your daily activities but you look better and feel better about yourself. Together with the improvement in cardiovascular efficiency, these benefits will give you increased energy for daily functioning, increased stamina, and greater resistance to fatigue.

■ *Reduced risk for injuries.* Strong muscles and supporting structures help reduce your overall risk for pulls, strains, and sprains, particularly in the back and legs.

■ *Improved sense of self-control, self-efficacy, and self-esteem.* By gaining some degree of control over your own health, you may feel better about yourself, feel that you have more strength to control potential difficulties in your life, and believe that you are capable of success. Such feelings and beliefs have the potential for a tremendous carryover effect to other areas of your life.

■ *Improved management and control of stress.* As a well individual, you are more likely to take positive action to control stress and to change perceptions that may lead to unnecessary stress. In addition, you may recover more quickly from a stressful event and find that you have more physical resources available to withstand prolonged stress.

■ *Improved outlook on life.* You will be better equipped to face life's challenges, setbacks, and opportunities and view them as growth experiences rather than as burdens to bear. When you are disappointed in a serious relationship and find yourself alone and lonely, focusing on the positive things you got out of the relationship and the many things you learned in the relationship will help your next relationship be a better one. This attitude is an example of an improved perspective on negative events in your life.

■ *Improved interpersonal relationships.* Although interpersonal relationships are complex, involving essential areas of physical, social, and psychological well-being, if you are striving to maximize your potential in each of these areas, you will be more ready to reach out to others as you begin to feel better about your own health.

■ *Decreased mortality (death) and morbidity (illness) from infectious and chronic diseases.* High levels of physical fitness and a body that is well rested, well fed, and cared for are directly related to a well-functioning immune system. *Host resistance* is a direct result of the health status of your body. Proper exercise and nutrition, stress management, adequate rest, and psychological well-being can all assist the body in its battle to fight off any potential threat. Proper checkups and sound "body awareness" will help you spot problems before they become serious threats.

Influences on Health and Wellness

Clearly, many factors influence how well you are. Some of these are positive—such as a family history with no heart disease—and some are negative—such as a body type that is prone to overweight. Some of these factors you can change or compensate for, and some you can't. A realistic appraisal of the factors that affect your health and wellness—that put you at risk or that constitute barriers to well-being—is an important first step in achieving a wellness lifestyle. Use the Wellness Inventory in Laboratory 1.1 at the end of this chapter to learn more about the factors that influence your health.

Predisposing Factors

Unfortunately, some of us are endowed with genetic traits that appear to put us at risk for significant physical and mental health problems. For example, having diabetic parents or a family history of abnormally high cholesterol levels may mean that you are more likely to experience these problems yourself. In such cases, although you cannot avoid your genetic legacy, you may be able to make lifestyle changes that will reduce or postpone its negative effects. Recognizing how your own family history may affect your health or the health of your children, and taking reasonable actions to reduce your risks, is part of a comprehensive health and wellness program. In addition to biological influences, many other predisposing factors influence your health. These are strongly related to the social and environmental conditions in which you were raised. In so many ways, we are products of our own past.

Perhaps now more than ever, researchers are examining the delicate threads of interpersonal life and those factors that may influence one person to be a loving, well-adjusted individual and another to be a drug abuser or rapist. Clearly, the more positive the social influences, the greater the likelihood that the individual will function on the positive side of the wellness continuum. One such area that has gained widespread attention is the effect that alcoholic parents may ultimately have on their children as the children enter adulthood. Research shows that these individuals are at much greater risk of becoming alcoholic themselves. Often, simply acknowledging the

MYTHS & CONTROVERSIES

Myth 1   **Behaviors during the college years don't matter.** In fact, the young adult years are a time when habits are formed that will last a lifetime. If you develop healthy habits like eating well, exercising, managing your level of stress, and drinking alcohol responsibly, they are likely to stay with you for years to come. You'll reap the benefits of your healthy behaviors now as a greater sense of well-being, and as you grow older, you'll be rewarded with a reduced risk of heart disease, some form of cancer, and other diseases. On the other hand, if you spend your college years eating poorly, being sedentary, or drinking too much alcohol, you will feel the consequences both now and in the future. The good news is that the college years are a great time to establish healthy habits and change unhealthy ones. Taking this course is a great first step.

Myth 2   **Genetics (or luck) determine who will get a disease.** Actually, lifestyle factors play a major role in all of the five leading causes of death in the United States. It is true that your heredity may put you at higher risk for getting certain diseases, but you may reduce your risk and/or have many more years of health through a healthy lifestyle. For example, if you have a genetic predisposition to diabetes, you may delay its onset for decades through diet and exercise. Likewise, heart disease, the leading killer of Americans, is influenced by diet, activity level, smoking, alcohol consumption, and stress management factors. Even if you have a family history of heart disease, you can tip the balance in favor of good health by eating well, exercising regularly, not smoking, and controlling your stress. Similarly, you can greatly reduce your risk of cancer, stroke, lung disease, and deadly injury by making changes in your behavior.

Source: U.S. Department of Health and Human Services, National Center for Health Statistics, 1997.

possibility that such a relationship exists has done much to help individuals with a history of interpersonal problems and parental drinking begin to understand the complex factors that may have contributed to their problems —the first step toward any behavior change.

Another example of how past influences may affect our present well-being is seen in the way values, attitudes, and beliefs about the importance of healthy lifestyle behaviors are instilled at an early age as a direct result of a person's external environment. Influences that are negative may hinder even the best intentions. For example, children whose families have a poor diet and are extremely sedentary are likely to continue such practices as adults. Again, many of these influences may be difficult for the individual to overcome alone, but good results have been achieved with school- and community-based prevention programs like those designed to prevent domestic violence.

In addition to values, attitudes, and beliefs, our entire range of emotional responses develop as a reaction to life experiences. But even though much of our emotional response to life is influenced by our social and genetic predispositions, it is important to recognize that well individuals are resilient beings, capable of rebounding from emotional trauma. As such, we are ultimately responsible for our emotional behaviors and appropriate or inappropriate responses. Remember: Just as many emotional responses and other behaviors are learned throughout your life, many of these can be unlearned once you begin to recognize which ones may influence you to be emotionally unhealthy or to behave in an unhealthy manner.

Reinforcing Influences

Just as certain influences predispose us toward various behaviors or make it more difficult for us to change a given behavior, reinforcing factors help us

Sound Decision Making

STAGES OF BEHAVIOR CHANGE

You have probably noticed that making lasting changes in your habits and behaviors is sometimes difficult. Why is it that some people are successful in maintaining an exercise program or stopping smoking while others struggle less successfully? One possible explanation for success relates to your "readiness" to make a change. Psychologists James Prochaska, John Norcross, and Carlo DiClemente studied individuals who had successfully changed health-related behaviors on their own to see what strategies were most helpful. They found that individuals progressed through distinct *stages of change* on their way to increased health wellness, and that different strategies are effective at different stages.

■ At the *precontemplation* stage, you either don't realize that you have a problem, or you deny it. Although you may have heard that a certain behavior is risky, you fail to really acknowledge your own problems and have no intention of changing your habits. In order to move to the next stage, you need to become convinced that there would be benefits to making behavior changes.

■ At the *contemplation* stage, you acknowledge that you have a problem and begin to think about doing something about it. You may struggle to understand your problem, what caused it, and why changing your behavior might be worthwhile. To move to the preparation stage, you can think about successful changes you've made in the past and list the short- and long-term benefits of making the change you're contemplating.

■ At the *preparation* stage, you are planning to make a behavior change within the next month and are putting together strategies and mobilizing your resources to put your plan into action. To move into the next stage, it may be helpful to make a written plan or contract and to talk with friends and relatives about your plan.

■ The *action* stage is the busiest stage and the one that requires the most commitment. You are putting your plan into motion, and changes made at this stage are most likely to be noticed by others. During the action phase, it is important to stick to your plan, use your friends for support, and reward yourself for progress toward your goal.

■ After the intense effort of the action stage, you move into the *maintenance* stage. At this point you work to keep up the changes you made and to avoid relapse to old problem behaviors. In some ways, maintenance is a lifelong process.

Although the stages of change represent one popular explanation for behavioral change, it is important to remember that behaviors are extremely complex and have many possible explanations. Your attitudes, beliefs, values, social support, perceived susceptibility for risks, perception of threat, and other factors influence what any of us will do or not do to help ourselves gain in "health" years.

In each chapter of this book the Sound Decision Making feature will focus on how students go through these stages of change in their quest to make decisions that will lead to a lifetime of wellness.

Source: Prochaska, J., J. Norcross, and C. DiClemente. *Changing for Good*. New York: William Morrow, 1994.

maintain our motivation to change; without them we may slide back toward negative wellness behaviors. For example, having a strong social support group to give you positive feedback, having a friend to call when you're craving a rich dessert, and knowing that others genuinely care about you and may actually help you continue on your diet or exercise program may reinforce your will to behave in a particular way. The extent to which you perceive yourself as feeling better or looking better and the feedback you receive from others following adoption of a given behavior may encourage or discourage your continuation of the behavior. Everyone is different and responds differently to reinforcing factors. Some people may participate in a 10K race for the T-shirt or prize that they get at the end of the race or because of the social atmosphere that such a race fosters; others will run the race and feel good because someone they care about encourages them or because they have set small goals and want to see how they have improved in each race they run. For others, peer pressure may motivate them to be participants: *Not* to participate may give the appearance of not supporting a particular group or activity. Each of us is prodded, pushed, reinforced, and influenced by different factors in our movements toward positive health behaviors. Some of these influences are internal; some are external.

It is important to determine what factors serve as negative reinforcement for you as you try to make a behavior change. If you are a very social person and you often meet friends over coffee and cigarettes, you may equate not smoking with not spending time with your friends. If so, the possibly negative thoughts about what not smoking means might keep you from beginning or staying on a program to stop smoking.

Enabling Influences and Barriers to Wellness

Practicing a wellness lifestyle is easier for some people than for others. Those experiencing more favorable socioeconomic and environmental conditions, better education, and a host of other positive variables can afford to purchase healthful foods, for example. They have greater access to health care facilities and health professionals, and these promote prevention and early intervention for health problems. They are more likely to be exposed to information about health and wellness and to have access to fitness and recreational facilities. By contrast, individuals who are educationally, socio-economically, or otherwise disadvantaged will often have more difficulty adopting a wellness lifestyle. As public health service data suggest, mortality rates for minority groups, for the working poor, and for elderly people on fixed incomes in comparison to white middle- and upper-class Americans provides stark evidence that the nation has an unequal system for promoting health and wellness. Similarly, exposure to pollution, workplace hazards, and street violence varies widely according to socioeconomic status. For all to reach their potential—physically, psychologically, and spiritually—a society must place the same value on all human lives and attempt to ensure that a mind-set of health and wellness for all prevails. If we are truly following a wellness lifestyle, we must look beyond our own emotional and physical status and become more directly involved in efforts to assist those who may not have the same opportunities for achieving health.

Although you can conceivably achieve a high level of individual wellness by focusing only on your own self-improvement, optimal wellness implies a much more comprehensive approach to each of the elements of the wellness continuum. Rather than just making choices based on how they will affect you, you must take a greater interest in how your actions affect others as well. Conditions that are difficult for individuals to change must be remedied through collective political action. Looking at the *micro* (individual) and the *macro* (societal) influences on health is an essential component of achieving optimal well-being.

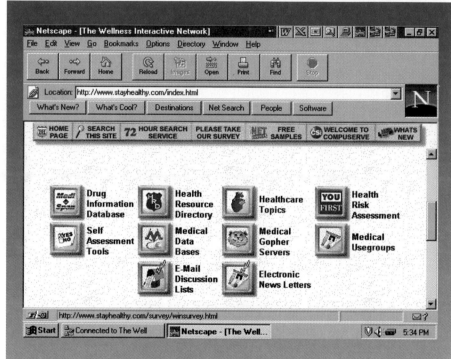

Wellness Interactive Network
http://www.stayhealthy.com/index.html

This wellness megasite includes thousands of Internet resources related to all areas of health and wellness. Users can start by taking a confidential online health risk assessment questionnaire that will pinpoint areas where behavior change can minimize current health risks. Additional assessment tools are available for cardiovascular health, weight control, and nutrition. There is a searchable database of drug information and links to sites on a wide variety of health and wellness topics, including sites on women's health, mental health, fitness, and aging. In addition, users can search medical information databases for additional information on specific diseases, subscribe to electronic newsletters on a variety of topics, or learn about mailing lists and newsgroups related to wellness.

Critical thinking: This Web site contains some advertisements. Do you think the ads change the value of the site? Can you think of any ways that the group that maintains this site might be influenced by its advertisers?

Source: From Avalon Group, Inc. 1998.

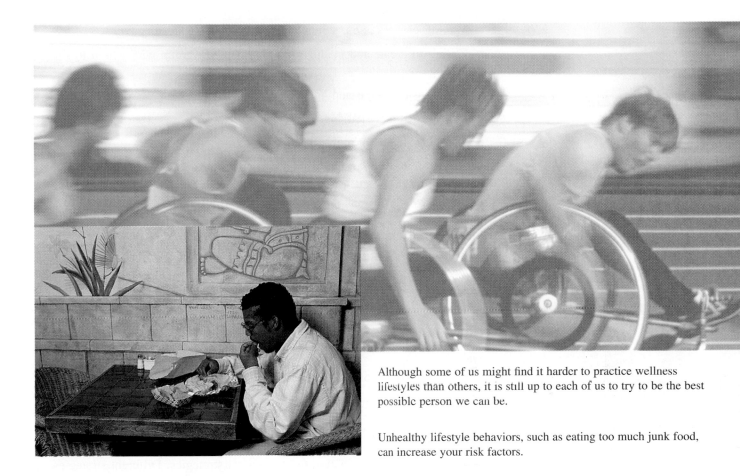

Although some of us might find it harder to practice wellness lifestyles than others, it is still up to each of us to try to be the best possible person we can be.

Unhealthy lifestyle behaviors, such as eating too much junk food, can increase your risk factors.

Lifestyle Influences

All these external factors have a significant role in determining whether you are predisposed, reinforced, and/or enabled to make positive behavioral changes; however, your own actions or lack of actions represent perhaps the single greatest influence on your overall health/wellness. The choices that individuals make from moment to moment, day to day, month to month, and year to year have been proven to have a significant, pervasive effect on both the quality and the length of life for people of all ethnicities and socioeconomic levels.

Certain **risk factors** are associated with an increased susceptibility to illness and premature death; these behaviors also interfere with high-level wellness. If you are practicing any of these behaviors you may want to assess their likely consequences and decide whether you need to make changes. Examples of risky behavior include the following:

- Smoking
- Consuming more than two alcoholic drinks per day or more than seven drinks per week
- Failing to exercise aerobically three times per week for a minimum of 20 minutes each time
- Eating and exercising such that body fat is above or below optimal levels
- Driving after drinking alcohol or riding with someone who has been drinking

risk factors factors associated with an increased susceptibility to an illness or premature death

- Making choices about sexual activity without regard to safety
- Failing to create and maintain a strong support group with whom to share feelings regularly
- Behaving in hostile and aggressive ways
- Acting extremely passive
- Adapting inappropriately to stress or not adapting at all

Risky behaviors are usually accompanied by delusional thinking: believing that you won't suffer from the consequences of such behaviors. If you think you will avoid the consequences or that an exception will be made for you, you aren't thinking clearly. "Ostrich" thinking is very risky; it's time for a reexamination.

Lifestyle Choices: Plan for Action

The whole notion of wellness offers exciting possibilities for each individual. As you strive to attain your own level of optimal health, you move closer to reaching your full potential—in how you look and feel, what you achieve, and how you cope with life's challenges.

For most people, changing existing behaviors can be a challenge that is best met with the systematic use of practical strategies. Different strategies may be helpful as you progress from initiating to maintaining and, finally, after a longer period of time, to "owning" a behavior change. The key is to try a variety of strategies and adopt those practices that you find most effective. These will certainly be based on your own needs, situation, and characteristics, but the following general principles should help you develop your own plan for change.

1. *Set realistic goals.* Identifying specific goals enables you to figure out the practical steps needed to achieve them and to measure your success. Your goals should be challenging but realistic and appropriate for you and your situation. You didn't, for example, gain 50 pounds in one month and you shouldn't expect to lose it in such a short time either. What you've been able to achieve in the past is a good gauge of where to start. Most important, you must care about achieving your goal and you must be sure that doing so will help you become the person you want to be. When you set your goals, think about a plan for achieving them, evaluate your goals, and write your goals down.

2. *Prioritize.* To be effective, you should develop a list of priorities that you would like to achieve in any program of change. What things do you need to change? What would you like to change? Which are most important to you right now? By assessing these areas, you may be able to come up with the one or two areas that are most important to you and most amenable to change within the framework of your present physical and social constraints. Approach these priorities one step at a time, with a clear vision of what you want to accomplish.

3. *Identify your resources.* What resources do you have that will help you reach your goals? Consider all that are available to you—time, money, skills, support from friends and family—and decide whether you have what you'll need. Germain suggests that encouragement and interest from significant persons in our lives may make a big difference in how long we continue a behavior pattern. Thus, one of the best ways to ensure your continued participation in any health activity is to find someone whom you enjoy being with, and to engage in the activity with that person. By doing so, you may actually be achieving two wellness goals: improving your physical health and improving your social and psychological wellness profile.

4. *Analyze barriers or potential problems.* Make plans to fill the gaps in your resources. Consult with others who may be able to help. Make a list of possible problems you might confront, and then list possible solutions. For example, if you love pizza but want to lose weight, don't eliminate pizza from your diet. Instead, try cutting back on the amount you eat, or forgo the sausage, pepperoni, or extra cheese. Feeling good about your choices is a key part of being able to stick with any behavior change strategy.

5. *Make a plan.* Taking principles 1–4 into account, decide which specific steps you'll take to reach your goal. Decide what criteria you'll use to determine that your goal has finally been met.

6. *Take action and continuously reevaluate.* If you've gotten this far, you're already well on the way toward achieving your goal. Once you've begun, don't be afraid to reevaluate your plan. And if it doesn't work, you'll have learned some lessons that will help you to make a new plan and begin again.

7. *Reward small successes and acknowledge setbacks.* If you find that you have achieved one of your goals, reward yourself with something you enjoy. If you have stopped exercising or slipped back into your old dietary habits, don't just decide to give up and negate all your previous successes. Health behavior change that works in the long run is interspersed with occasional setbacks. If you eat too much on the weekend, for example, acknowledge your behavior and make plans for resuming your positive dietary behaviors during the week. The more resilient you are, focusing on the good things you have accomplished, the more likely you are to succeed.

Once you have assessed the behaviors that you need to change and have analyzed the resources that are available to enable or reinforce your behavior, it is important to acknowledge that you may need help with certain behavior change activities. Friends, family members, or trained professionals should be contacted when necessary to assist you. Finding the right "cue to action" or factor that makes you really want to get going and will help keep you motivated and interested in your program is an important first step. Also, examining your personal priorities and the value you place on the outcome is an important part of any successful change. If you believe that you have a health risk, believe that what you do will make a difference in reducing your risk, value the health benefit that you might achieve, and are willing to be patient in finding the best approach, your chances of success will be greatly improved.

Readiness to change relates to your own motivation to begin working on a given behavioral change. The more you know about the risks, have assessed the options, and have considered the alternatives, the more likely you are to be successful. You also will be more ready to change and move from the contemplative to the active stage if you acquire the skills necessary to implement your change, feel good about the change, and sincerely value or want to achieve the specific behavior. In addition, recent research by Glanz suggests that behavior change strategies will be more likely to succeed if you observe the following:

1. *Consider individual differences.* The recipe for good health for one person is not necessarily your best recipe. As stated previously, wellness involves achieving your own level of optimal health in each of the various dimensions. Although you may never become an athlete, you may find that your vigorous walking program makes you feel better and allows you to function much more effectively on a daily basis.

2. *Follow a reasonable pace.* How many of you have made a New Year's resolution to lose weight, exercise more, stay away from beer and fast food, and study harder—all within a 24-hour period after a night of New Year's celebrating? Your chances of succeeding for more than a few hours are obviously not going to be high.

3. *Take time for yourself.* Perhaps one of the most important aspects of psychological health is to allow some time each day for some special attention to your own needs. It could be quiet time alone, time spent with someone you are close to, or time for a walk or bike ride. Often, we are much nicer to others than we are to ourselves. Sensitivity to your own needs is an important part of your spiritual, emotional, and environmental health.

Ideally, each of us will make choices in our behaviors that lead us to achieve the optimum balance among the physical, psychological, social, environmental, intellectual, and spiritual domains. One dimension should not be overemphasized, particularly if it means that another will be neglected. Thus, the fully healthy person will look his or her best, behave in a positive manner, and feel capable of meeting life's challenges, at least most of the time. In making lifestyle choices, the well person will consider each of the wellness dimensions, recognize areas that need improvement, acknowledge areas of strength, and act accordingly. Although we may occasionally stumble in our attempts to achieve optimum levels of wellness, becoming the best person possible remains the ultimate goal.

Your individual behaviors and actions, and the priorities and actions of society in general, will have a major impact on your overall well-being. For example, you may choose not to smoke, but if you live where smoke-free environments are virtually nonexistent, you may suffer the health consequences of breathing smoke-filled air. You will have to make special efforts to avoid secondhand smoke. In addition, although you cannot change your genetic predisposition to some diseases, you can dramatically influence the number of months or years that you can postpone disease symptoms and live a reasonably illness-free existence. Thus, avoiding cigarettes, controlling hypertension, eating a low-fat diet, and exercising regularly may reduce your risk of cardiovascular disease, even though your family may be predisposed to cardiovascular problems. Likewise, regular checkups, attention to body

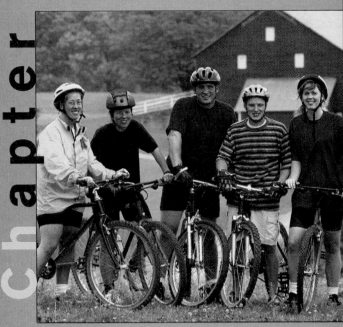
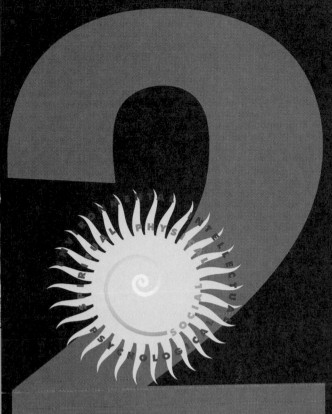

Becoming Physically Fit

One Student's View

Coming into college, I had many concerns about gaining the "freshman fifteen."
I heard rumors about the late night pizzas and beer guts. I made a solemn
promise to myself that I wasn't going to lead that lifestyle. In fact, as soon as I
got to college, I began regularly exercising three times a week, and I started
choosing healthy, low-fat foods. I'm happy to report that I've beaten the
"freshman fifteen" and gotten into the best shape of my life while doing it.

—Becky Guyer

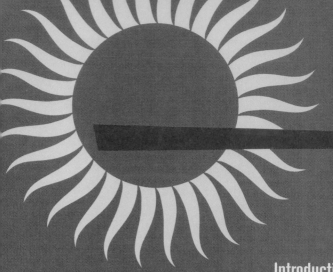

Introduction

When you were younger, you probably took your physical condition for granted. Playing Frisbee, riding your bike, or going for a swim may have been all in a day's activity for you. You might even have participated in organized sports such as soccer, softball, or track. The time you spent in physical activity was not only fun, but it kept you fit and healthy.

For most people, opportunities for regular physical activity become much more limited once they finish high school. Working a job, attending college, starting a family, or any combination of these drastically curtails the amount of time you have for physical activity. Labor-saving innovations such as cars, elevators, and even gas-powered lawn mowers also contribute to a decline in physical fitness by making it possible for you to do work with a minimal expenditure of energy.

As a result, you probably are not in the shape you used to be. Perhaps you've noticed that you are out of breath after climbing a flight of stairs, that the muscles in your back seem stiff and inflexible when you move, or that you have increasing difficulty keeping your weight down. Most people are not happy about these changes, but they accept them with resignation, thinking that being out of shape is an inevitable part of getting older. In fact, it's not uncommon to hear people in their twenties and thirties say that they are over the hill!

The fitness you enjoyed when you were younger was a result not of your youth but of your active lifestyle. By the same token, you may be out of shape as an adult not because you are older but because you are inactive. Research shows that middle-age and elderly people who are physically active can have a functional age well below their chronological age. Men and women in their forties and fifties who jog regularly, for example, can have a level of fitness that equals or exceeds that of inactive people in their teens and 20s. By lowering your

Objectives

After reading this chapter, you should be able to

- **Define the four health-related components of physical fitness and explain the importance of each to your overall fitness and health**

- **Identify the three training principles that describe the body's responses to exercise**

- **Describe the three phases of an exercise training program and the rate of progression**

- **Identify the people who can safely begin an exercise program and those who should consult their doctor and be tested first**

- **Identify the three energy pathways used during exercise and the pathways most associated with different forms of exercise**

expectations and equating aging with physical decline, you fail to recognize the control you have over your own fitness. Fortunately, as is the case with all other aspects of wellness, the lifestyle choices you make about physical fitness are better predictors of your health than your age. You can be physically fit at any age if you choose to be.

Your physical fitness is a major determinant of your wellness, and physical fitness is achieved through a regular habit of physical activity. In this chapter, you will discover what it means to be physically fit, what the four health-related components of physical fitness are, and why it is important to develop each component to improve your overall fitness and well-being. You will also learn the training principles that describe how the body responds to physical demands placed on it. The chapter concludes with an explanation of the energy systems muscles use to generate the forces needed for physical activity. As you read Chapters 3–5 and 8, you will have an opportunity to apply the training principles and your understanding of the energy pathways when developing a wellness lifestyle to enhance your aerobic fitness, muscular fitness, flexibility, and body composition.

The Components of Physical Fitness

Generally speaking, **physical fitness** is the ability to be physically active on a regular basis. But why is being physically fit so important? One of the best reasons for becoming physically fit is that it can lead to an improved quality of life. Physical fitness can help you maintain your ideal body weight, manage your stress levels, and generate the energy to perform your daily activities easily and quickly. It can also reduce your risk of developing chronic diseases such as coronary artery disease, diabetes, cancer, and osteoporosis, which are responsible for a reduced quality of life, to say nothing of premature death, for thousands of Americans each year. (See Chapter 13 for further discussion of chronic diseases.)

Physical fitness can be divided into skill-related and health-related components. The skill-related components of physical fitness such as speed, balance, agility, coordination, and power relate primarily to athletic performance and do not affect your overall health as much as the health-related components do. This book emphasizes the health-related components of fitness because of the many benefits associated with their development. The health-related components include aerobic fitness, muscular fitness, flexibility, and body composition. Skill-related and health-related fitness are not mutually exclusive, for many people achieve and maintain their health-related fitness through their regular participation in skill sports such as tennis or basketball. But skill is not a prerequisite for health-related fitness. Many of the activities that promote health benefits—for example, walking, running, cycling, stairstepping—do not require that you be blessed with special physical talents. An active lifestyle is the key to achieving physical fitness and wellness.

Aerobic Fitness

Aerobic fitness is the ability to engage in exercise that uses the large muscle groups in a rhythmic pattern of contraction and relaxation for an extended

physical fitness ability to be physically active on a regular basis

aerobic fitness ability to engage in exercise that uses the large muscle groups in a rhythmic pattern of contraction and relaxation for an extended period of time, usually between 15 and 60 or more minutes

period of time, usually between 15 and 60 or more minutes. Examples of aerobic activities include walking, jogging, cycling, swimming, cross-country skiing, in-line skating, aerobic dance, and step aerobics. The term *aerobic* (literally "with oxygen") is used to describe these activities because our muscles draw on oxygen to release the energy contained in carbohydrates and fats. Aerobic activities involve increased use of the lungs, heart, blood vessels, and muscles in the process of transporting oxygen from the air we breathe to the contracting muscle fibers. For this reason, aerobic fitness has also been called cardiorespiratory or cardiovascular fitness.

Aerobic fitness brings numerous health benefits—the reason it is an essential component of any personal fitness program. The high rate of energy use that occurs when you engage in aerobic exercise helps to reduce body fat, increase the levels of high-density lipoproteins (the beneficial form of cholesterol), and reduce your chances of developing diabetes by making the muscles more sensitive to insulin (the hormone that promotes the removal of glucose from the blood). For some people with high blood pressure, aerobic exercise may lower it. In addition, the increased energy levels, capacity to do work, and resistance to stress that come with aerobic fitness can improve your enjoyment of life and enhance your self-image. All these beneficial changes combine to give an aerobically fit person a greatly reduced risk of coronary heart disease, the major cause of death in the United States. (Programs to develop aerobic fitness are described in Chapter 3.)

Muscular Fitness

Muscular fitness is the strength and endurance of specific muscles or muscle groups. In this context, strength and endurance reflect two slightly different capacities of our skeletal muscles (muscles that are attached to our skeleton and move a part of the body when they contract). **Muscular strength** is the ability to generate force with a muscle, whereas **muscular endurance** is the ability to perform repeated contractions of a muscle group. The difference between muscular strength and muscular endurance can be better understood by considering how each is evaluated. Muscular strength is tested by determining the maximal amount of weight you can lift one time, such as with a bench press or biceps curl. Muscular endurance is evaluated by counting how many times you can repeat lifts with some fixed weight, such as bench-pressing 80 pounds, or how many sit-ups, push-ups, or pull-ups you can perform.

Both muscular strength and muscular endurance can be developed with resistance training. Using weights to stress the muscles is termed resistance training because muscles are made to contract against a resisting force. Resistance can be imposed in a variety of ways: by using free weights (barbells and dumbbells), by using sophisticated weight-training equipment, or by taking the low-tech approach of using your own body weight, as when performing push-ups or pull-ups. We recommend that you incorporate some form of resistance-training in your exercise program to promote both muscular strength and muscular endurance. This will help to maintain or develop muscle mass and bone strength, both of which often decline with age. Resistance training can also help you guard against low back pain, a common problem for many adults that has been linked to weakness in the abdominal muscles. (Muscular fitness and exercises for the back are discussed further in Chapter 4.)

muscular fitness muscular strength and endurance of specified muscles or muscle groups

muscular strength ability to generate force with the muscles

muscular endurance ability to perform repeated contractions of a muscle group

Flexibility

Flexibility is the ease of movement and range of motion we have when moving parts of our body. These movements take place at the various joints, such as the ankle, knee, hip, shoulder, or elbow. The ease and extent of motion at any joint is determined by the structure of the bones, the connective tissue, and the overlying muscles and skin. This structure can be modified with flexibility exercises—such as stretching or yoga. A lack of flexibility is often implicated in the occurrence of low back pain. Being flexible makes movement more enjoyable and may reduce the incidence of muscle or tendon injuries. Stretches to improve flexibility are frequently incorporated in the warm-up and cool-down phases of a workout. (Flexibility and stretching programs are covered in Chapter 5.)

Body Composition

Body composition refers to the relative proportions of fat (adipose) and lean (muscle, bone, water, organs) tissues in the body. Body composition is a health-related aspect of physical fitness because high percentages of body fat are associated with a greater incidence of heart disease, diabetes, high blood pressure, gout, gall bladder disorders, and certain forms of cancer. College-age males and females average 15% and 23% body fat, respectively, and the level at which males and females are considered obese is 25% and 32%, respectively. Conveniently, the activities that promote aerobic fitness (running, swimming, cycling, and so on) also help to reduce body fat because they entail a large expenditure of energy. (Techniques for measuring body composition and the principles of weight management are presented in Chapter 8.)

The Training Principles

Many centuries ago, Hippocrates, the father of medicine, made this observation: "That which is used, develops; that which is not used, wastes away." Chances are you have heard the modern-day version of this quote, "Use it or lose it." Both of these statements convey one of the basic truths that guide all exercise programs: You must pursue fitness in order to gain fitness.

Three general training principles describe the fundamental way the body responds to a program of exercise: the progressive overload principle, the specificity-of-training principle, and the reversibility-of-training principle. These principles apply to people of both sexes and all ages, and they apply to all forms of exercise training. When you design your exercise program, you will be applying these training principles when selecting the types and amounts of activity to use to achieve your wellness goals.

Progressive Overload Principle

There are two aspects to the progressive overload principle: the **principle of overload** and the principle of progression. The principle of overload states that the body must be subjected to a form of overload in order to improve a physical capacity. In simple terms, overload means that the body is being

flexibility ease of movement and range of motion we have when moving parts of the body

body composition relative proportions of lean tissue (muscle, bone, water, organs) and fat tissue in the body

principle of overload rule that the body must be subjected to a form of overload to improve a physical capacity

forced to do more than it's used to doing. Overload can be explained by the stress-adaptation response to exercise. According to this model, exercise is a stress—or demand placed on the body—that causes the body to respond or adapt. As the amount of exercise increases (overload), the body responds either by adapting to this higher level of stress or by failing to adapt, in which case injury may result (see Figure 2.1).

For example, when you lift a barbell, you place a very specific demand on your body, particularly the muscles performing the lift. When you run around a track, you stress your body in a different way—your lungs work harder, your heart beats faster, and your muscles contract in a rhythmic pattern. One episode of either of these activities will not result in any appreciable change in your physical condition, except perhaps for some temporary fatigue or soreness. But if you regularly engage in weight lifting or running, your body adapts to make it easier for you to perform the exercise. Eventually, your strength increases, so lifting weights becomes easier, or your endurance improves, so running around the track becomes easier. These changes brought about by a consistent program of regular exercise are termed **training effects.** In the above examples, the weight lifter's muscle fibers grow larger and contain more of the special proteins involved in muscle contraction. The runner develops a larger, stronger heart and the leg muscles become more energy efficient, enabling him or her to exercise for long periods without fatigue.

The **principle of progression** states that once the body has adapted to one level of exercise stress, a new overload must be initiated to stimulate further improvements in physical fitness. For example, suppose you do strength training and can perform biceps curls with 20 pounds. Once you have adapted to this weight, you will need to overload your muscles further by increasing the weight in order to gain strength. If you jog and want to further increase your aerobic fitness, you can do so by increasing the intensity, duration, or frequency

training effects changes in the body that are brought about by a consistent program of regular exercise

principle of progression rule that the body must be subjected to a new overload to stimulate further improvements in physical fitness after it has adapted to one level of stress

Figure 2.1

The relationship between stress and adaptation follows an inverted U. The absence of stress does not promote adaptation, whereas increasing stress stimulates adaptation up to an optimal level, beyond which a failure in the adaptive process occurs (injury, chronic fatigue). Optimal fitness represents a maximizing of fitness gains for the time spent in exercise. Additional exercise increases the risk of injury.

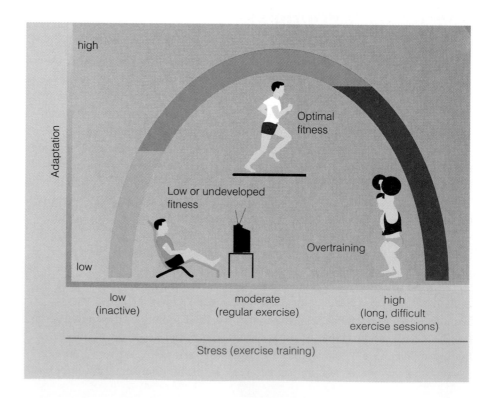

of your runs. You can jog the same distance faster (intensity), jog the same speed for a longer distance (duration), jog the same pace and distance as you have been but increase the number of times per week you run (frequency), or you can change two or more of these variables at the same time.

Specificity-of-Training Principle

The stress-adaptation model also describes the **specificity-of-training principle,** which states that the body systems stressed by exercise will be the ones that adapt. Different forms of exercise place specific, unique demands on the body. For example, swimming, cycling, and running are all aerobic activities, so all of them develop cardiorespiratory fitness. However, the specific muscle groups that develop aerobic endurance vary with each form of exercise. For instance, as swimming is predominantly an upper-body exercise, swimmers' shoulder and arm muscles are characteristically well developed. Even though running and cycling both use the leg muscles, they use them in different ways. Cyclists' thighs are usually more developed than are runners' because the work of cycling is concentrated on the thigh muscles, whereas running more evenly distributes work throughout the leg muscles.

Comparing bodybuilding with power lifting clearly illustrates the specificity-of-training principle. Bodybuilders want to sculpt themselves by enlarging and clearly defining their muscles. They must work each of these muscles with resistance exercises to stimulate muscular hypertrophy (increase in size). Their workouts include a wide assortment of different lifts, which stress individual muscle groups (see Figure 2.2a). Power lifters, on the other hand, train specifically for strength development rather than for muscle hypertrophy (see Figure 2.2b). A power lifter will train with very heavy weights, performing just a few repetitions of each lift, whereas a bodybuilder will use somewhat lighter weights but perform more repetitions of the same lift. These two approaches to resistance training produce different specificity-of-training results.

The specificity-of-training principle also illustrates which health benefits result from each type of exercise. As an example, look at the way the different

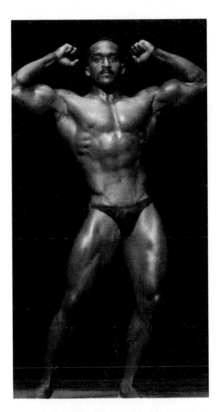

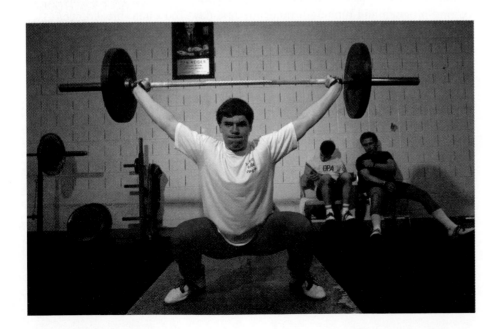

Figure 2.2

(a) A bodybuilder develops individual muscles all over the body for increased size and definition.

(b) A power lifter develops the major muscle groups for their maximal strength, without concern for definition or appearance.

specificity-of-training principle rule that systems stressed by exercise will be the ones that adapt

components of physical fitness affect coronary artery disease (CAD). Aerobic exercise greatly increases the heart's pumping efficiency and the body's fat-burning ability. For these reasons, it is associated with beneficial changes in CAD risk factors, such as lowering high blood pressure and high blood cholesterol, reducing the effects of diabetes, and fighting obesity. (For further discussion, see Chapter 13.) Whereas aerobic exercises challenge the heart to circulate blood at a rapid rate, resistance training primarily challenges the muscles to generate force. As a result, resistance training is not as effective in reducing CAD risk factors but is more effective in off-setting the muscle deterioration that accompanies inactivity. Flexibility exercises are generally low-energy activities that do not place any significant demand on the cardiovascular system, so they also are not an effective way to increase aerobic fitness or reduce CAD risk factors. Instead, stretching the muscles through their range of motion is the most effective way to develop joint range of motion, which helps to prevent injury.

Reversibility-of-Training Principle

The flip side of the overload principle is the **reversibility-of-training principle,** which states that the improvement in fitness gained through an exercise training program will be lost when the training is discontinued. Coyle and his colleagues at the University of Texas reported that competitive runners and cyclists experienced a 6% to 7% decline in their aerobic fitness within as little as 2 to 4 weeks after they stopped training. After 12 weeks of being sedentary, their aerobic fitness was 16% below their trained levels. Whether you are a competitive athlete or simply an individual who exercises in order to maintain your fitness, the same rule applies: Fitness cannot be stored. To receive the benefits of exercise for a lifetime, you need to exercise for a lifetime.

One of the most common reasons for discontinuing an exercise program and then experiencing reversibility of training involves sport injuries. Injuries are often the result of doing too much too soon. Instead of gradually increasing the intensity, duration, or frequency of activity, people try to increase their training overloads faster than their bodies can adapt to them, such as starting a jogging program and running 5 miles the first day. Too often, breakdowns result. Common breakdowns include strained muscles, inflamed tendons (tendonitis), small fractures of the bone (stress fractures), and chronic fatigue.

When training injuries occur, you must reduce or stop your training to allow them to heal. Continuing to exercise while you are injured will compromise your training and prevent the injury from healing—and may make it worse. During injury rehabilitation, you can expect to lose some of your fitness. To minimize this loss, you can switch to another activity that does not stress the injured part of the body. For example, competitive runners who have a foot or leg injury often will wear a flotation vest and simulate the running motion in a swimming pool. This activity works the leg muscles without subjecting the limbs to the forces of impact.

When you do sustain an injury, try to determine its cause so you can avoid reinjuring yourself later. Also, when you resume your exercise program after recovery, do it slowly. Do not rush the retraining process. Most injuries should be regarded only as temporary setbacks, not as reasons to abandon fitness activities. (Exercise-related injuries and their prevention and treatment are discussed more completely in Chapter 6.)

reversibility-of-training principle rule that the improvements in fitness gained through an exercise training program will be lost when the training is discontinued

Other reasons people start and then stop exercising include a lack of time or motivation. Keep in mind, though, that fitness can be improved with as little as 15 to 20 minutes of exercise just three times per week! Setting aside a specific time or exercising with a friend are some of the ways that people manage to make exercise a regular part of their lives. As you continue to exercise, you may also discover why others have turned to exercise to improve their lives—because exercise leads to a better self-image, increased strength and endurance, better ability to manage stress, and a more active and vigorous life, among other things. And these are only the short-term benefits; a lifetime of exercise may also help you decrease your risk for cardiovascular disease, osteoporosis, and cancer. These healthful physical and psychological outcomes constitute major features that define a state of personal wellness.

Designing a Fitness Program

People vary considerably in their fitness levels. Some people can run a marathon; others get tired walking around the block. Some people lug furniture without any help; others have trouble bringing in a bag of groceries. Some people can bend and move with ease; others strain to reach down and tie their shoes. One of the best ways to improve your fitness level is to start an exercise program that helps you realize your goals and individual potential in each of the health-related fitness components. The first step in designing an exercise program is to identify your current level of fitness. You will develop a complete profile of your fitness by taking the fitness tests described in the laboratories in Chapters 3, 4, and 5.

The next step in designing your program is to identify your personal fitness goals. When you establish goals, a helpful step is to include both short- and long-term goals. Short-term goals are steps you take toward achieving your long-term goals, and they can be changed or rewritten to reflect your progress. For example, if you decide that you would like to start a fitness program with the long-term goal of losing 15 pounds in 6 months, your short-term goals might include activities such as walking or swimming for a specific period of time to help you increase the number of calories you expend. Some examples of long-term fitness goals are presented in Table 2.1.

When writing your goals, try to include specific, quantifiable objectives. One way to do this is to specify a frequency, intensity, and duration for your activities. As noted in the previous section, *intensity* reflects the level of effort required by the exercise; *duration* is the length of time you spend in an exercise session; *frequency* is the number of times you exercise each week. For example, if your long-term goal is to increase your aerobic fitness through walking, you might start by establishing an intensity of 3 miles per hour (mph) for a duration of 30 minutes, at a frequency of two times per week. As you progress, you might decide to walk at 3 mph for 50 minutes, three times per week. By controlling the frequency, intensity, and duration of your workouts, you can control the amount of exercise you do and, subsequently, the progress of your fitness program.

As you develop your fitness goals, remember that you do not need to reach the highest levels of fitness to obtain health benefits. In fact, in studies conducted by the Institute for Aerobics Research in Dallas, Blair and colleagues (1989) demonstrated that only a moderate level of fitness is necessary

TABLE 2.1

Sample Long-Term Fitness Goals for an Exercise Program

1. Reduce my risk factors for heart disease (high blood pressure, high blood cholesterol levels, obesity, sedentary lifestyle) through aerobic exercise.

2. Achieve or maintain my appropriate body weight and physique through exercise.

3. Reduce my risk for developing lower-back pain by maintaining the strength and flexibility of my abdomen, back, and upper-leg muscles.

4. Increase my energy level and my confidence in my body's ability to remain active and strong and to handle physical challenges.

5. Prepare myself for a specific athletic event such as a fun run, triathlon, body-building contest, 10-kilometer or marathon race, Ultimate Frisbee competition, mountain climb, or bicycle trip.

6. Develop my endurance for continuous exercise through running, swimming, cycling, stair-stepping, or rowing.

7. Build my arm and shoulder strength and endurance through resistance training.

to attain a lower risk of death from all causes, including heart disease, stroke, and cancer. The researchers measured the aerobic fitness of over 13,000 people and then followed their health history for an average of 8 years. They found that the mortality rate was dramatically lower for those with at least moderate levels of fitness, whereas the rate for those with high levels of fitness was only slightly better than that of the moderately fit. The men and women with the lowest levels of fitness had the highest mortality rate. In another study, Blair and co-workers (1995) discovered that people who once had a low level of fitness and then became moderately fit had a 64% reduction in their rate of mortality compared to those who remained unfit. These studies demonstrate that you can reap the benefits of good health simply by keeping yourself out of the low-fitness group. In the chapters that follow, you will learn how to develop goals and select appropriate activities for improving each of the health-related components of physical fitness. You will discover that your wellness will be enhanced with the inclusion of relatively modest amounts of physical activity in your lifestyle.

Phases of a Training Program

A motivating training program that builds on your current level of fitness and gradually develops it to meet your long-term goals has three distinct phases: beginning, progression, and maintenance.

Beginning Phase

In the beginning phase of training, you gradually introduce yourself to regular exercise by engaging in small amounts of it. This builds the foundation for future training, preparing you for more vigorous activity and helping reduce the risk of exercise injuries. Your first goal is to become able to exercise for a desired amount of time before increasing the intensity of the exercise.

For example, your goal for the beginning phase of a running program might be to jog continuously for 10 to 15 minutes. You could begin with 100- to 200-yard jogs alternating with periods of 100- to 200-yard walks. Gradually, you would increase the length of the jogging intervals and decrease the length of the walking intervals. Similarly, if you were to begin a weight-training program, you would start by using relatively light weights to perform the lifts. This would allow you to concentrate on learning the proper techniques for the lifts. The easy jogging and use of light weights represent small overloads that initiate the stress-adaptation process.

Progression Phase

The progressive overload principle is most apparent in the progression phase of training. Because the overloads are very small in the beginning phase, it doesn't take the body long to adapt. In the progression phase, however, the overloads are somewhat larger, so more time is required for adaptation. Again, these increases are accomplished by increasing either the intensity, duration, or frequency of your workouts.

For example, you might increase the length of time you run from 15 to 20 minutes, or you might run four times per week instead of three, or you might increase your running speed. As you can see in Figure 2.3, the pattern of increasing the training overload and then staying at that level for 2 to 4 weeks for adaptation gives the progression phase of training a staircase appearance. This is appropriate because, in effect, you are climbing step-by-step toward a higher fitness level during this phase. If you are over 30 years of age, the process of adaptation takes a little longer, so you should allow 3 to 5 weeks for each step of adaptation.

Your level of fitness as you start an exercise program will influence the rate at which your fitness improves. The training effects of regular exercise will be most noticeable if you have been very inactive because you will have considerable room for improvement. In this case a small amount of exercise is all you will need to produce an improvement in fitness. If you are already somewhat fit, you will enter the training curve at a higher point, closer to your upper limit for fitness. The closer you are to your upper limits of fitness, the more exercise it will take to produce noticeable training improvements. The relationship between exercise session workloads and the resulting fitness gains is depicted in Figure 2.4.

Although the overall pattern of improvement in fitness is similar for everyone, there are individual as well as some group differences in fitness capacities. For example, males, as a group, can achieve a higher aerobic capacity and greater muscular strength than can females, while females often exhibit greater flexibility than males. The same is true when comparing young adults to the elderly. The rate of improvement or the ultimate level achieved may differ, but improvement is possible for all.

Maintenance Phase

As you enter the maintenance phase of training, your goal will be to hold steady with your current program rather than to increase your exercise intensity, duration, or frequency continually. Whereas athletes involved in compe-

Figure 2.3

The phases of a training program include beginning, progression, and maintenance. The weekly exercise level represents the combined effects of the frequency, intensity, and duration of the workouts each week.

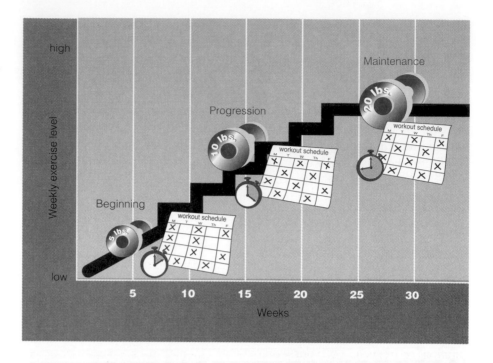

Figure 2.4

The training improvement curve has three phases: rapid gains in fitness (high yield of improvement for the amount of exercise performed), diminishing returns (less improvement in fitness with further increases in exercise), and approaching physical limits (further improvement is not possible).

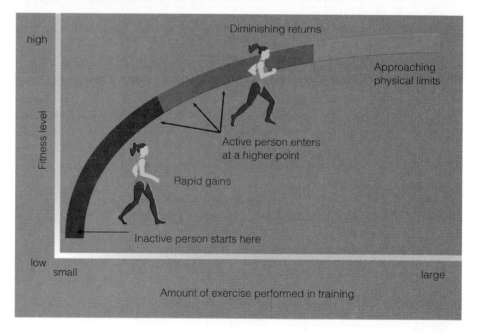

tition invest the time and effort to find their physical limitations in training, you need only increase your fitness to an acceptable level and then step off the progression staircase to achieve the health-related benefits of fitness. Although you may no longer be creating new overloads in your training program, you will likely want to keep your program interesting by varying your workouts. There are many ways you can add variety to your exercise routine. For example, if you have access to a fitness facility, you can work out on different exercise equipment (stair-stepper, treadmill, cycles, swimming pool, rowing machines, resistance equipment) or take aerobics classes. But you don't have to belong to a fitness club to achieve variety in your exercise program; you can vary activities on your own (walk, run, cycle, do in-line skating), vary the intensity and/or duration of your workouts day-today, or vary where you work out (city streets, river path, wood trails, on the beach, hills or flat lands).

Exercising Caution

Although exercise, particularly aerobic exercise, has many health benefits, it also carries some risks. For example, during vigorous exercise (such as running), the risk of a cardiac arrest is slightly elevated. This is because during exercise your heart contracts more frequently and pumps more blood with each contraction than when you are at rest. To perform this additional work, the myocardium (muscular layer of the heart) needs more oxygen, which means the coronary arteries must expand to allow an increased flow of oxygen-rich blood to the myocardium. A person whose coronary arteries have been narrowed by *atherosclerosis,* the accumulation of lipid and plaque in the lining of the blood vessels, may be unable to increase blood flow

Sound Decision Making

GETTING BACK IN THE GAME

While he was in high school, Keith would gather with other kids from the neighborhood almost every evening for a game of pickup basketball. Keith enjoyed the camaraderie and the competition, but when he got to college, there never seemed to be time for basketball or any other sport. During his sophomore year, Keith took a required physical activity class and was shocked to find that he could not complete the Cooper 1.5-mile run test without stopping to walk. He realized that in his commitment to put academics first, his body had come out last.

Keith began thinking about the benefits of starting a fitness program. He knew that he had gained some weight since starting college, and he didn't want that trend to continue. He also wanted to avoid having an early heart attack, as had several men in his family. Finally, Keith really missed playing basketball and thought a friendly game a few times a week would be a great study break.

Keith had already assessed his current level of fitness in his activity class, so his next step was to identify his personal long- and short-term fitness goals. He identified his long-term goals as losing 15 pounds, decreasing his stress level, and reducing his risk of heart disease. His short-term goals were to play basketball for an hour three times per week, and to go the gym to lift weights and to use the aerobic exercise machines three days a week when he wasn't playing basketball.

The first time Keith joined the informal game of basketball on his college court, he was pleased to see that he still had some of his old moves on the court, but he got winded after only 10 minutes and had to stop to catch his breath before he could reenter the game. He loved playing again, and within a few weeks his endurance had increased almost to its old levels—and Keith found that his weight-lifting routine at the gym also helped his basketball game.

Six weeks into his fitness routine, Keith sprained his wrist and had to take a rest from basketball for a few weeks. He went jogging on his normal basketball days to stay in shape and was still able to work his legs at the gym. Keith's doctor suggested that he do some stretches before and after exercise in the future to minimize the possibility of muscle pulls.

Today, Keith is back on the court and describes himself as healthier and happier than ever. He has even made some new friends at the gym. Making time for exercise isn't much of a problem because he sees it as an important part of his overall goal to be a happy, well-balanced person.

enough to meet the myocardium's need for oxygen. If cardiac muscle fibers are deprived of oxygen for any length of time, they cease to function and die, which is what happens in a heart attack (myocardial infarction). Thus, exercise can be a risk for someone with heart disease. For this reason, people with heart disease should have medical clearance prior to beginning an exercise program and, in many cases, are advised to exercise in medically supervised settings.

In weighing the risks of exercise, remember this: Even though the risk for a heart attack is slightly elevated during the time of exercise, the overall risk for a heart attack for physically active people is only 40% of that for sedentary people. In effect, when you repeatedly subject your heart to the stresses of exercise, the possibility that you will have a heart attack during rest or during exercise becomes much less likely. (See the Stats-at-a-Glance.)

The best way to evaluate the risks associated with exercise is to complete an exercise stress test (EXT). Administered by a physician and an exercise physiologist in a hospital or clinic, the EXT consists of a bout of exercise that begins at a low intensity and gradually increases to higher intensities until the person is too fatigued to continue. The EXT can indicate whether you have coronary artery disease and can also determine the safest level of exertion for your exercise program. The EXT is usually conducted on a treadmill, and the workrate is increased every second or third minute by increasing the speed of walking/jogging and/or by elevating the front end of the treadmill, making you go uphill. During the test the electrical signal from each heart beat is monitored by an electrocardiograph (ECG), and blood pressure is taken at 2- to 3-minute intervals.

It is neither necessary nor practical for everyone to have an EXT prior to beginning an exercise program. The American College of Sports Medicine (ACSM) has established guidelines concerning the need for a medical exam and an EXT prior to involvement in an exercise program. Their recommendations are given according to the following risk classifications:

1. *Apparently healthy.* If you are apparently healthy, with no symptoms of heart disease, and with no more than one major coronary risk factor (see Table 2.2), you can participate in moderate exercise without prior exercise stress testing. Moderate exercise is defined as a level of exertion that can be comfortably sustained for 60 minutes or more. The ACSM recommends exercise stress testing for males over age 40 and females over age 50 prior to beginning a vigorous exercise program, which is defined as exercise that represents a substantial challenge and would ordinarily result in fatigue in 20 minutes. Apparently healthy men under 40 and women under 50 years of age may participate in vigorous exercise without prior exercise stress testing.

2. *Individuals at higher risk.* Exercise stress testing is recommended if you have two or more of the major coronary risk factors listed in Table 2.2 or any of the signs or symptoms listed in Table 2.3. If you are at higher risk because of the presence of major coronary risk factors but without any of the symptoms listed, you can engage in moderate exercise without prior exercise testing, but you should be tested prior to engaging in vigorous exercise.

3. *Individuals with disease.* You should have an exercise stress test prior to starting an exercise program if you have cardiac, pulmonary, or metabolic disease.

STATS-AT-A-GLANCE
The Risks of Vigorous Exercise

■ When people who seldom exercise engage in vigorous exercise, their risk for a heart attack is 107-fold greater than when at rest (Mittleman et al.).

■ When people who regularly exercise engage in vigorous exercise, their risk for a heart attack is 2.4-fold greater than when at rest. Overall, they have a 40% lower risk for having a heart attack, at rest or during exercise (Mittleman et al.).

Because most people can be classified as apparently healthy, experts in the field believe most can safely participate in a program of moderate exercise without consulting their physician or having an EXT. As a minimum test for the safety of participation in an exercise program, you should complete the Physical Activity Readiness Questionnaire (PAR-Q) (see Laboratory 2.1). If for any reason you are unsure of the safety of undertaking an exercise program, or if you answered "yes" for any of the questions in the PAR-Q, consult your physician.

Physical activity is a crucial component in achieving your long-term goal of wellness. The process of reaching this goal begins first with a determination of your ability to exercise safely and then your progression through a sequence of short-term goals which will bring you to the maintenance stage of your exercise program. Not only is wellness your long-term goal, it is to be your lifelong condition. The weeks or months it takes to initiate and progress in your exercise program is a small amount of time compared to

TABLE 2.2

Coronary Artery Disease Risk Factors

POSITIVE RISK FACTORS	DEFINING CRITERIA
1. Age	Men > 45 years; Women > 55 years
2. Family history	Heart attack (myocardial infarction) or sudden death before age 55 in father, brother, or uncle or age 65 in mother, sister, or aunt
3. Current cigarette smoking	
4. Hypertension	BP ≥ 140/90 mmHg, confirmed by measurement on at least 2 separate occasions, or currently taking antihypertension medication
5. Hypercholesterolemia	Total serum cholesterol > 200 mg/dL (5.2 mmol/L) (if lipoprotein profile is unavailable) or HDL < 35 mg/dL (0.9 mmol/L)
6. Diabetes Mellitus	Persons with insulin dependent diabetes mellitus (IDDM) who are > 30 yrs of age or have had IDDM for > 15 yrs, and persons with noninsulin dependent diabetes mellitus (NIDDM) who are > 35 yrs of age
7. Sedentary lifestyle/ physical inactivity	Persons in the least active 25% of the population, as defined by the combination of sedentary jobs involving sitting for a large part of the day with no regular exercise or active recreational pursuits

NEGATIVE RISK FACTOR	COMMENTS
1. High serum HDL cholesterol	> 60 mg/dL (1.6 mmol/L)

If HDL is high, subtract one risk factor from the sum of positive risk factors, as high HDL decreases CAD risk.

Source: From Kenny et al., 1995.

TABLE 2.3

Signs or Symptoms Suggestive of Cardiopulmonary Disease

1. Pain or discomfort in the chest, neck, jaw, or arms, consistent with ischemia (insufficient blood flow to the heart muscle)

2. Shortness of breath at rest or with mild exertion

3. Dizziness

4. Episodes of difficult breathing while sleeping

5. Swelling of the ankles

6. Episodes of rapid heart rates at rest

7. Pains in the leg muscles with light exertion

8. Known heart murmur

9. Unusual fatigue or shortness of breath with usual activities

Source: Kenny et al., 1995.

the years and years you will be maintaining your wellness. Therefore, there is no need to rush. Start slowly, progress gradually, and enjoy the process of being active and achieving wellness.

The Energetics of Exercise

An exercise session is often referred to as a "workout" and, indeed, we do work when we exercise. Work is defined as the product of force times distance. Generally, the force being moved some distance is your body weight as you run, walk, swim, cross-country ski, or in-line skate. When you row or cycle, you move not only your body weight but the weight of the boat or bike as well. In weight lifting, the force is the weight being lifted. With stationary exercise equipment, it might seem as if no work is performed because you do not cover any distance. However, even though your body does not change its location when you pedal the stationary cycle, your pedaling moves the flywheel of the cycle, which accounts for the distance factor. Other stationary equipment, such as the rowing machine, cross-country skiing simulator, or stair-stepper, operate on a similar principle.

Doing work requires an expenditure of energy, which is referred to as the energetics of exercise. The more work you do, the more energy you expend. Your muscles generate the forces necessary for your exercise, so they require a steady supply of energy. **Adenosine triphosphate (ATP)** is the high-energy compound that provides energy for muscle contraction and the other reactions in cells that require energy. Muscle fibers generate this energy using three pathways: immediate, anaerobic, and aerobic (see Figure 2.5). Each pathway is particularly well suited to specific types of activities and exercise.

adenosine triphosphate (ATP) high-energy compound that provides the energy for muscle contraction and other reactions in cells that require energy

Immediate Energy Pathway

At the beginning of any activity, some ATP is already formed and available for immediate use in muscle contraction. To fuel contraction, ATP splits to release the energy needed for the activity. As ATP is used, creatine phosphate, another high-energy compound, restores the ATP that has been split during contraction. Together, the ATP that is present at the start of muscle contraction and the creatine phosphate that replenishes the ATP supply constitute the **immediate energy pathway,** which provides the energy needed to perform very quick and powerful movements. However, the supply of the ATP and creatine phosphate is quite limited. The immediate energy pathway can supply enough ATP for only a few seconds of intense activity. After that, the other energy pathways must supply additional ATP.

All-out, high-intensity, short-duration activities such as spiking a volleyball, smashing a forehand return in tennis, sprinting 100 meters, dunking a basketball, dashing up a flight of stairs, or lifting a heavy object rely on the immediate energy pathway. During these activities, muscles contract so rapidly that the anaerobic and aerobic pathways cannot form ATP fast enough to play a significant role. As a training adaptation, people who regularly engage in these activities will experience an increase in their ATP and creatine phosphate supplies so that their immediate energy pathways can fuel longer bouts of intense activity.

Anaerobic Energy Pathway

A second energy pathway to power high-intensity activities is the **anaerobic energy pathway,** so-called because it does not use oxygen in forming ATP. Although it cannot generate ATP rapidly enough to match the rate of ATP use during your most powerful or fastest muscle contractions, the anaerobic energy pathway provides much of the energy needed to sustain high-intensity activities for up to several minutes.

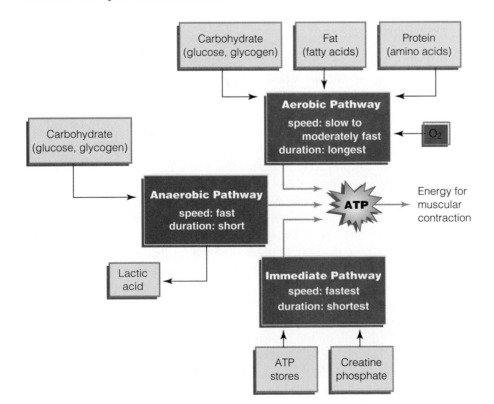

Figure 2.5

Three energy pathways produce the ATP that powers muscular contraction.

immediate energy pathway
route for the energy needed to perform very quick and powerful movements

anaerobic energy pathway
route for the energy needed to sustain high-intensity activities for up to several minutes

The source of energy for the anaerobic pathway is glucose, the form of carbohydrate that is available to the muscles from circulating blood. In addition, the anaerobic pathway draws on **glycogen,** which is glucose stored in the muscles and liver. Glycogen consists of clusters of glucose molecules from which individual glucose units can be split off and utilized during times of muscular activity, so the anaerobic energy pathway is not supply-limited in the way the immediate energy pathway is.

The sequence of chemical reactions that create ATP from the anaerobic breakdown of glucose is referred to as **glycolysis.** Anaerobic glycolysis produces ATP and **lactic acid,** which, at high concentrations in muscle fibers, interferes with muscle contraction and ultimately causes fatigue. The speed of glycolysis allows us to race a 200-, 400-, or 800-meter distance, cycle up a long hill, run up several flights of stairs, sustain a long volley in tennis, apply a full-court press in basketball, or perform multiple repetitions of a weight lift. However, the buildup of lactic acid interferes with continued muscular contraction and causes the stinging muscle fatigue you feel as you complete a quarter-mile race, run up a hill, or attempt one final repetition of a weight lift. High-intensity exercise that relies on the anaerobic energy pathway can be sustained for up to several minutes before lactic acid accumulates and you begin to experience the fatigue that has been popularized in the "feel the burn" refrain of aerobic classes. It is ironic that "aerobic" instructors often push you to exercise at intensities that heavily involve the "anaerobic" energy pathway.

Aerobic Energy Pathway

The **aerobic energy pathway** is the primary route for energy in activities of a lesser intensity than those relying on the immediate or anaerobic energy pathways. It uses oxygen to provide the energy for activities that take from 5 minutes up to several hours. Because it involves numerous reaction sequences in the cell, the aerobic is the slowest of the three energy pathways. However, the aerobic energy pathway can efficiently provide ATP for a prolonged period of time. Because most daily activities such as doing housework and yardwork, walking, studying, or working a desk job are low-intensity activities, you rely on the aerobic energy pathway for almost everything you do.

In the immediate and anaerobic energy pathways, individual muscle fibers act in virtual isolation because they have what they need to produce ATP. Such is not the case with the aerobic energy pathway, which requires a steady supply of oxygen to form ATP. In the aerobic pathway, carbohydrates and fats are broken down in the presence of oxygen to yield carbon dioxide, water, and ATP. The site of the aerobic reactions is the **mitochondria,** the energy-generating organelles of all cells. The source of carbohydrate is the same as for the anaerobic energy pathway: glucose and glycogen. Adipose (fat) tissue and, to a lesser extent, the muscle fibers store the fat that is used in the aerobic pathway. Protein can also be broken down to generate aerobic energy, but studies have shown that protein is only a minor source of energy during exercise unless a person is undernourished or engaged in very prolonged exercise.

The proportions of carbohydrate and fat used in forming ATP during aerobic exercise depend on the intensity of the exercise and the individual's aerobic fitness. The higher the intensity of exercise, the greater the contribution of carbohydrates to the energy production. However, individuals who are aerobically trained can use fat as an energy source even at high intensi-

glycogen glucose stored in the muscles and liver

glycolysis sequence of reactions that form ATP from the anaerobic breakdown of glucose

lactic acid end product, along with ATP, of anaerobic glycolysis; at high concentrations in the muscle fiber, it interferes with muscle contraction and causes fatigue

aerobic energy pathway route, using oxygen, that provides the energy for activities that take from 5 minutes up to several hours

mitochondria site of aerobic reactions; the energy-generating organelles of all cells

DESIGNING ◆ A
FITNESS ◆ PROGRAM

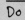 Do

▲ Start by identifying your current level of fitness.

▲ Write out specific short- and long-term fitness goals.

▲ Be realistic about the frequency, intensity, and duration of your workouts, especially in the beginning.

▲ Design a fitness program around activities you enjoy.

▲ Consider having a stress test done if you are at risk of cardiopulmonary disease.

▲ Plan to reward yourself for sticking with your program.

Don't

▼ Plan to have a "whole new body" in a matter of weeks.

▼ Adopt someone else's goals for you as you design an exercise program.

▼ Plunge into an exercise program without first assessing your current level of fitness, getting the proper equipment and training, and assessing any health risks you may have.

▼ Feel stuck with an exercise program you dislike. If your program turns out to be unpleasant or unrealistic, revise your plan.

▼ Expect to be a dynamo every time you exercise. On some days, you'll feel very energetic, and on others you'll have to drag yourself to finish your activities.

ties of exercise. An enhanced ability to use fat during exercise is advantageous, as it reduces the rate at which you are using your muscle glycogen. The muscle has a limited ability to store glycogen, and when its supply is depleted during prolonged exercise, fatigue results. Slowing the rate of muscle glycogen use during exercise postpones the point at which the supply of glycogen runs out, thus delaying fatigue.

Because aerobic exercise involves the lungs, heart, blood, and blood vessels in the transport and delivery of oxygen to the muscle fibers, and it uses the muscles in the performance of the activity, the training effects of an aerobic exercise program can be found in many of the body's systems. (See Chapter 3 for a discussion of these training effects.)

The three energy pathways have been described individually, but they are not used discretely, one at a time, as you use first, then second, then

MYTHS & CONTROVERSIES

Myth 1   **"No pain, no gain."** Exercise requires some effort, but pain during a workout is a warning sign you should not ignore. If you have continuing pain during an exercise, stop and rest, and don't continue with that exercise until you can do it painlessly. If you have pain in your neck or chest, see a doctor immediately, because you may be experiencing a heart attack.

      Muscle soreness after exercise is another matter; it usually means you are working too long or hard, or that you are not warming up sufficiently before your workout. Regard sore muscles as a sign to slow down a little, but don't quit exercising.

Myth 2   **Exercise affects only the body.** Most regular exercisers find that exercise can have a profound effect on mood and mental state, and research is providing evidence to support this belief. While the mechanism is not yet fully understood, studies show exercise improves mild to moderate depression, stimulates creativity, provides an outlet for aggression, improves cognitive functioning, and improves body image. Exercise is important to all dimensions of wellness, not just physical health.

Controversy 1   **How much exercise is enough?** Fitness experts recently published new, less stringent guidelines on how much exercise people need to stay healthy. They had previously recommended that Americans work out strenuously for at least 20 minutes 3 to 5 times per week; the new guidelines, however, suggest that accumulating at least 30 minutes of moderate exercise over the course of most days is enough. Do these new guidelines mean that high-intensity workouts are not worth the effort? Probably not.

      The new recommendations were made with the knowledge that more than half of Americans are completely sedentary. This inactivity is as bad for the nation's health as smoking and high cholesterol levels. Engaging in everyday physical activities such as gardening and walking to the store may be enough to improve the health of those who are currently sedentary. If you are already somewhat active, however, getting at least 20 minutes of high-intensity exercise 3 to 5 times per week will give your heart and lungs a good workout, and will further enhance your wellness.

Source: U.S. Department of Health and Human Services, Surgeon General's Report, 1996.

third gear when driving your car. Instead, they can be used simultaneously. Whenever you move from one level of exertion to another (for example, rest to exercise, or low-intensity exercise to high-intensity exercise), you utilize both the immediate and anaerobic energy pathways at the same time the slower responding aerobic energy pathway increases its contribution to energy production. Whereas the immediate energy pathway will be engaged for only a matter of seconds, the anaerobic and aerobic pathways can be simultaneously engaged for an extended time. The proportional contribution of either is dependent on the exercise intensity: at lower intensities, the aerobic pathway predominates, and exercise can continue for a long time before glycogen depletion occurs; at high intensities, the anaerobic pathway is substantially involved, and fatigue will occur when lactate levels get very high in the muscle fibers.

      Physical fitness is a major component of wellness; therefore, physical activity is an essential element in your wellness lifestyle. The next chapters will cover the various dimensions of physical fitness (aerobic fitness, muscular fitness, flexibility, body composition). With your understanding of the training principles and the energy pathways, you will now be able to predict what training effects will result from specific forms of exercise and what types of fitness they will promote. You now know the general principles for developing an exercise program. You will next deal with the specifics of developing a program that meets your needs and interests.

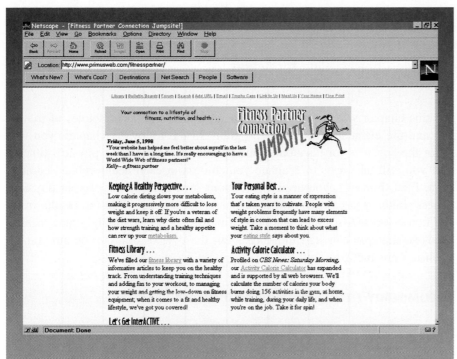

Fitness Partner Connection Jumpsite
http://www.primusweb.com/fitnesspartner/

This may be the biggest fitness-related site on the Web. Its search-able library contains information on getting active and staying motivated, choosing fitness equipment, weight management and nutrition, book reviews, and fitness in the news. In addition, there is a collection of pages on all kinds of specific activities, and special topics like kids and fitness. The Activity Calorie Calculator allows you to calculate how many calories your body will burn for over 150 different activities. Finally, there are links to hundreds of other sites related to all aspects of fitness and health.

Critical thinking: The Activity Calorie Counter calculates how many calories you will burn per activity according to your weight and how many minutes you spend in the activity. What other factors help determine how many calories a given individual will burn during an exercise session?

Source: From Pierson, 1998.

Lifestyle Choices: Plan for Action

In this chapter you have been introduced to the general principles of training and the elements of a fitness program. In the following chapters you will learn the specifics for developing the various components of physical fitness, and you will take tests to evaluate your fitness in each health-related component. First, however, you need to rate your own perceptions of your physical fitness. Later, you can see how your perceptions compare to the results from the fitness tests. Also, now is a good time to begin developing your fitness goals so that you can start thinking about the type of fitness program you wish to construct for yourself.

PRELIMINARY FITNESS PROFILE AND GOALS

WHERE I AM NOW

Aerobic fitness:	low	average	high
Muscular strength:	low	average	high
Muscular endurance:	low	average	high
Flexibility:	poor	average	good
Body composition:	fatter than I'd like to be	about right	thinner than I'd like to be

WHERE I WOULD LIKE TO BE

Aerobic fitness:	low	average	high
Muscular strength:	low	average	high
Muscular endurance:	low	average	high
Flexibility:	poor	average	good
Body composition:	fatter than I am	about the same	thinner than I am

THREE POTENTIAL FITNESS GOALS

_____

_____

_____

THREE POTENTIAL FITNESS ACTIVITIES

_____

_____

_____

Summary

An exercise program to develop the health-related components of physical fitness is an essential element of a wellness lifestyle. Aerobic fitness, muscular fitness, flexibility, and body composition all have a direct effect on your health and well-being. As most people age, they fall into a pattern of reduced physical activity. A direct consequence of this inactivity is a decline in the health-related aspects of physical fitness, a pattern that will continue unabated unless you take steps to prevent it. Being well is an active process. Your wellness is under your control; you can achieve it and maintain it by choosing the appropriate types and amounts of exercise.

Understanding the general training principles, the phases of a training program, and the ways in which energy is generated during exercise provide the foundation for developing your personal exercise program. The chapters that follow will show you how to implement your fitness program as part of your livable lifestyle choices. By doing so, you can use exercise to transform your body into a state of physical fitness.

Key concepts that you have learned in this chapter include these:

- The health-related components of physical fitness are aerobic fitness, muscular fitness, flexibility, and body composition.

- The progressive overload principle describes the way the body responds and adapts to all forms of exercise training.

- The specificity-of-training principle explains that the adaptations of the body to exercise are unique to the specific type of exercise being performed.

- The reversibility-of-training principle describes the way the body loses its training effects when the exercise program is discontinued.

- Each training program has a beginning phase, in which exercise is gradually initiated and increased; a progressive phase, in which the exercise levels are increased in larger increments and at regular intervals; and a maintenance phase, in which the level of exercise is held constant to maintain the fitness that has been developed.

- Apparently healthy individuals can start a moderate or vigorous exercise program without undergoing an exercise test beforehand; apparently healthy men over age 40 and women over age 50 should have an exercise test prior to beginning a vigorous exercise program; individuals with cardiac, pulmonary, or metabolic disease, or signs or symptoms of disease should have an exercise test and a doctor's approval before beginning any exercise program.

- Three major energy pathways generate the form of energy (ATP) used in muscle contractions: immediate, anaerobic, and aerobic.

- Each energy pathway differs from the others in its speed of ATP formation and the type of activities it powers.

- Carbohydrates and fats are the two primary sources of energy for ATP formation.

- Physical fitness is an essential component of wellness, and it is promoted through physical activity.

References

American College of Sports Medicine. *Guidelines for Exercise Testing and Prescription,* 5th ed. Baltimore: Williams & Wilkins, 1995.

Blair, S. N., et al. Physical fitness and all-cause mortality. *Journal of the American Medical Association,* 262: 2395–2401, 1989.

Blair, S. N., et al. Changes in physical fitness and all-cause mortality: A prospective study of healthy and unhealthy men. *Journal of the American Medical Association,* 273: 1093–1098, 1995.

Coyle, E. F., M. K. Hemmert, and A. R. Coggan. Effects of detraining on cardiovascular responses to exercise: Role of blood volume. *Journal of Applied Physiology,* 60: 95–99, 1986.

Coyle, E. F., et al. Time course of loss of adaptations after stopping prolonged intense endurance training. *Journal of Applied Physiology,* 57: 1857–1864, 1984.

McArdle, W. D., F. I. Katch, and V. L. Katch. *Exercise Physiology: Energy, Nutrition, and Human Performance,* 4th ed. Baltimore: Williams & Wilkins, 1996.

Mittleman, M. A., et al. Triggering of acute myocardial infarction by heavy physical exertion—protection against triggering by regular exertion. *New England Journal of Medicine,* 329: 1677–1683, 1993.

Siscovick, D. S., et al. The incidence of primary cardiac arrest during vigorous exercise. *New England Journal of Medicine,* 311: 874–877, 1984.

U.S. Department of Health and Human Services. *Physical Activity and Health: A Report of the Surgeon General.* Atlanta, GA: U.S. Department of Health and Human Services, Centers for Disease Control and Prevention, National Center for Chronic Disease Prevention and Health Promotion, 1996.

Laboratory 2.1

PAR-Q: The Physical Activity Readiness Questionnaire

Regular physical activity is fun and healthy, and increasingly more people are starting to become more active every day. Being more active is very safe for most people. However, some people should check with their doctor before they start becoming much more physically active.

If you are planning to become much more physically active than you are now, start by answering the seven questions below. If you are between the ages of 15 and 69, the PAR-Q will tell you if you should check with your doctor before you start. If you are over 69 years of age, and you are not used to being very active, check with your doctor.

Common sense is your best guide when you answer these questions. Please read the questions carefully and answer each one honestly: check YES or NO.

YES   NO

❑   ❑   1. Has your doctor ever said that you have a heart condition and that you should only do physical activity recommended by a doctor?

❑   ❑   2. Do you feel pain in your chest when you do physical activity?

❑   ❑   3. In the past month, have you had chest pain when you were not doing physical activity?

❑   ❑   4. Do you lose your balance because of dizziness, or do you ever lose consciousness?

❑   ❑   5. Do you have a bone or joint problem that could be made worse by a change in your physical activity?

❑   ❑   6. Is your doctor currently prescribing drugs (for example, water pills) for your blood pressure or heart condition?

❑   ❑   7. Do you know of any other reason you should not do physical activity?

IF YOU ANSWERED

YES to one or more questions

Talk with your doctor by phone or in person BEFORE you start becoming much more physically active or BEFORE you have a fitness appraisal. Tell your doctor about PAR-Q and which questions you answered YES.

You may be able to do any activity you want—as long as you start slowly and build up gradually. Or, you may need to restrict your activities to those that are safe for you. Talk with your doctor about the kinds of activities you wish to participate in and follow his or her advice.

Find out which community programs are safe and helpful for you.

NO to all questions

If you answered NO honestly to all PAR-Q questions, you can be reasonably sure that you can:

■ start becoming much more physically active. Begin slowly and build up gradually; this is the safest and easiest way to go.

■ take part in a fitness appraisal. This is an excellent way to determine your basic fitness so that you can plan the best way for you to live actively.

If you are not feeling well because of a temporary illness such as a cold or fever, wait until you feel better. If you may be pregnant, talk to your doctor before you start becoming more active.

Please note: If your health changes so that you answer YES to any of the above questions, tell your fitness or health professional. Ask whether you should change you physical activity plan.

Informed Use of the PAR-Q: The Canadian Society for Exercise Physiology, Health Canada, and their agents assume no liability for persons who undertake physical activity, and if in doubt after completing this questionnaire, consult your doctor prior to physical activity.

Source: From the Canadian Society for Exercise Physiology, 1994.

You are encouraged to copy the PAR-Q but only if you use the entire form.

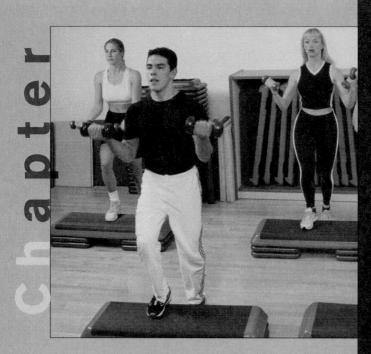

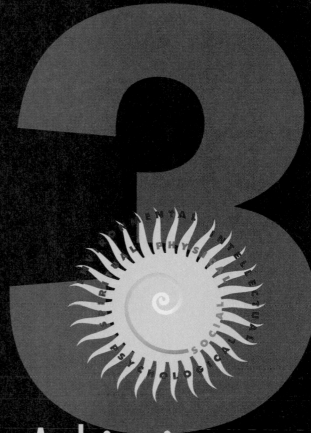

Achieving Aerobic Fitness

One Student's View

I feel so much better on days that I do work out. It gives me a feeling of invincibility and high self-confidence. After working out, I feel as if I can do anything.

Not working out tends to depress me, and I find that I don't have as much energy. It seems as though I don't have the same quality of effort in everyday activity without working out. For instance, I am not as alert in class if I have not adequately trained. Aerobic fitness keeps me alert and much more energetic, thus I am better prepared to put forth a strong effort in my activities.

—Brett Gerch

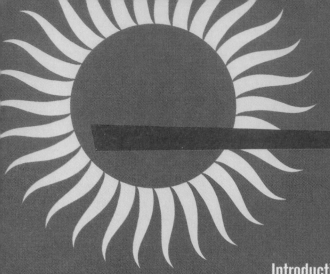

Introduction

Despite the so-called fitness boom of recent years, which gave us "designer workouts" and spawned a multibillion-dollar fitness apparel industry, many people still have not made exercise a part of their lives. An estimated 40% of Americans currently participate regularly in low- to moderate-intensity physical activities, such as walking; even fewer participate in activities that require more effort. Furthermore, 25% of all adults are inactive and the level of participation in activity decreases with increasing age (Centers for Disease Control). The decline in physical function commonly associated with aging is in fact largely a result of lack of exercise.

As you begin looking for ways to improve your overall wellness, you will want to consider how to best maintain or improve your aerobic fitness. Aerobic fitness has been referred to by some as the single most important component of physical fitness. For example, keeping aerobically fit throughout your lifetime can have such far-reaching health benefits as reducing your chances of developing coronary artery disease (CAD), cancer, and diabetes (Sharkey).

In addition to physical benefits, aerobic exercise can have a beneficial effect on the other dimensions of wellness—psychological, social, even spiritual. You may have noticed that activities such as going for a walk, riding a bike, or swimming can help lift your spirits if you are feeling somewhat out of sorts. More important, engaging in regular aerobic exercise can help you reduce your stress level, forestall anxiety or depression, and generally feel better about yourself.

Although aerobic fitness is clearly an important component of physical fitness, it sometimes has been overemphasized as the one aspect of fitness worth pursuing. However, the great popularity of

Objectives

After reading this chapter, you should be able to

- **Define aerobic fitness**

- **Describe the physiological systems at work during aerobic fitness training**

- **Explain the structure of the cardiovascular system**

- **Define the acute responses to aerobic exercise activities**

- **Define the chronic adaptations to aerobic fitness training**

- **Describe the benefits of aerobic fitness**

- **Explain how to improve aerobic fitness**

- **Plan a training program to improve aerobic fitness**

- **Describe the different ways to monitor intensity**

- **Discuss the importance of warm-up and cool-down**

- **Describe new approaches to achieving health benefits from activities**

aerobic fitness activities should not obscure the importance of the other components of fitness. Muscular fitness, flexibility, and body composition (defined in Chapter 2) all have important health ramifications as well, particularly as you age. Of what benefit, for instance, is aerobic fitness to an older person who does not have adequate strength to get out of a chair easily? In addition, a marathoner may have very high aerobic fitness but be prone to back pain as a result of weak abdominals and poor low back flexibility. In other words, a balanced program of exercise is the key to wellness.

In this chapter, you will become acquainted with all aspects of aerobic fitness. In addition to learning about health benefits, you will learn how to design a program of aerobic fitness training and identify ways to incorporate the plan into your lifestyle.

Defining Aerobic Fitness

As you move quickly up a flight of long stairs, your body systems must work together to allow you to reach the top. The more aerobically fit you are, the easier it will be for you to make that climb without discomfort. As discussed in Chapter 2, aerobic fitness can be defined as the ability of your cardiovascular and muscular systems to provide the necessary energy to sustain activity that uses the large muscle groups over an extended period of time. Dr. Kenneth Cooper, the physician who coined the term *aerobics,* defines aerobic exercise activities as those that use plenty of oxygen, thereby stimulating the heart and lungs for a time long enough to promote beneficial changes in the body. Jogging, swimming, cross-country skiing, and cycling are examples of aerobic exercise activities. Thus, **aerobic exercise** is any activity that uses a large percentage of muscle mass, can be maintained for a prolonged period, is rhythmical, and stimulates the heart, lungs, and muscles.

Also as discussed in Chapter 2, aerobic exercise is fueled by the aerobic energy pathway, which requires oxygen to produce the needed fuel for the body. The most accurate way to determine your level of aerobic fitness is to measure your **maximal oxygen consumption,** or VO_2max (pronounced vee-oh-two-max)—the maximal amount of oxygen that the body can use to generate energy while engaged in heavy exercise. By measuring your VO_2max, you can determine how well your cardiovascular and respiratory systems are working together to provide oxygen to your muscles.

VO_2max generally is measured while you exercise on a treadmill or a cycle ergometer (Figure 3.1a). As you gradually increase your intensity, or work rate, a corresponding increase in oxygen consumption occurs to support the increased rate of energy production in the muscles. The air you exhale is collected and analyzed to determine how much oxygen you are using at specific intensities. Eventually, you reach a point at which there is an increase in intensity without an accompanying increase in oxygen consumption; this is your VO_2max (Figure 3.1b).

As you engage in a regular program of aerobic exercise and experience its training benefits, your VO_2max increases. This, in turn, increases your capacity for aerobic exercise. As you become more aerobically fit, you can choose either to exercise at a higher intensity or to maintain at the same intensity as before but for a longer duration.

aerobic exercise any activity that uses a large percentage of muscle mass (50% or greater), can be maintained for a prolonged period, is rhythmic, and stimulates the heart, lungs, and muscles

maximal oxygen consumption (VO_2max) the maximal amount of oxygen the body can use to generate energy while engaged in heavy exercise

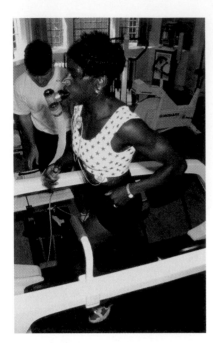

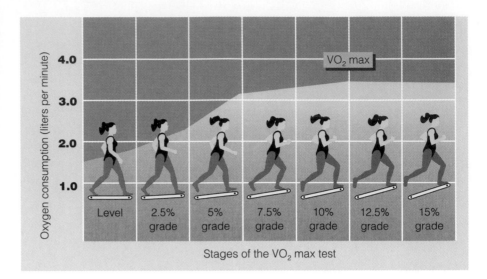

Figure 3.1

(a) Measurement of gases exhaled during an exercise stress test can be used to determine maximal oxygen consumption. **(b)** Oxygen consumption changes during an exercise stress test. The leveling off of the oxygen consumption in spite of an increase in exercise levels defines the VO_2max.

Source: From McArdle, Katch, and Katch, 1991.

Figure 3.2 illustrates the differences in aerobic fitness between Olympic-caliber athletes and sedentary individuals. As you can see, athletes who engage in rhythmic, continuous activities such as cross-country skiing, running, and cycling have the highest aerobic fitness as measured by their maximal oxygen consumption.

For both men and women, aerobic fitness declines with age at the rate of about 1% per year after age 25 (see Figure 3.3). However, you can see from Figure 3.3 that overall, men and women differ markedly in their levels of aerobic fitness. This is primarily due to the fact that, on average, men are larger than women. As a result of their greater size, men also have larger hearts, greater lung capacities, and more muscle mass, all of which contribute to a greater capacity for oxygen uptake.

Research by Niemann has shown that age-related declines in aerobic fitness are, at least to some degree, preventable. People who remain aerobically fit throughout their lifetime tend to experience much less of a decline than do sedentary individuals. Further, studies have shown that older adults are "trainable." That is, after 8 to 12 weeks of aerobic exercise, improvements in aerobic fitness can be achieved (Heath et al.; Pollock et al.) Nevertheless, the decline in aerobic fitness that comes with age cannot be stopped altogether. With advancing age there is a decrease in **maximal heart rate (MHR)**—the maximum number of beats per minute that the heart can achieve during exercise, estimated by the formula $220 - age$. As a result, the amount of blood that can be delivered to the working muscles is reduced. Thus, even with high levels of aerobic fitness training, aerobic fitness is somewhat lower in an older person because of a decreased MHR.

Physiology of Aerobic Fitness

To understand more fully the changes that occur to your body as you bike, jog, swim, or walk, you should be familiar with the body systems involved. Three important systems work together to provide energy for aerobic activities: pulmonary, cardiovascular, and muscular.

maximal heart rate (MHR)
the maximum number of beats per minute the heart can achieve during exercise, estimated by the formula $220 - age$.

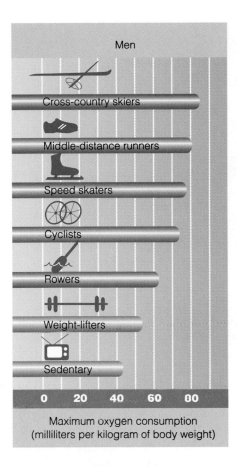

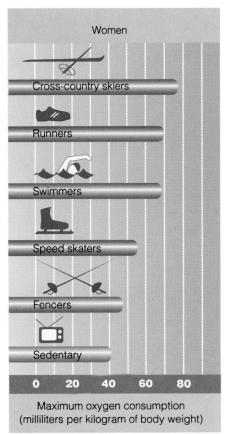

Men — Maximum oxygen consumption (milliliters per kilogram of body weight)

Cross-country skiers
Middle-distance runners
Speed skaters
Cyclists
Rowers
Weight-lifters
Sedentary

0 20 40 60 80

Women — Maximum oxygen consumption (milliliters per kilogram of body weight)

Cross-country skiers
Runners
Swimmers
Speed skaters
Fencers
Sedentary

0 20 40 60 80

Figure 3.2

Maximal oxygen consumption differs between elite athletes and inactive individuals. Even though you are not aiming for the Olympics, regular aerobic exercise will ensure that you have VO₂max levels well above those of a sedentary person.
Source: From McArdle, Katch, and Katch, 1991.

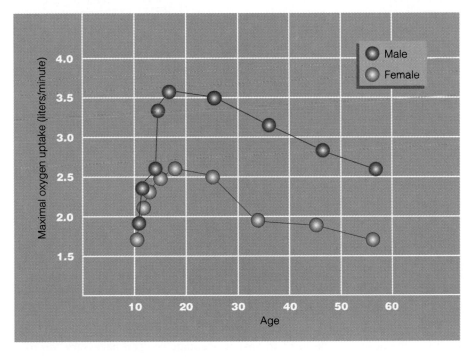

Figure 3.3

Maximal oxygen consumption changes with age and also differs by gender.
Source: From Larson, 1974.

The Body Systems

The **pulmonary system,** comprising the air passageways and lungs, brings oxygen from the atmosphere into the lungs. This oxygen is distributed throughout the tiny air sacs in the lungs called alveoli; it then rapidly moves from the alveoli into the blood through a process called diffusion.

pulmonary system the air passageways and lungs; it brings oxygen from the atmosphere into the lungs

Figure 3.4

The heart has four chambers. The right and left atria are holding tanks and pass blood through the valves into the right and left ventricles, which pump blood into the pulmonary system and to all body tissues. Source: From Marieb, 1992.

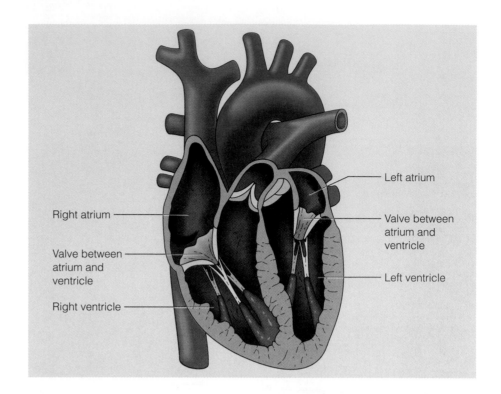

Right atrium

Valve between atrium and ventricle

Right ventricle

Left atrium

Valve between atrium and ventricle

Left ventricle

STATS-AT-A-GLANCE

Heart Disease and Physical Activity

■ Individuals who began activities such as running, swimming, cycling, or playing tennis between the ages of 15 and 25 had a 67% lower risk of stroke than adults who had never exercised. Those who started early and continued into their 60s had the lowest risk (Shinton and Sagar).

■ In a study of 3,000 men, a consistent inverse relationship was found between aerobic fitness and risk factors for coronary artery disease (CAD). As aerobic fitness increased, risk factors for CAD decreased (Cooper et al).

■ Individuals with low aerobic fitness are three times more likely to die than subjects with higher aerobic fitness (Blair).

cardiovascular system the heart and a network of arteries and vessels; it pumps blood throughout the body

atria the heart's "receptacles" that receive blood and then pass it into the ventricles

ventricles the main pumps of the cardiovascular system; they send blood to the lungs and other body tissues

stroke volume the amount of blood pumped with each contraction of the left ventricle

cardiac output the total amount of blood delivered into the cardiovascular system per minute

muscular system muscle fibers that receive and then use the oxygen supplied by the pulmonary and cardiovascular systems

The **cardiovascular system,** comprising the heart and a network of arteries and veins, pumps blood throughout the body. The heart functions as a muscular pump; every time it contracts, it sends blood either to the pulmonary system to pick up oxygen or to other body tissues (including itself) to deliver oxygen.

The heart contains four chambers: the right and left atria, which have relatively thin muscular walls, and the right and left ventricles, which are larger and have thick muscular walls (see Figure 3.4). As the heart's "receptacles," the **atria** receive blood and then pass it into the ventricles. As the main pumps of the cardiovascular system, the **ventricles** send blood to the lungs and other body tissues. Oxygen-poor blood enters the right atrium, where it is held until it flows through a valve into the right ventricle. This blood is then pumped into the pulmonary system to release carbon dioxide and pick up oxygen. The blood is returned to the left atrium, where it flows through a valve into the left ventricle. Oxygen-rich blood is then pumped to all body tissues. With each heart beat this cycle repeats itself. The passage of blood through the heart, lungs, and rest of the body is depicted in Figure 3.5.

The amount of blood pumped with each contraction of the left ventricle is called the **stroke volume.** The total amount of blood delivered into the cardiovascular system per minute is called the **cardiac output,** which is a product of the stroke volume and heart rate, or number of cycles the heart pumps per minute. During maximal exercise, cardiac output can be up to eight times faster than the resting rate.

The coronary arteries on the outside of the heart deliver oxygen-rich blood to the heart muscle itself to ensure adequate oxygen necessary to produce energy for contraction. If a coronary artery is narrowed by the buildup of cholesterol and fats, oxygen supply to the heart muscle is reduced. This reduced oxygen supply can result in gripping chest pains (angina) and, in severe cases, heart attack. (See the Stats-at-a-Glance on this page).

The **muscular system** is made up of the muscle fibers that receive and then use the oxygen supplied by the pulmonary and cardiovascular systems

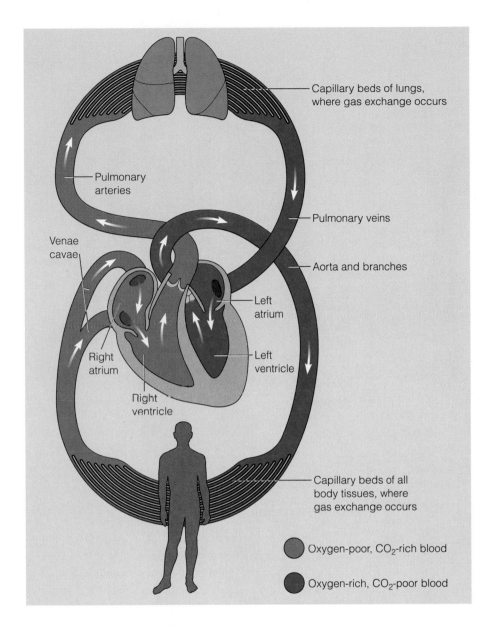

Capillary beds of lungs, where gas exchange occurs

Pulmonary arteries

Pulmonary veins

Venae cavae

Aorta and branches

Left atrium

Right atrium

Left ventricle

Right ventricle

Capillary beds of all body tissues, where gas exchange occurs

● Oxygen-poor, CO₂-rich blood

● Oxygen-rich, CO₂-poor blood

Figure 3.5

The heart pumps blood to the rest of the body. The right ventricle pumps blood into the pulmonary system and the left ventricle pumps blood into the system at large, supplying all body tissues with oxygen-rich blood. Source: From Hales, 1994.

to produce body movements. Carbon dioxide and other metabolic waste products are carried away from the muscles, allowing them to continue producing movement during aerobic exercise. The anatomy of the muscular system is illustrated in Figure 3.6.

Physiological Responses to Aerobic Fitness Training

The human body has a remarkable ability to adapt to changes in activity levels over both the short and the long term. These responses may be either acute or chronic.

Acute Responses. When you engage in aerobic exercise, your body systems respond immediately. This **acute response** refers to those changes that occur in the pulmonary, cardiovascular, and muscular systems during exercise. For example, when you begin to jog around the block, your body responds quickly to deliver more blood to the active muscles. The depth and frequency

acute response changes that occur in the pulmonary, cardiovascular, and muscular systems during exercise

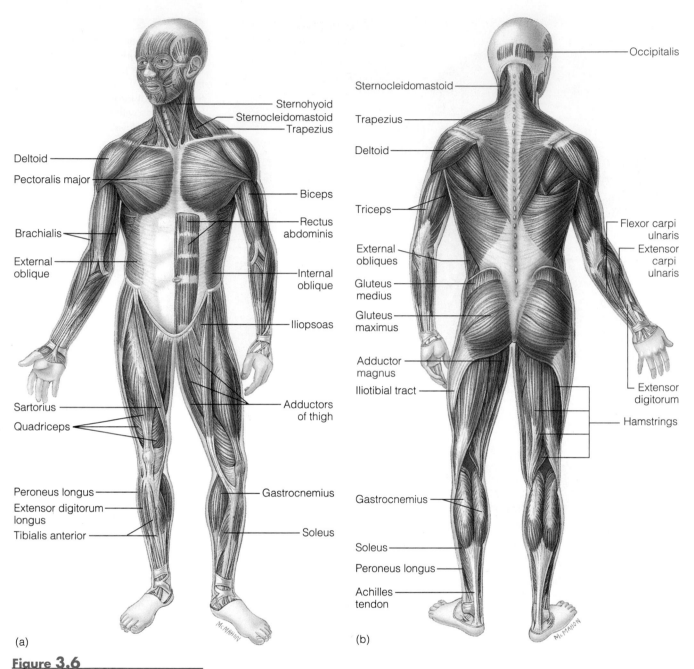

Occipitalis
Sternocleidomastoid
Trapezius
Deltoid
Triceps
External obliques
Gluteus medius
Gluteus maximus
Adductor magnus
Iliotibial tract
Flexor carpi ulnaris
Extensor carpi ulnaris
Extensor digitorum
Hamstrings
Gastrocnemius
Soleus
Peroneus longus
Achilles tendon

Sternohyoid
Sternocleidomastoid
Trapezius
Deltoid
Pectoralis major
Biceps
Brachialis
Rectus abdominis
External oblique
Internal oblique
Iliopsoas
Sartorius
Adductors of thigh
Quadriceps
Peroneus longus
Extensor digitorum longus
Gastrocnemius
Tibialis anterior
Soleus

(a)

(b)

Figure 3.6

Anatomy of the muscular system. Muscles that activate movement at major joints are shown at the front **(a)** and back **(b)** of the body. Source: From Alters and Schiff, 1998.

ventilation the depth and frequency of your breathing

systolic blood pressure the pressure exerted in the arteries when the heart contracts

of your breathing, termed **ventilation,** increases and your heart beats faster and pumps more blood (increases stroke volume) in order to increase the supply to your working muscles. As a result of the increase in cardiac output, **systolic blood pressure**—the pressure exerted within the arteries when the heart contracts—also increases to move blood through your body more rapidly. Oxygen is more quickly extracted from the blood by body tissues.

With the exception of heart rate, women have lower values than do men for each of these acute responses to exercise because of their generally smaller size. Heart rate is the only factor that is not governed by physical size; it is controlled by the nervous and endocrine systems. Thus, heart rate does not differ according to gender.

Chronic Responses. When you work out consistently, you demand more from your body. As you repeatedly overload your systems, an adaptation to training occurs. This **chronic response** (or training response) refers to changes in the pulmonary, cardiovascular, and muscular systems as a result of aerobic fitness training. For example, suppose you have not been exercising and decide to begin a walking/jogging program. For 8 weeks, you work out 3 days per week, beginning with 10 minutes per session during the first week and increasing to 30 minutes per session by the eighth week. As time passes, the workouts become easier and you can exercise harder and longer. Your body systems have responded by adapting to the new demands you have placed on them.

If you had taken a VO_2max test before and after your 8-week exercise program, the tests would have shown an improvement in maximal oxygen consumption. This result would mean that your aerobic fitness had improved, as work requiring less than maximum, or submaximal, effort had become easier. Thus, **submaximal exercise** is work performed at levels below maximal effort.

To understand better the concept of submaximal exercise, think back to the procedure involved in a VO_2max test on a treadmill, discussed earlier. This test involves walking and/or running to keep pace with the treadmill as it gradually speeds up and its slope increases. Your heart rate rises steadily as the work, measured by the speed and slope of the treadmill, increases. In fact, your heart rate may increase to as many as 200 beats per minute or more. At this point, you stop the test because of fatigue. In other words, you are performing **maximal exercise,** the highest level of work that you can perform. All work up to the point of maximal effort is referred to as submaximal.

As you continue to engage in aerobic exercise over time, your heart becomes more efficient. At rest, your heart rate is lower than it was before training because your stroke volume has increased. Therefore, your heart can beat fewer times in order to maintain cardiac output. A reduction of only five beats per minute can save your heart 2,628,000 beats per year! During submaximal exercise, your ventilation and heart rate are lower and your muscles are more efficient in removing and using oxygen to generate energy. At maximal exercise levels, you can perform more work because you can ventilate more air, your cardiovascular system can pump greater amounts of blood and distribute more blood to active muscles, and your muscle fibers are able to remove more oxygen from that blood. The end result is that you have a higher maximal oxygen consumption (VO_2max) and therefore improved aerobic fitness.

Benefits of Aerobic Fitness

Aerobic fitness is associated with physical as well as psychological wellness. It has been identified as an important factor in the prevention of chronic diseases, especially coronary artery disease, and also is effective in helping reduce psychological stress.

Cardioprotective Mechanisms. Dr. Brian Sharkey has described the "cardioprotective mechanisms" of aerobic fitness (see Table 3.1). The term *cardioprotective* refers to the physiological changes that occur with aerobic fitness training and that help to protect the cardiovascular system from disease. Keep in mind that other factors (for example, inherited tendencies, smoking, alcohol consumption, diet, stress) also contribute to overall health. The importance of the cardioprotective mechanisms relative to these other factors has yet to be established.

chronic response adaptations by the pulmonary, cardiovascular, and muscular systems as a result of aerobic fitness training

submaximal exercise work performed at levels below maximal effort

maximal exercise the highest level of work that can be performed

TABLE 3.1

Cardioprotective Mechanisms Resulting from Aerobic Fitness Training

MECHANISM	EFFECT OF AEROBIC FITNESS TRAINING
Fat metabolism	Enhances fat metabolism by increasing caloric expenditure; reduces body fat; reduces blood lipids
Lean body mass	Preserves lean body mass, particularly during dieting
Blood lipids	Lowers serum fat levels; lowers cholesterol
Blood vessels	Improves circulation within the heart (coronary circulation); develops collateral pathways within the heart
Blood pressure	Decreases systolic blood pressure in individuals with high blood pressure (hypertensives)
Heart	Reduces the workload of the heart by lowering resting and submaximal heart rate; increases blood volume, which contributes to a greater stroke volume

Source: From Sharkey, 1991.

The amount and intensity of exercise necessary to protect against heart disease is also unknown. The most beneficial amount of exercise for each individual likely depends on that person's particular risk factors. For instance, research has shown that moderate physical activity helps protect against diabetes, whereas higher levels of aerobic fitness training are more effective for reducing total cholesterol.

Psychological Effects. The potential effect of aerobic exercise activities on psychological health has sparked much research interest over the past 15 years. Although aerobic exercise appears to reduce psychological stress, the reasons for this are not clear. Psychological stress is a physical stressor and produces the same physiological responses that are associated with exercise, such as increases in heart rate, breathing rate, and oxygen consumption. Some reasons exercise may be an effective stress reducer include its ability to (1) induce actual physiological changes, (2) dissipate hostility and frustration, (3) provide a diversion that may help a person relax, and (4) improve self-concept.

Some evidence suggests that chemical changes in the brain during aerobic exercise induce a feeling of euphoria similar to a drug-induced high. For example, reports of a postexercise high from people who exercise aerobically led to speculation that these feelings may be caused by a morphine-like substance that is released into the bloodstream (Thoren et al.). The investigators theorized that, when stimulated by muscle stretching or muscle contraction, small receptors in the muscle tissues transmit impulses to the brain to control pain. In fact, their research has shown that prolonged, submaximal aerobic exercise increases beta-endorphin levels. **Beta-endorphins** are natural opioids that are produced in the brain and contribute to the regulation of blood pressure, pain perception, and control of body temperature. Some researchers attribute improvements in mood to higher concentrations of

beta-endorphins natural opioids produced in the brain that contribute to the regulation of blood pressure, pain perception, and control of body temperature

beta-endorphins. However, not all improvements in mood have been associated with a rise in beta-endorphins. More research is needed to help define the mechanisms by which exercise alters mood.

Aerobic exercise has also been found to increase alpha brain waves, which are associated with a relaxed state of mind. Research has shown that alpha waves appear 20 minutes into a 30-minute jog and can still be measured after exercise has stopped (Wiese, Singh, and Yeudall). (Chapter 10 discusses in detail brain waves, their association with stress, and ways to alter them with stress-reduction methods.)

In general, the positive attributes of personality such as self-concept, well-being, and mood improve with aerobic exercise, and unhealthy traits such as rapid increases in heart rate and blood pressure (which produces stress), depression, and anxiety tend to decrease (Niemann). These benefits are important reasons to consider taking steps to develop and maintain your aerobic fitness.

Designing an Aerobic Fitness Program

In designing an aerobic fitness program, you must focus on three phases: (1) assessment and/or definition of goals, (2) choice of exercise, and (3) exercise prescription, which includes frequency, intensity, duration, and rate of progression.

MYTHS & CONTROVERSIES

Myth 1 — **If I don't conform to a program of high intensity, I will not protect myself from heart disease.** There is evidence that being moderately active provides significant protection from heart disease and that consistency and commitment to an "active lifestyle" is of great benefit with respect to reducing your risk for heart disease.

Myth 2 — **Walking isn't really exercise.** In fact, walking is an excellent way for less active people to get into shape. It is convenient, involves no special equipment, can be done alone or with a friend, and has a very low injury rate. Briskly walking at 3.5 to 4 miles per hour burns about as many calories as running a comparable distance and has similar fitness benefits. And walking is a form of exercise many people find they can stick with for life. Once your fitness level starts to improve, you can vary your walking routine by going up and down hills, choosing varied terrain such as gravel or sand, or striding with your arms swinging freely. You can even make walking into a sport by taking up racewalking.

Controversy 1 — **Should you use hand and ankle weights?** You may notice people in the gym or on the track with small weights around their wrists or ankles. Do these weights actually improve your workout? Studies show that using these weights provides only small gains in heart rate and number of calories burned; similar gains can be made by exercising a little longer or harder—and the weights can increase your chances of injury during exercise, especially during aerobic dance or running. Unless you have complete control over them, using weights can lead to muscle sprains and damage to tendons and ligaments. For most people, the disadvantages of wearing weights during aerobic workouts outweigh any possible advantages.

Controversy 2 — **Working out for 45 minutes a day is more beneficial than 4, 10-minute bouts spread out over the day.** There is some evidence that shorter periods of exercise throughout a day carry health benefits (Blair et al.). However, there is no proof that this approach will significantly improve aerobic fitness. Research by Dr. Blair at the Cooper Institute is continuing to investigate these questions.

Assessment and Goal Setting

Before you begin your program, you need to assess your level of aerobic fitness, either objectively with a test of fitness, or subjectively, based on knowledge of your own physical activity habits. Assessment can help you in three ways: (1) in setting your goals, (2) in individualizing your exercise prescription, and (3) in evaluating your progress.

The most accurate way to assess aerobic fitness is by measuring maximal oxygen consumption (VO_2max). Other more practical but less accurate estimates of aerobic fitness include a bench-stepping test, a 1-mile walking test, and a 1.5-mile run/walk test, all of which are submaximal measures (see Laboratory 3.1). For both the walking test and the run/walk test, you move as quickly as you can over the designated distance. The faster you are able to cover the distance, the better is your aerobic fitness level. Although these tests yield only estimates of your true maximum, they offer a good alternative to VO_2Max testing.

Once you have determined your aerobic fitness level, it's time to define short- and long-term goals. Your short-term goals should be realistic and achievable even though your long-term goals may seem somewhat unattainable at the outset. Remember: Your goals are not carved in stone; they can change as you progress.

Suppose you are a 22-year-old woman and your results from the 1-mile walking test in Laboratory 3.1 indicate that your aerobic fitness falls in the category labeled "needs extra work." Subjectively, it was difficult for you to cover the 1-mile distance quickly. Because your fitness "needs extra work," you should develop a progressive training program to improve your aerobic fitness. You might decide to set your goals as follows:

SHORT-TERM GOAL
After 8 weeks, be able to jog 1.5 miles without stopping

LONG-TERM GOAL
In 6 months be able to run 3 miles comfortably without stopping

If your score had placed you in the category of "good" and you were already engaged in an exercise program, you might simply want to maintain your current habits. Or you might want to define goals to achieve other types of health-related benefits, such as reducing your blood pressure, lowering your total cholesterol, or losing weight. (Goals related to body weight and fat loss are discussed in Chapter 7.)

A good time to monitor these health-related changes is during your annual physical checkup. A health-related benefit you can monitor yourself is resting heart rate (see Laboratory 3.2). The most important change, however, is that you feel better and incorporate aerobic exercise into your lifestyle.

Choice of Exercise

The type, or mode, of exercise that you choose will be related to the goals you set. In the previous example, the type of exercise (walking progressing to jogging) was selected as part of the goal itself. In many cases, any type of aerobic exercise activity could help you accomplish the goal of simply becoming more active.

One of the most important considerations in deciding what type of exercise to choose is finding an activity or combination of activities that you enjoy. Some people roller-blade, some walk, some jog, some swim, and some take aerobic fitness classes. Table 3.2 identifies some aerobic activities based on their value for developing and maintaining aerobic fitness. You may prefer to vary our exercise choices. For example, even though your goal might be to walk 1 mile, you could add bike riding or stair-stepping to your walking program. Using different types of activity in an aerobic exercise program is called **cross-training.** Choosing two or more aerobic activities that each stress your cardiovascular system helps you achieve your desired training effects while avoiding monotony and maintaining a high level of motivation for exercising. However, in keeping with the principle of specificity (discussed in Chapter 2), don't forget that to improve a walking time, your training needs to be specific to walking.

Exercise Prescription

You improve your aerobic fitness by consistently and deliberately placing demands on your cardiovascular system beyond those of your normal daily activities. Your degree of improvement depends on the exercise prescription you establish. In other words, you intentionally prescribe a program of exercise for yourself based on the principle of overload (discussed in Chapter 2)

Program Design. Success in achieving your fitness goals is a result of designing a program with the appropriate intensity, duration, and frequency to meet your individual needs. The following aerobic exercise prescription is recommended by the American College of Sports Medicine (ACSM) to achieve health- and fitness-related benefits.

TABLE 3.2

Value of Various Physical Activities for Developing Aerobic Fitness

HIGH VALUE	MODERATE VALUE	LOW VALUE
Aerobic dance	Basketball	Archery
Bicycling	Calisthenics	Baseball
Brisk walking	Dancing	Bowling
Cross-country skiing	Downhill skiing	Football
Jogging	Field hockey	Golf
Jumping rope	Handball	Martial arts
Rollerblading	Racquetball	Softball
Rowing	Soccer	Volleyball
Running	Squash	
Skating	Tennis	
Stair climbing		
Stair-stepping machine		
Stationary bicycling		
Swimming		
Uphill hiking/walking		

cross training using different types of activity in an aerobic exercise program

Sound Decision Making

DANCING THE HEADACHES AWAY

Lisa played volleyball on her high school team, but since she started college last year, she has felt that she was too busy to exercise. She hadn't thought too much about it until she realized she's gained about 15 pounds since she started college. She has also been getting headaches regularly, which she suspects may be due to stress. Lisa starts to think that regular aerobic exercise could help her with both these problems.

Lisa talks with her roommate Tracy about the idea of starting an aerobic exercise program. Tracy goes to aerobic dance class three times a week with two other friends and invites Lisa to join them the next week. Lisa agrees to try it—she's always loved to dance. Over the next few days she buys some aerobic shoes and reschedules a study date so she can have time to go to aerobics class with Tracy. She also learns some stretching exercises to do before she exercises and practices them.

Tuesday afternoon, Lisa meets Tracy and her friends at the gym for her first class. They start out with some gentle stretches and warm-up exercises. Soon the music gets faster and the pace gets more intense. Many of the other people in the class seem to be able to keep up perfectly with the instructor's energetic moves. Lisa feels a little awkward because she is unfamiliar with some of the dance steps, and she feels winded after just a few minutes. But she keeps at it, resting when necessary. She doesn't worry too much about perfectly replicating the instructor's steps and concentrates instead on having fun.

Soon Lisa is joining the aerobics class four times per week, and within a month she can keep up with them for the whole workout. She feels better about herself for this achievement, and she's lost a few pounds too. She finds she really loves aerobic dance; all her problems seem to dissolve when she abandons herself to the music. And her headaches have almost completely disappeared.

Frequency: 3–7 times (most days of the week)

Intensity: 40%–85% of heart rate reserve (calculated using the target heart rate)

Formula on page 70

Duration: 15–60 minutes

Let your current level of aerobic fitness guide your choice of exercise prescription. Note that the minimum recommendation is 15 minutes of exercise 3 times per week at an intensity that is 40% of **heart rate reserve (HRR),** defined as maximal heart rate minus resting heart rate. (See page 70 for instructions on how to calculate your HRR.) These guidelines reflect the smallest amount of activity needed to achieve health-related benefits without necessarily improving your fitness level. For example, taking a brisk 15-minute walk 3 times per week would probably satisfy the minimum aerobic prescription.

If you are very inactive, however, even the minimum amount of exercise can improve your aerobic fitness. For example, if you sit most of the day, take the elevator instead of the stairs, and watch television or read in your leisure time, you would be considered sedentary, or physically inactive. In this case, you will most likely observe changes in your aerobic fitness level if you embark on a program of brisk walking 15 minutes 3 times per week for 6 to 8 weeks.

By contrast, if your days are filled with activities, such as walking a lot at work, taking the stairs instead of the elevator, and doing all your own gardening and housework, the minimum exercise prescription just described will

heart rate reserve (HRR)
maximal heart rate minus resting heart rate

probably not improve your aerobic fitness level. Still, you would not choose the maximum exercise prescription of 60 minutes 7 times per week at 85% of HRR. These values would be appropriate only for a person who has been training consistently. Your program would begin with a moderate exercise prescription—for example, 20 minutes 3 times per week at 55% of HRR.

Intensity. An important point to remember in designing your program is to keep the intensity low, particularly in the beginning stages. If you select an intensity that is too high, you may become frustrated or injured and be forced to stop the activity and reduce the length of your workout. Thus, in the beginning, you want to combine low intensity with higher duration—for example, exercising for 20 to 30 minutes at 55% of your HRR. As you work out, watch for clues to overexertion such as soreness, lingering exhaustion, and declining interest, and modify your workout accordingly. Table 3.3 presents the exercise intensity prescriptions for various fitness levels.

Duration. The interplay between duration and intensity determines how much work is done at each session. Because duration and intensity are inversely related, as you increase the duration of your workout, you also need to decrease the intensity. This means that you will not be working as hard but will be able to maintain the activity for a longer period of time.

Suppose you are walking at a comfortable speed on a flat surface and are breathing easily. You may feel that you could walk for long distances at this pace. However, you suddenly encounter a steep hill and your speed begins to decrease; depending on the length of the hill, you may even have to stop and catch your breath. Because the intensity of your flat walk was fairly low, the duration could be greater. When the intensity increased, your speed decreased and it took you longer to reach your destination.

Frequency. The frequency of your workouts should begin with a minimum of 3 times per week on nonconsecutive days and can increase to between 5 and 7 times per week depending on your goals. Working out at the same time each day makes it easier to introduce a new exercise habit into your lifestyle.

Monitoring Intensity. To guide your effort as you exercise, you need to be aware of methods of monitoring intensity. Heart rate, rating of perceived exertion, and the talk test are valuable methods to help you rate the difficulty of your workout.

Heart Rate. Because it is easy to calculate and correlates well with oxygen consumption, heart rate has been widely used as a measure of the intensity of

TABLE 3.3

Recommended Percentages of Heart Rate (HR) Reserve Within Target Zones

TARGET ZONE	AEROBIC FITNESS LEVEL		
	LOW	AVERAGE	HIGH
Minimum HR	40%	55%	65%
Target HR	65	70	75
Maximal HR	75	80	85

an activity. The methods for taking resting and exercise heart rates are presented in Laboratory 3.2. A simple formula can be used to determine your **target heart rate (THR)**—the submaximal heart rate zone within which one should train during aerobic activity:

Maximal heart rate (MHR) = 220 − your age = _____

Heart rate reserve (HRR) = MHR − resting heart rate = _____

(HRR × 0.40) + RHR = THR for *low end* of zone = _____

(HRR × 0.60) + RHR = THR = _____

(HRR × 0.85) + RHR = THR for *high end* of zone = _____

This formula individualizes your THR by taking your resting heart rate into account. By calculating a specific as well as a lower- and higher-intensity THR, you obtain a target zone. As you exercise, you want to keep your heart rate within this zone. The preceding calculations use a sample THR of 60% of HRR with a target zone between 40% and 85% of HRR.

Applying the formula to a 22-year-old with a resting heart rate of 70 beats per minute (bpm), we arrive at the following target heart rates:

Maximal heart rate (MHR) = 220 − 22 = 198 bpm

Heart rate reserve (HRR) = MHR − resting heart rate = 128 bpm

(128 × 0.40) + 70 = THR for *low end* of zone = 121 bpm

(128 × 0.60) + 70 = THR = 147 bpm

(128 × 0.85) + 70 = THR for *high end* of zone = 179 bpm

The target heart rate in this example is 147 bpm within a target zone of 121 bpm at the low end and 179 bpm at the high end. These are very realistic intensity values for a healthy individual who has normal levels of activity throughout the day.

A sample of target zones for different ages is illustrated in Figure 3.7. These values are based on a resting heart rate of 70 bpm and intensities of 40% and 85% of HRR. Notice that target heart rate decreases with age because maximal heart rate also decreases with age.

Rating of Perceived Exertion. Another method of determining the intensity of your workout is simply to assess how you are feeling. This perception is not directed at a specific body area—for example, leg fatigue or shortness of breath—but rather an overall feeling of exertion. Dr. Gunner Borg has developed a subjective scale that corresponds to actual heart rate values at mild, moderate, and high intensities for subjective evaluation of intensity. His **rating of perceived exertion (RPE)** is a subjective scale of values for various intensities that correspond well to heart rate at given intensities (see Table 3.4). This valuable and reliable tool of monitoring intensity is used extensively in clinics and laboratory settings when individuals are undergoing submaximal and maximal exercise evaluations. If you were to use this scale, you would be instructed to evaluate how you feel at various stages of your exercise. For example, in a resting state your activity will feel "very, very light," which corresponds to an RPE value between 6 and 8. As effort increases, you progress to a point at which your workout feels "somewhat hard," corresponding to an RPE value of 13, but you are able to continue the activity. Increasing your intensity will push you into a feeling of "hard," which corresponds to an RPE value between 14 and 16. A

target heart rate (THR) a submaximal heart rate zone within which one should train during aerobic activity, usually between 40% and 85% of heart rate reserve

rating of perceived exertion (RPE) a subjective scale of values for various intensities that correspond well to heart rate

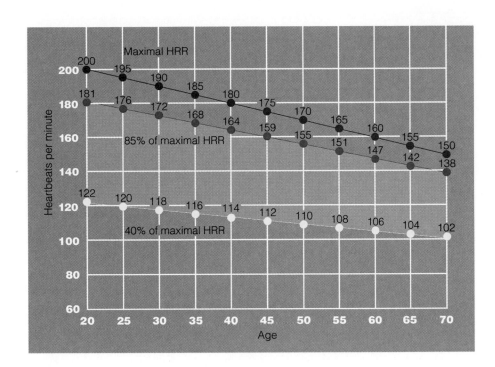

Figure 3.7
The proper exercise intensity should raise your heart rate between 40% and 85% of your maximal heart rate reserve (HRR). The target heart rate zone declines with age, due to the decline in maximal HRR. The graph depicts the training zone for a person with a resting heart rate of 70 bpm. Source: From Klug and Lettunich, 1992.

rating between 13 and 16 may correlate with the low and high ends of your target heart rate as identified previously in this section. At your very maximal effort, your exertion level becomes "very, very hard" and you would have to stop your activity. This represents the high end of the scale—an RPE value of 19—and thus your maximal exercise. Monitoring with this method is useful because it helps you become attuned to your body and does not require you to stop to take your pulse.

The Talk Test. Another method of determining how hard you are working is the "talk test," a simple approach that requires no stopwatch, scales, or memorization of numbers. Essentially, if you can talk comfortably while you are exercising, you are working within your target zone. When you are working at very high intensities, you need to breathe at high rates, which prevents you from being able to talk comfortably. The talk test is easy, uncomplicated, and fun because it means you are exercising with a partner.

Rate of Progression. How much and how quickly should you progress? This depends on a number of factors: current aerobic fitness level, age, health status, and desired goals. A sample program to achieve the short-term goal discussed previously (to be able, at the end of 8 weeks, to jog 1.5 miles without stopping) is presented in Table 3.5.

If you are just beginning an aerobic conditioning program, your rate of progression will include a beginning phase, progression phase, and maintenance phase (see Chapter 2). If you are already exercising and wish to improve your aerobic fitness level, you can bypass the beginning phase and start your program in the progression phase (see Table 3.6).

During the beginning stage, intensity, duration, and frequency are kept to a minimum in order to reduce the likelihood of soreness and encourage compliance with the program. Even though they are initially highly motivated, many people who start out too fast quit their programs after only a few weeks. After 4 to 6 weeks of the beginning stage, your cardiovascular

TABLE 3.4	
Scale for Rating Perceived Exertion (RPE)	
RPE VALUE	**ACTIVITY LEVEL**
6	
7	Very, very light
8	
9	Very light
10	
11	Fairly light
12	
13	Somewhat hard
14	
15	Hard
16	
17	Very hard
18	
19	Very, very hard

A rating between 13 and 16 correlates well with target heart rate.

TABLE 3.5

Rate of Progression for an Aerobic Exercise Program

Week 1:   Walk 1 mile at 50%–60% heart rate reserve (HRR) on flat terrain 3 times. (Either use a track or plan a 1-mile course in your neighborhood with your car.) Take exercise heart rate during and after your workouts.

Week 2:   Jog ¼ mile at 60% HRR, walk ½ mile at a brisk pace, jog ¼ mile at 60% HRR on flat terrain 4 times.

Week 3:   Jog ¼ mile at 60% HRR, walk ¼ mile at a brisk pace, jog ¼ mile at 60% HRR, walk ¼ mile at a brisk pace on flat terrain 4 times.

Week 4:   Jog ½ mile at 65% HRR, walk ¼ mile at a brisk pace, jog ½ mile at 65% HRR on flat terrain 4 times.

Week 5:   Jog ¾ mile at 65% HRR, walk ¼ mile at a brisk pace, jog ¼ mile at 65% HRR on flat terrain 4 times.

Week 6:   Jog 1 mile at 65% HRR, walk ½ mile at a brisk pace on flat terrain 4 times.

Week 7:   Jog 1 mile at 70% HRR, walk ¼ mile at a brisk pace on flat terrain 4 times.

Week 8:   Jog 1¼ miles at 70% HRR, walk ¼ mile at a brisk pace, jog ½ mile on flat terrain 4 times.

Week 9:   Jog 1½ miles to determine whether you have met your goal. Two days later, reassess your aerobic fitness level. Continue building duration into your program.

TABLE 3.6

The Three Phases of an Aerobic Exercise Program

STAGE	FREQUENCY	INTENSITY	DURATION	MONTHS
Beginning	3 times/wk	40% HRR[a]	15–20 min	1–12
Progression	Increase as body adapts	Increase as body adapts	Increase every 2 wks	4–5
Maintenance	3–5 times/wk	70–85% HRR	30–60 min/ session	At 6

[a]HRR = Heart rate reserve.

system will have adapted to the overload and you will be ready for the progression stage.

During the progression stage you will modify the duration and/or intensity of your activity. For example, if you are doing 20 minutes of aerobic conditioning three times per week, you will increase each session by approximately 5 minutes every 2 weeks. If an extra 5 minutes doesn't seem like enough, increase it by 10 minutes or work out 4 times per week instead of 3. Remember that all recommendations presented here are merely suggested guidelines. Only you know how you feel; therefore, you are the best judge of how to modify your program. (Be aware of the signs of overexercising, discussed in Chapter 6.) The American College of Sports Medicine (ACSM) recommends that people who work out on a daily basis alternate weight-bearing activities such as walking, jogging, and running with non-weight-bearing activities such as bicycling and swimming. This strategy reduces the impact to hip, knee, and ankle joints.

After 4 to 5 months at the progression stage, you may feel pleased with your progress. If so, you do not need to continue adding to your program. Instead, you can keep up what you have established by entering the maintenance phase. In this phase, your training levels off and the benefits of your efforts are achieved. Now it's time to stick with it for life!

Guidelines for Aerobic Exercise

Each exercise session should include three phases: (1) warm-up, (2) aerobic activity, and (3) cool-down. Often people overlook the warm-up and

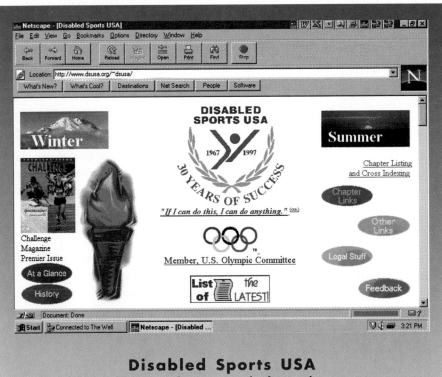

Disabled Sports USA
http://www.dsusa.org/~dsusa/#sports

This site contains lots of information of interest to disabled athletes and their supporters. It includes links to regional chapters of Disabled Sports USA (DS/USA) and other associations, and has information about upcoming events around the world for disabled athletes, including swimming, cycling, track, hockey, and skiing events plus much more. There is also legal information on the Americans with Disabilities Act.

Critical thinking: Does this site challenge any of your assumptions about disabled people? Do you think the disabled can reach high levels of wellness? Why or why not?

Source: From Disabled Sports, USA, 1995–1998.

cool-down phases in favor of the aerobic activity phase. Please take a minute to refer to question 3 from Section 11 of the Wellness Inventory you completed in Chapter 1; if you do not warm up or cool down, you are overlooking important parts of your workout. If you have chosen to join an aerobics class rather than plan your own program, the instructor has done the workout planning for you. However, to be able to critique the quality of instruction you receive, you still need to understand the three essential phases of an aerobic workout.

Warm-Up

The warm-up at the beginning of your workout should include specific exercises designed to prepare your body for aerobic exercise. Gradually increasing your heart rate until you reach your training zone is an important precaution to take; you don't want to "jump start" your heart. An adequate warm-up is important because it does the following:

■ Prepares the cardiovascular system for more strenuous activity

■ Increases blood flow and enhances the delivery of oxygen and fuel to exercising muscles

■ Provides a transition from rest to exercise, which may reduce muscle soreness

■ Increases the elasticity and temperature of muscles and connective tissues, resulting in safer, more effective performance

■ Enhances the mechanical efficiency and power of exercising muscles

A 10-minute warm-up prior to strenuous activity begins with a general form of exercise, such as a brisk walk. After this, your warm-up should become more specific to the aerobic activity you have chosen. Here is a sample warm-up for a running workout:

General: 5 minutes of brisk walk

Specific: 5 minutes of light, held stretches for the entire body with emphasis on hips and legs (see Figure 5.3 for examples). All stretches should be held for 10 to 30 seconds and repeated 2 to 3 times.

Aerobic Activity

This is the activity component of your workout—the time in which you focus on intensity and duration. Remember, the ACSM recommends that you achieve a minimum of 40% of your heart rate reserve for at least 15 minutes. For most, this represents a brisk walk. Others who are more fit will reach for a higher intensity for a longer duration. It is during this component of your workout that you are placing greater demands on your body and working toward achieving the many benefits of aerobic activity.

Cool-Down

One of the biggest mistakes many people make following a workout in which target heart rate levels reach between 140 and 150 bpm is to stop moving. In fact, cardiovascular problems most commonly occur during an inadequate cool-down period. Frequently, aerobics instructors ask people to sit down and begin stretching immediately following aerobic activity. This is a dangerous practice because blood cannot as easily be returned to the heart without the pumping action of leg muscles.

When you stop exercising in the standing or sitting position, blood that needs to return to the heart can pool in your lower extremities. Those with a weak heart may develop problems if not enough blood gets back to the heart. Although young, healthy college students are unlikely to suffer any abnormality, it is good practice to ease back to resting, just as you geared up for activity.

Your cool-down needs to be dynamic; that is, your feet should be moving in order to help blood flow back to your heart. Before you stop moving or sit down, your heart rate should be at most 120 bpm or 20 beats in a 10-second time period. For a person over age 50 this value should be 100 bpm or less. The easiest cool-down method following strenuous activity is a 5 to 10 minute walk at a comfortable pace (see the Do's and Don'ts box).

AEROBIC ◆ EXERCISE

Do

▲ Set realistic goals.

▲ Identify your barriers to exercise and work toward replacing them with activity.

▲ Choose activities that you enjoy.

▲ Begin slowly and ease into your progression phase.

▲ Include a warm-up and cool-down in each of your exercise sessions.

▲ Find a friend to work out with 1 or 2 times per week. It helps if she/he has a similar fitness level.

▲ Reward yourself when you reach your goals.

▲ Vary your program to reduce boredom and improve adherence—for example, alternate walking with bicycling, or play a game of racquetball.

▲ Be patient with yourself.

Don't

▼ Begin an activity just because somebody else likes it.

▼ Start out with high-intensity levels.

▼ Overestimate the time you can exercise.

▼ Begin your activity session without a proper warm-up.

▼ End your activity session without an appropriate cool-down.

▼ Get frustrated if you are not progressing as fast as you'd like.

Lifestyle Choices: Plan for Action

In the Wellness Inventory you completed in Chapter 1, Section II was devoted to fitness. If you are satisfied with your aerobic fitness level and training program, you may choose to move on to Chapters 4 and 5, which deal with muscular fitness and flexibility. Remember that a balance of all fitness components is important for wellness. However, if you answered "some of the time" or "never" to question 2 in Section 11 of the Wellness Inventory in Laboratory 1.1, you may want to examine your exercise habits and consider incorporating more activity into your daily routine.

How much exercise is enough? Research suggests that only 15 minutes of activity 3 times per week at a moderate level of intensity is enough to result in health benefits. Convincing evidence from research directed by Blair at the Cooper Institute of Aerobics in Dallas suggests that high levels of aerobic fitness do not offer an extra measure of protection. As a result of this evidence, the ACSM has reduced the recommended duration and intensity of aerobic exercise for achieving health benefits. The new exercise prescription was presented earlier in this chapter.

From another angle, Blair is investigating a unique approach to the challenge of convincing the American population to exercise. He theorizes that short bouts of activity "pulsed" into a day may result in the same health benefits as one longer session of exercise. In other words, four brisk 10-minute walks would serve the same purpose as one 40-minute brisk walk. In fact, as a result of his work and that of other experts, the U.S. Centers for Disease Control and Prevention and the ACSM recently released a new recommendation on the types and amounts of physical activity needed for maintenance and promotion of health. In summary, everyone should accumulate at least 30 minutes of moderate-intensity physical activity most days of the week (see Table 3.7). Thus, activities such as taking the stairs, walking to work or class, and raking leaves can be added together over the course of the day to meet the 30-minute minimum. This minimum translates into burning approximately 150 calories. Table 3.8 identifies activities that vary in intensity level, but all require about 150 calories of energy output (Surgeon General's Report on Physical Activity and Health, 1996). Notice that the activities requiring 30 minutes are categorized as "moderate intensity"—that is, at the mid-point of vigorous activity.

As you become more active, remember that some exercise is always better than none. Small amounts of physical activity can be beneficial even if they are below the ACSM recommendations for duration and intensity discussed previously. Blair recommends the 2-minute walk as a way to move out of the habit of nonactivity. As he says, "Small changes can make a big difference." You will find ideas to "get yourself moving" in Table 3.7 and to burn 150 calories in Table 3.8.

Getting started is often the most difficult part of an aerobic fitness training program. After you have completed the aerobic assessments for this chapter (Laboratories 3.1 and 3.2), you can create a plan of action for yourself by filling out the following goal-setting form. Use Tables 3.7 and 3.8 to select the activities that will help you to meet your goals for aerobic fitness.

My aerobic fitness classification is _____

Based on this classification of aerobic fitness and my personal interests, I have chosen the following short- and long-term goals:

SHORT-TERM GOALS

_____

_____

_____

I will achieve my short-term goals on _____ *(date)*

_____   _____

(signature)   *(witness)*

LONG-TERM GOALS

_____

_____

_____

I will achieve my long-term goals on _____ *(date)*.

_____   _____

(signature)   *(witness)*

Make a list of benefits you would gain from doing aerobic exercise. Then list any potential barriers that make it difficult for you to exercise.

POTENTIAL BENEFITS   POTENTIAL BARRIERS

_____   _____

_____   _____

_____   _____

Now, identify one barrier that you need to overcome in order to add *at least one session* of aerobic exercise to your schedule: _____

TABLE 3.7

On the Move: Ten Ways to Add Activity to Your Week

1. Take a 10-minute walk as a study break.
2. Jog 5 minutes as a study break.
3. Play Frisbee with a friend.
4. Clean your room.
5. Walk to the store or to school.

6. Volunteer at a local preschool.
7. Take a short bicycle ride.
8. Watch one less television show.
9. Go window shopping.
10. Take your dog or a friend's dog for a walk.

Fill out the following daily aerobic activity exercise log as you work toward your goals over the next 2 weeks.

At the end of 2 weeks, review your progress. What worked? What didn't work? If you need to start over, choose a new barrier to overcome. If you were successful, increase the duration of your exercise session or add another session per week. As your number of short sessions increases every week, you will develop a new habit of choosing activity over inactivity, which can only improve your wellness profile.

TABLE 3.8
Every Day Choose at Least One

ACTIVITY	AMOUNT OF TIME (MINUTES)
■ Washing/waxing car	45–60
■ Washing windows/floors	45–60
■ Volleyball	45
■ Touch football	30–45
■ Gardening	30–45
■ Wheeling self in wheelchair	30–40
■ Walking 1¾ miles (20 min/mile)	35
■ Basketball (shooting baskets)	30
■ Bicycling 5 miles	30
■ Dancing (fast)	30
■ Pushing a stroller 1½ miles	30
■ Raking leaves	30
■ Walking 2 miles (15 min/mile)	30
■ Water aerobics	30
■ Swimming laps	20
■ Wheelchair basketball	20
■ Basketball (playing a game)	15–20
■ Bicycling 4 miles	15
■ Jumping rope	15
■ Running 1½ miles (10 min/mile)	15
■ Shoveling snow	15
■ Stairwalking	15

Source: Surgeon General's Report on Physical Activity and Health.
http://www.cdc.gov/nccdphp/sgr/sgr.htm

DATE	ACTIVITY	INTENSITY	DURATION	WARM-UP	COOL-DOWN	HOW I FELT
————	————	————	————	————	————	————
————	————	————	————	————	————	————
————	————	————	————	————	————	————
————	————	————	————	————	————	————
————	————	————	————	————	————	————
————	————	————	————	————	————	————
————	————	————	————	————	————	————
————	————	————	————	————	————	————
————	————	————	————	————	————	————
————	————	————	————	————	————	————
————	————	————	————	————	————	————
————	————	————	————	————	————	————

Summary

Aerobic fitness is the key to wellness and is a choice that you can make for yourself. In this chapter you have learned how to make lifestyle choices that you can live with and modify according to your personal goals and enjoyment.

Key concepts that you have learned in this chapter include these:

- A measure of maximal oxygen consumption (VO_2max) best indicates levels of aerobic fitness.

- The pulmonary, cardiovascular, and muscular systems work together to provide energy for aerobic activities.

- Physiological responses to aerobic fitness training are both acute (immediate) and chronic (long term).

- Aerobic exercise yields both health-related and psychological benefits.

- Designing a personal aerobic fitness training program involves self-assessment, goal setting, choice of exercise, and exercise prescription.

- Exercise prescription includes designing the program and monitoring intensity and rate of progression.

- Any aerobic workout should include warm-up and cool-down as well as the aerobic activities themselves.

- Current research indicates that as little as 15 minutes of moderate aerobic activity 3 times per week provides substantial health benefits.

References

American College of Obstetricians and Gynecologists. *Exercise During Pregnancy and Postnatal Period.* ACOG Home Exercise Programs. Washington, DC: ACOG, 1985.

American College of Sports Medicine. *Guidelines for Exercise Testing and Prescription.* Philadelphia: Lea & Febiger, 1991.

Blair, S. N. Dose of exercise and health benefits. *Archives of Internal Medicine,* 157(2): 153–157, 1997.

Blair, S. N. Living with Exercise. *American Health,* 1991.

Blair, S. N., et al. Physical fitness and all-cause mortality: A prospective study of healthy men and women. *Journal of the American Medical Association,* 262: 2395–2401, 1989.

Borg, G. A. V. Psychophysical bases of perceived exertion. *Medicine and Science in Sports and Exercise,* 14: 377–387, 1982.

Casperan, C. J., K. E. Powell, and G. M. Christenson. Physical activity, exercise and physical fitness: Definitions and distinctions for health-related research. *Public Health Reports,* 100: 126–131, 1985.

Centers for Disease Control. *A Report of the Surgeon General: Physical Activity and Health.* Washington, DC: U.S. Department of Health and Human Services, 1996.

Cooper, K. *The New Aerobics.* New York: M. Evans, 1970.

Cooper, K., et al. Physical fitness levels vs. coronary risk factors: A cross-sectional study. *Journal of the American Medical Association,* 236: 1660–1669, 1976.

DeVries, H. A. *Physiology of Exercise for Physical Education and Athletics,* 4th ed. Dubuque, IA: Wm. C. Brown, 1986.

Farrell, P. A., et al. Enkephalins, catecholamines, and psychological mood alterations: Effect of prolonged use. *Medicine and Science in Sports and Exercise,* 19: 347–353, 1987.

Fernhall, B., and F. S. Daniels. Electroencephalographic changes after a prolonged running period: Evidence for a relaxation response. *Medicine and Science in Sports and Exercise,* 16: 181, 1984.

Getchell, B. *Physical Fitness, a Way of Life,* 4th ed. New York: Macmillan, 1992.

Heath, G. W., et al. A physiological comparison of young and older endurance athletes. *Journal of Applied Physiology,* 51: 634–640, 1981

Howley, E. T., and B. D. Franks. *Health/Fitness Instructor's Handbook,* 2nd ed. Champaign, IL: Human Kinetics Press, 1992.

Janal, M. N., et al. Pain sensitivity, mood, and plasma endocrine levels in man following long-distance running: Effects of naloxone. *Pain,* 19: 13–25, 1984.

Kampert, J. D., S. N. Blair, C. E. Barlow, and H. W. Kohl. Physical activity, physical fitness, and all-cause mortality: A prospective study of men and women. *Annals of Epidemiology,* 6(5): 452–457, 1996.

Klug, G., and J. Lettunich. *Exercise and Physical Fitness.* Guilford, CT: Dushkin, 1992.

McArdle, W. D., F. L. Katch, and V. L. Katch. *Exercise Physiology,* 4th ed. Philadelphia: Lea & Febiger, 1996.

Niemann, D. C. *Fitness and Sports Medicine.* Palo Alto, CA: Bull, 1990,

Pollock, M. L., et al. Effect of age and training on aerobic capacity and body composition of master athletes. *Journal of Applied Physiology,* 62: 725–731, 1987.

Sharkey, B. J. *New Dimensions in Aerobic Fitness.* Champaign, IL: Human Kinetics Press, 1991.

Shinton, R., and G. Sagar. Lifelong exercise and stroke. *British Medical Journal,* 307(6898): 231–234, 1993.

Thoren, P., et al. Endorphins and exercise: Physiological mechanisms and clinical implications. *Medicine and Science in Sports and Exercise,* 22: 417, 428, 1990.

Wiese, J., M. Singh, and L. Yeudall. Occipital and parietal alpha power before, during and after exercise. *Medicine and Science in Sports and Exercise,* 14: 117, 1982.

Laboratory 3.1

Determining Aerobic Fitness

Assessing your current level of aerobic fitness will help you define goals, develop a personalized exercise prescription, and monitor your progress. One or all of the following three tests can be used to classify your fitness level.

BENCH-STEP TEST

The bench-step test consists of 3 minutes of stepping up and down on a bench and then determining your recovery pulse rate at intervals during the 3.5 minutes immediately following the exercise. This test does not predict VO_2max. Instead, the sum of the pulse counts is used to classify your aerobic fitness level. The recovery heart rate (HR) is a function of both the extent of HR elevation during the period of exercise and the rate at which HR returns to resting once the exercise is over. Both factors are influenced by your level of aerobic fitness. The more quickly your HR "recovers," the better your cardiovascular function.

PROCEDURE

1. Find a bench 16–18 inches high.

2. Perform the step in a four-step cadence: up-up-down-down. Standing before the bench, step up with your lead foot, raise yourself onto the bench, straighten your lead leg completely, and step up with your other foot. Then lower yourself to the floor with one foot and bring the other foot back down to the floor.

3. Repeat this process for 3 minutes, performing 30 stepping cycles each minute. The instructor will lead you in the four-step cadence per cycle (up-up-down-down) which gives 120 steps per minute.

4. At the end of 3 minutes, sit down on the bench. Recovery HR is counted three times, at 1-, 2-, and 3-minute intervals. Prior to each count, gently palpate your carotid, radial, or temporal artery, and then check your pulse for 30-second intervals. (Laboratory 3.2 explains how to take your pulse.) Your instructor will direct you when to start and stop counting.

TABLE 3.9

Aerobic Fitness Based on Recovery Index from Step Test

	RECOVERY INDEX	
	WOMEN	MEN
Super	95–125	97–121
Excellent	126–140	122–136
Good	141–157	137–151
Average	158–175	152–166
Fair	176–192	167–181
Needs work	193 and above	182 and above

Source: From Getchell, 1992.

TABLE 3.10

Aerobic Fitness Based on Rockport Walking and Cooper 1.5-Mile Run/Walk Tests

AGE	VO$_2$MAX (ML/KG/MIN)		1.5-MILE RUN TIME (MIN:SEC)	
	FEMALE	MALE	FEMALE	MALE
GOOD				
15–30	> 40	> 45	< 12	< 10
35–50	> 35	> 40	< 13:30	< 11:30
55–70	> 30	> 35	< 16	< 14
AVERAGE				
15–30	33–40	38–45	12–14:30	10–12:30
35–50	28–35	33–40	13:30–16	11:30–14
55–70	23–30	27–35	16–18:30	14–16:30
BELOW AVERAGE				
15–30	25–32	30–37	14:30–17	12:30–15
35–50	20–27	25–32	16–18:30	14–16:30
55–70	15–22	20–26	18:30–21	16:30–19
NEEDS EXTRA WORK				
15–30	< 25	< 30	> 17	> 15
35–50	< 20	< 25	> 18:30	> 16:30
55–70	< 15	< 20	> 21	> 19

Source: Adapted from E. T. Howley and B. D. Franks, *Health/Fitness Instructor's Handbook*, 2nd ed. (Champaign, IL: Human Kinetics Press, 1992).

5. Record your pulse count from each 30-second interval. Add them together to compute your Recovery Index.

Recovery HR (1) _____ + (2) _____ + (3) _____

= _____ Recovery Index

6. Consult Table 1 to determine your fitness evaluation.

Fitness classification from Table 3.9 (circle one):

super   excellent   good   average   fair   needs work

ROCKPORT WALKING FITNESS TEST

The object of this test is to walk as fast as you can for 1 mile and record your time and 15-second pulse count immediately following the walk.

Time to walk 1 mile = _____ (min:sec)

15-second pulse count at completion of the walk = _____ beats

HR (pulse count × 4) = _____ bpm

VO$_2$max can be estimated from the following calculation:

$$VO_2max = 132.853 - [0.0769 \times \text{body weight (lbs)}]$$
$$- [0.3877 \times \text{age (yr)}] + (6.3150 \times \text{gender})$$
$$- (3.2649 \times \text{time}) - (0.1565 \times HR)$$

where gender = 0 for female and 1 for male; time = walk time to the nearest hundredth of a minute; and HR = heart rate (bpm) at the end of the walking test.

Fitness classification from Table 3.10 (circle one):

good   adequate for most activities   below average   needs extra work

COOPER 1.5-MILE RUN/WALK FITNESS TEST

The object is to run (or run/walk) as fast as you can for 1.5 miles. Try to achieve an even pace, but you may walk for a time if you become too tired to keep running. It is important to pace yourself at the beginning of the run so that you do not start out too fast. You need to record your time at the end of the test to the nearest second.

1.5 mile time = _____ (min:sec)

Fitness classification from Table 3.10 (circle one):

good   adequate for most activities   below average   needs extra work

Laboratory 3.2

Assessing Heart Rate

RESTING HEART RATE

Resting heart rate (RHR) is simply the beats per minute of your heart at rest. Because RHR is used to determine your exercise HR and monitor improvements in fitness, it's important that you obtain an accurate reading. RHR is best taken upon waking, without an alarm, after a restful night's sleep. If it is not possible to do so, then you should rest quietly for 5–10 minutes prior to counting. You will be measuring your heart rate by finding your pulse in 2 of 3 arteries and counting the pulse for 15 seconds. You will then multiply your pulse rate by 4 to get beats per minute. You may take your pulse at one of the following sites: (a) carotid artery, (b) radial artery, or (c) temporal artery (see photos below).

TIPS FOR AN ACCURATE READING

1. Use the tip of your middle and index fingers. Don't use your thumb because it has a pulse of its own.

2. If you are taking your pulse at the carotid artery, use light pressure. The carotid arteries contain special receptors that reflexively slow the heart rate when heavy pressure is sensed.

3. Start your stopwatch (or use the second hand of your watch or clock) as you feel the beat of the pulse. Count the first beat as zero. Continue counting for 15 seconds and then multiply that value by 4 to obtain your RHR.

4. Take your pulse rate at least 3 times and average the values.

Pulse Rate #1 _____ × 4 = _____ (RHR #1)

Pulse Rate #2 _____ × 4 = _____ (RHR #2)

Pulse Rate #3 _____ × 4 = _____ (RHR #3)

RHR #1 _____ + RHR #2 _____ + RHR #3 _____

= _____ ÷ 3 = _____ (RHR)

EXERCISE HEART RATE

To determine whether you are exercising within your target heart rate zone, you need to measure your heart rate during exercise. The sites most commonly used are the carotid and radial arteries, although the temporal artery is a quick and easy alternative. In recording your exercise heart rate, it is important that you record your pulse quickly because, in a well-trained individual, heart rate can drop very quickly when activity is stopped. Your method of counting is the same as for RHR, except that you typically count for 10 rather than 15 seconds.

TIPS FOR AN ACCURATE READING

1. Although intensity is reduced, do not stop moving altogether. Learn to walk and take your heart rate at the same time.

2. If you are suing the carotid artery, be sure to maintain light pressure.

3. Begin counting at zero and count for 10 seconds. Multiply by 6 to obtain your exercise heart rate in beats per minute.

Pulse rate #1 _____ × 6 = _____ (Exercise HR #1)

Pulse rate #2 _____ × 6 = _____ (Exercise HR #2)

Pulse rate #3 _____ × 6 = _____ (Exercise HR #3)

Practice taking your exercise heart rate after one of the following activities: (1) a lap around the track or gym, (2) 2–3 minutes of bicycling, stair-stepping, rowing, running on the treadmill, or jump-roping, or (3) 1–2 minutes of calisthenics such as jumping jacks. Practice exercising at different intensities and monitor the changes in your heart rate.

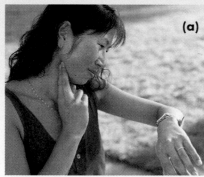 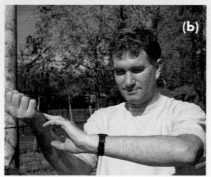 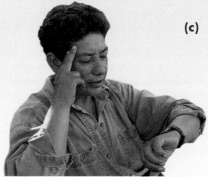

(a) To take the pulse at the carotid artery, the first and second fingers are placed gently on either side of the throat. (b) For the radial pulse, place the first and second fingers at the wrist, just below the thumb. Apply firm pressure. (c) The temporal pulse can be found just to the side of the eye socket. Apply gentle pressure using the first and second fingers.

YMCA Submaximal Bicycle Ergometer Test for Estimating Maximal Aerobic Capacity (VO_2max).

This protocol uses three or four consecutive 3-minute workloads on the bicycle ergometer for you to reach 85% of your estimated maximum heart rate based on age (calculate below). The initial workload is 150 kg meters/minute and the heart rate is taken during the last minute of the initial workload and used to determine subsequent loads (see Figure 3.9). This system provides individualized settings depending on the person's initial fitness, and values are used to estimate maximum aerobic capacity. From *The Y's Way to Fitness* by L. A. Golding, C. R. Myers, and W. E. Sinning (Eds.), 1989, Champaign, IL: Human Kinetics Publishers.

   Goal: To record heart rate values for the last 2 workloads during a submaximal bicycle test and use these to estimate your maximal aerobic capacity.

Directions:

1. Set first workload at 150 kgm/min (0.5 kp) and pedal at 50 revolutions per minute.

2. Take heart rate (HR) at the radial or carotid artery during the last 30 seconds of the third minute. If HR is

   ■ less than 80 beats per minute (bpm), set the second load at 750 kgm (2.5 kp)

   ■ 80–89 bpm, set the second load at 600 kgm (2.0 kp)

   ■ 90–100 bpm, set the second load at 450 kgm (1.5 kp)

   ■ greater than 100 bpm, set the second load at 300 kgm (1.0 kp)

3. Set the third and fourth (if required) loads according to the loads in the columns below the second loads (refer to Figure 3.8). Take HR during the last 30 seconds of minutes 2 and 3. If these heart rates differ by more than 5 bpm, then extend the workload for 1 minute until HR stabilizes.

Estimating Maximum Aerobic Capacity on Recording Form (see sample, Figure 3.8)

1. Draw a line across the graph (parallel with the x axis) at your age-adjusted maximum heart rate (220 − your age = _____).

2. On the graph, plot your heart rate from the workloads of your bicycle test with heart rates of greater than110 (workload is on the x axis, heart rate on the y axis).

3. Draw a diagonal line through both points and extend to the maximum heart rate line (drawn in #1 above).

4. Draw a line from the point of intersection with the maximum heart rate line, parallel to the y axis, to the baseline and determine predicted maximal oxygen uptake in liters per minute (L/min).

5. Multiply your value (L/min) by 1,000 to obtain ml/min, then divide this number by kilograms of body weight to obtain aerobic capacity in ml/kg/min. Compare this value to the norms in Table 3.11.

TABLE 3.11

Standards for Evaluating Aerobic Capacity (VO_2max)

	VO_2MAX (ML $\cdot$ KG^{-1} $\cdot$ MIN)$^{-1}$	
AGE[a]	**FEMALE**	**MALE**
GOOD		
15–30	> 40	> 45
35–50	> 35	> 40
55–70	> 30	> 35
ADEQUATE		
15–30	35	40
35–50	30	35
55–70	25	30
BORDERLINE		
15–30	30	35
35–50	25	30
55–70	20	25
NEEDS IMPROVEMENT		
15–30	< 25	< 30
35–50	< 20	< 25
55–70	< 15	< 20

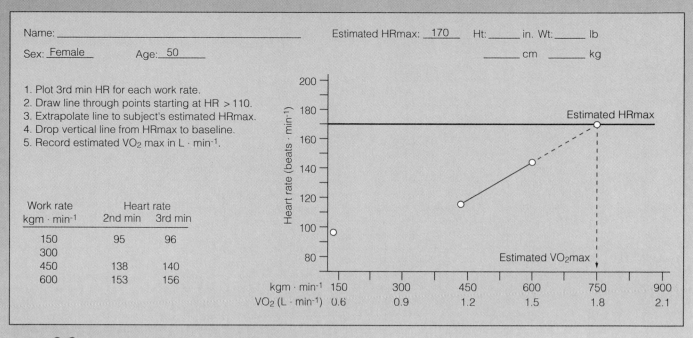

Name: _____   Estimated HRmax: __170__ Ht: _____ in. Wt: _____ lb

Sex: _Female_   Age: _50_____   _____ cm _____ kg

1. Plot 3rd min HR for each work rate.
2. Draw line through points starting at HR > 110.
3. Extrapolate line to subject's estimated HRmax.
4. Drop vertical line from HRmax to baseline.
5. Record estimated VO_2 max in $L \cdot min^{-1}$.

| Work rate | Heart rate | |
kgm · min⁻¹	2nd min	3rd min
150	95	96
300		
450	138	140
600	153	156

Figure 3.8

Sample recording form for estimating maximal aerobic capacity (VO_2max).

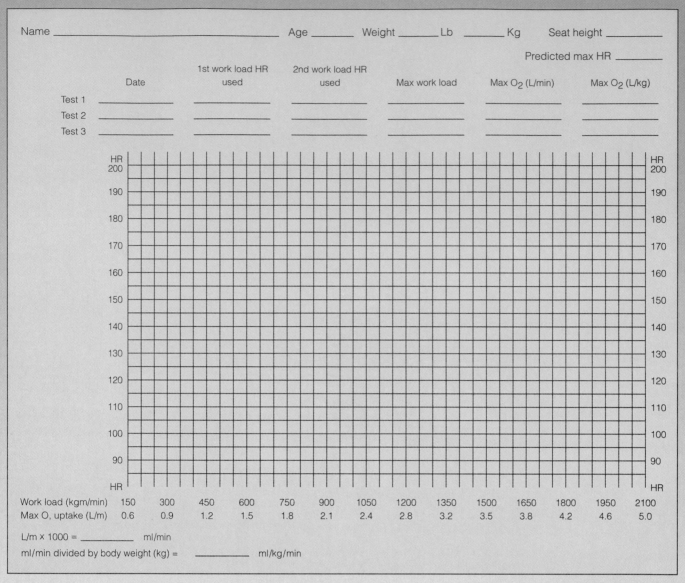

Name _____ Age _____ Weight _____ Lb _____ Kg   Seat height _____

Predicted max HR _____

	Date	1st work load HR used	2nd work load HR used	Max work load	Max O₂ (L/min)	Max O₂ (L/kg)
Test 1	_____	_____	_____	_____	_____	_____
Test 2	_____	_____	_____	_____	_____	_____
Test 3	_____	_____	_____	_____	_____	_____

Work load (kgm/min)	150	300	450	600	750	900	1050	1200	1350	1500	1650	1800	1950	2100
Max O, uptake (L/m)	0.6	0.9	1.2	1.5	1.8	2.1	2.4	2.8	3.2	3.5	3.8	4.2	4.6	5.0

L/m x 1000 = _____ ml/min

ml/min divided by body weight (kg) = _____ ml/kg/min

Figure 3.9

Recording form for maximal aerobic capacity (VO₂max)

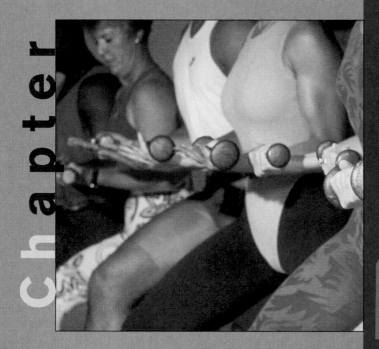

chapter

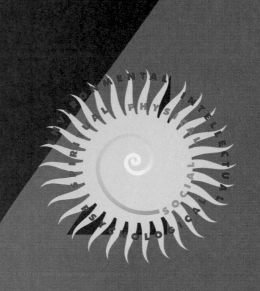

4

Building Muscular Strength and Endurance

One Student's View

Working out to develop my muscles is a very important part of my weekly schedule. However, it is not always easy to motivate myself to go to the gym on a constant basis. I, like most other people, often find myself tired and wanting to lay around and watch television instead of working out. This is why I have set a time with a couple of friends for us to work out at this time, no matter what. We have a set time, four days a week, that we adhere to. I find that having other people to push me and motivate me is the best way to stick to my goal.

—Jake Pascale

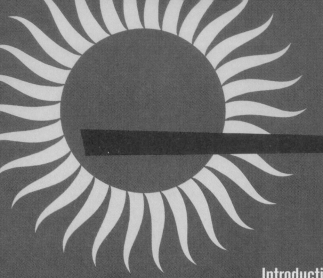

Introduction

In today's world of automation, we can accomplish most of our daily tasks with minimal physical effort. As a result, our muscle development tends to fall short of the standards required for optimal health. If, however, we want the benefits of muscular fitness—if we are interested in building stronger, healthier bodies and reducing the risk of injury—we need to make a conscious effort to develop our muscular strength and endurance.

When planning an exercise program for wellness, you need to include training for all the health-related components of fitness. This means incorporating activities that improve aerobic fitness, muscular fitness, flexibility, and body composition. Any form of physical activity is better than none; however, emphasizing one type of fitness over another limits your potential for improvement. For example, being aerobically fit will certainly help you bicycle up a hill, but you probably won't make it unless you also have strong leg muscles. By developing all aspects of health-related fitness, you should find it much easier to do all the things you want or need to do.

Although primarily associated with the physical dimension of wellness, muscular fitness carries psychological and social benefits as well. Physical strength can translate into inner strength in a variety of ways. For example, it can help you feel better about yourself—more self-confident and more self-reliant. And whether it's helping a friend move, carrying in the groceries, or whatever, you will always have many opportunities to put your strength to use.

In this chapter, we will examine the basics of muscular fitness and its associated health benefits. You will learn how to design an appropriate training program for muscular fitness based on your own personal goals. You also will develop an action plan to incorporate muscular fitness activities into your daily routine.

Objectives

After reading this chapter, you should be able to

- Define muscular fitness, muscular strength, and muscular endurance

- Explain the structure of muscle and differentiate among muscle fiber types

- Describe the energy systems for muscular strength and endurance

- Identify the types of muscle actions

- Describe gender differences in muscle strength

- Outline benefits of training for muscular fitness

- Describe physiological adaptations to weight training

- Compare and contrast weight training, bodybuilding, and weight lifting

- Define the appropriate mode frequency, intensity, and duration for muscular fitness

- Develop a personalized beginning weight training program

Defining Muscular Fitness

In Chapter 2, we introduced the concept of muscular fitness. To review: Muscular fitness refers to the strength and endurance of your muscles relative to your body weight; in other words, it includes the components of both muscular strength and muscular endurance. Muscular strength is the maximum force that a muscle or muscle group is capable of exerting against resistance or the maximum amount of force that can be exerted by those muscles at one time. Muscular endurance is the amount of force that can be generated by a muscle or muscle group over a prolonged period of time.

In a program of exercise to develop muscular fitness, your strength is determined by the amount of weight you can lift; your endurance is determined by the number of repetitions you can perform at a given weight. Although these two components of muscular fitness are defined separately, in practice they are closely related. One way to visualize this relationship is to consider the heaviest object you have ever lifted—perhaps a box packed full of books, a small refrigerator, or a room air conditioner. Could you have lifted it more than once? How about more than 10 times in a row? If you couldn't lift it more than once at a given time, then the weight of that object represents your muscular strength. If you could lift it two or more times in succession, then the weight was not heavy enough to determine your maximum strength; instead, the number of repeated lifts would represent your muscular endurance.

Muscular strength and endurance can be pictured on a continuum (see Figure 4.1). The relationship between strength and endurance is an interplay of two factors: intensity (the amount of weight used) and duration (the number of repetitions). Intensity and duration as they apply to muscular fitness will be discussed in greater detail in the exercise prescription section of this chapter.

Keep in mind that strength and endurance overlap. Thus, for example, if you have very low levels of strength, a muscular fitness training program that emphasizes low weights and high repetitions will likely result in both strength and endurance improvements. Similarly, if you have done extensive strength training, you are unlikely to have poor muscular endurance.

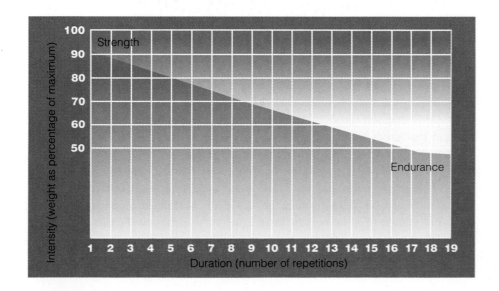

Figure 4.1

Muscular strength and muscular endurance exist on a continuum and are dependent upon intensity, or amount of weight used as a percentage of maximum, and duration, or number of repetitions. Strength training uses higher intensity for fewer repetitions than endurance training.
Source: From Klug and Lettunich, 1992.

Figure 4.2

Muscle fibers are organized into bundles that are wrapped within connective tissue. The connective tissue meshes with the tendon, which attaches the muscle to the bone.
Source: From Marieb, 1992.

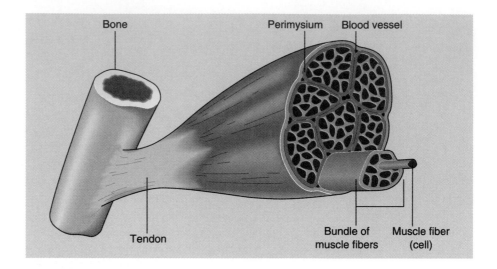

Muscle Structure and Physiology

In order to move, your muscles must shorten or lengthen while generating force. To understand how muscles develop force, you should be familiar with the basic principles of muscle structure and physiology.

Muscles comprise countless numbers of muscle cells, commonly referred to as muscle fibers. These **muscle fibers** are arranged in bundles that together form a larger muscle and that serve as the basic unit of force production. The muscle is wrapped in connective tissue that holds the bundles in place and also forms the tendons for attachment to bones. Blood vessels run between the muscle bundles, and extensive capillary networks branching off the blood vessels feed nutrients to each muscle fiber (see Figure 4.2).

Each muscle fiber contains thousands of thick and thin protein filaments, which produce muscle action. The **thick protein filaments** are long strands of contractile proteins that, when stimulated, activate placement of thin filaments. The **thin protein filaments** are long strands of contractile proteins that contain active sites for muscle action, pulling closer together during development of maximal force and moving apart during relaxation (see Figure 4.3).

Muscle Fiber Types

Through the use of a specialized technique called muscle biopsy, different types of skeletal muscle fibers have been identified. During a muscle biopsy a needle is inserted through the skin into the muscle and a "slip" of tissue is cut and extracted. Upon microscopic examination three distinct muscle fiber types can be observed. **Slow-twitch oxidative fibers,** or fatigue-resistant fibers, which derive energy from the oxidative pathway, respond relatively slowly to a nerve stimulus, and allow the muscle to sustain activity for a long period of time. The muscles that maintain posture in humans have a large percentage of slow-twitch fibers in order to generate the almost continuous muscle tension needed to hold an upright stance. These muscle fibers are red because they contain a lot of oxygen-carrying myoglobin, the "muscle" form of hemoglobin, and mitochondria, the energy-generating structure

muscle fibers (cells) a long multi-nucleated cells comprised of many myofibrils

thick protein filaments long strands of contractile proteins that, when stimulated, activate placement of thin protein filaments

thin protein filaments long strands of contractile proteins that contain active sites for muscle action, pulling closer together during development of maximal force and moving apart during relaxation

slow-twitch oxidative fibers muscle fibers that derive energy from the oxidative pathway, respond relatively slowly to a nerve stimulus, and allow the muscle to sustain activity for a long period of time

in cells, both of which are important to aerobic metabolism.

Fast-twitch fibers are characterized by their high speed of response to stimulus. They are classified into two groups according to their energy supply. **Fast-twitch glycolytic (FG) fibers,** which use only glycolytic energy release pathways, have a high glycogen content and a rapid rate of fatigue. Structurally, these fibers are large, have low myoglobin stores, contain very few mitochondria, and are fed by fewer capillaries than are slow-twitch fibers. A high percentage of FG fibers are found in the gastrocnemius muscles of the lower legs, enabling rapid activation of these muscles for a quick getaway. **Fast-twitch oxidative glycolytic (FOG) fibers** possess characteristics of both slow-twitch and FG fibers: They generate force quickly but are also more resistant to fatigue, and they derive energy from both oxidative and glycolytic pathways. Like slow-twitch fibers, FOG fibers contain a high percentage of myoglobin, mitochondria, and capillaries, and use aerobic metabolism for energy. The gastrocnemius muscles in the lower legs also contain FG fibers, enabling you to jog for extended periods of time.

Muscles contain all three types of fibers, but the percentages of these types in each muscle vary according to the function of the muscle. This variation is an important factor in determining athletic potential. For example, in a study that examined muscle biopsies in athletes, endurance athletes (marathon runners, cross-country skiers) had a much higher percentage of slow-twitch fibers than did speed or power athletes (sprinters, weight lifters), who had a higher percentage of fast-twitch fibers (Powers and Howley). Genetics play an important role in determining the fiber distribution within your muscles, which helps explain why some individuals become world-class marathoners whereas others, no matter how hard they train, could never reach such status.

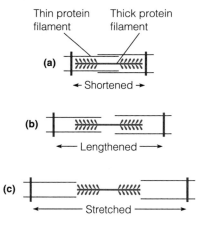

Figure 4.3

Sliding filaments produce shortening, lengthening, and stretching of muscle fibers.
(a) During shortening the tiny projections on the thick protein filaments cause the thin protein filaments to slide across on another and create a shortening of the muscle fiber.
(b) In the lengthened state there is a small gap between the thin filaments.
(c) When excessively stretched, the gap between the thin filaments widens.

Types of Muscle Actions

For many years, the term *contraction* was used to define the tension a muscle produces as it shortens. Research has shown, however, that tension also develops as a muscle lengthens. Thus, all muscle tension is now referred to as "muscle action."

Different types of muscle actions allow you to function effectively throughout the day. These can be classified as isometric, concentric, or eccentric.

Isometric. Muscle tension without visible joint movement is referred to as **isometric muscle action.** An example of isometric muscle action would be holding a heavy bag full of books on your arm. In this instance, your muscles (primarily biceps brachii) maintain constant tension so that you can support the book bag in one position. In general, your muscles have adapted to isometric actions required for your normal daily activities. However, if one day you add a heavy textbook to your bag or try to carry a huge stack of papers to the recycling center, you likely will have some difficulty.

fast-twitch glycolytic (FG) fibers muscle fibers that use only glycolytic energy release pathways and have a high glycogen content and a fast rate of fatigue

fast-twitch oxidative glycolytic (FOG) fibers muscle fibers that possess characteristics of both slow-twitch and FG fibers: They generate force quickly but are also more resistant to fatigue

isometric muscle action muscle tension without visible joint movement

Muscular fitness programs usually do not use isometric muscle actions because training muscles on only one joint position tends to have less carry-over to daily activities.

Concentric and Eccentric. Muscle actions that produce visible joint movement are classified as either concentric or eccentric. **Concentric muscle actions** occur when a muscle shortens; **eccentric muscle actions** occur as a muscle lengthens. In each case, the muscle or muscle group overcomes a resistance (a weight or heavy object) and movement is produced. To illustrate these two types of muscle actions, think of performing a bench press using a Universal Gym. In the upward phase of the bench press, your triceps (muscles on the backs of your arms) shorten as they produce force to extend your arms and lift the weight stack. This is a concentric muscle action. With a weight machine, you can do as much or as little of the eccentric activity as you want. You can let the weight down slowly as your triceps lengthen and control the movement, or you can let the weight stack crash down onto the machine without any eccentric muscle activity in your triceps. Research has shown that the eccentric muscle actions produce the greatest amount of force, followed by isometric and concentric muscle actions. In order to maximize results, be sure to include eccentric muscle action in your muscular fitness program,

Because concentric and eccentric muscle actions are central to activities of daily living, they are the focus of most muscular fitness programs. Most weight equipment, such as free weights, Universal, and Nautilus, is designed to provide resistance for these types of muscle actions.

Energy for Muscle Actions. Muscular actions associated with aerobic exercise are fueled by the aerobic pathway; by contrast, energy for muscular strength development is generated by the immediate energy pathway. The immediate energy system provides fuel for the quick, powerful bursts of activity involved in lifting heavy weights. Energy for muscular endurance, where many repetitions of a lift are performed, is generated primarily by the anaerobic pathway. (These energy pathways were discussed in detail in Chapter 2.)

The Training Effect

As you may recall from Chapter 2, the training effect refers to the changes in the body that result from a program of regular exercise. As with aerobic training, muscle-training causes distinct physiological adaptations and leads to important health benefits.

Physiological Adaptations

Muscle fibers adapt to accommodate the loads imposed on them in two distinct stages: the neuromuscular and the hypertrophic and metabolic.

Neuromuscular Response. The initial stage, known as the **neuromuscular response,** involves both the nervous and muscular systems, as motor nerve cells send signals to the muscle fibers telling them to contract (shorten) (see Figure 4.4).

---

concentric muscle action action that occurs when a muscle shortens

eccentric muscle action action that occurs when a muscle lengthens

neuromuscular response action that occurs when motor nerve cells send signals to muscle fibers telling them to contract

Adaptation in the neuromuscular system accounts for most of the improvements in strength observed during the first 2–4 weeks of training. When you lift an object heavier than you would normally lift over a given period of time, the stress of overload creates an adaptation in the neural system that stimulates the recruitment of more muscle fibers. Neuromuscular improvement in strength follows an increase in the number of muscle fibers that develop force when stimulated by a nerve signal. This, in turn, allows for lifting of heavier loads. (This is in accordance with the stress adaptation concept presented in Chapter 2.)

To illustrate, imagine that a friend lends you a computer but that you have to carry it to and from your home each day. The first day you go to pick the computer up, your arm muscles contract when they receive a nerve impulse from your brain telling them to lift the object. At first, the nerves that signal muscle action cause only a limited number of muscle fibers to develop force. However, with daily lifting, more and more fibers are stimulated, which results in more fibers sharing the load and a resultant increase in strength. Thus, after a week or two, you find the task of lifting and carrying your friend's computer to be much simpler than in the first few days. You have become stronger.

Hypertrophic and Metabolic Response. The next stage in strength improvement results from structural and metabolic changes within the muscle fibers due to progressive weight increases. The structural changes, known as the **hypertrophic response,** reflect an increase in contractile protein within the muscle fibers. Although these microscopic increases in protein may not be outwardly apparent, they can markedly increase strength through greater force production from contraction. In the case of your friend's computer, after 4–6 weeks of progressively overloading by daily carrying, your arm muscles probably will not have gotten noticeably larger. However, microscopic increases in the size of muscle fibers in your arms will result from an adaptation to the daily resistance of the computer.

Researchers have observed this response in muscle biopsy studies of individuals who have been weight training. Under a microscope, a significant increase in the cross-sectional area of the fast-twitch fibers can be observed when compared with a pretraining cross-sectional area (cross-sectional area is strongly associated with strength). A study from Stanford University reported that an increase of 22% in the cross-sectional area of fast-twitch leg muscle fibers was associated with a 120% increase in leg strength in older women (Charette et al.)

Metabolic changes that occur as a result of strength training include increases in the enzymes that enhance immediate and anaerobic energy production and that help store and mobilize carbohydrates to fuel the energy systems. In addition, the number of mitochondria and capillaries in the muscle tissue can decrease with training. The fact that these changes are different from those produced by aerobic exercise points to the importance of training that specifically focuses on muscular development to improve muscular fitness.

Progressive Resistance Exercise

The term progressive resistance exercise appropriately describes the process of training to improve muscular fitness. **Progressive resistance exercise (PRE)**

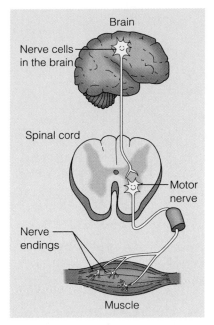

Figure 4.4

The motor unit. To move your muscles, nerve cells in the movement center of your brain are excited and send signals to motor nerves in your spinal cord. These signals are relayed to the muscle by a chemical called acetylcholine which signals your muscles to contract.
Source: From V. Patteson Lombardi, Beginning Weight Training. Copyright © 1989 Wm. C. Brown Communications, Inc., Dubuque, IA. All rights reserved. Reprinted with permission of the McGraw-Hill Companies.

hypertrophic response an increase in the contractile proteins within muscle fibers

progressive resistance exercise (PRE) exercise characterized by gradual increases in resistance (weight) over time, resulting in increases in muscular strength and/or endurance

STATS-AT·A·GLANCE
Muscular Fitness and Aging

■ Muscle strength declines 30%–40% between ages 30 and 80 (Grimby and Saltin).

■ One in three people over age 75 who is living independently has trouble climbing 10 steps (Fiatarone et al.).

■ After age 74, 28% of men and 66% of women in the United States cannot lift objects heavier than 10 pounds (Jette and Branch).

■ Resistance training in the elderly (75–94 yrs old) has been shown to improve measures of balance and function up to 35% (Protiva et al.).

is characterized by gradual increases in resistance (weight) over time resulting in increases in muscular strength and/or endurance. There are three types of PRE: weight training, bodybuilding, and weight lifting.

Weight training is a noncompetitive form of PRE training that people practice to improve their muscular strength and endurance as well as to realize its general health- and fitness-related benefits. By contrast, bodybuilding and weight lifting are primarily competitive sports with more highly focused goals. Bodybuilders work with weights at a variety of intensities and repetitions to achieve muscular enlargement. Shortly before a competition, they typically begin a very restrictive diet to lose body fat and to achieve the conspicuous muscular definition characteristic of bodybuilders.

The goal of weight lifting, including Olympic and power lifting, is to increase muscular strength. This is accomplished through training sessions that accentuate few repetitions (up to 3) of very heavy weights. Olympic lifters can be massive and can lift more than 1,000 pounds—up to 5 times their body weight—but they are not necessarily as well defined as bodybuilders. In keeping with the focus of this text on activities that can be performed on a lifetime basis, weight training—rather than bodybuilding or weight lifting—is the form of PRE most highly recommended for improving muscular fitness. (See the Myths and Controversies box.)

Benefits of Muscular Fitness

Weight training improves muscular fitness by increasing both muscular strength and endurance. These changes are particularly meaningful as methods for preventing chronic diseases, offsetting muscle deterioration associated with the aging process, and enhancing the quality of your life. (See the Stats-at-a-Glance.) Specifically, they produce health benefits in three major areas: the musculoskeletal system, body composition, and the cardiovascular system.

Protecting the Musculoskeletal System. With respect to the musculoskeletal system, improved muscular fitness can reduce chronic back problems by protecting the back from injury. Jackson and Brown found that individuals who are free of back pain have stronger abdominal and back musculature than those with back pain. Further, stronger muscles are associated with higher bone mineral density (Snow et al.). In the normal population of generally sedentary individuals, muscular strength and bone mineral density decline by approximately 30% between ages 30 and 80. Thus, the magnitude of this age-related decline could possibly be prevented if more young men and women participated in weight training to enhance muscular fitness. Additional research is needed to test this theory.

Yet another way that weight training contributes to a reduction in low back pain is by increasing flexibility. In a recent study by Adams, competitive weight lifters were observed to have greater low back flexibility than a group of noncompetitive athletes. These differences likely were a result of weight training because none of the subjects were training for flexibility. It is important to note, however, that improved flexibility comes about only when a lift is performed through the full range of motion of the joint. This training principle, referred to as FROM, enhances flexibility because the lift is performed from full extension to full flexion.

Another benefit of improving muscular fitness is the increased ability of muscles to relax during rest. Although muscle tension due to daily stress is

MYTHS & CONTROVERSIES

Myth 1 **Because I am a woman, weight training will make me "bulk up" like a man**. Without the high blood levels of the hormone testosterone, women do not develop the strength and size that men can with weight training.

Myth 2 **If I weight train specific areas of my body, I can lose the fat and therefore improve definition**. Unquestionably, you can improve muscular definition by weight training. However, weight training will not provide "spot reduction" in areas where you wish to be fat free. People often believe that by doing hundreds of abdominal curl-ups, they will lose fat on the abdomen. Not so! A well-rounded program of weight training and aerobic exercise (for increased calorie expenditure) will help you achieve that desired muscular definition and tone.

Myth 3 **If I stop weight training, my muscle will turn to fat**. Muscle and fat are completely different in structure and biochemical makeup; therefore, they cannot convert back and forth. What often happens to weight trainers who stop training is that their subcutaneous (under the skin) fat increased as a result of decreased activity and unchanged diet. This imbalance of caloric expenditure and intake results in fat gain.

Source: National Center for Health Statistics, 1996.

common among untrained individuals, training can help muscles maintain a more relaxed state. For example, if you tend to "bunch up" in the neck and shoulder area, after a session of weight training with overhead lifts you may find your neck and shoulders resting in a more natural posture.

Improving Body Composition. With respect to body composition, weight training increases the amount of muscle or lean mass on your body. In addition, the calories burned during a workout can contribute to the loss of body fat. In a study of older women, resistance training resulted in a 3% increase in lean mass and an 8% decrease in fat mass in the legs (Shaw and Snow). This same phenomenon can be observed in young adults who begin weight training at their local facility and observe shifts in body composition specific to the areas that are overloaded. This change occurs if caloric intake remains stable. (Weight management and body composition are discussed in detail in Chapter 8.)

Enhancing Cardiovascular Health. The effect of weight training on cardiovascular health has not been found to be as pronounced as that of aerobic exercise. Nevertheless, some studies have shown that weight training reduces systolic and diastolic blood pressures (Hagberg et al.). In addition, there is evidence that resistance training may counteract other risk factors for coronary heart disease—for example, by increasing high-density lipoproteins, which exert a protective effect on the cardiovascular system (Hurley & Kokkinos; Hurley et al.).

Designing Your Muscular Fitness Program

The basic ingredients of your muscular fitness program are (1) assessment and/or definition of goals, (2) choice of exercises and equipment, and (3) exercise prescription, which includes programming of resistance, repetitions, sets, rest intervals, frequency, and rate of progression.

Assessment and Goal Setting

If possible, you should determine your current level of muscular fitness prior to defining your goals and developing a program of exercise. You can assess your muscular fitness using the measurement of dynamic strength known as the **one repetition maximum (1-RM):** the maximum amount of weight that can be lifted only one time. A repetition refers to the number of times you perform that lift. (In Laboratory 4.1 you will use a variant of the 1-RM test to measure your muscular fitness.)

Because it requires considerable skill and increases the chance of injury, the 1-RM test is generally used only by experienced weight trainers. For these reasons, Laboratory 4.1 suggests you estimate your maximum strength using a 6-RM—the amount of weight you can lift 6 times, no more and no less. You derive your 6-RM through trial and error. This value is plugged into an equation from which your estimated maximum strength is calculated. Because strength is directly related to body weight, this value is then divided by body weight to determine your relative strength.

The test for muscular endurance is the maximum number of times you can lift a weight that is less than your maximum capacity. This weight, known as a submaximal lift, is derived as a certain percentage (25%–100%) of body weight (see Laboratory 4.2). When your testing is complete, you rank both your strength and endurance scores against a table of normative values.

Once you know your current level of muscular fitness, you can set specific short- and long-term goals. If, for example, your muscular fitness assessment scores for your upper body (arms and shoulders) are in the lowest ranking for both muscular strength and endurance, you may want to set the following short- and long-term goals:

SHORT-TERM GOAL
Improve muscular endurance of the arms and shoulders by 50% in 8 weeks

LONG-TERM GOAL
Improve muscular strength of the arms and shoulders by 50% in 4 months

Because you need both strength and endurance training, you may decide to focus initially on muscular endurance exercises with lighter weights. When you build sufficient strength and learn proper lifting techniques, you can begin training with heavier weights. You may choose to evaluate your strength/endurance at 2 to 3 week intervals in order to readjust the resistance.

Remember, however, that assessment is not a prerequisite for goal setting. Perhaps your goal is to be able to perform one pull-up. Your program then would emphasize shoulder and arm strength.

Gender Differences in Strength and Response to Training

In general, women exhibit about two-thirds the *absolute* amount of strength and power of men (Holloway & Baechle). This is not surprising given that women have smaller bodies and less lean tissue overall; thus, unit for unit, women generally have force output similar to that of men. More recent evidence com-

one repetition maximum (1-RM) the maximum amount of weight a person can lift only one time

paring muscle strength, muscle cross-sectional area, and muscle biopsies between men and women demonstrate that women were approximately 52% and 66% as strong as men in the upper and lower body, respectively. Further, strength and muscle cross-sectional area were associated with each other; women had significantly smaller muscle cross-sectional areas than did men, particularly in the upper body (45% less in upper versus 25% less in lower). The main difference between genders that accounted for lower strength in women was that they had smaller muscle fibers compared to men. Women also tended to have a lower proportion of their lean mass distributed in the upper body, which helps explain why women have markedly lower strength values in their upper bodies (Miller et al.). Gender differences in lean tissue and also hypertrophy response to weight training is largely due the higher amounts of testosterone in men than in women. Because of these differences, some women have used anabolic steroids to improve their muscle response to weight training. This topic is discussed in more detail in Chapter 11.

Choice of Equipment

For maximum development of muscular strength, you need to use some type of resistance equipment that allows you to add weight. There are two basic kinds of resistance equipment: machine weights and free weights (that is, dumbbells and barbells).

Machine Weights. Machine weights include both isotonic and isokinetic equipment. With **isotonic weight equipment,** you control the speed of movement as you perform the lift. Older machine weights and those with pulley systems employ constant resistance. That is, the amount of weight or

work load does not change throughout the range of motion, so the resistance does not vary.

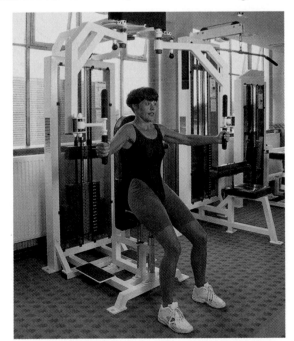

When using this type of equipment, you are limited by what is known as the "sticking point." This typically occurs at the beginning and end of the range of motion because mechanical advantage is low at these points. The greatest force can be generated at the middle range of motion where leverage is optimal. For example, during a biceps curl, you may be able to hold a 100-lb weight at a 90-degree angle but be unable to move the same weight from an extended arm position to a 90-degree angle.

The newer machine weights employ variable resistance and maximize muscular tension throughout the range of motion. By the use of mechanical devices such as cams or levers, these machines reduce the resistance early in

Machine weights are often safer for beginners than free weights, because they help maintain correct form.

isotonic weight equipment
equipment on which you control the speed of movement as you perform the lift

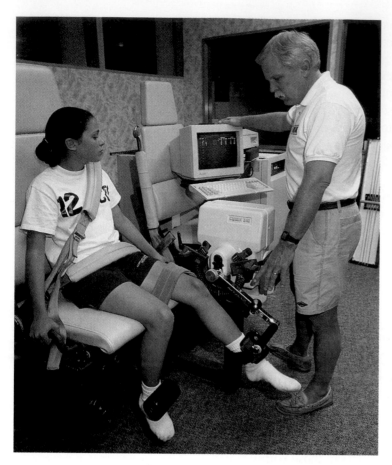

This isokinetic weight machine builds strength by controlling the speed of movement so that muscles contract at or near maximal tension throughout the entire range of motion. This equipment is most often seen in rehabilitation and research settings.

the movement (the sticking point), thereby allowing you to get past the weakest joint angle more easily than do standard machines. Further, resistance is increased at those points in the range of motion where there is greater mechanical advantage. The resulting smoothness in performance is felt during a lift. Although there is an improved comfort zone associated with the variable-resistance machine weights, they have not yet been proven superior to standard machines. In any case, both constant-resistance and variable-resistance machine weights effectively promote strength of isolated muscle groups.

Isokinetic weight equipment controls the speed of movement throughout most of the range of motion during a lift. For example, when you are performing a biceps curl using isokinetic machine weights, your arm moves at a constant speed and your biceps muscle can develop force at near maximal tension during the entire exercise. Whatever force you generate, the machine will match; thus, the term *accommodating resistance* is used to describe isokinetic weight equipment. Although speed is not purely constant, because your arm accelerates early in a biceps curl and decelerates at the end of the curl, this type of equipment eliminates the sticking point associated with isotonic weight equipment.

Free Weights. Free weights are not attached to a pulley or lever system. Like standard machine weights, they offer a constant load resistance and have the limitation of the sticking point. However, free weights have an advantage over machine weights in that they more closely mimic real-life activities and more effectively train both the neural and muscular systems. When you are performing a lift using free weights, your muscles must stabilize your body. This necessity leads to an improvement in overall strength and balance rather than in just isolated muscle groups, as can occur with machine weights. Also, free weights offer more variety and are much less expensive.

From a safety standpoint, free weights represent a higher risk than machine weights, but this can be overcome by technique mastery, use of the appropriate amount of weight, and consistent use of spotters. The spotter is the person who sees that you position yourself correctly, execute a proper lift, and then return the weight safely to its resting position. This person is there to grasp the weight if it is too heavy or if it slips. With certain lifts, such as the bench press and the squat, it is important that a spotter always assist you to ensure safety.

Most facilities offer a variety of machine and free-weight equipment. Your choice of equipment depends on your muscular fitness level and personal goals as well as your choice of exercises. Both types of weight equipment improve muscular strength and endurance. We recommend that you begin your muscular fitness program with machine weights and then move to free weights once you gain familiarity and confidence.

isokinetic weight equipment
equipment that controls the speed of movement throughout most of the range of motion during a lift

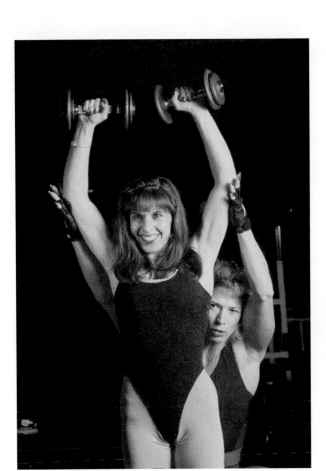

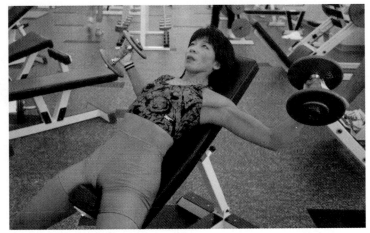

(a) Spotting is a very important component of weight training. A spotter promotes good form, increases safety, and provides a positive motivating force.

(b) Free weights (shown here) and machine weights—types of equipment found in gyms and clubs—promote strength but the movement speed is controlled by the lifter.

Choice of Exercises

It is not uncommon when beginning a weight-training program for a person to give little or no thought to an overall program of exercises. More often than not, the emphasis is on lifting greater amounts of weight for a specific area rather than systematically choosing exercises to develop overall strength, endurance, and balance. For example, people often work only the biceps (front of arm) and quadriceps (front of thighs) without incorporating exercises for the triceps (back of arm) and hamstrings (back of thigh). This imbalance in the legs is one potential cause of knee injury.

Table 4.1 outlines eight basic exercises to use in your muscular fitness program. These exercises are designed to work all three segments of the body: the lower body, upper body, and abdomen and lower back. You'll notice that exercises have been included using both free weights and machine weights. Some of the exercises can be adapted to either free or machine weights; these include the bench press, biceps curl, and triceps extension. All the exercises should be performed using light weights in the initial stages of your program.

In the order presented, the exercises progress from those that use large muscle groups to those using smaller muscle groups. As you train, be aware of this order in your program. Based on your fitness assessment and your training goals, your program will include some or all of these basic exercises. If you begin the entire set but find that this is too much for you, reduce the number of exercises and then restore exercises when you feel that you are ready. Illustrations and instructions for performing these exercises are provided in Figure 4.5a–h.

TABLE 4.1

Basic Exercises for Development of Muscular Strength and Endurance

EXERCISE	MAJOR MUSCLES WORKED
LOWER BODY	
1. Leg extension	Quadriceps
2. Leg curl	Hamstrings
UPPER BODY	
3. Bench press	Pectoralis major and minor, triceps
4. Lateral pull	Latissiumus dorsi, deltoids, biceps
5. Triceps extension	Triceps
6. Biceps curl	Biceps, brachialis
ABDOMEN AND LOWER BACK	
7. Back extension	Erector spinae, quadratus lumborum, gluteus maximus
8. Curl-up	Rectus abdominis, internal and external obliques

Exercise Prescription

Planning the design and progression of your muscular fitness program is important for maintaining motivation and ensuring attainment of your goals. This is the time when you develop your overload schedule by prescribing frequency, intensity, and duration to improve fitness. If you are overzealous in your planning and do too much too soon, you may experience burnout and/or injury, and not achieve your goals (as discussed in Chapter 2). If you underprescribe, you also will not achieve your goals. However, it is better to start too light than too heavy. The following is a sensible prescription for muscular fitness:

■ Mode: Resistance provided by free weights or weight machines

■ Frequency: 2 to 3 times per week on nonconsecutive days

■ Duration: For strength, 3 sets of 5 to 7 repetitions; for endurance, 3 sets of 12 to 15 repetitions

■ Intensity: For strength, 60% to 85% of 1-RM; for endurance, 50% of 1-RM or 15-RM

■ Rest intervals: For strength, 3 to 5 minutes between sets; for endurance, 15 to 60 seconds between sets

As outlined in Chapter 2, overload, which is determined by exercise frequency, duration, and intensity, is the key to developing fitness. In Chapter 3, the principle of overload was applied to aerobic fitness. Although the concept of overload is the same for muscular fitness as for aerobic fitness, some of the terminology has a slightly different meaning. In the case of muscular fitness, intensity also refers to difficulty and describes the amount of weight you are using whereas duration is defined as the number of repetitions and sets you perform.

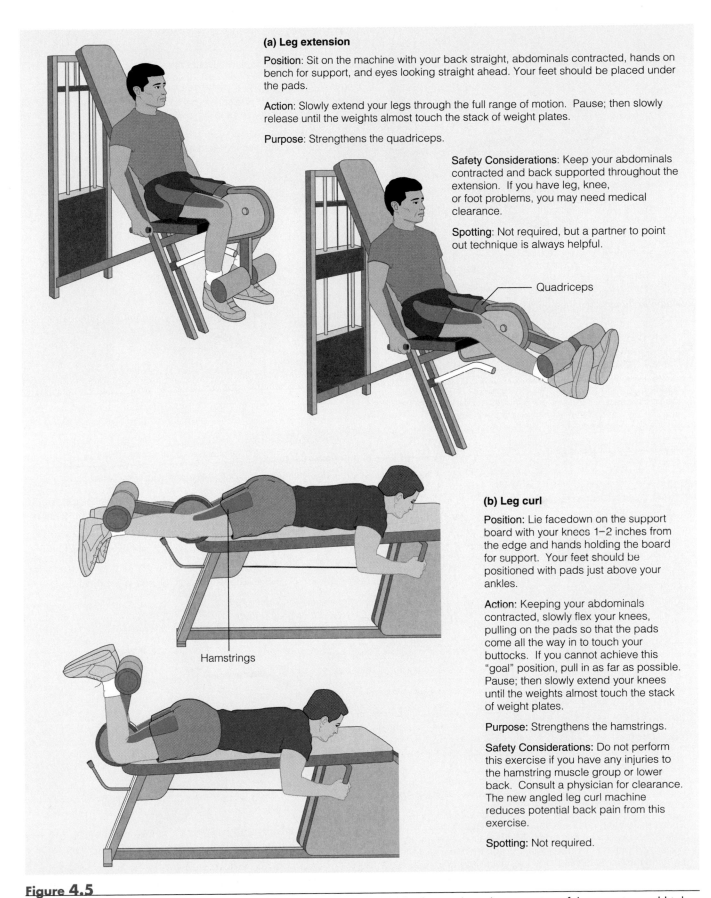

(a) Leg extension

Position: Sit on the machine with your back straight, abdominals contracted, hands on bench for support, and eyes looking straight ahead. Your feet should be placed under the pads.

Action: Slowly extend your legs through the full range of motion. Pause; then slowly release until the weights almost touch the stack of weight plates.

Purpose: Strengthens the quadriceps.

Safety Considerations: Keep your abdominals contracted and back supported throughout the extension. If you have leg, knee, or foot problems, you may need medical clearance.

Spotting: Not required, but a partner to point out technique is always helpful.

Quadriceps

Hamstrings

(b) Leg curl

Position: Lie facedown on the support board with your knees 1–2 inches from the edge and hands holding the board for support. Your feet should be positioned with pads just above your ankles.

Action: Keeping your abdominals contracted, slowly flex your knees, pulling on the pads so that the pads come all the way in to touch your buttocks. If you cannot achieve this "goal" position, pull in as far as possible. Pause; then slowly extend your knees until the weights almost touch the stack of weight plates.

Purpose: Strengthens the hamstrings.

Safety Considerations: Do not perform this exercise if you have any injuries to the hamstring muscle group or lower back. Consult a physician for clearance. The new angled leg curl machine reduces potential back pain from this exercise.

Spotting: Not required.

Figure 4.5

These illustrations (parts a–h) of a basic exercise set for improving muscular fitness show the execution of the exercise and highlight the primary muscles affected during the specific lifts.

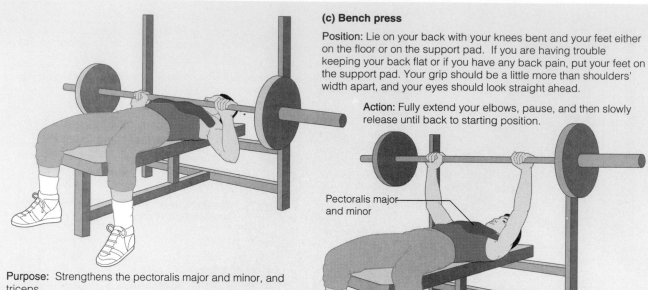

(c) Bench press

Position: Lie on your back with your knees bent and your feet either on the floor or on the support pad. If you are having trouble keeping your back flat or if you have any back pain, put your feet on the support pad. Your grip should be a little more than shoulders' width apart, and your eyes should look straight ahead.

Action: Fully extend your elbows, pause, and then slowly release until back to starting position.

Pectoralis major and minor

Purpose: Strengthens the pectoralis major and minor, and triceps.

Safety Considerations: Do not perform this exercise if you have injured your chest, shoulders, or any part of your arms. Consult a physician for clearance.

Spotting: For machine weights, not required. For free weights, the spotter should stand about 6 inches from the lifter's head and help guide the bar only if assistance is needed.

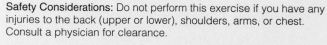

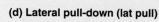

Latissimus dorsi

(d) Lateral pull-down (lat pull)

Position: Sit or kneel with a wide grip on the bar and your arms extended. Your body should be directly beneath the bar so that the cable is perpendicular to the ground.

Action: Slowly flex your elbows and pull the bar to one of two positions: (1) behind your head until the bar is low on your shoulders or (2) in front of your head to a point high on your chest. Pause; then slowly extend your arms until the weights almost touch the weight stack.

Purpose: Strengthens the latissimus dorsi, deltoids, biceps, and brachialis.

Variations: With a shoulder-width grip or short grip, pull the bar down in front of your face. These variations emphasize the lateral and upper back more than does the wide grip.

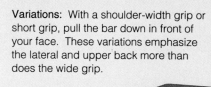

Safety Considerations: Do not perform this exercise if you have any injuries to the back (upper or lower), shoulders, arms, or chest. Consult a physician for clearance.

Spotting: Spotting can be helpful with the lat pull because it is commonly performed incorrectly and because, even though it is performed with machine weights, the spotter can assist with bringing the bar to the lifter and taking it away.

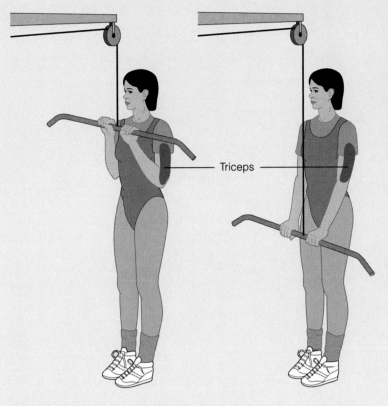

Triceps

(e) Triceps extension

Position: Use the lat station for this exercise. Stand and grip the bar two fingers' width apart with your palms down. Your knees should be slightly bent with your feet at shoulders' width apart. Bring your elbows in and "pin" them to your waist so that your forearms are parallel to the floor. *Free-weight adaptation:* Lie on your back with your arms bent overhead and the weight in both hands; then extend your arms up overhead so that you can see them, and slowly release.

Action: With your eyes focused ahead and abdominals contracted, slowly extend your arms at the elbows until they are fully extended. Pause; then slowly return to the 90° flexed position.

Purpose: Strengthens the triceps.

Safety Considerations: Do not perform this exercise if you have any injuries to the shoulders, elbows, forearms, or wrists. Consult a physician for clearance.

Spotting: *For machine weights*, spotting is not necessary but helps with correcting technique. *For free weights*, the spotter should stand above the lifter. If needed, press on the bar lightly from beneath.

(f) Biceps curl

Position (bottom figure): Stand with your feet at shoulders' width apart and your knees slightly bent. Pick up the bar with a "palms up" grip, bringing the bar to midthigh. For machine weights, use the biceps station.

Action (top figure): With your elbows "pinned" to your waist and your knees bent, slowly flex at the elbows and pull the bar into your shoulders. Pause; then slowly extend to the starting position. Cautionary note: It is essential that the knees stay bent and that movement be restricted to the arms. If back involvement begins, stop the lift and rest.

Purpose: Strengthens the biceps and brachialis.

Safety Considerations: Do not perform this exercise if you have any injuries to the shoulders, elbows, forearms, or wrists. Consult a physician for clearance.

Spotting: For machine weights, the spotter should stand in a position to check for back involvement during the lift. For free weights, the spotter should stand about 2 feet away from the lifter. If needed, press on the bar lightly from beneath. At the end of the completed set, the lifter may need assistance returning the bar to the rack or the floor.

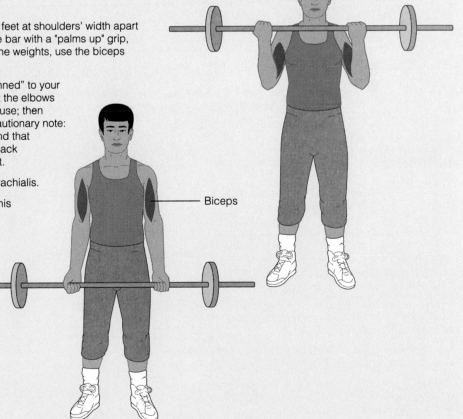

Biceps

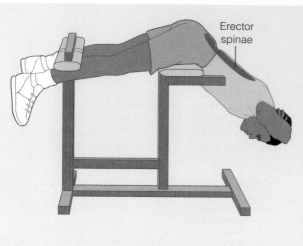

Erector spinae

(g) Back extension

Position: Lie facedown with your hips comfortably resting on the support pad of the Universal or similar device and your ankles underneath the foot supports. Your hands should be clasped and placed behind your head while your trunk is hanging over the end of the hip support. (See Chapter 5 for recommended back exercises to help build the strength necessary to perform this more advanced lift. For a beginner, it is advisable to begin with back lifts from a prone position on the floor.)

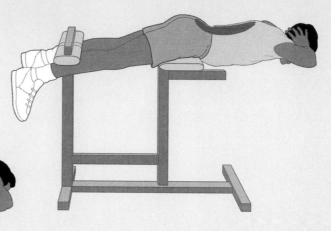

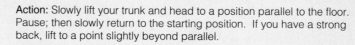

Action: Slowly lift your trunk and head to a position parallel to the floor. Pause; then slowly return to the starting position. If you have a strong back, lift to a point slightly beyond parallel.

Purpose: Strengthens the erector spinae, gluteus maximus, and hamstrings.

Safety Considerations: Do not perform this exercise if you have any acute or chronic back problems. Consult a physician for clearance.

Spotting: Not required.

(h) Curl-up

Position: Lie on your back with your hands on your neck lightly supporting your head and your knees bent at approximately 110°.

Action: For middle abdominals: Lift your head, arms, and chest off the floor until you feel a strong contraction in your abdominal region. Do not pull your head forward; rather, look up to the ceiling. Pause; then release. For waist abdominals (obliques): Twist your head, chest, and left elbow to the right, keeping your right elbow on the floor. Pause; then release. Perform to the left, keeping your left elbow on the floor.

Purpose: Strengthens the rectus abdominis and internal and external obliques.

Safety Considerations: Consult a physician if you have any acute or chronic back problems that may be aggravated by this exercise.

Spotting: Not required.

Rectus abdominis

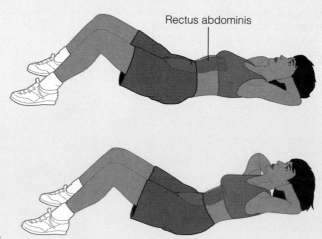

Program Design. The terms *resistance, repetitions,* and *sets* are key words in discussing muscular fitness training. Resistance is defined as the amount of weight used in a lift or exercise; repetitions are defined as the number of times that you perform the lift or exercise. Once you have established the number of repetitions you want to perform for a given exercise, you overload that muscle group by performing "groups" of repetitions, or sets. Completing that number of repetitions constitutes a set. By grouping your repetitions into sets, you can add rest periods between sets. Therefore, a set may be considered complete when you reach a predetermined number of repetitions or when you are too fatigued to continue.

Training for Strength. The primary difference between programming for strength and for endurance is in determining intensity, repetitions, and rest intervals. When muscular strength is your goal, your program design should emphasize greater resistance with fewer repetitions. As noted previously, the recommended range for intensity is 60% to 85% of 1-RM; thus, you will start at 60% of 1-RM. For example, if your 1-RM for the biceps curl is 30 pounds, your starting resistance (weight) would be 60% of 30 pounds, or 18 pounds.

If you are not able to estimate or assess your 1-RM, use the trial resistances outlined in Table 4.2. These values represent conservative free-weight estimates for apparently healthy 20-year-old male and female beginners of average body weight. For strength development, use the higher-end intensity and keep your repetitions between 5 and 7. If this is too easy, add weights, but keep the repetitions low. For endurance, use the lower-end intensities so that you can perform 12 to 15 repetitions. If this is too difficult, reduce the weight. Also, the number of sets you complete will vary depending on your fitness level.

If you choose to begin with these resistance guidelines, use trial and error to match them with your own strength level. Notice that no resistance is suggested for back extensions (Figure 4.5g) and abdominal curl-ups (Figure 4.5h). These endurance exercises should be central to your program because they improve trunk strength and endurance. Weight machines built

TABLE 4.2

Resistance Selection Guidelines for Basic Exercises

EXERCISE	TRIAL RESISTANCE FOR WOMEN (LBS)	TRIAL RESISTANCE FOR MEN (LBS)
Leg extension	10–20	40–60
Leg curl	10–20	40–60
Bench press	20–25	60–90
Lateral pull	20–40	50–80
Triceps extension	10–20	30–50
Biceps curl	15–20	35–50
Back extension	0	0
Curl-up	0	0

specifically for these areas are generally not available in gyms or clubs, so we suggest that you perform these on incline boards or flat surfaces and add 3- to 5-pound weights as your body adapts.

Training for Endurance. When muscular endurance is your goal, begin your training with a program of high repetitions and low resistance. For example, suppose that in assessing your muscular endurance you did 4 repetitions of each exercise using the chosen percentages of body weight and that your goal is to do 15 repetitions at the given intensity. In designing your exercise program you begin by performing three sets of 4 repetitions for each exercise with a rest period of 15 to 60 seconds between sets. This style of training will allow you to overload your muscular system in a way that is compatible with your current fitness level. The rest period between sets allows you time to recover before another set of repetitions. In this way you gradually build up until you reach your goal of 3 sets of 15 repetitions.

For endurance training, intensity can be established in one of two ways. The first is to use 50% of the 1-RM you already assessed; however, this method is appropriate only if you already know your 1-RM. The second is to determine your **15-repetition maximum (15-RM),** which is the maximal weight that can be lifted 15 times without stopping. This amount of weight is going to be far less than your 1-RM. For instance, if your 1-RM for a biceps curl is 30 pounds, your 15-RM will probably be between 10 and 15 pounds. If the machine weight plates or free-weight bars are too heavy for you to perform 15 repetitions, then you will not be able to measure your 15-RM. Instead, you can begin by using no weight (only the weight of your body) or handheld weights of 3 to 5 pounds. Use these light weights until you can perform at least 8 repetitions, and then work up to 15 repetitions.

Rate of Progression. Your rate of progression, or the rate at which you build up over time in order to reach your goal, should allow you to adapt comfortably to increased workloads. For example, the progression in Table 4.3 can help you attain a short-term muscular endurance training goal of three sets of 15 repetitions. Note, however, that your rate of progression may be faster than this if you are a strong beginner.

Once you have reached your goal of an increase of 50% in muscular endurance (as in the earlier example), you have probably developed enough muscular strength to move into a strength training program using fewer repetitions with heavier weights. However, at this point you may want to change your long-term goals and continue working on muscular endurance by slowly increasing the weights but maintaining repetitions at 10 to 15. If you increase weight, you may need to drop back to one or two sets for a week until your body can adapt to three sets at a higher weight. The only basic exercises discussed in this chapter for which this pattern does not apply are the abdominal curl-ups and back extensions. Initially, these should be performed with no weights until you can easily complete three sets of 15 repetitions. You can then add light weights for increased resistance.

When you are training for muscular strength, your program plan is similar in progression to that for endurance training, but the intensity is increased and the repetitions either remain the same or are decreased. Typically, repetitions stay in the range of 5 to 7 until you reach very high levels of intensity, that is, 90% to 95% of 1-RM. Rest intervals should be a minimum of 3

15 repetition maximum (15-RM) the amount of weight that can be lifted only 15 times; 15-RM is used in designing muscular endurance training

TABLE 4.3
Rate of Progression for Endurance Training

Week 1:   2 sets of 15 repetitions using 3-lb weights

Week 2:   3 sets of 15 repetitions using 3-lb weights

Week 3:   3 sets of 15 repetitions using 5-lb weights

Week 4:   3 sets of 15 repetitions using 5-lb weights

Week 5:   2 sets of 10 repetitions using the lowest resistance on the weight machine or free weights

Week 6:   3 sets of 10 repetitions using the lowest resistance on the weight machine or free weights

Week 7:   3 sets of 12 repetitions using the lowest resistance on the weight machine or free weights

Week 8:   3 sets of 15 repetitions using the lowest resistance on the weight machine or free weights

Week 9:   Assess muscular endurance to determine whether goal has been reached

TABLE 4.4
Rate of Progression for Strength Training

Week 1:   2 sets of 7 repetitions with weights set at 60% of 1-RM

Week 2:   3 sets of 7 repetitions with weights set at 60% of 1-RM

Week 3:   2 sets of 7 repetitions with weights set at 65% of 1-RM

Week 4:   3 sets of 7 repetitions with weights set at 65% of 1-RM

Week 5:   2 sets of 7 repetitions with weights set at 70% of 1-RM

Week 6:   3 sets of 7 repetitions with weights set at 70% of 1-RM

Week 7:   2 sets of 7 repetitions with weights set at 75% of 1-RM

Week 8:   3 sets of 7 repetitions with weights set at 75% of 1-RM

Week 9:   Assess muscular strength to set a new 1-RM

minutes and maximum of 5 minutes between sets. An example of an 8-week strength-training program is presented in Table 4.4. (Note that repetitions do not change.)

Note that this sample program does not progress to the use of 85% of 1-RM because its progression is designed to sustain motivation by prescribing overload at a steady, manageable pace. At this rate, you will be able to achieve your long-term goal of 50% increase in strength in 4 months. As with aerobic fitness training, remember that your prescription is not set in stone but can be adjusted depending on your individual response.

Cyclic Training. Another method for planning strength training programs that has become popular among weight trainers is periodization, or cyclic training: a macrocycle of training comprising four phases—base, load, peak, and recovery. This training design is for the motivated person who is willing to put in the time required to train over a 9- to 12-month period. Cyclic training has an advantage over straight progressive training programs because it helps prevent the trainer from reaching a plateau where no additional improvements are realized. Because cyclic training is more varied, it also enhances motivation. An example of the progression for cyclic training is illustrated in Table 4.5.

During the base phase your neuromuscular system has time to accommodate to the exercise and to overload. Your goal during this cycle is to perfect your form by doing many repetitions and sets at a fairly low intensity. This type of workout is often termed "high volume" because the weight lifted is low but the number of repetitions and sets is fairly high. If you are a beginner, this period should last 10 to 12 weeks.

The load phase, which lasts 6 to 8 weeks, is characterized by higher-intensity workouts and dramatic strength gains. The volume is still relatively high because the number of sets increases to between 4 and 6, even though the repetitions decrease to between 4 and 8. As illustrated in Table 4.5, the intensity of the workouts should vary between 70% and 80% of 1-RM. A 1-week recovery period is recommended before moving into the peak phase to allow time for the muscles to rest prior to an increase in intensity.

High workloads during the peak phase are intended to maximize strength gains. When you are using intensities of 80% to 90%, it is important for you to decrease the volume of training to avoid overtraining. Sets and repetitions drop to 1 to 5 and 2 to 5, respectively. As with the other phases, workout intensities vary from low to medium to high and then back to low again. The peak phase typically lasts 3 to 4 weeks.

As its name suggests, the recovery phase is intended to provide your muscular system a needed break from intensity. Lasting 2 to 4 weeks, this phase is marked by low resistance, moderate volume, and a frequency of only 2 times per week. Following full recovery, your body will be ready to either begin a new base phase or continue on a maintenance schedule as outlined in Table 4.5.

TABLE 4.5

Sample Cyclic Weight Training Plan

VARIABLES	BASE[a]	LOAD[b]	PEAK	RECOVERY
Duration (weeks)	6–8	6–8	3–4	2–4
%		80–90	60	
Sets/exercise	3–4	4–6	1–5	2–3
% variation	60–65–70	70–75–80	80–85–90	60–60
	12–10–8	8–6–4	5–3–1 or 2	to-low

[a]This phase may last up to 10–12 weeks depending on the progress of the individual.

[b]1-week recovery period of low intensity is appropriate to introduce between the load and peak phases in order to allow for the delayed training effect.

Guidelines for Weight-Training

To maximize strength gains and minimize injury, you should adhere to certain safety considerations as you train. The following guidelines provide you with information to use when planning and executing your program.

1. **Warm up and cool down.** Your body needs preparation for weight training activity. The methods as well as benefits of warm-up for weight training are similar to those discussed in Chapter 3 for aerobic exercise. We recommend that you warm up with 5 minutes of walking, slow jogging, or bicycling. This should be followed by light, active stretching in which only slight tension is placed on the muscle groups. Examples of warm-up stretches can be found in Chapter 5 (see Figure 5.3).

   The cool-down is similar to the warm-up in that it includes dynamic activity such as walking, slow jogging, or cycling. For muscular fitness training, deep stretching for specific muscle groups should follow the exercises that use those muscle groups because the muscles are warm and pliable at this time. For instance, after your sets of leg curls, you should perform 2 to 3 repetitions of hamstrings stretches (see Figure 5.3d) and hold each for 15 to 30 seconds. Examples of other appropriate stretches for cool-down can be found in Chapter 5.

2. **Use equipment properly.** A thorough orientation to all equipment should precede your training program. Facilities generally have a supervisor or instructor who can explain how to use the equipment and can provide periodic consultation as you develop your program design. If an instructor is not available or you have an in-home gym, it is even more important that you acquaint yourself with the equipment prior to initiating your program.

   Proper use of equipment is an ongoing priority for weight training. To prevent injury caused by equipment failures, always make sure that all machines are working properly and all pieces are secure before attempting your lift.

3. **Use spotters.** In the beginning stages of weight training, even with machine weights, it is a good idea to have a spotter. Spotters are especially important when you are using free weights because you risk injury if you are lifting alone and a weight slips. A spotter should be thoroughly familiar with the exercise in order to guide you in perfecting your form and should be able to lift more than the maximum weight you are attempting to lift. When performing maximal lifts, two or three spotters are recommended.

4. **Breathe continuously.** Holding your breath and bearing down during a lift greatly increases pressure within your chest and abdomen, thus reducing the return of blood to your heart and increasing your risk of fainting. By breathing constantly throughout the lift, you can minimize this pressure response and reduce stress on your heart. This is called the Valsalva maneuver. We recommend that you exhale during the concentric work and inhale during the eccentric work. For example, when performing a biceps curl, you exhale as you bend your arms and inhale as you straighten them.

Sound Decision Making

BEYOND THE 10K

Gita started running three years ago with her older sister, and since then she has continued to run three to five miles several times a week. She loves the freedom of the open road, and welcomes the time to herself to digest the events of the day. Recently, Gita saw a flyer for a 10-kilometer race to benefit a local charity. She has never run in a race but she is interested in the idea of running competitively. Gita takes a couple of books out of the library on physical conditioning and realizes that, in addition to gradually increasing her mileage, she can increase her competitive edge by incorporating weight training into her fitness routine.

Gita arranges to meet with a weight-training instructor at her school gym to go over safety issues, learn how to use the equipment, and plan a weight-training program to meet her needs. Gita had thought she just needed to work on her legs, but she learns that a strong upper body and abdominal muscles are important to runners too. She puts together a plan concentrating on muscular endurance, in which she will lift three days a week, alternating between concentration on her legs and her abdominals and upper body. On the advice of her instructor, Gita decides to train with weight machines instead of with free weights to minimize her chance of injury before the race. Gita's short-term goal is to increase her muscular endurance by 50% in the 10 weeks before the 10-K run.

Gita spends her first weight-training session with the instructor at the gym to be sure she uses the equipment correctly. The instructor shows her how to warm up with 5 minutes on an exercise bike followed by a few light stretches. She does 2 sets of 12 to 15 repetitions at about 50% of her repetition maximum at each weight machine. She finishes with a cool-down period of more stationary biking and a longer period of stretching. The next week she adds another set of repetitions to each exercise without changing the weight.

Gita notices the change in her running soon after she begins the weight-training routine. She finds she feels stronger and requires less exertion to finish her route. She didn't win the 10-K race, but she is hooked on competitive running. She continues slowly to progress in her endurance training and to increase her running speed and distance. Who knows? Maybe next year she'll try running a marathon!

5. Emphasize form, not weight. There is a tendency to become "gung-ho" in a weight training program, focusing on the amount of weight rather than appropriate form and progression. Without correct form, maximum strength gains are not possible, safety is compromised, and muscle soreness and/or injury can result. To maintain good form, remember to bend your knees, to contract your abdominal muscles when standing, and to use your lower body and abdominal muscles instead of your back muscles during a lift.

Correct form can be enhanced in two ways. The first is to have a partner assist and watch you execute the lifts. The second is to use a mirror to help you self-correct. Either way, once you have perfected form, your body will "program" the movement so you are able to self-correct without the use of a partner or a mirror.

6. Keep movements slow and controlled. The maximum amount of tension is developed within a muscle when a movement is performed slowly with control. This results in the greatest possible strength gains. By contrast, rapid, jerky movements not only are associated with a high dropout rate but can lead to injury. When using machine weights, the weight should be lifted slowly during the concentric loading phase and then released slowly during the eccentric loading phase. You can gauge your degree of control by listening for the "banging" sound of the weights and working to

reduce the noise as needed. One way to ensure a controlled lift is to count 2 seconds for the concentric and 2 to 3 seconds for the eccentric phases—for example, Up: One-one thousand, two-one thousand; Down: Three-one thousand, four-one thousand. (See the Do's and Don'ts box.)

Improving Muscular Fitness Without Weight Training

Undoubtedly, some of you have no interest in going to a weight room but do want to improve your muscular fitness. Perhaps you associate weight

WEIGHT ◆ TRAINING

Do

▲ Breathe freely and rhythmically while performing all exercises.

▲ Begin slowly with light weights or no weight to encourage correct lifting technique.

▲ Emphasize form, not weight.

▲ Move through the full range of motion of the joint (FROM principle).

▲ Control the weight to avoid sudden release.

▲ Include sufficient warm-up and cool-down.

▲ Practice spotting techniques, particularly with free and/or heavy weights.

Don't

▼ Hold your breath while performing a lift.

▼ Attempt a lift without proper instruction.

▼ Use weights that are too heavy.

▼ Bang the weights.

▼ Progress too quickly.

▼ Work out when you have a fever, respiratory infection, or other systemic illness.

▼ Work out when you are injured.

rooms with an intimidating, unfriendly environment. Maybe your primary goal is muscular endurance, in which case a weight room is not as important to your program as it would be to someone whose goal is muscular strength.

The exercises illustrated in this chapter using weights can all be performed at home or in a gym without weights or with light wrist and ankle weights. Using this approach, gains in muscular endurance will be most dramatic if you continue to increase repetitions and weight. Other ways to achieve your goal include attending specialty muscle-conditioning classes. You can find such "body toning" or "body sculpting" classes at your local parks and recreation department, YMCA, health club, or school athletic center.

In addition, most aerobics classes include specific conditioning exercises to promote muscular endurance. Many people have achieved marked increases in muscular fitness as a result of attending these classes and performing many repetitions of the exercises. Step aerobics classes, which use a short bench for moving on and around, offer a challenge and promote endurance in the upper

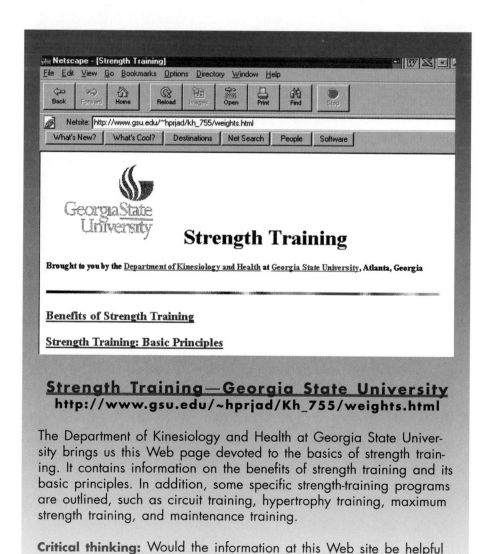

Strength Training—Georgia State University
http://www.gsu.edu/~hprjad/Kh_755/weights.html

The Department of Kinesiology and Health at Georgia State University brings us this Web page devoted to the basics of strength training. It contains information on the benefits of strength training and its basic principles. In addition, some specific strength-training programs are outlined, such as circuit training, hypertrophy training, maximum strength training, and maintenance training.

Critical thinking: Would the information at this Web site be helpful to you in planning a strength-training program? What additional information or features would make it more helpful?

Source: From Georgia State University, Department of Kinesiology, 1998

and lower body. Remember, you must choose some type of program if you wish to improve your muscular fitness. The key is to make it "livable" for you—to select a program that suits your own goals, lifestyle, and schedule. (See the Perspectives box.) Beginning a program now will provide you both the success of building strength and the positive pattern of implementing this program into your lifestyle.

Perspectives

Weight-Training & Older Adults

Over the years, young men have dominated weight rooms and been the primary participants in this type of exercise, which gave rise to the belief that weight training was only for a specific body type, age, and gender. Times have changed, however, and so has the thinking on weight training activities. Given the significant decline in strength most people experience with age, the American College of Sports Medicine now promotes strength training as part of a well-balanced exercise program for all adults.

Older individuals, in particular, can participate successfully in weight training programs and improve their ability to function in daily life. Research examining the effectiveness of strength-building exercises for the elderly has found tremendous strength gains. For example, Fiatarone and colleagues reported increases of well over 100% in nonagenarians (90-year-olds) who trained with weights for 3 months; Charette and colleagues observed an increase in muscle fiber size in 65-year-old women who lifted weights for 12 weeks.

Older adults interested in muscular fitness need not be intimidated by outmoded ideas about strength training. They can develop a program to suit their individual goals using guidelines similar to those outlined in this chapter. However, we recommend that they receive physician clearance prior to beginning a strength-training program.

Lifestyle Choices: Plan for Action

In your wellness journey it is critical to find ways to incorporate activities that improve muscular fitness into your lifestyle. If you already perform muscle-building exercises on a regular basis, good for you! You undoubtedly are reaping the benefits of improved levels of muscular strength and endurance. However, if muscular fitness activities are not part of your program, or if you answered "some of the time" or "never" to questions 9 and/or 10 in Section 11 of the Wellness Inventory in Chapter 1, you may want to examine your exercise habits as they apply to muscular fitness.

Table 4.6 presents a variety of ways to increase muscular fitness as you go about your daily life. How many of these do you do regularly? What can you choose to do in the future? After completing Laboratories 4.1 and 4.2 to assess muscle strength and endurance, create a plan of action for yourself by filling out the following goal-setting form. Use Table 4.6 to select the activities that will allow you to meet your goals for muscular fitness.

My rating for muscular strength: _____

My rating for muscular endurance:

    Bench press: _____

    Lateral pull: _____

    Biceps curl: _____

    Leg press: _____

Based on the ratings of my muscular fitness, I have chosen the following short- and long-term goals:

SHORT-TERM GOALS

_____

_____

_____

I will achieve my short-term goals on _____ *(date).*

_____   _____

(signature)　　　　　　　　　　　　　　*(witness)*

LONG-TERM GOALS

_____

_____

_____

I will achieve my long-term goals on _____ *(date).*

_____   _____

(signature)　　　　　　　　　　　　　　*(witness)*

Now, consider whether you are really willing to commit to your goals. As with aerobic exercise, begin by making a list of the benefits you would gain from doing this type of training. Also list any barriers that make it difficult for you to exercise

POTENTIAL BENEFITS　　　　　　**POTENTIAL BARRIERS**

_____   _____

_____   _____

_____   _____

Now, identify one barrier that you need to overcome in order to add *at leaset one session* of weight-training to your schedule: _____

_____

Weekly Weight Training Diary

WEEK 1

From _____ *(date)* to _____ *(date)*

Weight-Repetitions

	____ *day*	____ *day*	____ *day*	____ *day*	____ *day*
Set 1	_____	_____	_____	_____	_____
Set 2	_____	_____	_____	_____	_____
Set 3	_____	_____	_____	_____	_____
Set 4	_____	_____	_____	_____	_____
Set 5	_____	_____	_____	_____	_____
Set 6	_____	_____	_____	_____	_____

WEEK 2

From _____ *(date)* to _____ *(date)*

Weight-Repetitions

	____ *day*	____ *day*	____ *day*	____ *day*	____ *day*
Set 1	_____	_____	_____	_____	_____
Set 2	_____	_____	_____	_____	_____
Set 3	_____	_____	_____	_____	_____
Set 4	_____	_____	_____	_____	_____
Set 5	_____	_____	_____	_____	_____
Set 6	_____	_____	_____	_____	_____

WEEK 3

From _____ *(date)* to _____ *(date)*

Weight-Repetitions

	____ *day*	____ *day*	____ *day*	____ *day*	____ *day*
Set 1	_____	_____	_____	_____	_____
Set 2	_____	_____	_____	_____	_____
Set 3	_____	_____	_____	_____	_____
Set 4	_____	_____	_____	_____	_____
Set 5	_____	_____	_____	_____	_____
Set 6	_____	_____	_____	_____	_____

WEEK 4

From _____ (date) to _____ (date)

Weight-Repetitions

	_____ day	_____ day	_____ day	_____ day	_____ day
Set 1	_____	_____	_____	_____	_____
Set 2	_____	_____	_____	_____	_____
Set 3	_____	_____	_____	_____	_____
Set 4	_____	_____	_____	_____	_____
Set 5	_____	_____	_____	_____	_____
Set 6	_____	_____	_____	_____	_____

At the end of 4 weeks, review your progress. What worked? What didn't? If you need to start over, choose a new barrier to overcome. If you were successful, increase the duration of your exercise session or add another session per week. Was the muscular fitness training an aid in other choices for wellness, such as nutrition, sleep patterns, positive behaviors?

TABLE 4.6

Ten Ways to Improve Muscular Fitness Through Daily Activities

1. Climb stairs instead of taking the elevator.
2. Carry your own groceries.
3. When you shop, use pull doors instead of automatic.
4. Do your own housework
5. Scrub floors on your hands and knees.
6. Help a friend with small children.
7. During break times, do 10 deep knee bends.
8. During break times, do 10 push-ups off a desk top or counter top.
9. During TV commercials, do as many abdominal curl-ups as possible.
10. Dig, weed, and plant in your garden or in a friend's or parent's garden.

Summary

Muscular fitness is often overlooked when people plan exercise programs. However, having greater muscular fitness improves your ability to perform daily activities, increases independence, and can have positive effects on your self-esteem, body image, social life, and health. These are all very important components of wellness. In order to achieve optimal wellness, your strength and endurance program should accompany or be built into aerobic exercise and flexibility training. Most important, make sure it works for you and blends well into your lifestyle.

Key concepts that you have learned in this chapter include these:

- Muscular fitness involves both muscular strength and muscular endurance.

- Skeletal muscles develop tension through the interplay of thick and thin protein filaments.

- Three distinct muscle fiber types generate force for specific activities: slow-twitch oxidative, fast-twitch glycolytic, and fast-twitch oxidative glycolytic

- Muscle actions are either isometric, concentric, or eccentric.

- In the concentric, muscles shorten as they produce force; in the eccentric, they lengthen.

- Muscles respond to training in two stages: the neuromuscular and the hypertrophic and metabolic.

- Gender differences in muscle strength are due mainly to differences in total amount of lean mass and also the muscle cross-sectional area.

- Training for muscular fitness prevents chronic diseases and back pain, offsets muscle deterioration, and enhances self-image.

- Designing a program of muscular fitness involves assessing current fitness, setting realistic goals, and choosing the right equipment and exercises.

- An effective training program considers safety and proper technique.

References

Adams, K. Bone mineral density. Strength, Power, and Flexibility in Nonlifters and Competitive Lifters. Dissertation, Oregon State University, 1992

Brooks, G. A., and T. D. Fahey. *Exercise Physiology: Human Bioenergetics and Its Applications.* New York: Wiley, 1984.

Charette, S., et al. Muscle hypertrophy response to resistance training in older women. *Journal of Applied Physiology, 70*: 1912–1916, 1991.

Fiatarone, M. A., et al. High-intensity strength training in nonagenarians: Effects on skeletal muscle. *Journal of the American Medical Association, 65*: 1147–1151, 1990.

Gonyea, W. J. Role of exercise in inducing increases in skeletal muscle fiber number. *Journal of Applied Physiology, 48*: 421–426, 1980.

Grimby, G., and B. Saltin. The aging muscle. *Clinical Physiology, 3*: 209–218, 1983.

Hagberg, J. M., et al. Effect of weight training on blood pressure and hemodynamics in hypertensive adolescents. *Journal of Pediatrics, 104*: 147–151, 1984.

Holloway, J. B., and T. R. Baechle. Strength training for female athletes. A review of selected aspects. *Sports Medicine 9*:216–228, 1990.

Hurley, B. F., and P. F. Kokkinos. Effects of weight training on risk factors for coronary artery disease. *Sports Medicine, 4*: 213–238, 1987.

Hurley, B. F., et al. Resistive training can reduce coronary risk factors without altering VO_2 or percent body fat. *Medicine and Science in Sports and Exercise, 20*: 150–154, 1988.

Jackson, C. P., and M. D. Brown. Is there a role for exercise in the treatment of patients with low back pain? Analysis of current approaches and a practical guide to exercise. *Clinical Orthopedics and Related Research, 179*: 39–54, 1983.

Jette, A. M., and L. G. Branch. The Framingham disability study: Physical disability among the aging. *American Journal of Public Health, 71*: 1211–1216, 1981.

Kraemer, W. J. Involvement of eccentric muscle action may optimize adaptations to resistance training. *Sports Science Exchange, 4*(41): 1992.

Lombardi, V. P. *Beginning Weight Training.* Dubuque, IA: Wm. C. Brown, 1989.

MacDougall, J. D., et al. Muscle ultrastructural characteristics of elite power lifters and bodybuilders. *European Journal of Sports Medicine, 48*: 117–126, 1982.

Miller, A. E., J. D. MacDougall, M. A. Tarnopolsky, and D. G. Sale. Gender differences in strength and muscle fiber characteristics. *European Journal of Applied Physiology, 66*: 254–262, 1993.

Powers, S. K., and E. T. Howley. *Exercise Physiology.* Dubuque, IA: Wm. C. Brown, 1990.

Reid, C. M., R. A. Yeater, and H. Ullrich. Weight training and strength, cardiorespiratory functioning and body composition of men. *British Journal of Sports Medicine, 21*: 40–44, 1987.

Samson, J., and J. Yerles. Racial differences in sports performance. *Canadian Journal of Sports Science, 13*: 109–116, 1988.

Shaw, J., and C. Snow. Weighted vest exercise improves indices of fall risk in older women. *Journal of Gerontology, XX,* 1998.

Snow-Harter, C., et al. Bone mineral density, muscle strength and recreational exercise in men. *Journal of Bone and Mineral Research, 7*: 1291–1296, 1992.

Snow-Harter C., et al. Muscle strength as a predictor of bone mineral density in young women. *Journal of Bone and Mineral Research, 5*(6): 589–595, 1990.

Laboratory 4.1

Assessing Muscular Strength

One way to measure strength is by using a one-repetition maximum, or 1-RM, to determine the amount of weight with which you can perform only one complete lift. Because 1-RM testing is not recommended for the beginning student, we suggest that you estimate your 1-RM by measuring your 6-RM—that is, the weight at which you can perform only six repetitions and no more. After you have begun your strength-training program and wish to assess your 1-RM, be sure to consider the following safety guidelines, adapted from Lombardi, for performing a 1-RM test:

1. Do not administer more than once every two months.

2. Warm up for 5–10 minutes before the trial.

3. Have at least one spotter for each attempt. In the case of free weights, two spotters are advised.

4. Do not count lifts that deviate in form.

5. Have the first trial be as close to estimated maximum as possible, but avoid overestimating 1-RM on the first trial.

6. Conduct a maximum of three trials.

7. Vary the rest period according to the individual, but keep it at 3–5 minutes between trials.

Your instructor will demonstrate each of the lifts you will be performing—the bench press, lateral pull, and biceps curl—according to starting position, finishing position, spotting, breathing, and back safety. For this laboratory, it is best to work with a partner. One of you will be performing the lift; the other will be spotting for correct form and recording 6-RM values.

Prior to attempting your 6-RM, you should take five practice trials at the lowest weight on the machine. When you are ready to measure strength, you should begin at a fairly high weight so that you do not get fatigued. It is best to try to obtain your 6-RM using three or fewer trials.

Estimating Your 1-RM

The equation used to calculate 1-RM is

$$\text{1-RM}_{estimated} = 1.2 \times \text{weight in pounds lifted}$$

For example, if you completed six repetitions of the biceps curl at 10 pounds, the equation would then look like this:

$$\text{1-RM}_{estimated} = 1.2 \times 10 \text{ lbs} = 12.0 \text{ lbs}$$

Estimate your 1-RM for each lift below.

	6-RM Lifted	Coefficient	Estimated 1-RM
Leg press	_____	× 1.2	_____
Bench press	_____	× 1.2	_____
Lateral pull	_____	× 1.2	_____
Biceps curl	_____	× 1.2	_____

Record your estimated 1-RM below. Then determine "ratio" by dividing your value by your body weight. Refer to Table 4.7 to determine points from the ratio for lifts 1–4. Add all points together for a total, then find your strength fitness category in Table 4.8.

	Estimated 1-RM	Ratio (1-RM/Body Wt)	Points
Leg press	_____	_____	_____
Bench press	_____	_____	_____
Lateral pull	_____	_____	_____
Biceps curl	_____	_____	_____
Total points			_____
Your strength fitness category			_____

TABLE 4.7
Points for Strength/ Body Weight Ratios

MEN

BENCH PRESS	BICEPS CURL	LATERAL PULL	LEG PRESS	POINTS
1.5	0.70	1.20	3.00	10
1.4	0.65	1.15	2.80	9
1.3	0.60	1.10	2.60	8
1.2	0.55	1.05	2.40	7
1.1	0.50	1.00	2.20	6
1.0	0.45	0.95	2.00	5
0.9	0.40	0.90	1.80	4
0.8	0.35	0.85	1.60	3
0.7	0.30	0.80	1.40	2
0.6	0.25	0.75	1.20	1

WOMEN

BENCH PRESS	BICEPS CURL	LATERAL PULL	LEG PRESS	POINTS
0.90	0.50	0.85	2.70	10
0.85	0.45	0.80	2.50	9
0.80	0.42	0.75	2.30	8
0.70	0.38	0.73	2.10	7
0.65	0.35	0.70	2.00	6
0.60	0.32	0.65	1.80	5
0.55	0.28	0.63	1.60	4
0.50	0.25	0.60	1.40	3
0.45	0.21	0.55	1.20	2
0.35	0.18	0.50	1.00	1

TABLE 4.8
Strength Fitness Category

TOTAL POINTS	STRENGTH FITNESS CATEGORY
32–40	Excellent
25–31	Good
18–24	Average
10–17	Below average
0–9	Need to start strength training

Source: Adapted from Heyward, V. *Advanced Fitness Assessment and Exercise Prescription* (Champaign, IL: Human Kinetics, 1991).

Laboratory 4.2

Assessing Muscular Endurance

Muscular endurance training is characterized by the use of low-resistance weights with many repetitions. In this laboratory, you will be determining the endurance of specific muscle groups using a defined percentage of body weight. For example, on the bench press, the weight for women to use for testing is 50% of body weight; for men it is 66%. You need to calculate these percentages for every lift.

Your instructor will demonstrate each of the lifts you will be performing—the bench press, lateral pull, biceps curl, and leg press—according to starting position, finishing position, spotting, breathing, and back safety. For this laboratory, it is best to work with a partner. One of you will be performing the lift; the other will be spotting for correct form and recording values.

Prior to this assessment, you should have a 5- to 10-minute general body warm-up. Prior to actual testing, you should take five practice trials at the lowest weight on the machine. When you are ready to measure endurance, you should begin at the predetermined weight and then execute the lift as many times as possible up to a maximum of 15 repetitions. For each of the exercises listed, find the specific percentages of body weight to use from Table 4.9. Then record them on the following form using Table 4.10 as a guide.

Appropriate Weight and Number of Repetitions

	Pounds Lifted	Repetitions	Category
1. Bench press	_____	_____	_____
2. Lateral pull	_____	_____	_____
3. Biceps curl	_____	_____	_____
4. Leg press	_____	_____	_____

Muscular endurance fitness categories

>12 repetitions You have great muscular endurance and should work to maintain it.

8–12 repetitions You have good muscular endurance but could improve it still more.

5–7 repetitions You have average muscular endurance and should work to improve it.

<5 repetitions You have poor muscular endurance and need to start a muscular endurance training program.

TABLE 4.9

Percentages of Body Weight to Use for Muscular Endurance Assessment

STATION	MEN	WOMEN
Bench press	66%	50%
Lateral pull	66%	50%
Biceps curl	33%	25%
Leg press	100%	75%

Source: From Heyward, 1991.

TABLE 4.10

Guidelines for Body Weight and Weight Percentages

BODY WEIGHT	WEIGHT PERCENTAGES (LBS)				
	25%	33%	50%	66%	75%
200	50	66	100	132	150
190	48	63	95	125	142
180	45	60	90	120	135
170	43	56	85	112	127
160	40	53	80	106	120
150	38	50	75	100	112
140	35	46	70	92	105
130	33	43	65	86	97
120	30	40	60	80	90
110	28	36	55	73	82
100	25	33	50	66	75

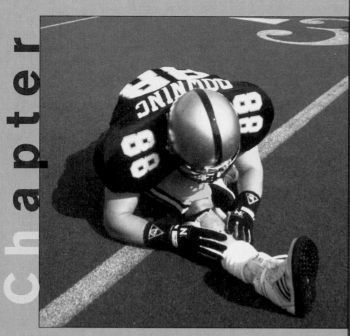
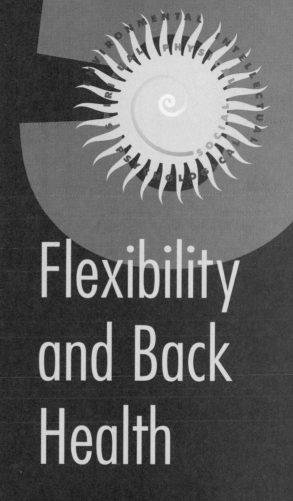

chapter 5

Flexibility and Back Health

One Student's View

Wellness to me means being capable of achieving anything that I strive for mentally, emotionally, and physically, yet also being able to cope with setbacks along the way. It means enjoying simple pleasures like a walk on the beach at sunset. It means achieving goals like completing a marathon. It even means surviving personal tragedies like the death of a loved one. To me, wellness means that the mental, emotional, and physical aspects of my life are all in balance. And when one of these aspects is "out of kilter," the other two are strong enough to keep me in good health.

—Julie Liudahl

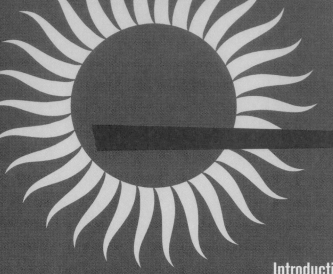

Introduction

Have you ever admired the remarkable ability of dancers and gymnasts to move their bodies in almost any way they want? This ability is due largely to greater-than-average flexibility—that is, to an increased range of motion in their joints. Most of us do not need to make flying leaps or do deep back bends, but we need some degree of flexibility to perform everyday tasks such as reaching a can on the top shelf at the supermarket, getting in and out of a car, or bending over to pick up a box. Because many of us take these abilities for granted, we make little effort to maintain and develop our flexibility. Thus, flexibility may decline, making everyday tasks more difficult to perform.

Reduced flexibility not only makes free body movement difficult but can also lead to neck and upper and lower back pain. Low back pain, in particular, can significantly reduce your quality of life and predispose you to injuries as you age. Most individuals with back pain are inflexible, and (as discussed in Chapter 4) they tend to have weak abdominal and back muscles.

You make many choices (how you sit, stand, and move) throughout each day that play an important role in determining the flexibility of your joints and the health of your back. Habitual body positions and movement patterns influence body mechanics so that, over time, your joints become less mobile. For example, if your shoulders are usually rounded, sooner or later you will probably notice that your neck and upper back have become tight and that the movement in your shoulder joints is more limited.

Fortunately, it is never too late to improve your flexibility and back health. Indeed, many studies have shown that for both the young and the old, flexibility and back strength can be increased through stretching and strengthening exercises (Einkauf and colleagues; Etnyre and Lee; and Germain and Blair). Staying active throughout your life can offset the decreased range of motion that results naturally from the aging process (Gracovetsky, Farfan, and Helleur).

Improved flexibility can have a beneficial effect on the various dimensions of wellness, including both physical and psychological well-being. If you are flexible, you will find it easier to perform aerobic exercise. Flexibility is also an asset for most athletic endeavors and can help prevent sports injuries. And good posture can contribute to mental health by enhancing your appearance and self-image.

In this chapter, you will learn how to maintain or increase your flexibility and back health. You will learn about the joints in the body: where they are, how they work, and how to work with them. Specific exercises for promoting fluid movement, reducing muscular tension, and improving back health are included, as well as suggestions for developing a flexibility training program that will help you prevent injuries associated with decreased flexibility. Maintaining or increasing your flexibility will help you achieve the physical health you need to lead an active and productive life.

Defining Flexibility

Flexibility refers to the capacity of a joint to move easily through its full range of motion. (Throughout this chapter, you will find the terms *flexibility* and *range of motion* used synonymously.) If you are very flexible, your body will move easily, but if you are inflexible, your joints may not be able to move through the full range of motion. For example, if you can easily bend down and touch your toes and hold the position, you have good flexibility in that part of your hip and lower back joints. However, if you experience considerable resistance and are unable to reach the position, then your movement in this specific joint is limited due to reduced flexibility.

Poor flexibility can interfere with your ability to perform simple daily tasks effectively. Moreover, a limited range of motion can lead to injuries while performing such activities as driving, vacuuming, or moving quickly. For instance, when driving a car, you must be able to turn your head fully from side to side to have good visibility. If you have a tight neck and upper back, you may not have an adequate view of traffic, and this lack could lead to accidents. Older adults who experience a reduced range of motion that limits their ability to perform daily activities can find themselves becoming increasingly dependent on others for assistance. Flexibility declines with age as the muscles, tendons, ligaments, and joint capsules become less pliable. In general, most people become less active as they grow older; disuse of their muscles leads to tightening of the tissues and a reduced range of motion. Women are generally more flexible than men. Men typically have greater muscle mass and less ligament laxity than do women, which limits their range of motion. However, both men and women can increase their flexibility at any age.

Stretching is the best method for improving flexibility. As part of their training, gymnasts and dancers perform many repetitions of stretching exercises in which stretches are held for long periods of time. Although flexibility

flexibility capacity of a joint to move easily through its full range of motion

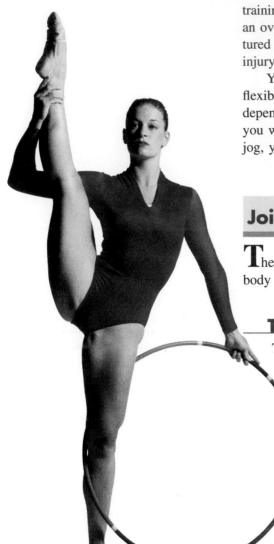

training is central to dance and gymnastics, it is often overlooked as part of an overall exercise program. Frequently, stretching exercises are simply featured as "tag-ons" at the beginning or end of a workout and used solely for injury prevention.

Your exercise program should include stretching exercises for general flexibility. You may also want to work on the flexibility of specific joints, depending on the forms of exercise you select. For example, if you swim, you will benefit from developing flexibility in your shoulders. If you run or jog, you might concentrate on stretching the hamstrings and other leg areas.

Joint Anatomy and Mechanics

The way your body moves is influenced by the type of joint found in that body part, which in turn dictates its function.

Types of Joints

The joints of the body can be grouped into three categories according to their function: diarthrodial, amphiarthrodial, and synarthrodial.

- Diarthrodial (dia: through, apart; arthro: joint) joints are freely movable and are found primarily in the knees, hips, fingers, ankles, and shoulders—areas where movement is emphasized. Diarthrodial joints have the following structural features: (1) cartilage (connective tissue) covering the opposing joint surfaces, (2) a joint cavity filled with fluid, (3) a capsule that encloses the joint, and (4) ligaments (tissue that joins bones with other bones) that surround and strengthen the joint (see Figure 5.1). Most flexibility training focuses on increasing the range of motion for diarthrodial joints.

- Amphiarthrodial (amphi: on both sides) joints are slightly movable joints that are found predominantly in the central skeleton—the chest, ribs, and pubic bones.

- Synarthrodial (syn: together) joints are immovable joints, such as those between most bones in the head.

The purpose of the reduced movement in both the amphiarthrodial and synarthrodial joints is to protect the internal organs, such as brain, kidneys, liver, and heart.

Joint Function

The structure of your joints dictates their movement; that is, they move in very specific ways based on their anatomy. Understanding the motion capabilities of primary joints is important in designing an exercise program that maximizes movement capability in the joint. The more freely movable joints of the arms, legs, and neck allow you to perform your daily activities with relative ease whereas those joints that move less freely provide stability and protection from internal injury as you move. Figure 5.2 illustrates some of the major joints in your body and their motion capabilities.

As you can see from Figure 5.2a, **flexion** refers to movement that brings two ends of jointed body parts closer to each other—for example, bending the arm, leg, or trunk. The opposite of flexion is **extension,** which refers to movement that carries two ends of jointed body parts away from each other—for example, straightening the leg, arm, or trunk. Flexion and extension can work together as you perform an action. For example, when you kick a ball, you flex your leg before the kick and extend your leg as you make contact. **Hyperextension** refers to the movement of jointed body parts beyond the normal range of motion. For example, when you lift your chin to the ceiling, you are hyperextending your head, and when you perform a backbend or arch your back, you are hyperextending your trunk (Figure 5.2a).

Flexion and extension have specific names when applied to motion at the ankle joint. For example, pointing your toes is referred to as planter flexion; pulling your toes up is called dorsiflexion (see Figure 5.2b). In broader terms, **circumduction** refers to special capability of the shoulder and hip joints that allows circular movement. **Abduction** is the capability of the shoulder and hip joints that allows the arms and legs to move away from the midline of the body; **adduction** is the capability of the shoulder and hip joints that allows the arms and legs to move toward the midline (see Figure 5.2c). Finally, body parts also **rotate,** which refers to the movement of the head, arms, and legs from side to side along an axis (see Figure 5.2d). For example, you rotate your head to look both ways at a stop sign when deciding whether it is safe to proceed into the intersection.

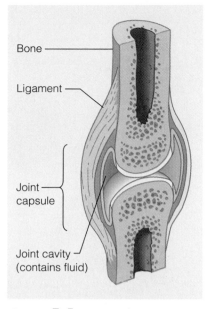

Figure 5.1

The diarthrodial knee joint permits joint motion through the interplay among ligaments, cartilage, and joint cavity and capsule.
Source: From Marieb, 1992.

The Training Effect

The capacity for a greater range of motion at many of your joints can be increased through a program of flexibility training.

Physiological Adaptations to Stretching

Many people believe that flexibility is strictly genetically determined, that some people are simply more flexible than others. Although genetics do, to some extent, determine the limits of your flexibility, your joints have the capacity to increase their range of motion. Stretching is the most effective type of training to improve your flexibility. Stretching focuses on reducing tightness in the muscles and, to a limited degree, the soft tissues surrounding the joints. The joint capsule, ligaments, and tendons (which attach muscle to bones) are made of **nonelastic tissue**—soft, nonpliable tissue that does not respond favorably to stretching. By contrast, muscle fibers are extremely elastic and therefore are the target tissue in flexibility training.

Benefits of Improved Flexibility and Back Health

Training to improve flexibility and back health is one key to preventing back problems and minimizing age-related declines in range of motion. Flexibility training can also improve your performance in aerobic and muscular fitness activities and help reduce sports-related injuries. As Heyward has demonstrated,

flexion movement that brings two ends of jointed body parts closer to each other

extension movement that carries two ends of jointed body parts away from each other

hyperextension movement of jointed body parts beyond the normal range of motion

circumduction special capability of the shoulder and hip joints that allows circular movement

abduction capability of the shoulder and hip joints that allows the arms and legs to move away from the midline of the body

adduction capability of the shoulder and hip joints that allows the arms and legs to move toward the midline of the body

rotate movement of head, arms, and legs from side to side along an axis

nonelastic tissue soft, nonpliable tissue that does not respond favorably to stretching

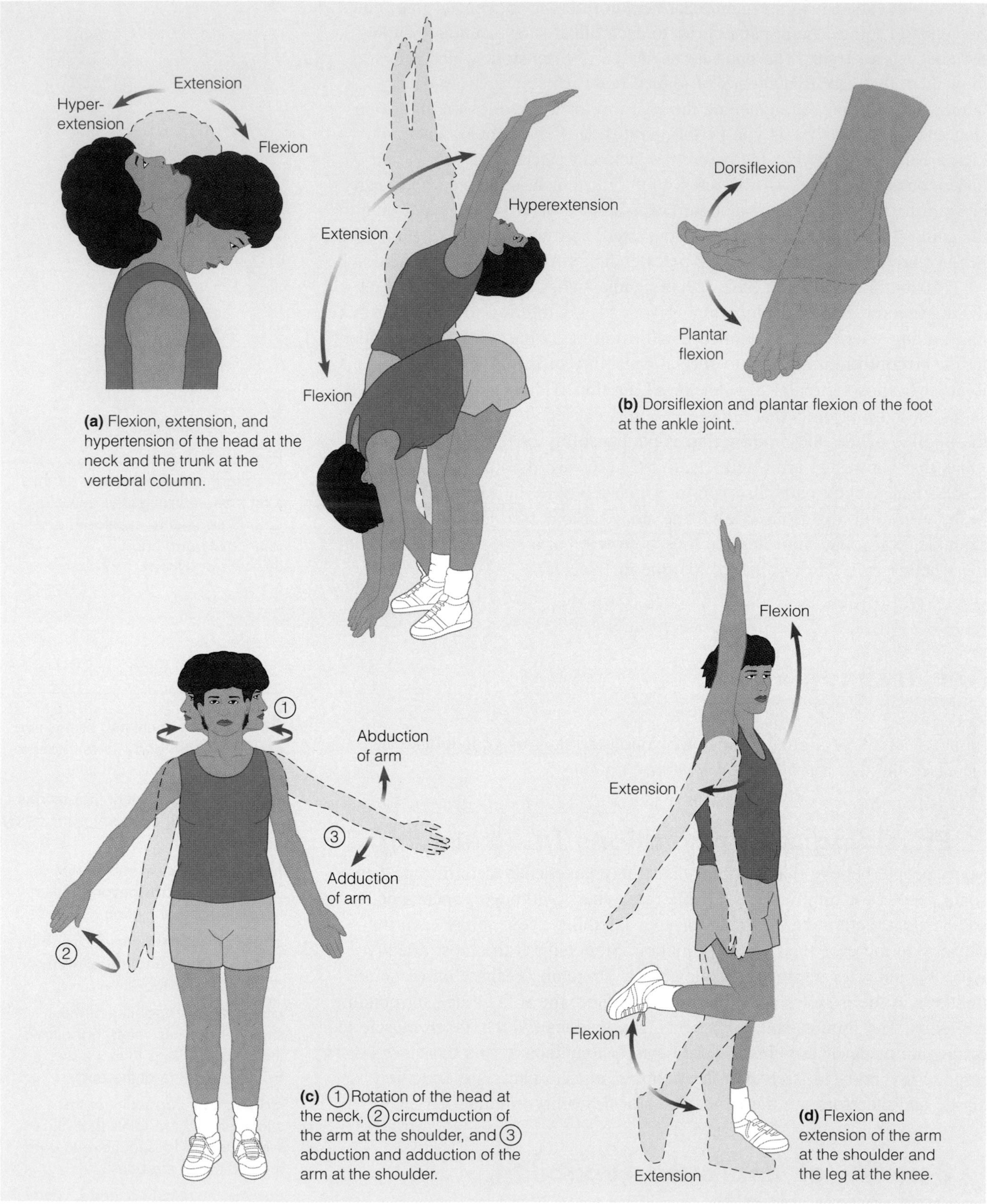

(a) Flexion, extension, and hypertension of the head at the neck and the trunk at the vertebral column.

Hyper-extension

Extension

Flexion

Extension

Hyperextension

Flexion

(b) Dorsiflexion and plantar flexion of the foot at the ankle joint.

Dorsiflexion

Plantar flexion

(c) ① Rotation of the head at the neck, ② circumduction of the arm at the shoulder, and ③ abduction and adduction of the arm at the shoulder.

Abduction of arm

Adduction of arm

(d) Flexion and extension of the arm at the shoulder and the leg at the knee.

Flexion

Extension

Flexion

Extension

Figure 5.2

Some major joints in the body enable a variety of movements.

Perspectives

Pregnancy and Flexibility

During the 9 months of pregnancy, a hormone called relaxin is secreted. This hormone helps prepare a woman for childbirth but also causes a general "relaxation" of all ligaments in her body. Thus, while it is important for a pregnant woman to maintain range of motion, she must be careful to avoid overstretching.

The dynamic stretches and the exercises for the back and neck (except those that require a facedown posture) presented in this chapter are suggested for pregnant women. During the third trimester (months 7–9), a pregnant woman should avoid lying on her back (supine). She should practice only the exercises that call for standing, sitting, or kneeling on hands and knees.

flexibility training leads to fewer injuries in active individuals; Jackson and Brown observed women over a 4-year period and found a higher incidence of injuries in subjects with imbalanced flexibility—that is, women who had a better range of motion in one leg than the other. (Injuries are discussed in detail in Chapter 6.)

Benefits can be derived just from the act of stretching itself. Yoga, which includes a great deal of stretching, has become increasingly popular because of its ability to reduce muscular and mental tension. A simple stretching routine that includes exercises for the neck, back, and shoulders is a very effective way to reduce the tension that often accompanies studying or desk work. (See the Perspectives box.)

Stretching Techniques

Stretching the muscles beyond their normal range—that is, overloading them—is the most effective way to improve flexibility. There are three types of stretching: ballistic stretching, static stretching, and proprioceptive neuro-muscular facilitation (PNF). Each of these techniques can increase range of motion, but static stretching is the safest and most practical and effective way.

Ballistic Stretching

Ballistic stretching involves repeated bouncing motion to stretch muscles. For example, suppose you want to improve the flexibility in the front of your shoulder joint. To stretch it ballistically you would stand with your arms stretched out from your sides and repeatedly swing your arms back as far as they could go. While this type of stretching does improve range of motion, its effectiveness is limited. This is because the muscle contains a sensory organ called a muscle spindle. When the muscle spindle senses a quick stretch, it immediately shortens to protect the muscle from overstretching and tearing. Therefore, when you stretch ballistically, you cannot stretch the muscle as far as it might go because it will shorten as soon as it senses the quick stretch. Drawbacks to ballistic stretching include the possibilities that the muscle spindle will not respond in time and that the stimulus (that is, the stretch) will be too great, causing the muscle to tear.

ballistic stretching repeated bouncing motion to stretch muscles

Static Stretching

Static stretching is the slow, gradual lengthening, holding, and releasing of specific muscle groups. If you wanted to stretch the front of your shoulder joint statically, you would slowly extend your arms behind your back until you could clasp your hands together, hold them there for at least 10 seconds, relax, and then repeat the process. During your static stretch of the shoulder, the muscles in the region are slowly lengthening due to the gradual motion of the stretch. In this case, the instinctive response of the muscle spindle is avoided, as there is no sudden stretch of the muscle. As a result, you can stretch the muscle more effectively. Remember, though, that because your shoulder has a wide range of motion (it is capable of circumduction), stretching the front of the shoulder will improve only one part of its motion capability. Therefore, your stretching program should include several different stretches for the shoulders

Proprioceptive Neuromuscular Facilitation (PNF)

Proprioceptive neuromuscular facilitation (PNF) refers to stretching of a muscle group facilitated by previous contraction of an opposite muscle group. PNF requires the assistance of a partner or therapist to help you contract and then relax your muscles. This technique is most commonly used by athletes, in clinical settings, and for rehabilitation purposes. Although an effective way of stretching, it is, according to Hall, more complicated and time-consuming to perform than static stretching.

If you were to complete the shoulder stretch using PNF, you would stand with your arms outstretched from your shoulders to the side and have a partner stand behind you and gently pull your arms behind you without any resistance from you. You would hold this position for at least 10 seconds and then release. Next, in the same position, you would resist your partner by trying to pull your arms together in front of you, contracting the front of your shoulder. After 6 to 10 seconds of isometric muscle action against resistance, you would relax again before your partner pulled your arms back as far as possible. This position would be held for 15 to 30 seconds.

Designing Your Flexibility Training Program

To increase your flexibility, you can develop an exercise program, much as you did in Chapters 3 and 4 for aerobic fitness and muscle fitness. To develop a flexibility training program, (1) assess your current flexibility and set goals, (2) choose exercises to help you achieve your goals, and (3) write an exercise prescription.

Assessment and Goal Setting

To design an appropriate training program and to monitor your progress as you train, you should be aware of your current level of flexibility. If possible, you should determine your flexibility prior to developing your goals and

static stretching slow, gradual lengthening, holding, and releasing of specific muscle groups

proprioceptive neuromuscular facilitation (PNF) stretching of a muscle group facilitated by previous contraction of an opposite muscle group

program of exercise. You surely have an idea of your current level of flexibility simply judging from the ways in which you move in daily activities. For example, how easily you are you able to pick up something off the floor? How much of a strain is it to reach overhead when grabbing for a book on the top shelf of your closet? If you hear an oncoming car while driving, is it a strain to quickly turn your head as far as possible to one side? Can you grab something from behind you without moving your torso? And last, if you have good flexibility, how consistently do you include sustained stretching exercises into your program of exercise in order to maintain your flexibility?

It certainly is valuable to conduct a quantitative assessment of your flexibility in order to measure your progress when undertaking a stretching program. A typical assessment for flexibility is the sit-and-reach test, which is part of Laboratory 5.1. This test evaluates the ability of the muscles in the back of your thighs (hamstrings) to stretch. It is commonly used as a screening test for low back flexibility Another flexibility assessment tool is the shoulder rotation test, also included in Laboratory 5.1.

After you have performed the assessments in Laboratory 5.1, rank your results against the normative values to determine your level of flexibility. Remember, however, if you feel you have a good sense of your own flexibility, an assessment may not be necessary. You know your own body and can set goals based on your own "flexibility sense."

Once you have evaluated your flexibility, you should set specific short- and long-term goals for maintaining or improving your range of motion. Suppose you scored high on all measures except shoulder flexibility, where you scored very low. You might decide to focus on improving this area while maintaining your overall flexibility Your goals might look like this:

SHORT-TERM GOAL
To improve shoulder flexibility by 25% in 8 weeks

LONG-TERM GOAL
To improve shoulder flexibility by 50% in 4 months

A goal sheet can help you define your goals. A sample goal sheet can be found in the Lifestyle Choices section. Once your goals have been established, you will want to choose exercises that can help you attain your goals.

Choice of Exercise

Whether you want to improve or simply maintain your range of motion, your training program should include flexibility exercises for every major joint, not just those you have targeted. Depending on your goals, you may choose dynamic range of motion exercises and light static stretches for maintenance and warm-up, and deep static stretching for improving specific areas. Figure 5.3 shows a set of basic stretching exercises.

Dynamic Range of Motion Exercises. Dynamic range-of-motion (ROM) exercises are recommended for maintaining flexibility, warming up joints, and easing muscle tension. *Dynamic* refers to the movement of a body part, and *range of motion* to the movement capability of the joint. An example of a dynamic ROM exercise for your shoulders would be to place your hands on your shoulders, touch your elbows in front of you, and then slowly draw one continuous circle up and around with your elbows (Figure 5.3a).

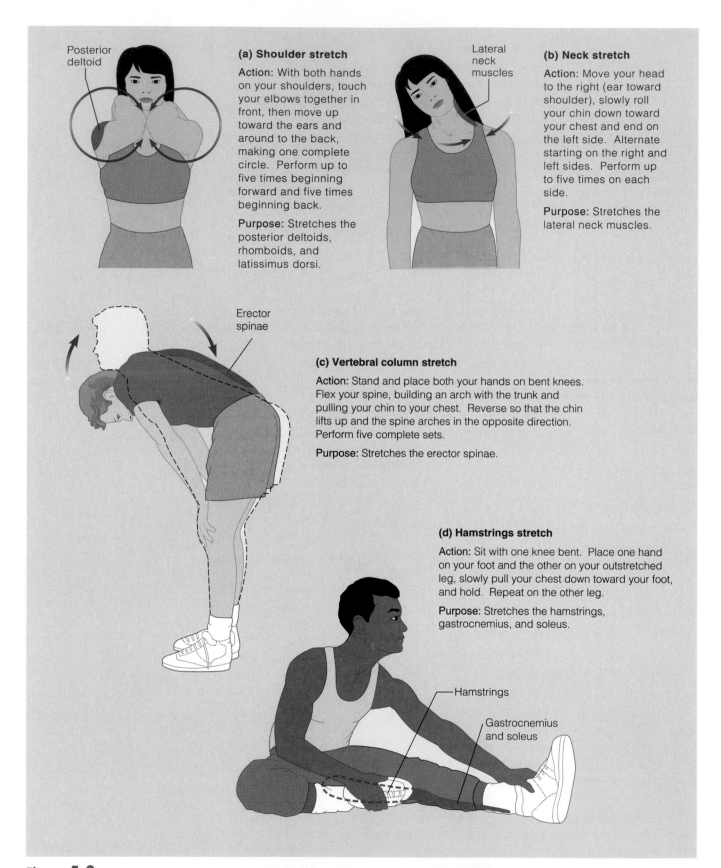

(a) Shoulder stretch

Posterior deltoid

Action: With both hands on your shoulders, touch your elbows together in front, then move up toward the ears and around to the back, making one complete circle. Perform up to five times beginning forward and five times beginning back.

Purpose: Stretches the posterior deltoids, rhomboids, and latissimus dorsi.

(b) Neck stretch

Lateral neck muscles

Action: Move your head to the right (ear toward shoulder), slowly roll your chin down toward your chest and end on the left side. Alternate starting on the right and left sides. Perform up to five times on each side.

Purpose: Stretches the lateral neck muscles.

(c) Vertebral column stretch

Erector spinae

Action: Stand and place both your hands on bent knees. Flex your spine, building an arch with the trunk and pulling your chin to your chest. Reverse so that the chin lifts up and the spine arches in the opposite direction. Perform five complete sets.

Purpose: Stretches the erector spinae.

(d) Hamstrings stretch

Action: Sit with one knee bent. Place one hand on your foot and the other on your outstretched leg, slowly pull your chest down toward your foot, and hold. Repeat on the other leg.

Purpose: Stretches the hamstrings, gastrocnemius, and soleus.

Hamstrings

Gastrocnemius and soleus

Figure 5.3

These illustrations (parts a-k) of a basic exercise set for flexibility show the execution of the stretch and highlight the primary muscle group affected

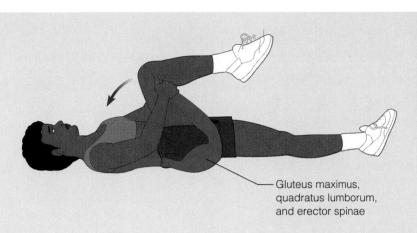

Gluteus maximus,
quadratus lumborum,
and erector spinae

(e) Knee pull

Action: Lie on your back and position your hand behind your knee. Slowly pull your leg toward yourself, and hold.

Purpose: Stretches the gluteus maximus, quadratus lumborum, and erector spinae.

(f) Ankle stretch

Action: With your right leg bent and tilted forward, and your left leg back and straight, lean forward against a wall and hold. Switch legs and repeat.

Purpose: Stretches the gastrocnemius and soleus.

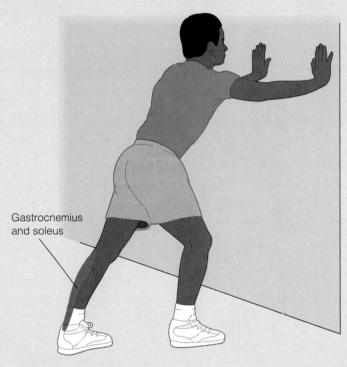

Gastrocnemius
and soleus

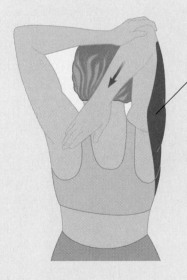

Triceps and
latissimus dorsi

(g) Shoulder and elbow stretch

Action: Bend one elbow and lift it so that it is up by your ear, and position the palm of your hand on your upper back. Place your opposite hand on your uplifted elbow, slowly pull, and hold.

Purpose: Stretches the triceps and latissimus dorsi.

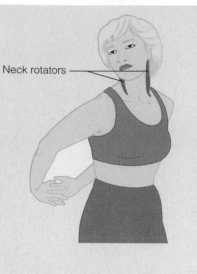

Neck rotators

(h) Chest stretch

Action: Lace your hands behind your back, pushing hands toward floor; straighten your arms, and hold. If possible, lift your arms and hold.

Purpose: Stretches the upper trapezius, pectoralis major and minor, and anterior deltoids.

(i) Ankle-to-hip stretch

Position: Right foot foward with knee bent at a 90 degree angle. Left leg is straight behind with heel on the floor.

Action: Hold the position above to stretch the calf and hip flexors on the left side. Then, place the left knee on the floor and bend at the knee to add a stretch to the quadriceps on the left. As this position becomes comfortable, hold the left foot with your right hand and gently pull. Hold the stretch then repeat on other side.

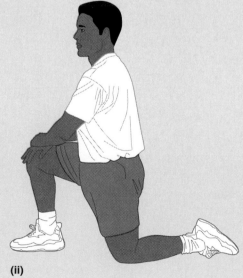

(i)

(ii)

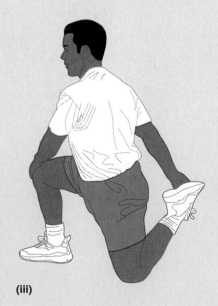

(iii)

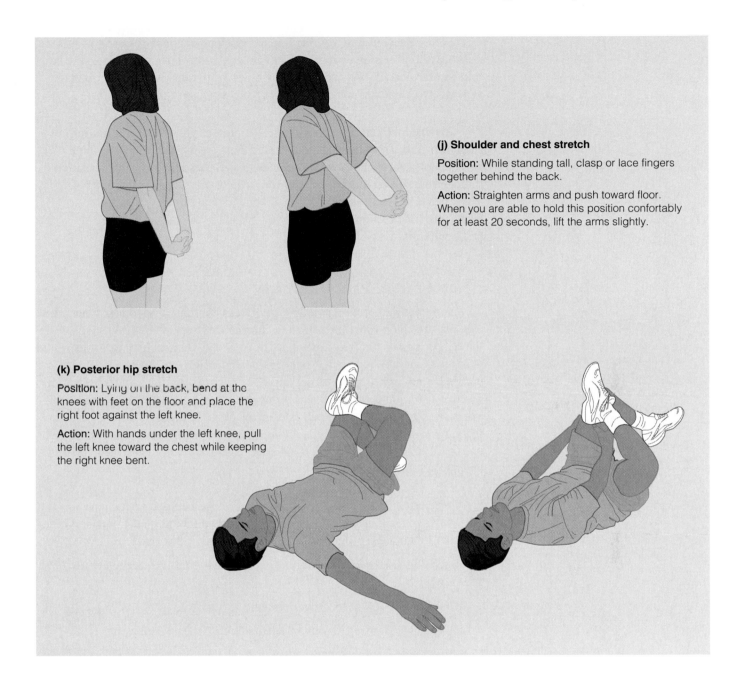

(j) Shoulder and chest stretch

Position: While standing tall, clasp or lace fingers together behind the back.

Action: Straighten arms and push toward floor. When you are able to hold this position confortably for at least 20 seconds, lift the arms slightly.

(k) Posterior hip stretch

Position: Lying on the back, bend at the knees with feet on the floor and place the right foot against the left knee.

Action: With hands under the left knee, pull the left knee toward the chest while keeping the right knee bent.

Dynamic ROM exercises do not lead to dramatic gains in flexibility because the muscles are not stretched to their limits; however, they are useful for warming up and for maintaining current flexibility levels. These exercises are also beneficial during sport or study breaks. Some common dynamic ROM exercises are illustrated in Figure 5.3a–c. Wrist and ankle rotations are good additions to this set of exercises.

Stretches. As mentioned previously, stretching is the most effective way of improving your flexibility. While all three techniques of stretching will produce significant changes in your flexibility, static stretching will yield the best results in most cases. Static stretches for various joint regions are presented in Figures 5.3d–k; the muscle regions being stretched are highlighted in each panel. Again, your choice of exercise will depend on your goals and current flexibility.

We recommend that you include at least one exercise for each joint in your flexibility training program. To enhance your performance and reduce injuries in your aerobic and muscular fitness programs, you should include at least two exercises for each joint in your stretching plan.

Contraindicated Stretches. To protect yourself from injuring a muscle or other soft tissue around your joints, you need to know which stretching exercises not to perform. Some stretches and stretching positions that are considered unsafe, or *contraindicated,* are shown in Figure 5.4. These stretches have more risks than benefits and should be avoided. By performing the recommended stretches instead, you can accomplish the same goals with less risk of injury.

Exercise Prescription

To significantly improve flexibility, you must continue to overload your muscles by stretching them beyond their normal limits more frequently and for longer periods of time. For example, to overload your hamstrings, you would need to sit on the floor with your legs extended in front of you, grasp as close to your ankles as possible, and hold the position for a minimum of 10 seconds. For you to observe an improvement, you would need to repeat this exercise at least once, and then perform it on a consistent basis at least three times per week. In other words, doing the stretch once per week for 10 seconds will not sufficiently "overload" the hamstrings muscles if your goal is to improve your flexibility

Program Design. The American College of Sports Medicine (ACSM) has recommended a specific intensity, duration, and frequency of exercise for training programs designed to improve flexibility:

Intensity: To the point of mild discomfort, but ensure the position can be held

Duration: 10–60 seconds per stretch

Frequency: 3–5 repetitions of each stretch, at least 3 days per week

Note that these recommendations apply to static stretching, which is the preferred method of improving flexibility, not to dynamic ROM exercises, which are used to warm up or to maintain flexibility

Intensity. The intensity of a stretch should be to the point of mild to moderate tension. When you stretch, you should definitely feel the stretch, but you should feel only mild discomfort when holding the position for the recommended length of time. Pain in the joint itself may indicate other problems. As you progress, gradually achieving greater ranges of motion, the intensity of your stretches should increase.

Duration. The duration of a stretch depends on your own limitations. A 10–second hold is an absolute minimum and is recommended for use in warm-up and for beginners. The longer a stretch is held, the greater the gains in range of motion. The exercise prescription recommends that you work up to a 60–second hold. After your first repetition, you should perform a minimum of two more repetitions at the same intensity and duration.

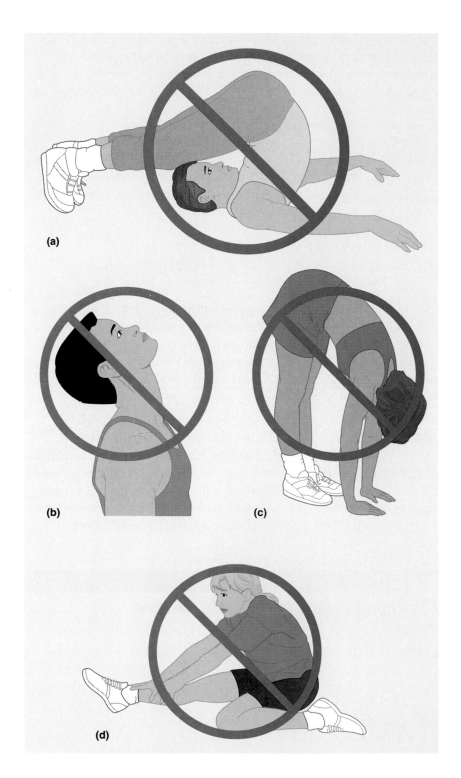

Figure 5.4
Contraindicated stretches.
(a) This stretch places undue stress on the neck. **(b)** The "collapsed neck" increases the compression in the back of the neck. **(c)** This standing hang is harmful to the lower back because of the hinge action at the lumbosocral joint. **(d)** The "hurdler's stretch" position puts great stress on the hip, knee, and ankle.

Frequency. The frequency of your stretching should be at least three times per week. A sample 9-week program for increasing shoulder range of motion, using shoulder stretches and performed a minimum of three times per week, is presented in Table 5.1.

Rate of Progression. When you reach the end of your 9-week training period, you should reassess your flexibility to determine whether you have met your short-term goal. If not, you should increase the number of stretches up to a maximum of five, but stick with 60-second duration and the initial intensity; then reassess after 2 weeks. If you have reached your short-term goal, you can continue to increase intensity and repetitions in progressing toward your long-term goal. For progressions, increase the intensity of the stretch and reduce the duration of the hold to 15 seconds, but add one more repetition up to a maximum of five.

Remember that you need to stretch at all major joints to maintain current flexibility. The assessments included in this text evaluate only a few major joints to provide an indication of overall flexibility. When you design your program you should include stretches for the joints mentioned as well as at least 8 to 10 additional stretching exercises to round out your routine.

Guidelines for Flexibility Training

As you train for improved flexibility, the following guidelines can help you stick with your program and integrate it into your lifestyle. These guidelines are specific to static stretching and provide important hints that can make stretching enjoyable as well as appropriate to your individual needs. Once these exercises have become second nature, you can look forward to including them in your weekly routine.

1. Don't overstretch. The primary reason most people don't stretch is because, when they do, it hurts. As with any other program of fitness, if you try to do too much too soon, you may become discouraged and fail to achieve your goals. Thus, you need to know your body's limitations and work with them. One of the cardinal rules for static stretching is not to overstretch. If you overstretch and can't hold the position because the pain is too great, you will not succeed in increasing your range of motion.

TABLE 5.1

Rate of Progression for Flexibility Training

Week 1: 3 repetitions of each exercise, holding each stretch 15 seconds to the point of mild discomfort

Week 2: 3 repetitions of each exercise, holding each stretch 25 seconds at the same intensity as in week 1

Week 3: 3 repetitions of each exercise, holding each stretch 30 seconds at the same intensity as in week 1

Week 4: 3 repetitions of each exercise, holding each stretch 40 seconds at the same intensity as in week 1

Week 5: 3 repetitions of each exercise, holding each stretch 50 seconds at the same intensity as in week 1

Week 6: Same as in week 5

Week 7: 3 repetitions of each exercise, holding each stretch 60 seconds at the same intensity as in week 1

Week 8: Same as week 7

Week 9: Reassess shoulder flexibility with shoulder rotation test

2. Breathe comfortably. As with all physical activities, breathing comfortably is important. An effective method of breathing during stretching is to inhale before beginning a stretch, exhale into the stretch, and then breathe comfortably as you are holding the stretch. Breathing in this manner will keep you from holding your breath.

3. Choose specific exercises. Remember that the principle of specificity applies to all areas of fitness. In developing flexibility, you need to choose exercises specific to each joint region in order to make improvements. In other words, stretching the neck region will improve flexibility of the neck joint, but it will not increase flexibility in your lower back.

4. Stretch warm muscles. For the best results, you should stretch when your muscles are warm. Warm muscles are less resistant to stretching; therefore, they will lengthen more easily and produce less discomfort. The best time to train for improved range of motion is after your aerobic or muscular fitness workouts.

5. Limit stretching during warm-up. When you use stretching as a warm-up for aerobic or muscular fitness activities, your stretch should be very gentle and slow. This is not a time to work on flexibility improvements, but rather a time to prepare your muscles and joints for movement. Use the dynamic ROM exercises described previously for this purpose.

As your flexibility improves, you will notice the increased ease with which you move through your day. You'll also have chosen a healthy habit to last you a lifetime.

Your Healthy Back

Often we hear about otherwise healthy people—even people in their 20s—experiencing back pain. Take the case of the 25-year-old woman who hobbled into her physician's office with debilitating back pain resulting from a work-related injury. A meat cutter at the local market, she had injured her back while improperly lifting objects too heavy for her. She was suffering so much pain she could not carry on her daily activities, much less perform her job. The physician found that outside her job she led a very sedentary lifestyle devoid of regular exercise. In other words, she did nothing to prepare her back physically for the demands of the meat-cutting job.

One of the main reasons for the current epidemic of poor back health in this country is the sedentary lifestyle that many people lead. Most people prefer to take the elevator instead of the stairs, want to park close to home or work so they have to walk only a few steps to reach their destinations, and avoid lifting heavy objects. Statistically, just about everyone is a candidate for experiencing back pain and/or injury at some time in his or her lifetime. (See the Stats-at-a-Glance.) This susceptibility can be explained, in part, by the decrease in physical activity for most people after their early 20s. In the majority of cases, the pain results from muscular, not disc, problems. Most people suffering from back pain have weak back muscles, suggesting that poor lifestyle choices are the primary culprit in back problems.

Back pain and injuries can be prevented, but the key is making lifestyle choices that you can fit into your daily routine. The health of your back is in

STATS-AT-A-GLANCE
Low Back Pain

■ An estimated 8 in 10 people will experience low back pain sometime in their lives.

■ An estimated $50 billion per year is the annual cost of lost productivity, medical and legal fees, and disability insurance and compensation from low back pain.

■ Low back pain is the number 1 symptomatic complaint by patients age 25 to 60 and the most frequent cause of activity limitation in individuals under age 45.

■ Low back pain is the second most common reason for absences from work and the most costly medical problem in our society for the 30 to 60 age group.

■ Although backache can signal a variety of diseases, an estimated 80% of all low back problems are muscular in origin.

■ Patients suffering from low back pain are found to have weak muscles in the back.

your hands and your commitment to a program of back exercise and body carriage will contribute to your wellness over your entire lifetime. It is up to you to improve your body mechanics (that is, your posture as you stand, sit, bend, lift, move, and sleep) and to incorporate exercises that strengthen and stretch your back. To learn how to care for your back, you first need to understand how it works.

Structure of the Vertebral Column

The vertebral column comprises 5 lumbar vertebrae, 12 thoracic vertebrae, and 7 cervical vertebrae (see Figure 5.5). The vertebrae can be distinguished both by location and by structure. In the neck region, the cervical vertebrae do not support a great deal of weight but have motion capabilities that the thoracic and lumbar vertebrae do not. Specifically, free rotation of the head is accomplished by the specialized architecture of the first and second cervical vertebrae. In the upper back, the thoracic vertebrae have less mobility than the cervical or lumbar vertebrae because they form a joint with the ribs. They are larger than the cervical vertebrae but not as large as the lumbar vertebrae. In the lower back, the lumbar vertebrae increase in size from the first through the fifth because they must support greater weight farther down the spinal column.

As each vertebra meets the other, a joint is formed providing the trunk with its primary motion capabilities of flexion, extension, and rotation. Between the vertebrae are discs that enhance the stability of the joints. You have probably heard of people having a "slipped" disc. The disc does not actually slip out of the joint space, but rather protrudes slightly. This can put pressure on the spinal nerves, creating a great deal of pain.

The Musculature

The abdominal muscles, comprising the rectus abdominis and obliques, provide the primary stabilizing support for the pelvis and control its position. The muscles in the **rectus abdominis** run from the sternum down to the pubic bone and flex and rotate the vertebral column. The **obliques,** or waist muscles, run diagonally and assist the flexion and rotation of the vertebral column. Both muscle groups need to be strengthened to provide maximum stability for the trunk. When strong, these muscles act as a girdle to hold the pelvis in alignment underneath the ribs.

On the other side of the trunk are the back muscles, which hold the trunk upright and move you from a position of forward bending to an upright posture. Strong back muscles hold the vertebrae in proper position and help prevent injury when performing lifting activities. Both of these muscle groups are often very weak, particularly among individuals with back pain. In the hip area, the hip flexors and the hip extensors are the key to back health. The **hip flexors** are the muscles that flex the thigh at the hip; they are a key to back health because they attach along the lumbar vertebrae. The **hip extensors** are the strong muscles that extend the thigh at the hip; they should be used during lifting activities. The primary hip extensor is the gluteus maximus (buttock muscle).

Causes of Back Pain

Back injury can sometimes be traced to a specific accident, but the causes of back pain are often less obvious. Chronic disuse of the trunk muscles and

rectus abdominis muscles that run from the sternum down to the pubic bone and flex and rotate the vertebral column

obliques waist muscles that run diagonally and assist in the flexion and rotation of the vertebral column

hip flexors muscles that flex the thigh at the hip; they are a key to back health because they attach along the lumbar vertebrae

hip extensors strong muscles that extend the thigh at the hip; they should be used during lifting activities

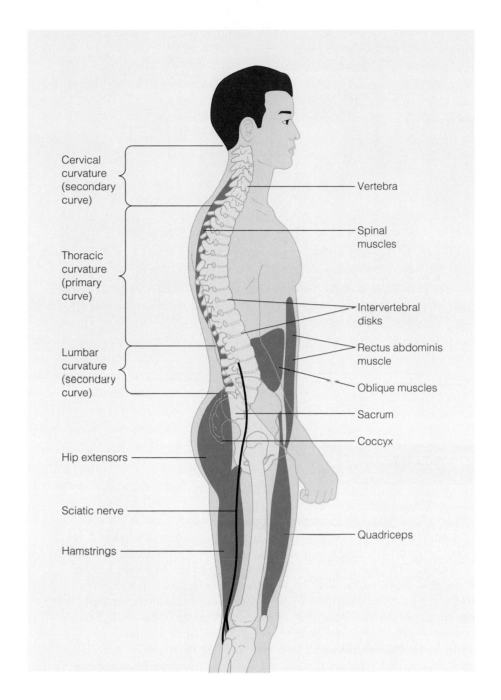

Cervical curvature (secondary curve)

Thoracic curvature (primary curve)

Lumbar curvature (secondary curve)

Hip extensors

Sciatic nerve

Hamstrings

Vertebra

Spinal muscles

Intervertebral disks

Rectus abdominis muscle

Oblique muscles

Sacrum

Coccyx

Quadriceps

Figure 5.5
The vertebral column has 7 cervical vertebrae that comprise the secondary curve in the neck, 12 thoracic vertebrae that comprise the primary curve in the upper back, and 5 lumbar vertebrae that comprise the secondary curve in the lower back.

poor posture or other body mechanics are the primary reasons for the onset of back pain. You can evaluate your posture in Laboratory 5.2.

In an unhealthy posture, the trunk is separated into two segments with the chest and pelvic areas broken at the waist. This causes an improper alignment of the trunk. When the pelvis is out of alignment, the vertebrae above it curve, putting pressure on the nerves between the vertebrae and leading to a "sway" back, often tagged as the culprit in low back problems. This type of problem also can occur in the neck area if you carry your head too far forward. When the secondary curves of the lumbar or cervical areas become disturbed, you experience reduced flexibility, muscular tension, and muscular weakness—all of which contribute to pain.

Figure 5.6 illustrates the relative pressure created by various postures on the third lumbar disc. You can see that pressure is greatest when sitting in the

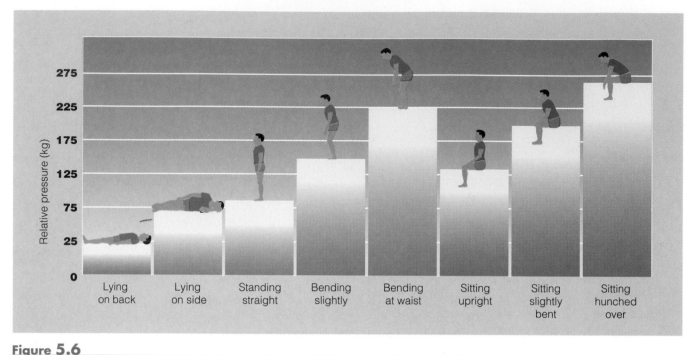

Figure 5.6

The critical third lumbar disc experiences different relative pressure in various body positions.

STRETCHING BODY AND SPIRIT

Sound Decision Making

It all started with an injury. Peter was helping some friends move and went to lift yet another box into the van. As he started to lift, he felt a sharp, tearing pain in his lower back. Peter spent the rest of the day lying on the couch with an ice compress on his back, taking aspirin to relieve some of the pain. The next day Peter was supposed to go to work, but he couldn't move without considerable pain, so he went to see the doctor instead. The doctor determined that no major damage had been done to Peter's back, and recommended that Peter continue to rest for a couple of days. He told Peter that when he felt up to it, he should begin a stretching program to increase his flexibility and help to avoid future back injuries.

The next week the pain in his back had subsided to a dull twinge. Peter really wanted to avoid future incidents of back injury, so he pulled out his old wellness textbook from college and looked over the flexibility exercises. He decided he wanted to work not only on his back but also on general flexibility so he wouldn't lose his range of motion in other parts of his body. His goal was to strengthen his back to avoid future injuries and to improve his overall flexibility.

For a couple of weeks, Peter went through the series of exercises outlined in the book every morning before work. However, he found the exercises boring, so he bought a video of stretches done to upbeat music. He got tired of that too, and his frustration at his difficulty in keeping with his program was high until he picked up a flyer from a nearby yoga studio. They offered an early morning beginning yoga class, and Peter decided to try it.

From his very first class, Peter loved yoga. The exercises were a little different from the ones he had been doing, but the stretches were deep and satisfying. And Peter was amazed at how calm and energetic he felt after class. Yoga turned out to be not just a way to increase his flexibility but also a way to connect with his body and spirit. Peter never suffered a repeat of his old back injury and was soon talking about the benefits of yoga to his friends who complained of back pain.

MYTHS & CONTROVERSIES

Myth 1

You need to reduce the curve in your lower back and keep it flat. Your spine has natural curves that provide resilience to the forces of gravity and daily activities. Therefore, the spine is able to withstand greater forces when the natural curves are maintained. This means that neither excessive lumbar curvature (lordosis) nor a flat back (inadequate lumbar curvature) is desirable.

Myth 2

Exercises that extend the spine are not good for you. Traditionally, experts such as Williams have prescribed "flexion only" exercises for the back. These exercises include those that pull the knees into the chest. However, Jackson and Brown have shown that strong back extensors reach fatigue more slowly and are protective of spinal ligaments. Furthermore, according to McKenzie, back extension is helpful for realigning protruding discs.

The best way to strengthen back muscles is to contract them by extending your back. An example of a back extension exercise is lying on your stomach and then lifting your head, chest, and arms off the floor. You will feel a strong contraction in your back. Keep in mind that the use of extension exercises, particularly hyperextension, should be done slowly and carefully; they are not recommended for anyone with an acute injury.

Controversy 1

You must maintain the lumbar curve when lifting objects. It is important to use the legs as much as possible during a lift, but Gracovetsky has demonstrated that reduction of lordosis (that is, flexing slightly at the waist) enables the large hip extensors to play a greater role in the lift. This also reduces compression forces on the discs. In Kishino's study, when back patients were told to lift an object the way that "felt right," the majority did not lift the way they had been taught in back clinics. This suggests that prescribed lifting techniques may have limitations. What is most important to remember while lifting is to keep the object as close to your body as possible and use your legs and glutei during the process.

Controversy 2

You should never perform an exercise for the neck by taking the head to the back. It is true that "collapsing" the neck is potentially damaging to intervertebral discs and arteries; however, there is no evidence that a controlled movement of the head to the back, where the neck does NOT collapse, but remains lifted, is damaging. In fact, there is no other way to stretch the front of your neck, an area that can become tight from a constant "head forward" posture. One way to practice this is to perform the neck press, outlined in the back exercise program.

flexed position and lowest when lying on your back. Minimizing pressure within the vertebral column will help reduce your risk of back problems.

The muscular imbalances that occur as a result of poor posture can be observed in the legs and trunk. Shorter and weaker muscles in the legs, hips, back, neck, and shoulders make it difficult to stand or sit correctly for any length of time because the muscles have not been trained for a new posture. For example, you may find that when you try to sit up straight you cannot hold an erect position. Due to the natural inclination to "give in" to gravity, your back muscles have become weak. Or, if you are accustomed to sitting with slumped shoulders, the muscles in the front of your shoulders will have shortened. When you try to assume an upright position, your trunk will be erect but your shoulders may still be rounded because the muscles are too short to allow your shoulders to drop back. (See the Myths and Controversies box).

Improving Your Back Health

There are three primary ways to improve the health of your back: (1) maintain correct posture, (2) perform specific strengthening exercises, and (3) perform specific stretching exercises. Together, these activities build a stronger, healthier back.

Correct Posture. The way in which a body is positioned throughout the day is as important as performing daily exercises if you want to enhance your back health. You need to make an effort to maintain correct sitting, standing, walking, and sleeping postures as well as using proper body mechanics when lifting and bending.

Correct sitting, standing, and walking postures are those in which there is no break at the waist. Rather, the trunk is held in an erect position and the shoulders are lifted so that they are in line with your pelvis. The head and chin are held high rather than tipped forward or back. This posture reduces pressure within the discs of the lumbar vertebrae, encourages relaxed shoulders, and helps maintain a normal secondary curve of the neck. In the standing and walking postures, the secondary curve in the lumbar region is normal when the abdominal muscles position the pelvis directly under the ribs (see Figure 5.7a).

For sleeping, the best positions are either on your side or back. Avoid sleeping on your stomach, as this position exaggerates the lumbar curve and increases tightness of the muscles and pressure within the discs. A firm mattress is also recommended.

When lifting, you should always maintain a straight back and keep the object as close to your body as possible (see Figure 5.7b). Remember the phrase "Lift with your legs!" If you think the object is too heavy for you, don't attempt the lift on your own.

Strengthening Exercises. Your spine will benefit most from strengthening exercises for the abdominals—both rectus abdominis and obliques—back muscles (including upper region), and hip extensors.

Stretching Exercises. Stretching exercises also should be performed to relieve muscular tension throughout the back and neck, to allow for correct alignment, to improve mobility of the trunk during bending and twisting activities, and to encourage adequate spacing between vertebrae. The most important areas to stretch include the hip flexors, hip extensors, and back muscles.

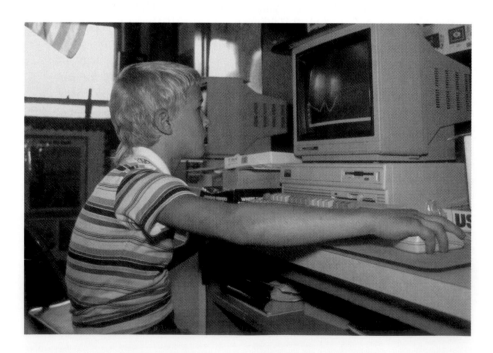

Good posture (or lack thereof) is a habit that can start at any age.

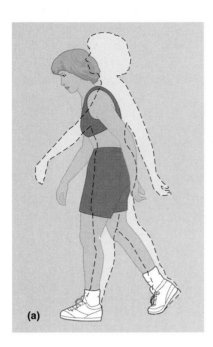

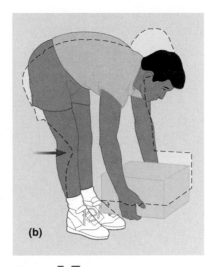

Figure 5.7

(a) Compare incorrect and correct walking postures. **(b)** Compare incorrect and correct lifting postures.

Back Exercise Program for Life

As discussed in the last section, the stability of your back relies heavily on the condition of the muscles, tendons, and ligaments that move and attach to it. The abdominals flex the vertebral column and the back extensors extend it. Flexibility in the joints and strength of the muscles are necessary for stabilization and prevention of back problems. Improving muscular fitness in these areas will transfer to your posture throughout the day.

The back exercise program illustrated in Figure 5.8a–o is designed to strengthen and stretch the muscles of your abdominals, back, and neck and improve your posture. Notice that it promotes the secondary curves in your neck and low back regions. Many back programs overlook the neck area; this is unfortunate as it often carries a great deal of muscular tension associated with poor muscle tone.

This program should be performed at least 3 times a week for maximum benefits. Included in the program are both stretching and strengthening exercises. All stretching exercises are denoted by an asterisk. The *goal* for the stretching exercises is to hold for a maximum of 60 seconds and perform each exercise 3 times. Initially, you may begin with a minimum 10-second hold and perform each exercise twice. For the strengthening exercises, the prescription is 1 set of 4–8 repetitions. In the beginning you will want to start with 1 set of 4 repetitions, then build to a maximum of 8 repetitions. Your progression should add 1 repetition per week, if comfortable. Otherwise, wait to add repetitions for 2–3 weeks. You will notice that some of the exercises have more than one position. You should begin with position I, then progress to the alternate, more advanced positions when maximum repetitions of position I can be completed. If you experience pain or significant discomfort, discontinue the exercise. It is important that you perform the exercises in a slow, controlled manner. After you are experienced with the program and can do the maximum repetitions of the strengthening exercises

(a) Pelvic tilt and lift

Position: Lying on the back, arms on floor with hands next to hips, knees bent and slightly apart, feet flat on floor.

Action: Begin by pressing the waist into the floor (pelvic tilt), then slowly "roll" the spine off the floor. Hold lift briefly, pressing the buttocks together tightly, then roll down one vertebra at a time.

Purposes: Strengthens gluteal (buttocks) and low back muscles. Develops and maintains secondary lumbar curve.

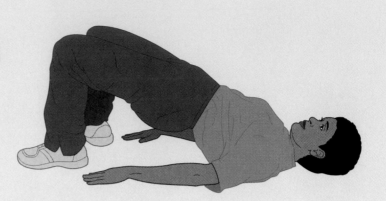

(b) Double knee-to-chest

Position: Lying on the back with knees bent and feet on the floor (hook lying position).

Action: Pull right knee, then left into chest. Place hands under knees and hold, then lower one leg at a time. Relax. Maintain back contact with floor during movement of legs.

Begin with position I below:

I. Head stays on floor.

II. Lift head

III. Lift head and shoulders, forehead toward knee.

Purpose: Strengthens abdominals (rectus) and stretches back.

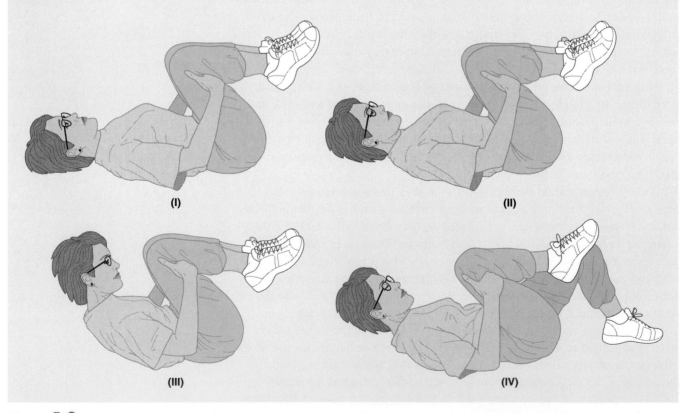

(I)   (II)

(III)   (IV)

Figure 5.8

These illustrations (parts a–o) show some stretching and strengthening exercises to improve back health and posture and highlight the primary muscle group affected.

(c) Lateral trunk stretch

Position: In hook lying position, finger tips behind ears, elbows on floor.

Action: Cross left leg over the right, then use the left leg to pull the right to the side without letting the elbows off the floor. Hold up to 60 seconds. Repeat on other side.

Purpose: Stretches the hips and trunk.

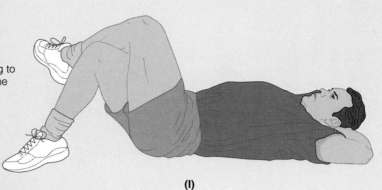

(I)

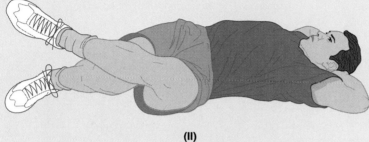

(II)

(d) Abdominal curl (head and shoulder lift):

Position: Hook lying.

Action: Press the low back into the floor and lift the shoulders off the floor. Begin with position I below.

I. Hand reach to knees. Support your neck with one hand, if necessary.

II. Hands crossed on chest.

III. Finger tips by ears, elbows out.

Purpose: Strengthens abdominals (rectus)

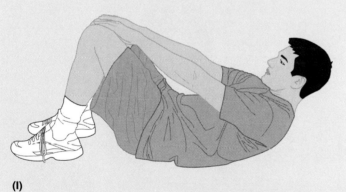

(I)

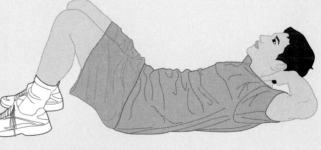

(III)

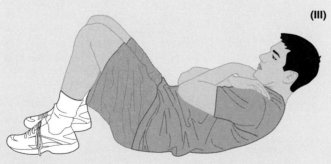

(II)

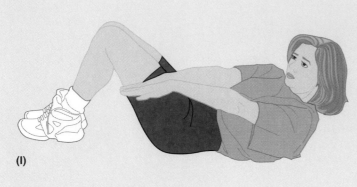

(I)

(e) Oblique abdominal curl (lateral head and shoulder lift):

Position I: Hook lying. Place your hands to the left side of your left knee.

Action: Lift as for the abdominal curl, but twist toward the left knee. Repeat to the right. Begin with position I below.

I. Hands reaching to knees.

II. Hands crossed on chest.

III. Finger tips by ears, elbows out, support one elbow on floor.

Purpose: Strengthens abdominals (obliques)

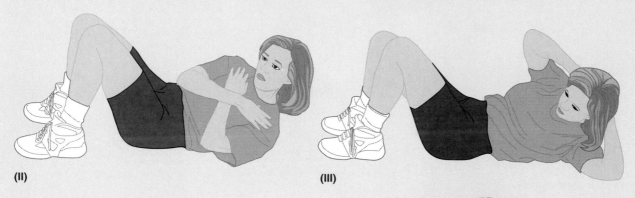

(II)

(III)

(f) Butterfly stretch

Position: Sitting, place the soles of feet together (about 6 inches away from the body) and knees out. Hands should rest lightly on the ankles or on the floor in front of the feet.

Action: Keeping the back straight, hinge at the hip and lean forward over the feet.

Purposes: Increases flexibility in the hips and promotes awareness of the trunk as a unit, i.e. not bent at the waist.

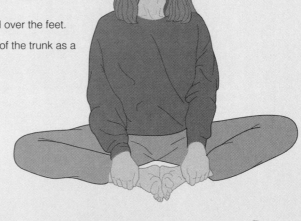

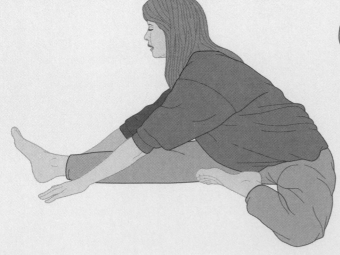

(g) Hamstrings stretch

Position: Sitting, with right leg extended, bend left knee, and place the sole of the left foot against the right knee. Hands reach out in front of the body, close to the floor.

Action: Keeping back straight, hinge at the hip and lean forward over the extended leg. Hold up to 60 seconds. Repeat with the left leg extended and right knee bent.

Purposes: Increases flexibility in the hips and promotes awareness of the trunk as a unit, i.e. not bent at the waist.

(h) Diagonal lift

Position: Lying on right side, right knee bent, resting the weight of the upper trunk on the right forearm. The left leg is extended back and the left arm is reaching forward as far as possible, chest and head rotated toward the floor.

Action: Lift the head, chest, left arm and leg together, using the right arm to help press the chest up. Hold for 5 seconds, then release.

Purposes: Strengthens extensors and lateral rotators of the entire vertebral column. Strengthens muscles of the shoulder.

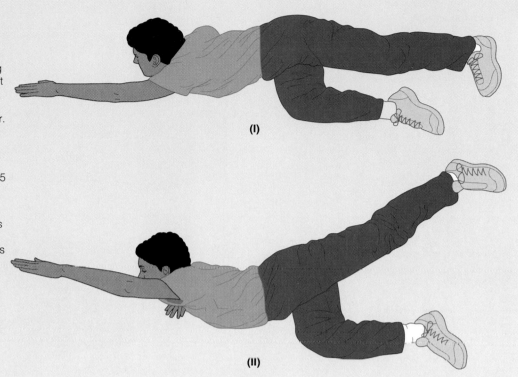

(I)

(II)

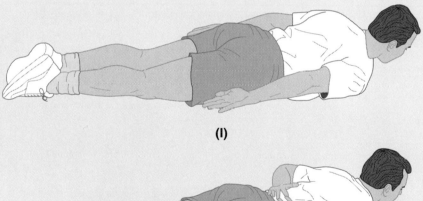

(I)

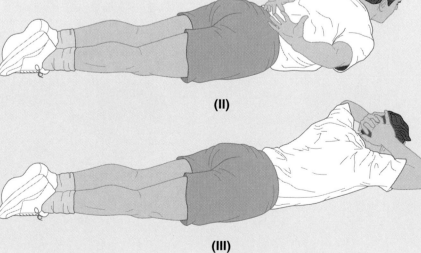

(II)

(III)

(i) Chest lift

Position: Lying face down, legs slightly apart, chin on the floor, hands next to the hips with palms turned toward the ceiling.

Action: Slowly lift the head and chest off the floor as high as possible, pressing the palms toward the ceiling and keeping the feet and thighs on the floor. Hold for 5 seconds, then release.

Begin with position I below.

I. Place your arms on the floor, hands close to hips with palms turned toward the ceilings.

II. Place tops of your hands on either side of your middle back (thoracic spine).

III. Place your hands (palms down) behind your head.

Purposes: Strengthens back, hip and arm extensors. Develops and maintains secondary curves.

(j) Leg and arm lift

Position: Lying prone, legs together, right arm stretched out on the floor over the head, left arm relaxed on the floor by the left hip.

Action: Slowly lift the head, right and left leg off the floor. Hold, then release.

Purposes: Strengthens back, hip and arm extensors. Develops and maintains secondary curves.

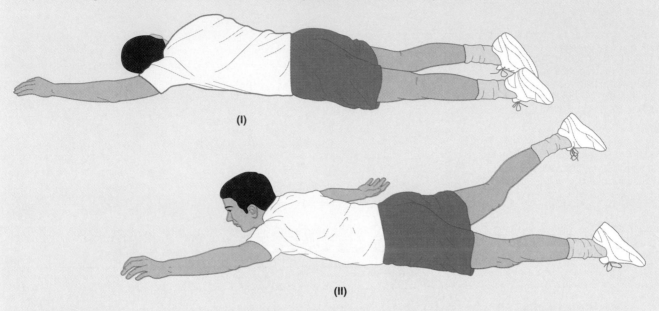

(I)

(II)

(k) Neck press

Position: Sitting or standing upright, hands placed on the back of the head *(not neck)* with fingers laced.

Action: Resisting with hands, slowly lift the chin toward the ceiling while pressing back against the hands, opening the elbows and looking up toward ceiling. Hold for 5 seconds.

Purposes: Strengthens the extensor muscles of the neck and upper back. Develops and maintains secondary curve of the neck region.

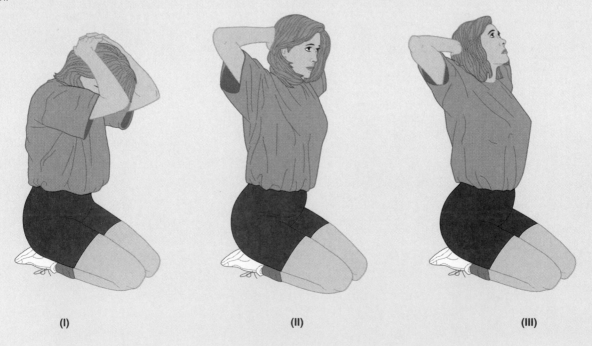

(I)   (II)   (III)

(m) Lateral neck stretch

Position: Standing or sitting with tall, upright torso.

Action: Move head toward the left shoulder, keeping chin lifted and ear facing shoulder. Hold a minimum of 10 seconds, then repeat on the right. Begin with position I below:

I. Arms rest quietly next to body.

II. As you move the head to the left, lift the left hand and gently place over the right side of the head. Repeat on the right side.

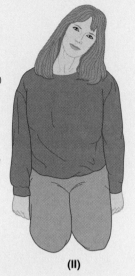
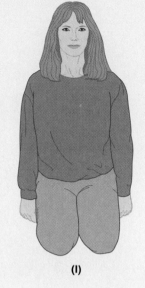
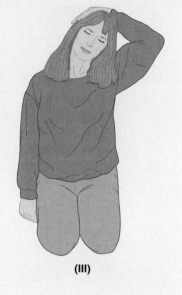

(II)   (I)   (III)

(n) Forward lunge

Position: Begin on hands and knees. Lift body up slightly, bring left leg forward, plant left foot directly between hands. Keeping the chest on the left thigh, extend the right leg back. Perform on opposite leg.

Begin with position I below.

II. Back knee continues to rest on the floor.

III. Back knee lifts up, but leg is still bent.

IV. Back leg extends completely. Press down with the hips.

Purpose: Stretches hip flexors.

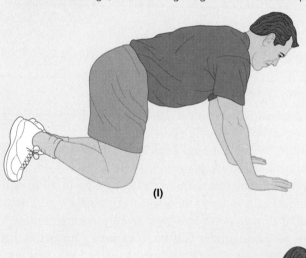

(I)

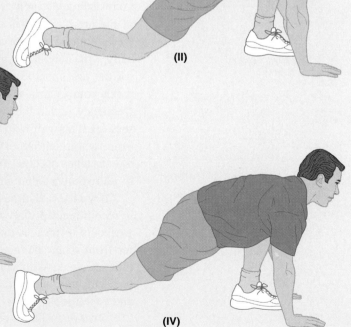

(II)

(III)

(IV)

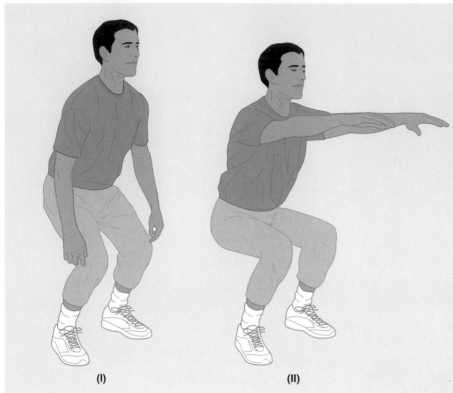

(I)   (II)

(o) Squat

Position: Stand with feet slightly greater than shoulder width apart, knees slightly bent, and abdominals contracted. Keep heels in contact with the floor. Use wall for support.

Action: With back straight, squat to a position where the thigh is parallel to the floor. Pause and press up to a standing position. Begin with position I below.

I. Arms relaxed next to body.

II. Arms extended in front of the body, parallel to the ground.

Purposes: Promotes awareness of trunk as a unit; strengthens back and legs

using the most advanced positions, you may want to add light weights at the ankles and/or wrists in order to build more strength.

Laboratories 5.1 and 5.2 provide the opportunity for you to evaluate the condition of your abdominals and back muscles as well as your posture. In your evaluation, you may find that you score in the low range in all or some of the areas. If this is the case, it is very important that you find ways to incorporate all exercises of this program into your weekly routine. Practically, you may begin by performing only half the exercises 3 times per week for the first month or two, then add 2 the third month, and so on until you reach your goal of the complete program. It is to your advantage to focus on frequency within the week rather than getting all the exercises in at each session. This will help make the program more habitual. Because stretching exercises are an important part of this program, you may want to begin with the stretches specific to the back program until you become more advanced to add stretches that were illustrated earlier in this chapter.

If your evaluation indicated that you are average or better in all areas, it is recommended that you include the back exercise program in your weekly workouts to prevent the onset of problems. Find exercises that do not transfer from other activities and be sure to fit them into your day at least 3 times a week. With your better physical condition, you should be able to perform the more advanced positions and begin at the highest number of sets and repetitions.

Overall wellness combines all dimensions of health and requires both an assessment of current condition and a responsibility to make adjustments where necessary. Your decision to improve and maintain back health is one which has potential to dramatically impact your daily life and well-being.

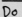

YOUR ◆ BACK

Do

▲ Stretch it from the lower back through the neck.

▲ Strengthen it from the lower back to the neck.

▲ Strengthen your abdominals, including obliques, with curls and cross curls.

▲ Stretch your hip flexors and hip extensors.

▲ Maintain your normal curvatures.

▲ Bend at the knees when bending and lifting in order to use leg muscles in the activity.

▲ Keep objects close to your body when lifting.

▲ Sleep on your back or side.

▲ Sit in an upright position.

Don't

▼ Perform full sit-ups with straight or bent knees.

▼ Perform straight-leg toe-touches.

▼ Sleep on your stomach.

▼ Sit, stand, or walk "bent" at the waist.

▼ Lift with straight legs.

▼ Stand with excessive lumbar curvature or, at the other extreme, a flat back.

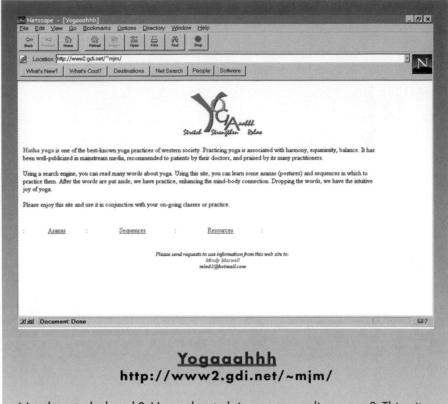

Yogaaahhh
http://www2.gdi.net/~mjm/

Need a study break? How about doing some on-line yoga? This site features instructions on how to do many yoga poses, complete with illustrations. It also lists suggested sequences of poses so you can put together a complete yoga session. There is also a list of resources related to yoga, including other Web pages, books, and videos.

Critical thinking: Which muscles feel like they are being stretched in each of the yoga poses? Does this workout seem to include all the muscle groups illustrated in Figure 5.3?
Source: From Maxwell, 1998.

Lifestyle Choices: Plan for Action

Now that you have a good understanding of the whys and hows of flexibility and back health, you are ready to begin your strategy for change. If you already perform exercises for flexibility and a healthy back, that's great! You probably have improved movement capabilities and do not suffer any twinges of discomfort in your back. However, if these types of exercises are not a part of your program or if you answered "some of the time" or "never" to questions 4, 5, 6, 7, or 8 in Section 11 of the Wellness Inventory in Laboratory 1.1, you may consider examining your exercise habits as they relate to flexibility and back health.

As you did in Chapters 3 and 4, after completing Laboratory 5.1 and 5.2 to assess your flexibility and back health, create a plan of action for yourself by filling out the following personal goal-setting form.

My sit-and-reach test rating: _____

My chin lift rating: _____

My shoulder test rating: _____

My abdominal endurance rating: _____

My back muscle endurance rating: _____

My posture evaluation: _____

Based on these ratings on flexibility and back health and my personal interest, I have chosen the following short- and long-term goals:

SHORT-TERM GOALS

_____

_____

_____

I will achieve my short-term goals on _____ *(date)*.

_____   _____
(signature)   *(witness)*

LONG-TERM GOALS

_____

_____

_____

I will achieve my long-term goals on _____ *(date)*.

_____   _____
(signature)   *(witness)*

As in Chapters 3 and 4, begin by making a list of benefits you would gain from doing training for flexibility and back health. Then list any barriers that make it difficult for you to exercise.

POTENTIAL BENEFITS   **POTENTIAL BARRIERS**

_____   _____

_____   _____

_____   _____

Indentify one barrier that you need to overcome in order to add *at least 1 session* of exercise (including 4 stretches and 4 back exercises) to your schedule. You may decide to try this for 1 month using the recommendations provided in this chapter.

Use the following diary to record your progress toward your goals over the next 4 weeks.

FOUR-WEEK FLEXIBILITY TRAINING DIARY

Exercises for the 4-Week Period

_____

_____

_____

WEEK 1

From _____ *(date)* to _____ *(date)*

Frequency this week: _____

Duration of each exercise this week: _____

How I felt:

The intensity level this week was (check one):

❑ too high for me to hold the stretch

❑ just right

❑ not high enough

Other comments: _____

_____

WEEK 2

From _____ *(date)* to _____ *(date)*

Frequency this week: _____

Duration of each exercise this week: _____

How I felt:

The intensity level this week was (check one):

❑ too high for me to hold the stretch

❑ just right

❑ not high enough

Other comments: _____

_____

WEEK 3

From _____ *(date)* to _____ *(date)*

Frequency this week: _____

Duration of each exercise this week: _____

How I felt:

The intensity level this week was (check one):

❑ too high for me to hold the stretch

❑ just right

❑ not high enough

Other comments: _____

_____

WEEK 4

From _____ *(date)* to _____ *(date)*

Frequency this week: _____

Duration of each exercise this week: _____

How I felt:

The intensity level this week was (check one):

❑ too high for me to hold the stretch

❑ just right

❑ not high enough

Other comments: _____

_____

At the end of 4 weeks, review your progress. What worked? What did not work? If you need to start over, choose a new barrier to overcome. If you were successful, increase the duration of your exercise session or add another session per week.

DATE	ACTIVITY	INTENSITY	DURATION	WARM-UP	COOL-DOWN	HOW I FELT
_____	_____	_____	_____	_____	_____	_____
_____	_____	_____	_____	_____	_____	_____
_____	_____	_____	_____	_____	_____	_____

Summary

Flexibility training is often treated as a secondary aspect of fitness training. Exercises for back health typically are performed only as a result of injury or back pain. However, if you want to achieve a high level of wellness, you need to incorporate these important exercises into your lifestyle. A well-designed flexibility and back health program should accompany your aerobic and muscular fitness training. However, be sure that your choices work for you and fit into your weekly routine.

Key concepts that you have learned in this chapter include these:

- Flexibility is defined as the range of motion around joints and is important in allowing you to perform daily tasks and in protecting your body from injury.

- The three basic types of joints—diarthrodial, amphiarthrodial, and synarthrodial—have different movement capabilities.

- Specific sensory organs in muscles adapt to stretching.

- The three stretching techniques are ballistic, static, and proprioceptive neuromuscular facilitation.

- The basic components of designing a flexibility training program are assessment and goal setting, choices of exercises, and exercise prescription.

- The vertebral column is comprised of 5 lumbar vertebrae (lower back), 12 thoracic vertebrae (upper back), and 7 cervical vertebrae (neck).

- Correct posture can reduce the incidence of back pain and injury.

- The benefits of improved flexibility and back health include reduced incidence of injury, improved movement capability, reduced age-related declines in flexibility, and stress reduction.

- One way to help begin a program of flexibility and back exercises is to identify barriers to training, and then plan ways to overcome these barriers.

References

Einkauf, D. K., et al. Changes in spinal mobility with increasing age in women. *Physical Therapy,* 67: 370–375, 1987.

Etnyre, B. R., and J. A. Lee. Chronic and acute flexibility of men and women using three different stretching techniques. *Research Quarterly for Exercise and Sport,* 59: 222–228, 1988.

Germain, N. K., and S. N. Blair. Variability of shoulder flexion with age, activity and sex. *American Corrective Therapy Journal,* 37(6): 156–160, 1983.

Golding, L., C. Myers, and W. Sinning. *Y's Way to Physical Fitness.* Chicago: YMCA, 1982.

Gracovetsky, S., H. Farfan, and C. Helleur. The abdominal mechanism. *Spine,* 10: 317–324, 1985.

Hall, H. *The Back Doctor.* East Rutherford, NJ: Berkeley Press, 1982.

Heyward, V. H. *Advanced Fitness Assessment and Exercise Prescription.* Champaign, IL: Human Kinetics Press, 1991.

Hochshuler, S. *Back in Shape.* Boston: Houghton Mifflin, 1991.

Howley, E. T., and B. D. Franks. *Health/Fitness Instructor's Handbook.* Champaign, IL: Human Kinetics Press, 1992.

Jackson, C. P., and M. D. Brown. Is there a role for exercise in the treatment of patients with low back pain? Analysis of current approaches and a practical guide to exercise. *Orthopedics and Related Research,* 179: 39–54, 1983.

Keim, H. A., and W. H. Krkaldy-Willis. Low back pain. *Clinical Symposia,* 39(6), 1987.

Knapik, J., et al. Preseason strength and flexibility imbalances associated with athletic injuries in female collegiate athletes. *American Journal Sports Medicine,* 19: 76–81, 1991.

Levine, M., et al. An analysis of individual stretching programs of intercollegiate athletes. *The Physician and Sports Medicine,* 15(3): 130–137, 1987.

Malmivaara, A., et al. The treatment of acute low back pain—bed rest, exercises, or ordinary activity. *New England Journal of Medicine,* 332: 351, 1995.

Mayer, T. G., et al. A prospective two-year trial of functional restoration in treating industrial low back injuries. *Journal of the American Medical Association,* 258: 1763–1767, 1987.

McArdle, W. D., F. I. Katch, and V. L. Katch. *Exercise Physiology.* Baltimore: Williams & Wilkins, 1996.

McKenzie, R. Prophylaxis in recurrent low back pain. *New Zealand Medical Journal,* 89: 22–23, 1979.

McQuade, K. J., J. A. Turner, and D. M. Buchner. Physical fitness and low back pain: An analysis of the relationships among fitness, functional limitations, and depression. *Orthopedics and Related Research,* 223: 198–204, 1988.

Melleby, A. *The Y's Way to a Healthy Back.* Piscataway, NJ: Century, 1982.

Nachemson, A. Towards a better understanding of back pain: A review of the mechanics of the lumbar disc. *Rheumatism Rehabilitation,* 14: 129–135, 1975.

Pollock, M. L., and J. H. Wilmore. *Exercise in Health and Disease.* Philadelphia: Saunders, 1990.

Raab, D., et al. Light resistance and stretching exercise in elderly women: Effect upon flexibility. *Archives of Physical Medicine and Rehabilitation,* 69: 268–272, 1988.

Ricci, B., M. Marchetti, and F. Figura. Biomechanics of sit up exercises. *Medicine and Science in Sports and Exercise,* 13: 54–59, 1981.

Rikli, R., and S. Busch. Motor performance of women as a function of age and physical activity level. *Journal of Gerontology,* 41: 645–649, 1986.

Sihvonen, T., K. Lindgren, O. Airaksinen, and H. Manninen. Movement disturbances of the lumbar spine and abnormal back muscle electromyographic findings in recurrent low back pain. *Spine,* 22: 289–295, 1996.

Williams, P. Examination and conservative treatment for disc lesions of the lower spine. *Orthopedics,* 5: 28–40, 1974.

Laboratory 5.1

Assessing Flexibility and Back Health

In this laboratory you measure posterior hip joint and shoulder joint flexibility and vertebral column extensibility. You also will assess the endurance of your abdominal and back extensor muscles.

The range-of-motion tests will give you an indication of your general flexibility; the muscular endurance tests will evaluate the condition of your trunk muscles. Keep in mind that these tests are evaluating only selected areas and that a well-rounded program of exercise to promote flexibility and back health needs to include a variety of exercises to improve overall range of motion.

Sit-and-Reach Test

This procedure measures your posterior hip flexibility. It requires a sit-and-reach box apparatus. To prepare for the test, remove your shoes and do a light warm-up consisting of easy stretches. Sit at the box with your feet flat against it and your arms outstretched with one hand on top of the other. Reach forward as far as possible while your partner checks that your knees remain straight. Perform two trials of this exercise and use the value from your best trial for rating. Use the norms in Table 5.2 to evaluate your score.

TABLE 5.2

Standard Values for Trunk Flexion (in centimeters)

	AGE (YEARS)		
RATING	**20–29**	**30–39**	**40–49**
MEN			
Excellent	56	53	51
Good	48–53	46–51	43–48
Average	33–46	30–43	28–41
Fair	25–30	23–28	20–25
Low	23	20	18
WOMEN			
Excellent	61	58	56
Good	56–58	53–56	51–53
Average	41–53	38–51	36–48
Fair	33–38	30–36	28–33
Low	30	28	25

Source: From Golding and Sinning, 1983.

Shoulder Rotation Test

Grasp one end of a rope with your left hand and, a few inches away, grasp the rope with your right hand. Extend both arms in front of your chest and rotate them overhead, keeping your elbows straight. As resistance is met, slide your right hand farther from your left hand along the rope until the rope can be lowered against your back. Measure the distance, in centimeters, between your thumbs. Perform two trials of this exercise and use the value from your best trial for calculating your shoulder flexibility.

To calculate your shoulder flexibility, have a partner measure your shoulder width across the back from shoulder to shoulder. Measure the distance of your right arm from the outside edge of your acromion (the bony part of your shoulder) to the tip of your longest finger. Add these two values and divide by 2. Subtract this number from your best trial (lowest number). Use the norms in Table 5.3 to evaluate your score.

TABLE 5.3

Shoulder Flexibility (in centimeters)

MEN	PERFORMANCE RATING	WOMEN
18.0 or less	Excellent	13.0 or less
29.0–18.25	Good	24.75–13.25
36.75–29.25	Average	33.0–25.0
50.0–37.0	Fair	45.0–33.25
50.25 or more	Low	45.25 or more

Source: From Johnson and Nelson, 1986.

Chin Lift Test

This test measures the extensibility of your vertebral column. Lie on your stomach on the floor and place your hands under your shoulders. Push your chest up off the floor while maintaining pelvic contact with the floor. Do not use your back muscles in this test. Have a partner measure the distance from the notch at the top of the sternum (chest bone) to the floor in centimeters. Perform two trials of this exercise and use the value from your best trial for rating. Use the norms in Table 5.4 to evaluate your score.

TABLE 5.4
Trunk Flexibility (in centimeters)

RATING	CHIN LIFT
Excellent	> 30
Good	20–29
Fair	10–19
Low	< 9

Source: From Howley and Franks, 1997.

TABLE 5.5
Ratings for Tests of Muscular Endurance (curl-ups and back-ups)

RATING	MEN		WOMEN	
	CURL-UPS	BACK-UPS	CURL-UPS	BACK-UPS
Excellent	≥ 69	≥ 71	≥ 69	> 71
Good	58–68	60–70	51–68	61–70
Fair	48–57	50–59	38–50	51–60
Low	≤ 49	≤ 49	≤ 37	≤ 50

Source: From Howley and Franks, 1997.

Curl-Up Test

The reason for using this test instead of the standard bent-knee sit-up test is that the hip flexors take over forward flexion after approximately 30 degrees. Because the hip flexors are attached to the lumbar vertebrae, bent-knee sit-ups are potential stressors on the lower back. Curl-ups (without the feet held) are the best alternative to the bent-knee sit-up. To perform the test, do the following:

1. Lie back on a mat, with your arms by your sides, your palms flat on the mat, your elbows locked, and your fingers straight. Bend your knees at a 90-degree angle (feet 12–18 inches away from your buttocks).

2. Curl your head and upper back upward, keeping your arms stiff. Reach forward along the floor to touch a line that is 3 inches away from the longest fingertip of each hand; then curl back down so that your upper back touches the floor. During the entire curl-up, your fingers, feet, and buttocks stay on the mat. The movement should be continuous and well controlled at a pace of 20 curl-ups per minute.

3. Have a partner check closely for form, deviations should not count in your final score.

The test score is the number of complete touches on the line up to a maximum of 75 repetitions. Use the norms in Table 4 to evaluate your score. Record your score on the form at the end of Laboratory 5.1.

Back Extension Test

The purpose of this test is to assess the endurance of your back muscles. To perform this test, do the following:

1. Lie facedown on a mat 4 inches from the measuring bench. On the bench a measuring device is taped 5 inches above the mat to guide the height of chest lift. For the beginning position, place your arms behind your head. Keep your legs together, with your knees bent at a 90-degree angle and feet crossed.

2. Lift your head, chest, and arms off the floor until your chest clears the 5-inch mark on the bench; then release completely to the starting position (your chin must return to the mat). The movement is paced at 20 back-ups per minute.

3. Have a partner check for correct form.

The test score is the number of complete lifts performed, up to a maximum of 75. Use the norms in Table 5.5 to evaluate your score. Record your score on the form at the end of Laboratory 5.1.

Recording Form for Flexibility and Back Health Assessments

1. Sit-and-reach test for posterior hip flexibility
Trial 1 _____ cm   Trial 2 _____ cm
   (use best of two values for rating Rating = _____

2. Shoulder rotation test for shoulder flexibility
Trial 1 _____ cm   Trial 2 _____ cm
   (use best of two values for rating)
Distance of biacromial width across the back = _____ cm (A)
Distance from outside edge of right acromion to the tip of the
   longest finger = _____ cm (B)
A + B = _____ (C)   C ÷ 2 = _____ = D
   Best trial _____ − D _____ = shoulder flexibility score
   Rating = _____

3. Chin lift test for trunk flexibility
Trial 1 _____ cm   Trial 2 _____ cm
   (use best of two values for rating)   Rating = _____

4. Curl-up test for abdominal endurance
Abdominal endurance: _____ repetitions (up to a maximum of 75)   Rating = _____

5. Back extension test for back muscle endurance
Back muscle endurance: _____ repetitions (up to a maximum of 75)   Rating = _____

Laboratory 5.2

Evaluating Posture

Have a partner evaluate your posture using the following posture score sheet.

Posture Score Sheet	Name			Scoring Dates			
	Good——10	Fair——5	Poor——0				
Head Left Right	Head erect, gravity line passes through center	Head twisted or turned slightly to one side	Head twisted or turned markedly to one side				
Shoulders Left Right	Shoulders level (horizontally)	One shoulder slightly higher than other	One shoulder markedly higher than other				
Spine Left Right	Spine straight	Spine slightly curved laterally	Spine markedly curved laterally				
Hips Left Right	Hips level (horizontally)	One hip slightly higher	One hip markedly higher				
Ankles	Feet pointed straight ahead	Feet pointed out	Feet pointed out markedly, ankles sag in (pronation)				
Neck	Neck erect, chin in, head directly above shoulders	Neck slightly forward, chin slightly out	Neck markedly forward, chin markedly out				
Upper Back	Upper back normally rounded	Upper back slightly more rounded	Upper back markedly rounded				
Trunk	Trunk erect	Trunk inclined slightly to rear	Trunk inclined markedly to rear				
Abdomen	Abdomen flat	Abdomen protruding	Abdomen protruding and sagging				
Lower Back	Lower back normally curved	Lower back slightly hollow	Lower back markedly hollow				
			Total Scores				

Source: From New York State Education Department, 1958.

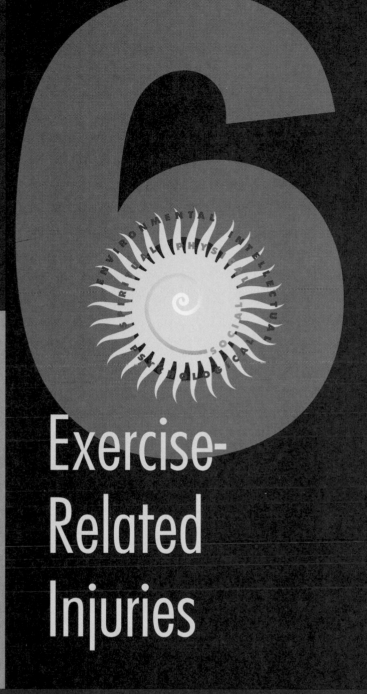

Exercise-Related Injuries

One Student's View

Over spring break my freshman year in college, I was playing basketball in my
friend's driveway. I twisted my knee and tore some cartilage. I ended up needing
arthroscopic surgery. I found out you do need to take things slowly at first when
you are in rehab. Don't try to do the same activities right after your injury. I tried
to go out and play basketball after my surgery and my leg was not ready for it.
You need to stick with a well-developed rehab schedule. Don't rush things.

—Eric Beck

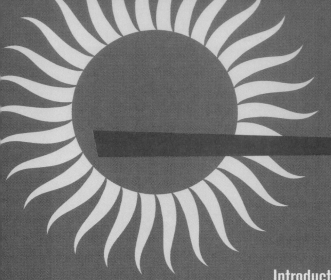

Introduction

In general, participation in fitness activities is associated with a relatively low frequency of injury. However, the more fitness activities you're involved in, the greater the opportunities you have for accidental injury. The type of exercise program you engage in determines your injury risk. For example, if you do aerobic walking, racquetball, and swimming as your main activities, you will have a different set of injury risks from someone who participates in distance running, weight training, and snowboarding.

Walking 30 minutes per day, five days per week, for example, would expose you to potential overuse injuries in the lower extremities, but not nearly to the same degree as distance running. Racquetball would expose you to potential injuries such as ligament sprains, muscle strains, and eye injuries, whereas swimming would put you at risk for swimmer's shoulder (overuse of the shoulder muscles) and swimmer's ear (a fungal infection of the outer ear). Certainly, the chance of suffering an injury while snowboarding is significantly greater than during daily activities. Approximately six of ten snowboarding injuries involve the lower body, with the ankle and foot being injured most frequently; wrist and hand sprains and fractures are the most common upper-body injuries (see Figure 6.1) (Elmqvist et al.). Finally, the greatest injury risk associated with weight training is soft-tissue injury to muscles, tendons, ligaments, and intervertebral discs. With proper instruction in the techniques of weight training, however, most of the injuries suffered by novice weight trainers can be prevented.

In general, popular recreational activities such as walking, jogging, bicycling, swimming, and tennis have much lower injury rates than do intercollegiate sports such as football and gymnastics or intramural sports like soccer, basketball, and softball. When selecting your fitness

Objectives

After reading this chapter, you should be able to

- **Identify the specific factors and conditions that may increase your risk of injury during exercise**

- **Differentiate between injuries caused by overuse and those caused by accidents**

- **Discuss the various training errors that will produce overuse injuries**

- **Describe the most common types of exercise-related injuries, and recognize the warning signs and symptoms associated with each**

- **Describe the appropriate first-aid treatment for acute exercise-related injuries**

- **Know when to seek medical treatment for an exercise-related injury**

- **Identify special concerns for exercise in various environmental conditions**

activities and developing a workout schedule, a lifetime of injury-free, enjoyable physical activity should be foremost in your mind. In this chapter, you will learn techniques for preventing injury as well as ways to recognize some of the most common fitness-related injuries (see Table 6.1) and methods for treating those injuries.

We now know that you can improve your health and decrease your risk of heart disease by engaging in regular (daily!) moderate-intensity physical activity (National Institutes of Health). During participation in fitness activities, you must pay close attention to identifying and avoiding situations that may needlessly cause injury, for this strategy is the best proactive measure for maintaining wellness. For those unfortunate enough to sustain an accidental or overuse exercise-related injury, obtaining proper medical treatment (and having patience while recovering) is the optimal way to restore wellness.

Injury Prevention

Consistent with the concept of maintaining all facets of one's health while leading an active life, injury prevention is a vital consideration within the physical activity component of wellness. Whether you're about to enroll in a beginning weight training class at your college or have just signed up for an intramural volleyball team, you should follow the injury prevention steps outlined in this chapter.

To prevent injury, you should take certain precautions, including the following six steps:

- obtaining a preparticipation medical screening examination
- using appropriate protective equipment
- wearing appropriate footwear
- wearing appropriate clothing
- warming up properly
- adopting a commonsense approach to exercise to avoid overtraining

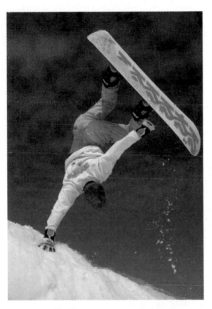

Figure 6.1
Snowboarders are vulnerable to a wrist injury when they trail the uphill hand while making an inside turn.

Medical Screening

Even for young people, annual physical examinations are a vital part of any wellness program. The major goal of a medical screening examination is to identify any predisposing risk factors that might cause sudden death or a debilitating injury during exercise. One way to guard against this possibility is to complete the Physical Activity Readiness Questionnaire (PAR-Q) included in Chapter 2. If you answered "yes" to one or more of the seven questions on the PAR-Q, talk with your doctor by telephone or in person before you start more physical activity and discuss the questions you answered "yes" (Thomas et al.). If risk factors are identified, your physician can recommend appropriate preventive measures (see the section "Exercising Caution" in Chapter 2).

If you already know your medical history includes high blood pressure, cardiovascular abnormalities, diabetes, obesity, respiratory ailments, or other health problems and you have been sedentary but recently decided to

TABLE 6.1

Common Injuries in Fitness-Related Activities

ACTIVITY	MOST FREQUENT INJURIES/CONDITIONS	MOST CATASTROPHIC INJURY
Baseball/softball	Upper-extremity strains and sprains; contusions	Head and chest injuries; eye injuries
Basketball	Lower-extremity musculotendinous injuries; stress fractures of foot and leg	Traumatic head and neck injuries
Cross-country skiing	Overuse injuries in lower extremity	Hypothermia
Cycling	Lower-extremity overuse injuries; nerve compression; wrist and hand injuries	Head injuries from falls or collisions with cars
Downhill skiing	Knee sprains; fractures; wrist and thumb sprains; severe sunburn; hypothermia	Severe head injury; death
Golf	Low back strains and sprains; wrist and hand injuries	Electrocution by lightning strike
In-line skating	Wrist and forearm fractures and sprains; abrasions; contusions	Severe head injury
Racquetball/squash	Lower-extremity musculotendinous injuries; eye injuries (90% preventable if protective eyewear with poly-carbonate lenses used)	Cardiac arrest
Running/jogging	Lower-extremity musculotendinous injuries; stress fractures; heat illnesses	Cardiac arrest
Snowboarding	Ankle and knee sprains; wrist and lower extremity fractures	Hypothermia; death
Step aerobics	Lower-extremity musculotendinous injuries; stress fractures of foot and leg; bursitis	Cardiac arrest
Swimming	Shoulder overuse injuries ("swimmer's shoulder"); ear fungal infections ("swimmer's ear")	Drowning
Tennis	Elbow injuries ("tennis elbow"); shoulder strains	Virtually none
Walking	Lower-extremity strains and sprains	Virtually none
Weight lifting	Low back strains and sprains; muscle soreness	Virtually none

Source: From Fahey, 1986.

become more active, you still should consult a physician before starting your fitness program (American College of Sports Medicine). Your physician will be familiar with information compiled by the American Medical Association or the American Academy of Pediatrics regarding physical conditions that would put you at risk if you decided to participate in certain fitness activities or intramural sports.

For example, if you have asthma, you may not be aware that 80% of persons with asthma experience *exercise-induced asthma* (EIA) attacks after just 6 to 8 minutes of strenuous exercise. Consult with your physician to set up a special plan for using your asthma medication before exercise and for choosing exercise times and environments that allow you to avoid situations almost certain to trigger EIA, such as an early morning jog on a cold winter day in the air pollution of rush hour traffic (Anderson and Hall).

Appropriate Equipment

Perhaps the most effective means of injury prevention for recreational fitness activities is the use of correctly fitted protective equipment. Some fitness activities, such as tennis, racquetball, and squash, require specific types of equipment for successful participation as well as injury prevention. In tennis, for example, proper equipment reduces the risk of developing *tennis elbow,* an inflammatory condition caused by excessive racquet string tension, repetitive use of the forearm muscles, and poor flexibility. An instructor or skilled salesperson can assist you in selecting the appropriate tennis racquet and string tension. In addition, formal tennis instruction, either through a college class or from a local tennis professional, can improve your stroke mechanics and reduce your chances of injury.

Eye injuries can occur in virtually all fitness-related activities, although the risk factor is higher in such activities as ice hockey, racquetball, and squash. However, recent studies indicate that as many as 90% of the eye injuries that occur in racquetball and squash can be prevented through the use of appropriate eye protection, such as protective goggles made with polycarbonate lenses. Similarly, wearing silicone earplugs while swimming and putting a dropperful of a nonprescription drying agent in each ear after swimming will help to prevent swimmer's ear.

Since its introduction in 1980, in-line skating has become one of the fastest growing recreational activities in the United States with approximately 23 million participants of all ages in 1995. About 100,000 of these in-line skaters were injured to the extent that they required hospital emergency room treatment. The most common site of injury is the wrist (37% of all injuries), with fractures comprising two-thirds of all wrist injuries (Centers for Disease Control and Prevention). Researchers recently have investigated the effectiveness of wrist guards, elbow pads, knee pads, and helmets in preventing injuries and found that 46% of the injured in-line skaters they interviewed wore no protective equipment whatsoever. The researchers concluded that wearing wrist guards could reduce the number of wrist injuries by 87%, wearing elbow pads could reduce the number of elbow injuries by 82%, and wearing knee pads could reduce knee injuries by about one-third (see Figure 6.2). An insufficient number of in-line skaters in this study sustained head injuries to draw any conclusions regarding the protection provided by helmets, but previous studies have demonstrated that helmets are highly protective against head injuries to bicyclists who are exposed to injury in environments similar to those of in-line skaters (Centers for Disease Control and Prevention).

Approximately 100 million Americans currently ride bikes for pleasure, fitness, or competition. Selecting the right-size bicycle frame, adjusting the seat to the proper height, wearing a bicycle helmet, using padded grips/handlebars, and wearing padded biking shorts and gloves can significantly reduce the number of biking injuries. In fact, helmets that meet the standards established by the American National Standards Institute (ANSI) should be worn by all cyclists. Recent estimates suggest that as many as 85% of the cycling fatalities caused by head injuries could be prevented by the use of an appropriate cycling helmet (Noakes).

Mountain bikes now account for over one-half of all new bicycle sales. Off-road biking differs from on-road cycling because, among other things, it places much more strenuous demands on the wrists and hands. In a recent

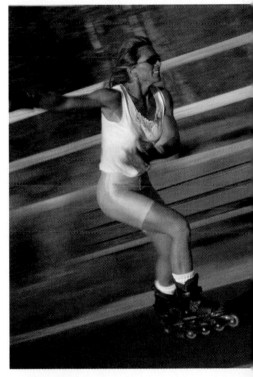

Figure 6.2

An example of an in-line skater not wearing appropriate protective equipment.

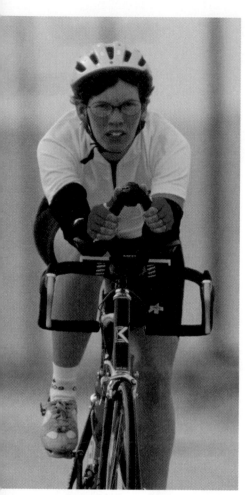

Figure 6.3

"Aero-bars" distribute the cyclist's body weight over the forearms and hands and decrease the risk of cyclist's palsy.

study of injuries at a major off-road bicycle race in California, falls were the main cause of injury. Abrasions were the most common injury, followed by contusions, lacerations, fractures, and concussions. Not surprisingly, 81% of the injuries occurred while the racers were going downhill (Kronisch et al.).

One common complaint among both recreational bikers and long-distance bicycle racers is a numbness and tingling in the ring and little fingers. This inflammatory condition, known as *cyclist's palsy,* is caused by prolonged compression of the nerves in the fourth and fifth fingers. Cyclist's palsy is linked especially to the use of conventional touring (road) bikes because their drop handlebars put the cyclist's weight forward onto the hands. Modified handlebars, known as aerodynamic bars ("aero-bars"), can reduce the risk of cyclist's palsy and are now commercially available. These handlebars have a triangular configuration that lets the cyclist choose between distributing weight all along the forearms or riding in the traditional manner (see Figure 6.3). However, even if you don't have the latest equipment, you can avoid cyclist's palsy by changing your hand position every few minutes and by using padded biking gloves and handlebars.

Appropriate Footwear

Forty years ago a limited number of athletic shoe companies manufactured canvas gym shoes, known as sneakers. Today, a myriad of athletic shoe companies market a wide variety of sport shoes. Specialty athletic shoes, some costing $150 or more per pair, are now made for virtually every sport and recreational activity. For the consumer, this overwhelming variety means that making an informed decision on sport shoe selection has become increasingly difficult.

What should you look for when purchasing a running shoe? Biomechanics research has taught us that running is a "collision" sport—that is, the runner's foot collides with the ground with a force 3 to 5 times the runner's body weight. Depending on stride length, the runner's feet will collide with the ground 800 to 2,000 times per mile. Thus, the 150-pound runner who takes 1,000 strides per mile, at a force 3 times his or her body weight, applies a cumulative force to the body of 450,000 pounds per mile! And the force not absorbed by the running shoe is transmitted to the feet, legs, and back, where injury to the muscles, tendons, bones, cartilage, and ligaments can result from the cumulative effects of these repetitive impacts.

Thus, a running shoe must have both good shock-absorbing qualities, at the midsole and the heel, and a flexible midsole. To evaluate the flexibility of the midsole, hold the shoe between the index fingers of your right and left hands. When you push on both ends of the shoe with your fingers, the shoe should bend easily at the midsole. If the force exerted by your index fingers cannot bend the shoe, its midsole is probably too rigid and may cause irritation of your Achilles tendon, among other problems (Brody). Running shoes also should have (1) a rigid plastic insert in the shoe's heel, known as a *heel counter* to control the movement of your heel; (2) a cushioned foam pad surrounding the shoe's heel to prevent Achilles tendon irritation; (3) a removable thermoplastic inner sole that uses your body heat to mold the shoe to the shape of your foot, and (4) at least one thumb-width of room between your longest toe and the end of the shoe. Figure 6.4 shows the components of a modern running shoe.

By purchasing a cross-training shoe you can avoid the expense of having to buy separate pairs of shoes for running, tennis, weight training, and so on.

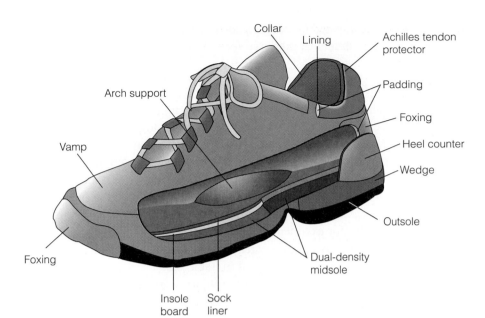

Collar
Lining
Achilles tendon protector
Padding
Arch support
Foxing
Vamp
Heel counter
Wedge
Outsole
Foxing
Dual-density midsole
Insole board
Sock liner

Figure 6.4
Today's running shoes are complex, scientifically designed athletic equipment.

The cross-training shoe can be used for participation in several different fitness activities by the novice or recreational athlete; however, a serious long-distance runner who runs 20–25 or more miles per week needs a pair of specialty running shoes to help prevent injury. Although running shoes can be quite expensive, they are the runner's most important equipment. If you're running 20 to 25 miles per week, you should consider replacing your running shoes every six months or 400 miles, whichever comes first.

Appropriate Clothing

Selection of activity-appropriate fitness and recreational clothing is as important as the choice of the proper footwear or equipment. With regard to injury prevention, the function of your athletic clothing is far more important than the fashion statement you make. For example, if you are running in hot weather, you should have clothing that allows for maximal body heat dissipation (for example, light-colored nylon shorts and a mesh tank top). If you are cross-country skiing, you should wear clothing that retains heat but keeps you from getting soaked with sweat (for example, various layers of polypropylene and/or wool clothing).

Proper Warm-Up

As you should know by now, prior to vigorous physical activity you need to warm up properly to reduce the chance of injury and increase the efficiency of your performance. As discussed in Chapter 3, the warm-up increases the temperature of your muscles and connective tissues so that they function more efficiently during exercise. When warmed up sufficiently, these tissues become more elastic and thus less prone to tearing—for example, when a ligament or muscle is rapidly stretched, or when a muscle is maximally contracted.

As in the age-old controversy of the chicken and the egg, there is some debate regarding which warmup activity should be performed first—a brief period of walking/jogging or static stretching. We recommend that your warm-up regimen include both a dynamic component (for example, walking, low-intensity cycling, jogging, or reduced-speed performance of the specific activity) and static stretching exercises for the muscles to be used.

Commonsense Approach

Because overtraining is the most frequent cause of injury in aerobic fitness activities, you need to adopt a commonsense approach to your fitness regimen. Often, enthusiastic but out-of-shape beginning exercisers are injured when they try to do too much, too soon. Participating in an hour-long step aerobics class six nights per week may be an enjoyable social activity as well as an effective means of weight control, but you may suffer a debilitating overuse injury in the lower or upper extremity as a result. Unfortunately, overtraining is also a major cause of injury for experienced participants (for example, runners, bicyclists, swimmers) who unwittingly increase their mileage too rapidly or commit one of the other training errors listed in Table 6.2.

To avoid overtraining, learn to read the injury warning signs your body gives you. Muscle stiffness and soreness, bone and joint pains, and general (whole-body) fatigue are some of the signs of an impending injury. If these signs go unheeded, the risk of significant injury, such as a stress fracture, increases dramatically. *Cross-training* is one method of preventing overuse injury to a particular muscle group or body part (see Chapter 3 for more on cross-training). By varying your fitness activities, you give specific muscles and joints a chance to rest and recover. For example, instead of swimming 25 laps 5 times per week and risking an overuse injury at the shoulder joint, you might swim 3 times per week and cycle or jog 2 times per week to exercise your leg muscles while resting the muscles and joints of your upper body.

TABLE 6.2

Factors Responsible for Overuse Injuries

FACTOR	EXPLANATION
Excessive impact forces	Walking generates impact forces 1 to 3 times body weight; running creates impact forces 3 to 5 times body weight; gymnastic landings and dismounts can generate impacts 10 to 15 times body weight.
Exercise on hard surfaces	This increases the impact forces transmitted to bone and soft tissues.
Improper or worn-out athletic shoes	Shoes should be in good condition and specific to the activity if possible; they must provide good shock absorption and support.
Changes in frequency, intensity, and duration of exercise regimen	Too rapid an increase in these exercise parameters may result in a stress fracture or associated soft-tissue injury.
Lack of flexibility	Poor flexibility is a particular problem in the Achilles tendon (calf muscle) and the hamstring muscle group.
Downhill running	Associated with lateral knee pain (iliotibial bond friction syndrome) and patellar tendonitis.
Overtraining	There is a delicate balance between being in "peak" physical condition and pushing too hard, which can lead to injury or illness.
Running more than 25 miles per week	A relatively high incidence of injury (approximately 50%) exists for runners who run more than 25 miles (40 km) per week.
Muscular imbalance or weakness	There needs to be a good balance in any fitness or weight training program so as not to neglect or overuse any particular muscle group; the concept of cross-training addresses this factor.

Source: From Roy and Irwin, 1983.

Another way to prevent an overtraining injury is to set appropriate short- and long-term training goals. A short-term goal for a beginning runner might be to run a mile without stopping to walk. An appropriate long-term goal might be to complete a 3-mile race while running at an 8-minute per mile pace. However, take care not to be over-ambitious and overload your muscles and joints by doing too much, too soon.

The bottom line is that an over-eager, underprepared approach to physical activity, fitness training, or sports could have the opposite effect on wellness than you intended: Instead of becoming more fit, you might actually become weaker or more exposed to injury. By following the injury prevention guidelines in this chapter you will dramatically reduce your risk of injury.

Common Exercise-Related Injuries

There are two basic causes of injury in fitness-related activities: microtrauma and macrotrauma. **Microtrauma** refers to injuries that occur as a result of cumulative, day-after-day stress placed on body parts (for example, inflamed tendons, stress fractures, fatigued muscles) during exercise. Individuals who sustain this type of injury typically cannot pinpoint the specific time or place of injury. The forces that are normally applied during physical activity are not sufficient to cause a sprain or strain, but when applied on a daily basis for weeks or months, they can cause an injury. Common sites for this type of problem are the leg, knee, shoulder, and elbow.

Macrotrauma refers to injuries that occur as a result of an accident. Sometimes accidental injuries are unavoidable, as when, for example, you sprain the ligaments in your ankle by landing on another person's foot after jumping for a rebound while playing basketball. Wearing a protective ankle brace might have reduced the severity of your injury, but the circumstances that caused the injury were accidental. Errors in judgment can also be responsible for macrotrauma injuries. The fatigued, out-of-shape downhill skier who wants to make one last run down the slope may sustain an injury while taking that ill-advised final run. (See the Stats-at-a-Glance.)

Your body responds to repetitive microtrauma (overuse) and macrotrauma (accidental injury) by producing inflammation. Many different body parts can be affected by inflammation. The Latin suffix *itis* means inflammation; thus, **tendonitis** refers to inflammation of a tendon, **arthritis** refers to inflammation of a joint, and so on. Table 6.3 summarizes the five easily recognized signs and symptoms—pain, swelling, local heat, redness, and loss of function—produced by an inflammatory response at one of these sites.

Fitness-related injuries occur most often in repetitive-motion activities such as swimming, running, dance aerobics, and bicycling. Because the majority of these activities involve locomotion, the lower extremities (foot, ankle, knee, and hip) are most prone to injury. However, there are a few exceptions, such as swimming and baseball/softball, in which the frequency of injury is distributed between the upper and lower regions of the body.

Literally hundreds of different musculoskeletal injuries are possible from physical activity. We have grouped our presentation of these into five categories, based primarily on the anatomical structure involved: (1) muscle strain, (2) ligament sprain, (3) tendonitis, (4) stress fracture, and (5) general inflammatory conditions.

STATS-AT-A-GLANCE
Exercise-Related Injuries

■ The typical snowboarder who sustains an injury is a 19-year-old male who has just started snowboarding (Elmqvist et al.). Most snowboarding injuries are caused either by impact (56% to 63%), such as shoulder dislocations; whiplash-type neck injuries; or by twisting (32% to 34%), such as sprains to the extremities or fractures (Van Tilburg).

■ Approximately 85% of all injuries to the ankle are sprains, of which more than 80% involve the lateral ligament complex. Ankle injuries account for 40% of the injuries to basketball players (Nike).

■ Tennis elbow is common among tennis players, but lower-extremity injuries occur more frequently. In a study of more than 1,000 tennis players, leg and hip pain were most prevalent (42%), followed by pain in the upper extremities (32%) (Nigg and Segesser).

■ The shoulder is dislocated more frequently than any other human joint, causing pain and limiting motion in athletes and nonathletes of all ages (Nevasier, Nevasier, and Nevasier).

■ A recent study of more than 4,000 running injuries ranked the location of the problems as follows: knee (48%), lower leg (20%), foot (17%), hip (6%), upper leg and thigh (4%), and low back (4%) (MacIntyre et al.).

microtrauma injury that occurs as a result of cumulative, day-after-day stress placed on body parts during exercise

macrotrauma injury that occurs as a result of an accident

tendonitis inflammation of a tendon

arthritis inflammation of a joint

TABLE 6.3
Signs and Symptoms of Inflammation

SIGN OR SYMPTOM	PHYSIOLOGIC CAUSE
Pain	Due to direct injury to a nerve or to pressure applied to pain receptors from swelling or compression (for example, sprain, fracture, joint dislocation)
Swelling	Due to the internal accumulation of blood after trauma or to the release of substances from damaged or dead cells, which causes bodily fluids to travel outside the vascular system
Local heat	Due to increased metabolic activity in the area of injury or irritation and to increased blood flow to the skin surface
Redness	Due to dilation of arterial blood vessels permitting increased blood flow to the injured or irritated area
Loss of function	Due to damage to a bone (fracture), ligament (sprain), or muscle (strain), or to swelling into a joint making normal movement painful or impossible

Source: From Booher and Thibodeau, 1994.

Strains

A **strain** is a partial or complete tear of the fibers of a muscle and/or tendon caused by sudden or repetitive overload (see Figure 6.5). Together, the muscle and tendon are referred to as the **musculotendinous unit**—the functional unit of a muscle and its tendons of attachment to bone. The most frequent exercise-related strains occur to the hamstring muscle group on the posterior thigh, the muscles of the low back that extend from the spine, and the muscles of the calf that converge to form the Achilles tendon.

Strains can be classified according to three degrees of severity: mild, moderate, and severe. With a mild strain, microscopic tears of the tendon and/or muscle fibers occur. The injured person has some pain and tenderness at the site of the injury but suffers little swelling or loss of function. For example, you can suffer a mild muscle strain during weight training if the repetitive overloading intended to produce hypertrophy causes muscle damage. In this case, you may experience **delayed-onset muscle soreness**—muscle pain that occurs 24 to 48 hours after intense physical activities such as weight lifting and downhill running. With appropriate rest periods between workouts, the microscopic muscle tears will heal without medical treatment. Delayed onset muscle soreness can also occur if you arbitrarily increase intensity and duration during an aerobic activity.

It is often difficult to distinguish between mild and moderate strains. A moderate muscle strain is associated with significant pain, swelling from internal bleeding, and spasm of the injured and surrounding muscles—all of which contribute to temporary loss of strength and function in the affected muscle. Several days of rest and then gentle range-of-motion exercises generally are the treatment prescription for this type of injury. When you are able to move your injured muscle through its full range of motion without pain,

strain a partial or complete tear of the fibers of a muscle and/or tendon caused by a sudden or repetitive overload

musculotendinous unit the functional unit of a muscle and its tendons of attachment to bone

delayed-onset muscle soreness muscle pain that occurs 24–48 hours after intense physical activities such as weight lifting and downhill running

EXERCISE ◆ SAFETY

Do

▲ Warm up properly before you exercise.

▲ Be sure you understand how to use equipment safely.

▲ Be sure your shoes and other equipment fit correctly, and you have the appropriate helmets, pads, and so on.

▲ Have a medical screening done before starting an exercise program if you have any risk factors.

▲ Develop the right technique. An improperly executed move is often the cause of injury.

▲ Counter muscle imbalances. For example, if your calf muscles are strong from running, strengthen the opposing shin muscles to avoid injury to the Achilles tendon.

▲ Monitor your body as you exercise for any abnormal sensations.

▲ Stop exercising if you feel any sharp or intense pain.

▲ Remember RICE (rest, ice, compression, elevation) as the first treatment for almost any injury. Start icing as soon as possible after the injury.

▲ See a physician if pain is very intense, involves numbness or tingling, or persists for more than a couple of days.

Don't

▼ Overdo it. Injuries are more likely when muscles are fatigued.

▼ Think that ignoring an injury is a sign of toughness.

▼ Ignore a slow onset of pain; it may be a sign of an overuse injury.

▼ Leave an ice pack directly on the skin; either keep it moving or wrap it in a towel.

▼ Leave an ice pack on for too long; remove it once the skin is numb.

▼ Use ice on blisters or open wounds.

▼ Put off seeing a doctor if pain persists for more than a couple of days.

▼ Start exercising again before an injury has had a chance to heal completely.

Figure 6.5

A muscle strain injury occurs when a sudden overload or a series of repetitive loads tears muscle and/or tendon fibers. It is helpful to view the muscle and the tendons that attach it to the bone as a unit (the musculotendinous unit).
Source: From Hunter-Griffin, 1991.

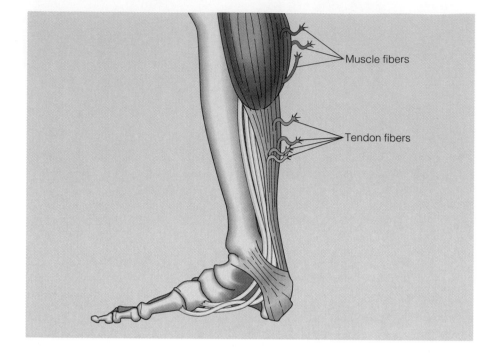

Muscle fibers

Tendon fibers

you should begin a specific program of resistance exercises to restore muscular strength and endurance. Consult a physician or certified athletic trainer for the proper activities and rate of progression for your rehabilitation program.

A severe strain is a complete tearing of the musculotendinous unit into two parts. This type of injury is extremely rare (and extremely painful) and will leave no doubt in the injured person's mind as to what has occurred. Often the torn muscle rolls up at each end like a windowshade, creating an easily observed deformity. An injury of this severity requires immediate medical treatment. Depending on the muscle or tendon involved, as well as one's age and activity level, surgery might have to be performed to reattach the torn ends of the muscle or tendon and restore normal function.

Muscle strains are best prevented through performance of appropriate warm-up activities prior to your selected fitness activity, as well as a regular program of stretching exercises designed to improve your flexibility.

Sprains

A **sprain** is a partial or complete tear of the fibers of a ligament or joint capsule caused by a sudden overload. Like muscle strains, sprains can be classified according to three degrees of severity: mild, moderate, and severe. With a mild sprain the ligament is stretched, but no significant tearing of its fibers occurs. With a moderate sprain the ligament is partially torn, resulting in a less stable joint. A severe sprain is one in which the ligament is completely torn, significantly weakening and temporarily disabling the joint involved. In many instances, complete tearing of the ligaments that stabilize a joint will result in **dislocation,** the temporary displacement of a bone from its normal position in a joint.

In virtually all cases, sprains are accidental injuries resulting from excessive force applied to the ligaments of a joint. By far the most common fitness-related sprain is the sprained ankle, although the knees, shoulders, and joints of the fingers and toes can also be sprained. If a fitness activity

sprain a partial or complete tear of the fibers of a ligament or joint capsule caused by a sudden overload

dislocation the temporary displacement of a bone from its normal position in a joint

does not involve collisions or direct body contact with other participants (for example, swimming, jogging, cycling), the chances of sustaining a sprain or dislocation are relatively small.

Approximately 90% of all ankle sprains occur to the lateral (outside) ligaments of the ankle (see Figure 6.6). Lateral ankle sprains are generally caused by an unexpected, forceful turning of the foot inward during weight-bearing activities that require rapid starts, stops, and changes in direction (for example, basketball, tennis, snowboarding, step aerobics). Many ankle sprains can be avoided or minimized with the use of prophylactic ankle braces available at most sporting goods stores.

In general, sprains are treated initially with rest and ice (to reduce pain and swelling), followed by a systematic program of therapeutic exercise to restore full function. If you suffer a sprain that causes considerable pain and disability, you should see a physician.

Tendonitis

Tendonitis is an inflammation of a tendon resulting from overuse. In each of the over 600 muscles of the body, there are two tendons that attach that muscle to bone. Therefore, the potential locations for tendonitis are numerous. Three of the most common sites are the heel *(Achilles tendonitis)*, the knee *(patellar tendonitis),* and the elbow *(tennis elbow)* (Curwin and Stanish).

Tendonitis involving the Achilles, the largest tendon in the body, is often caused by sudden changes in the quantity or type of fitness activity, leading to overuse. For runners and joggers, a different style of athletic shoe, the addition of sprinting or hill workouts, or a sudden increase in mileage can produce an inflamed Achilles tendon. Runners should increase their mileage gradually in increments of 10% or less per week to reduce the chances of creating tendonitis (Ballas et al.).

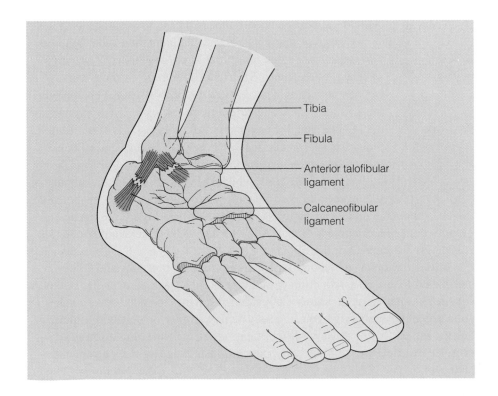

Tibia

Fibula

Anterior talofibular ligament

Calcaneofibular ligament

Figure 6.6

The two most commonly injured ankle ligaments are the anterior talofibular and the calcaneofibular.

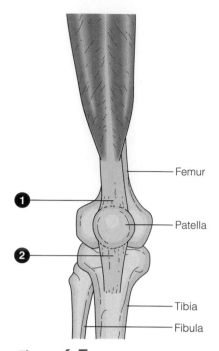

Figure 6.7

Patellar tendonitis occurs in two places: (1) above the patella, in what is sometimes referred to as "quadriceps tendonitis," and (2) below the patella, the most common site.

Another area that frequently becomes irritated during fitness activities is the tissue around the **patella,** or kneecap. Patellar tendonitis is an inflammatory condition resulting from overuse of the tendon that attaches the quadriceps, a group of four muscles that run from the thigh to the **tibia,** or shin bone (see Figure 6.7). Women are more susceptible than men to patellar tendonitis if they participate in activities that require frequent jumping with great force, such as basketball and volleyball (Arendt). Repetitious endurance activities such as cycling, running, and step aerobics also can produce this inflammatory condition.

The pain associated with patellar tendonitis is most commonly felt above and below the kneecap. People who suffer from patellar tendonitis often complain of stiffness if they keep their knee in one position for any length of time. As with any inflammatory condition, if you experience a significant loss of function you should be treated by a physician.

More than 25 painful elbow conditions have been categorized as "tennis elbow." Different factors, such as age and experience level, appear to be responsible for the onset of tennis elbow. The high incidence of this condition in the 35- to 50-year-old group suggests that age-related degenerative changes in the elbow structure are a prime cause. Beginning tennis players are more likely than expert players to develop this condition (Curwin and Stanish). Thus, according to this theory, experienced players who use proper stroke techniques would not be expected to suffer from tennis elbow. However, a study of 2,500 players revealed a 45% incidence rate among world-class players and a 47% incidence rate in average players (Priest et al.).

In broad terms, **tennis elbow** is an inflammation of the muscles and tendons that attach to the elbow. Technically, this condition is known as *lateral epicondylitis,* because the inflammation actually involves the tendons of the wrist extensor muscles where they attach to the **humerus,** the bone extending from the shoulder to the elbow. Lateral epicondylitis is the more accurate term because many carpenters, painters, and other laborers as well as tennis players suffer from this type of pain, caused by the repeated gripping required in their work-related activities. The main symptoms of lateral epicondylitis are pain during strong gripping and a loss of grip strength in the affected hand. For players of racquet sports (for example, tennis, squash, racquetball), elbow pain occurs during backhand strokes and sometimes during slice or twist serves. A faulty backhand stroke in which the elbow is flexed at impact of the ball on the racquet ("leading elbow backhand") is responsible for this condition in many novice players (see Figure 6.8). Any elbow pain severe enough to cause you to hit weaker backhands or serves is grounds for consulting a physician.

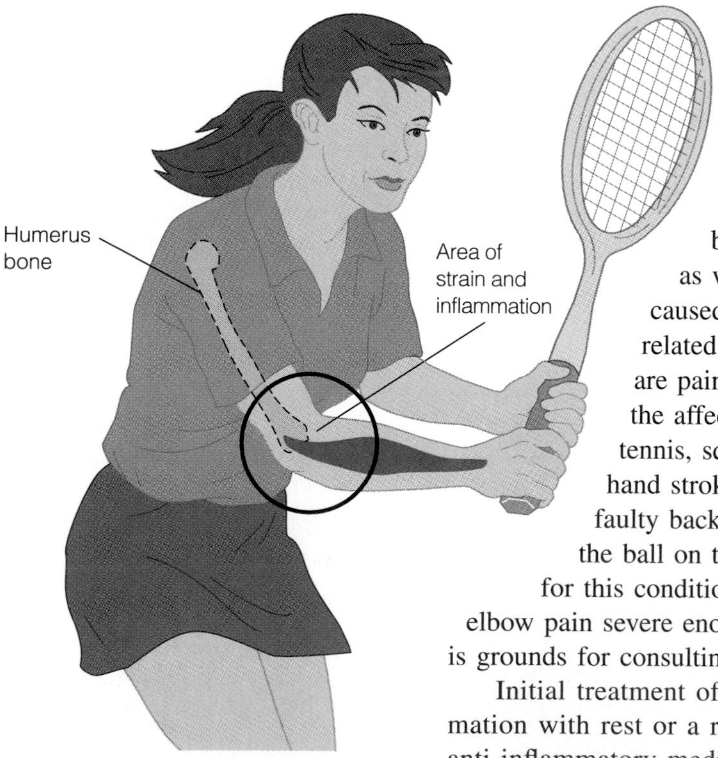

Initial treatment of tendonitis involves treating the pain and inflammation with rest or a reduction in activity and the use of over-the-counter anti-inflammatory medications (ibuprofen, aspirin). In more severe cases, your physician will refer you to a physical therapist or certified athletic trainer for treatment (e.g., with ice, heat, or electrical stimulation) and exercises to heal the injured body part while preventing a recurrence of injury.

Figure 6.8

"Leading elbow" backhand is the most common cause of "tennis elbow" (*lateral epicondylitis*) in novice racquet sport participants

Stress Fractures

A **stress fracture** is a hairline (superficial) fracture that is produced by repetitive forces that eventually exceed a bone's normal limits and that occurs without any sign of soft-tissue injury. Stress fractures generally occur in bones of the lower extremities and are quite common among runners (see Figure 6.9).

In a classic example of the detrimental effects of overtraining, a 27-year-old competitive triathlete (swimming, running, and cycling) sustained a stress fracture of his **femur,** or thigh bone (Jackson). This triathlete's regular training program involved running more than 40 miles, cycling 150 miles, and swimming nearly 10 miles every week. It should come as no surprise that he suffered a stress fracture to the largest bone in his body! Although this is an extreme case, aerobic fitness participants suffer stress fractures with far less intensity and duration of exercise.

Typical symptoms associated with stress fractures in the lower extremities are pain during weightbearing activities (for example, walking and running) and the absence of the pain with rest. Stress fractures must always be considered as a possibility when you experience pain in a bone but not in the surrounding soft tissues. New stress fractures are difficult to diagnose with regular X rays, but a bone scan can confirm the presence of a stress fracture.

A stress fracture takes several weeks to heal. Depending on its location, your physician may or may not place the broken bone in a cast. For stress fractures in the lower extremities, partial weight-bearing walking with crutches can help the healing process.

General Inflammatory Conditions

The final category of fitness-related injuries is a series of overuse injuries that occur most frequently in the lower extremities but may also be found in the upper extremities. Four of the most common general inflammatory conditions created through microtrauma during exercise are (1) plantar fasciitis, (2) shin splints, (3) runner's knee, and (4) swimmer's shoulder.

Plantar Fasciitis. The **plantar fascia** is a broad band of tough, inelastic tissue (fascia) located on the bottom of the foot that protects the muscles, blood vessels, and nerves from injury. In repetitive, weight-bearing activities such as step aerobics and jogging, the plantar fascia is subjected to microtrauma and may become inflamed. Recall that the suffix *-itis* means inflammation; thus, plantar fasciitis is an inflammation of the plantar fascia (see Figure 6.10).

Common signs and symptoms of this condition include pain and tenderness at the heel, under the ball of the foot, or at both locations, particularly when first stepping out of bed in the morning. If not treated properly, this injury may become so severe that weight-bearing exercise is too painful to endure. Uphill running is not advised if you have this condition because each uphill stride stretches and irritates the inflamed area.

This injury can often be prevented by regular stretching of the plantar fascia prior to exercise and by wearing athletic shoes that support the arches and absorb shock. The plantar fascia may be stretched by slowly pulling all five toes toward your head (hyperextension), holding for 10 to 15 seconds, and repeating 3 to 5 times on each foot prior to exercise.

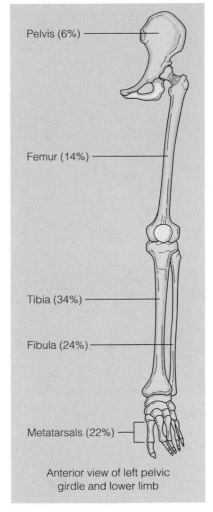

Pelvis (6%)
Femur (14%)
Tibia (34%)
Fibula (24%)
Metatarsals (22%)

Anterior view of left pelvic girdle and lower limb

Figure 6.9

The tibia is the most common site for stress fractures in the lower extremities followed by the fibula. Source: From Marieb, 1992.

patella kneecap

tibia shin bone

tennis elbow inflammation of the muscles and tendons that attach to the elbow

humerus the bone extending from the shoulder to the elbow

stress fracture a hairline (superficial) fracture produced by repetitive forces that eventually exceed a bone's normal limits and that occurs without any sign of soft-tissue injury

femur thigh bone

plantar fascia a broad band of tough, inelastic connective tissue on the bottom of the foot that protects the muscles, blood vessels, and nerves from injury

Figure 6.10

Plantar fasciitis is caused by inflammation of the plantar aponeurosis. This burning or aching pain occurs on the bottom of the foot, particularly at the heel (shaded area)

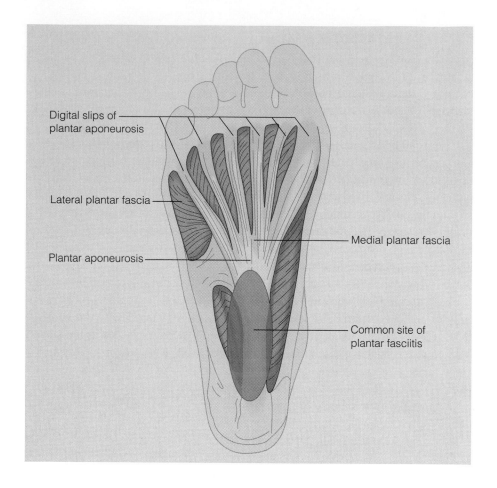

Digital slips of plantar aponeurosis

Lateral plantar fascia

Plantar aponeurosis

Medial plantar fascia

Common site of plantar fasciitis

Shin Splints. The term **shin splints** is used to classify any of the more than 20 conditions that cause pain below the knee and above the ankle. These problems range from a stress fracture of the tibia to severe inflammation in the muscular compartments of the lower leg that can interrupt the flow of blood and nerve impulses to the foot. Shin splints usually occur along the back and inner *(posteromedial)* tibia and are a combination of tendonitis and irritation of the tibia. Typically, there is pain and swelling along the middle third of the posteromedial tibia in the soft tissues, not on bone. Sometimes, shin splint pain occurs on the front and outer *(anterolateral)* aspect of the tibia (see Figure 6.11).

Out-of-shape individuals who start new weight-bearing exercise programs are most at risk for shin splints; however, well-conditioned aerobic exercisers (walkers, joggers, runners) who rapidly increase their distance or pace are also likely to develop shin splints. Running is the most frequent cause of shin splints, but those who do a great deal of walking (for example, food servers and infantry soldiers) may also develop this condition.

Wearing athletic shoes that absorb shock well and provide good arch support can help prevent shin splints. Other preventive measures include improving the strength and flexibility of your leg muscles and tendons, doing warm-up stretches before exercising, and exercising on soft surfaces, not on asphalt or concrete.

If shin splints become so severe that you cannot comfortably complete your desired fitness activity, you should see a physician. Specific pain on the tibia or the adjacent, smaller **fibula,** the bone extending from the knee to the

shin splints any of the more than 20 conditions that cause pain below the knee and above the ankle

fibula bone extending from the knee to the ankle

Figure 6.11
The pain from shin splints more frequently occurs in the posterior-medial region of the lower leg, but also can be located anteriorly (shaded areas).

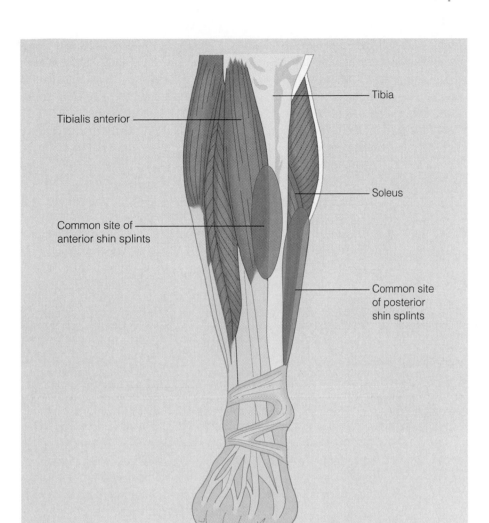

Tibialis anterior

Common site of anterior shin splints

Tibia

Soleus

Common site of posterior shin splints

ankle, should be examined for a possible stress fracture. Reduction of the frequency, intensity, and duration of weight-bearing exercise may be required. A non-weight-bearing activity such as swimming may be substituted for weight-bearing exercise during your period of recovery.

Runner's Knee. The single most common problem associated with running is abnormal movement of the patella (Brody). Like the catch-all term *shin splints*, **runner's knee** describes a group of overuse injuries involving the muscles, tendons, and ligaments around the patella. The patella glides up and down in the groove at the distal end of the femur during normal knee flexion and extension. Anomalies such as quadriceps muscle imbalance, the shape of the patella, and abnormal hips, knees, and foot biomechanics all may contribute to runner's knee.

Women are more prone than men to this condition due to their wider pelvis and the increased angle at which their quadriceps muscles act at the knee (Arendt). An imbalance between two of the quadriceps muscles can also cause problems if one muscle exerts a stronger lateral pull, causing the cartilage on the underside of the patella to be damaged.

The main symptom of runner's knee is pain when downward pressure is applied to the patella after the knee is fully straightened. Additional symptoms include swelling, redness, and tenderness around the patella, and a dull,

runner's knee a group of overuse injuries involving the muscles, tendons, and ligaments around the patella

aching pain felt in the center of the knee. If you have these symptoms, your physician may recommend that you stop running or doing aerobics for a few weeks and reduce activities that put compressive forces on the patella (for example, kneeling or exercising on a stair-climbing machine). You may substitute swimming or water exercise during the rehabilitation period. After all symptoms have cleared up, exercise may be resumed gradually under your doctor's or therapist's supervision.

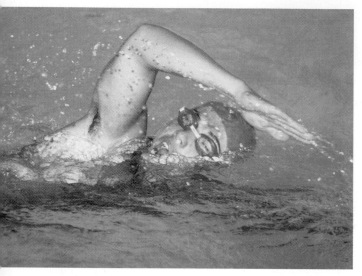

Figure 6.12

Swimmer's shoulder is an inflammatory condition that results either from overuse of the muscles of the shoulder (tendonitis) or an irritation of the shoulder bursa (bursitis).

Swimmer's Shoulder. The shoulder is the most commonly injured anatomical region among swimmers. The repetitive motions associated with swimming, particularly the overhand strokes used in the crawl and the butterfly, subject the shoulder joints to thousands of cycles in any given workout. **Swimmer's shoulder** is the painful condition that results from impingement of the muscles, tendons, and other structures during the overhand forward swimming stroke (see Figure 6.12). Specifically, it refers to inflammation of the musculotendinous structure and the **bursae**—the fluid-filled sacs found in connective tissue that help reduce friction between anatomical structures of the shoulder joint.

Pain and inability to perform the desired pool workout are the most common symptoms associated with swimmer's shoulder. The pain is usually nonspecific but typically occurs during the pull-through phase of the swimming motion, just after the hand enters the water, or during the recovery phase of the stroke. Swimmer's shoulder, like other overuse injuries, is treated initially with ice, rest or modified exercise levels, and anti-inflammatory medications; in more severe cases, a visit to your physician is warranted.

This overuse condition can be prevented through static stretching exercises for the shoulder muscles before and after swimming, use of a proper warm-up swimming period prior to any vigorous workout, and variation in swimming strokes during extended workouts.

First Aid and Medical Treatment for Exercise-Related Injuries

There is an old medical saying that "a person who treats himself or herself has a fool for a patient and a fool for a doctor." Although this axiom is true in many instances, a number of minor fitness-related injuries and conditions can be treated adequately with standard first-aid procedures. However, any injury serious enough to cause a noticeable loss of function should be evaluated by a physician. The wellness-minded individual is conscious of proper evaluation and treatment of fitness injuries that do occur.

swimmer's shoulder the painful condition that results from impingement of the muscles, tendons, and other structures during the overhand forward swimming stroke

bursae fluid-filled sacs found in connective tissue that help reduce friction between anatomical structures

RICE (Rest, Ice, Compression, Elevation)

To treat virtually all musculoskeletal injuries, simply remember the acronym RICE: *R*est, *I*ce, *C*ompression, and *E*levation (see Table 6.4).

The first component, rest, is used to eliminate irritation or to avoid further injury. For many fitness-minded people rest is the worst four-letter word a physician can utter. However, complete rest is often crucial for proper

TABLE 6.4

When to Apply RICE* with Acute Injuries

SEVERITY OF INJURY	APPLY RICE
Minor, no loss of function	First 24 hours post-injury
Moderate, some loss of function	24–48 hours post-injury
Severe, major loss of function	48–72 hours post-injury

*RICE = rest, ice, compression, elevation

healing to occur. In some cases, physicians will place an injured limb in a plaster or fiberglass cast to ensure complete rest.

Cold application is used as an anesthetic to reduce pain and as an agent to constrict the blood vessels so that swelling and **hemorrhaging,** or internal or external bleeding, is slowed or stopped. Swelling is caused by the accumulation of blood and damaged tissue cells at the injury site; cold is applied to reduce the blood flow to facilitate clotting and to slow the metabolic rate of the affected tissues. Ice comes in various forms (ice cubes, reusable gel cold packs, single-use chemical cold packs) and should not be applied directly to the skin. A layer of wet toweling or elastic bandage will transmit the cold to the injured area more readily than a dry towel or bandage. When treating an injury at home, you can use a bag of frozen peas or corn; it will thaw in about 20 minutes, can be refrozen, and will not leak like a melting ice bag invariably does! If you use this form of cold, be sure not to eat the repeatedly thawed and refrozen vegetables. Even more convenient are reusable gel cold packs that are widely available and very user friendly. Regardless of the source of the cold, the duration of an individual treatment should be about 20 minutes on, 40 minutes off, with this pattern repeated throughout the day.

Compression of the injured body part helps stop internal hemorrhaging. A 4-inch or 6-inch wide elastic bandage, wrapped in a figure-8 or spiral pattern, can be used to apply indirect pressure to damaged blood vessels. You must be careful, however, that the compression wrap does not interfere with normal blood flow. A throbbing limb is an indication that the compression wrap was applied too tightly and should be loosened.

Elevation of the injured extremity above the level of the heart also helps control hemorrhaging by making the blood work harder (by forcing it to flow "uphill") to get to the injured area. Pillows can be used to create a soft, comfortable surface to support the elevated part.

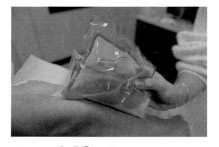

Figure 6.13
Easy-to-use cold gel packs can fulfill the "ICE" portion of RICE.

Treatment of Overuse Injuries

Virtually all overuse injuries can be divided into four categories based on level of pain and disability. This classification system can be used to determine the appropriate level of medical care (see Table 6.5). The RICE protocol is appropriate for fitness-related overuse injuries of all levels of severity.

For most overuse injuries, nonprescription (over-the-counter) anti-inflammatory medications such as aspirin and ibuprofen will relieve mild pain and reduce inflammation. If you use these medications, however, you need to be aware of their limitations and potential side effects. For example, aspirin and ibuprofen should always be taken with food or milk to avoid

hemorrhaging internal or external bleeding

TABLE 6.5

Classification of Overuse Injuries

SEVERITY	SYMPTOMS	TREATMENT
Grade 1	Pain occurs after activity only.	Reduce/modify activity level; evaluate athletic equipment (running shoes worn out? too much tension on tennis racquet strings? bicycle seat height too high or low?); RICE* after the workout.
Grade 2	Pain occurs during and after activity without a significant loss of function.	Same as Grade 1, with the addition of ice massage of the inflamed area; use over-the-counter anti-inflammatory medications (aspirin, ibuprofen) to control inflammation.
Grade 3	Pain occurs during and after activity with a significant loss of function.	Rest; same as Grades 1 and 2, but consult a physician for more potent (prescription-strength) anti-inflammatory medication, and a proper rehabilitation program.
Grade 4	Pain occurs before, during, and after activity and the person is unable to complete the workout.	Combine Grades 1, 2, and 3 treatments; surgery may be indicated in selected cases.

*RICE = rest, ice, compression, elevation
Source: From Roy and Irwin, 1983.

stomach upset. Also, these medications should not be taken for pain for more than 10 days or for fever for more than 3 days, unless directed by a physician. Unfortunately, some individuals use massive doses of these medications to mask pain in their effort to continue exercising. Remember, rest is an essential aspect of the healing process and enables the anti-inflammatory medication to act on the inflamed tissues.

Only rarely will fitness activities result in a situation that is a true medical emergency. Concussions, suspected skull or neck fractures, cardiac emergencies, or internal injuries that appear serious or life threatening *should not be treated with the RICE protocol.* If you are trained in standard or advanced first aid or have current cardiopulmonary resuscitation (CPR) certification, you can provide basic life support to the injured person. If you are not trained in first aid or CPR, you should immediately contact emergency medical services.

Injuries Caused by Environmental Conditions

Regardless of the climate where you live and exercise, seasonal conditions such as temperature, humidity, and wind chill may put you at risk for environmentally related injuries such as hyperthermia and hypothermia. However, If you are in good physical condition and wear appropriate clothes, you can safely withstand a wide range of ambient temperatures and humidity levels (Brooks et al.).

Hyperthermia

Hyperthermia is a potentially fatal excessive core body temperature. Hyperthermia should be a concern when you are exercising or working in humid, warm-to-hot weather, because your body's rate of heat production will often be greater than its ability to cool itself in these conditions.

hyperthermia potentially fatal excessive core body temperature

Sound Decision Making

A CRUCIAL DECISION

I hadn't been downhill skiing in a couple of years, but I thought I was in pretty good shape," says Robin. "I was tired by the afternoon, but my boyfriend wanted to do one last run from the top of the mountain." As they started down the trail, Robin hit a patch of ice and the tips of her skis crossed. The next thing she knew she was flat on her back in the snow, and there was a sharp pain in her knee. The ski patrol came and whisked her down the mountain in a sled to the first-aid hut, where a nurse had Robin lie down with an ice pack on her knee.

That evening the pain had subsided, but Robin's knee was very swollen and she couldn't put any weight on it. Although Robin was hesitant to go to the doctor, her boyfriend insisted that they go to an urgent care facility right away. There, a physician took some X rays to be sure no bones were broken and gave Robin a brace and crutches. She was to stay off her feet as much as possible, continue to use an ice pack, and see an orthopedic specialist as soon as possible.

Over the next few days, the swelling in Robin's knee went down, but the joint still felt strangely loose. She kept her promise to see an orthopedist, who told her she had torn her anterior cruciate ligament (ACL). The doctor explained that the ACL normally stabilizes the front to back and rotation movement of the knee. She could live fairly normally with a torn ACL, though she would have a hard time with sports like soccer, basketball, and skiing that require rapid starting and stopping or changes in direction. And she would face a risk of early arthritis in that knee. Or she could have surgery to reconstruct the ACL. The surgery would be difficult in the short run but would assure her of full functioning in her knee in the future.

Robin decided to have the surgery. "I figured that it was worth it, since I am young and active. And the idea of getting arthritis in my knee kind of scared me. The first couple of weeks after the surgery were pretty difficult, but now I'm glad I did it. The physical therapist really helped me strengthen my knee and the muscles around it. My knee doesn't really bother me any more, but I haven't gotten up the nerve to try skiing again."

There are three types of heat injuries: heat cramps, heat exhaustion, and heat stroke. You can prevent each of these illnesses by taking the following precautions. First, acclimatize yourself properly to hot and/or humid climates through gradual exposure, avoiding exercise during the hottest parts of the day. The process of heat acclimatization causes physiological changes (increases) in the body's cooling efficiency and occurs after about 7 to 14 days of exercising in a hot environment. Second, avoid dehydration through proper fluid (water) replacement following exercise. Third, wear clothing appropriate for the fitness activity and environmental conditions. Finally, use common sense when exercising in hot and humid conditions.

The three types of heat illness are progressively more severe, with *heat cramps* being the least severe. The cause of muscle cramps while exercising in hot weather is not clearly understood. In any case, this condition is easily prevented through adequate fluid replacement and a diet that includes the electrolytes lost during sweating (for example, sodium and potassium).

Heat exhaustion is caused by excessive water loss through intense or prolonged exercise or work in a warm and/or humid environment. Symptoms of heat exhaustion include nausea, headache, fatigue, dizziness and faints, and, paradoxically, "goose bumps" (hair follicle erections) and chills. If you were suffering from heat exhaustion, your skin would appear pale or gray and be cool and moist to the touch. Heat exhaustion actually is a mild case of circulatory system shock, in which the blood pools in the arms and legs, away from the brain and major body organs.

Heat stroke, often called "sunstroke," is a life-threatening emergency condition with reported mortality rates ranging from 20% to 70% (Hafen and Karren). Heat stroke occurs during vigorous exercise when the body's rate of heat production significantly exceeds its cooling capacities and the body becomes overheated. Body core temperature can increase from normal (99.6°F) to 105°–110°F within minutes after the body's cooling mechanism shuts down (normal body core temperature is 1°F higher than normal oral temperature). Rapidly increasing core temperatures can cause brain damage, permanent disability, and death. Common signs and symptoms of heat stroke are dry, hot, and usually red skin; very high body temperature; and a very rapid heart rate.

Heat illnesses may occur in situations where the danger is not obvious. Serious or fatal heat stroke may result from prolonged sauna/steam baths, prolonged total immersion in a hot tub/spa, or exercise in a plastic or rubber, head-to-toe "sauna suit." If while exercising outdoors you experience any of the symptoms or signs mentioned here, you should stop exercising immediately, move to a cooler spot to rest, and drink large amounts of cool fluids. The most important point to remember is that with a commonsense approach to exercise in hot, humid climates, heat illness need never occur.

Hypothermia

Hypothermia is a potentially fatal insufficient core body temperature. When exercising in cool-to-cold weather, especially in windy conditions, your body's rate of heat loss frequently is greater than its heat production, and hypothermia may result. However, bone-chilling cold weather is not a prerequisite for hypothermia. This often deadly condition can occur during prolonged, vigorous exercise in moderate temperatures (40° to 50°F) when combined with windy or rainy conditions.

In mild cases of hypothermia, as your body core temperature dropped from the normal 99.6°F to 93.2°F, you would typically experience cold hands and feet, shivering, poor judgment, apathy, and amnesia (Thornton).

hypothermia potentially fatal insufficient core body temperature

---

MYTHS & CONTROVERSIES

Myth 1

Bicycle helmets won't really protect you in an accident. In fact, helmets are a must, especially for children. According to two recent studies, wearing a helmet decreases the risk of head injury during a crash by 63% to 85%. Yet survey findings show that about 76% of bicycle riders never or almost never wear helmets, and helmet use is lowest among children. Bike helmets these days are lightweight, cool, and comfortable, and could very well save your life.

Myth 2

You can "run through" pain. In fact pain (beyond mild discomfort) is your body's way of warning you that something is wrong. Don't try to keep exercising through a pain; stop and rest. If the pain goes away quickly and you can exercise again without pain it is okay to do so, but if the pain persists, take the day off from your fitness routine and carefully monitor the painful area.

Controversy 1

Ice or heat? There is some confusion about when ice is the most appropriate treatment for an injury, and when heat is best. Most physicians, certified athletic trainers, and physical therapists recommend icing immediately after a sudden, wrenching injury that causes localized pain. This can relieve swelling and minimize spasm. Ice is the best treatment in the days following most injuries. However, chronic or widespread pain that gradually sets in hours after exercise may be soothed by a hot bath or heating pad. Of course, if any pain persists, see a physician.

Shivering ceases in most hypothermia victims as the body core temperature drops to a range between 87°F and 90°F, a sign that the body has lost its ability to generate heat. Death from hypothermia usually occurs at core temperatures between 75° and 80°F.

To prevent hypothermia, a number of commonsense guidelines are suggested. First, analyze the weather conditions and chances of hypothermia prior to your workout, remembering that wind and humidity are factors as important as temperature. Second, employ the "buddy-system": Have a friend join you for your cold-weather outdoor activities. Third, wear layers of appropriate clothing to prevent excessive heat loss (for example, polypropylene or woolen undergarments, Gore-Tex windbreaker, wool hat, and gloves). Finally, don't allow yourself to get dehydrated, particularly when engaging in recreational cycling, long-distance running, or cross-country skiing.

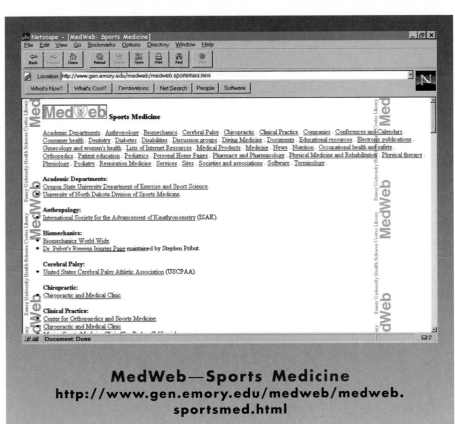

MedWeb—Sports Medicine
http://www.gen.emory.edu/medweb/medweb.sportsmed.html

This clearinghouse for information on exercise-related injuries is maintained by the Emory University Health Sciences Center Library. The searchable database includes lots of interesting and practical topics, including alternative sports medicine, diving medicine, orthopedics, physical therapy, and respiratory medicine.

Critical thinking: Although the focus of this chapter is on preventing exercise-related injury, most of the topics in this site address the treatment of injury. Why do you think this is? How could medical professionals do a better job of educating people about preventing injury in the first place?

Source: From Emory University, Health Sciences Center Library, 1998.

Lifestyle Choices: Plan for Action

As mentioned at the beginning of this chapter, your choice of fitness activities largely dictates your risk of suffering an injury. What types of physical activity do you enjoy? Do you prefer exercising by yourself as a break from your hectic day—for example, taking a long run to give yourself some quiet time for self-reflection? Or do you enjoy exercising with a group of people, perhaps in an aerobics class or a doubles match in tennis, for the social interaction and sheer fun of it? Whatever your fitness regimen, remember to vary your day-to-day activities, utilizing the cross-training principle to minimize your chances of sustaining an overuse injury

If you do sustain an exercise-related injury, you have many choices for medical care. Most often, your family/primary care physician is the medical professional to see first. Patients with more severe musculoskeletal injuries are commonly referred to orthopedists, physicians who specialize in treating injuries to bones, joints, and soft tissues. If your injury requires prolonged rest, you'll need a proper rehabilitation program prior to resuming your previous activity level. Physical therapists and certified athletic trainers employed at sports medicine centers care for recreational athletes to help them recover full function after injury or surgery. Depending on your personal philosophy (and medical insurance benefits), the services of nontraditional allied health practitioners such as chiropractors, licensed massage therapists, and acupuncturists may also be utilized in the healing process.

Prevention of fitness-related injuries is essential, for it is much more difficult and painful to recover from an injury than to prevent it in the first place. Use the information presented in this chapter as a foundation, but obtain additional information about injuries and their prevention and treatment by enrolling in first-aid and sports medicine courses offered at your school.

Summary

The injury frequency associated with fitness activities is relatively low. Numerous factors can increase your risk of injury during exercise, but by creating and following a workout schedule that incorporates the guidelines presented in this chapter you can prevent the majority of these from occurring.

Key concepts that you have learned in this chapter include these:

■ Prudent exercisers start their fitness program slowly; avoid sudden changes or increases in the frequency, intensity, and duration of their workouts; and vary their fitness activities to avoid overuse of muscles, tendons, and joints.

■ Injury prevention involves getting medical screening, using the right equipment, wearing appropriate clothing and footwear, warming up properly, and adopting a commonsense approach.

■ Microtrauma injuries result from cumulative stress placed on body parts; macrotrauma injuries result from accidents.

■ Musculoskeletal injuries generally involve muscle strains, ligament sprains, tendinitis, stress fractures, and general inflammatory conditions.

■ The warning signs and symptoms of common fitness related injuries include pain, swelling, and loss of function.

■ The appropriate procedure for first-aid treatment of most injuries is RICE—rest, ice, compression, elevation.

■ Professional medical care is warranted any time there is noticeable loss of function as a result of an injury.

■ Injuries related to environmental conditions include hyperthermia and hypothermia.

References

American Academy of Orthopaedic Surgeons. *Athletic Training and Sports Medicine,* 2nd ed. Park Ridge, IL: AAOS, 1991.

American College of Sports Medicine. *Guidelines for Exercise Testing and Prescription,* 5th ed. Philadelphia: Lea & Febiger, 1995.

American College of Sports Medicine. The Prevention of Thermal Injuries During Distance Running *(Position Stand).* Indianapolis, IN: ACSM, 1985.

Anderson, M. K., and S. J. Hall. *Sports Injury Management.* Baltimore: Williams & Wilkins, 1995.

Andrish, J., and J. A. Work. How I manage shin splints. *The Physician and Sportsmedicine,* 18 (December): 113–114, 1990.

Arendt, E. A. Common musculoskeletal injuries in women. *The Physician and Sportsmedicine,* 24 (July): 39–48, 1996.

Ballas, M. T., J. Tykyo, and D. Cookson. Common overuse running injuries: Diagnosis and management. *American Family Physician,* 55(7): 2473–2484, May 15, 1997.

Booher, J. M., and G. A. Thibodeau. *Athletic Injury Assessment,* 3rd ed. St. Louis: Mosby, 1994.

Brody, D. M. Running injuries: Prevention and management. *Clinical Symposia,* 390, 1987.

Brooks, G. A., T. D. Fahey, and T. P. White. *Exercise Physiology: Human Bioenergetics and its Applications,* 2nd ed. Mountain View, CA: Mayfield, 1996.

Centers for Disease Control and Prevention. *National Center for Injury Prevention and Control 1997 Fact Book.* Atlanta: U.S. Health and Human Services, 1997.

Clancy, W. G. Tendinitis and plantar fasciitis in runners. In R. D'Ambrosia and D. Drez, Jr., eds., *Prevention and Treatment of Running Injuries.* Thorofare, NJ: Charles B. Slack, 1982.

Curwin, S., and W. D. Stanish. *Tendinitis: Its Etiology and Treatment.* Lexington, MA: Collamore Press, 1984.

Elmqvist, L. G., P. A. F. H. Renstrom, and J. I. B. Pyne. Nordic and alpine skiing. In F. H. Fu and D. A. Stone, eds., *Sports Injuries: Mechanisms, Prevention, Treatment.* Baltimore: Williams & Wilkins, 1995; 481–500.

Erie, J. C. Eye injuries: Prevention, evaluation, and treatment. *The Physician and Sportsmedicine,* 19 (November): 108–122, 1991.

Hafen, B. Q., and K. J. Karren. *Prehospital Emergency Care and Crisis Intervention,* 4th ed. Englewood Cliffs, NJ: Prentice-Hall, 1992.

Hamill, J., and K. M. Knutzen. *Biomechanical Basis of Human Movement.* Baltimore: Williams & Wilkins, 1995.

Jackson, D. L. Stress fracture of the femur. *The Physician and Sportsmedicine,* 19 (July): 39–42, 1991.

Kronisch, R. L., T. K. Chow, L. M. Simon, and P. F. Wong. Acute injuries in off-road bicycle racing. *American Journal of Sports Medicine,* 24: 88–93, 1996.

MacIntyre, J. G., J. E. Taunton, D. B. Clement, D. R. Lloyd-Smith, D. C. McKenzie, and R. W. Morrell. Running injuries: A clinical study of 4,173 cases. *Clinical Journal of Sports Medicine,* 1: 81–87, 1991.

Munnings, F. Cyclist's palsy: Making changes brings relief. *The Physician and Sportsmedicine,* 19 (September): 113–119, 1991.

National Institutes of Health. *NIH Consensus Statement—Physical Activity and Cardiovascular Health,* 13 (3): December 18–20, 1995; 1–33.

Nevasier, R. J., T. J. Nevasier, and J. S. Nevasier. Concurrent rupture of the rotator cuff and anterior dislocation of the shoulder joint in the older patient. *Journal of Bone and Joint Surgery,* 7OA: 1308–1311, 1988.

Nigg, B. M., and B. Segesser. The influence of playing surfaces on the load on the locomotor system and on football and tennis injuries. *Sports Medicine,* 5: 375–385, 1988.

Nike, Inc. *Sports Research Review,* July/August, 1989.

Noakes, T. D. Fatal cycling injuries. *Sports Medicine.* 20: 248–362, 1995.

O'Connor, F. G., J. R. Sobel, and R. P. Nirschl. Five-step treatment for overuse injuries. *The Physician and Sportsmedicine,* 20 (October): 128–142, 1992.

Priest, J. D., V. Braden, and S. G. Gerberich. The elbow in tennis, Part 1: An analysis of players with and without pain. *The Physician and Sportsmedicine,* 8 (April): 80–91, 1980.

Schelkun, P. H. Swimmer's ear: Getting patients back in the water. *The Physician and Sportsmedicine*, 19 (July): 85–90, 1991.

Shea, K. G., B. Shumsky, and F. Shea. Shifting into wrist pain: DeQuervain's disease and off-road mountain biking. *The Physician and Sportsmedicine*, 19 (September): 59–63, 1991.

Thomas, S., J. Reading, and R. J. Shepard. Revision of the Physical Activity Readiness Questionnaire (PAR-Q). *Canadian Journal of Sport Science,* 17: 338–345, 1992.

Thornton, J. S. Hypothermia shouldn't freeze out cold weather athletes. *The Physician and Sportsmedicine,* 18 (January): 109–113, 1990.

Van Tilburg, C. Surfing, windsurfing, snowboarding and skateboarding: Medical aspects of board sports. *The Physician and Sportsmedicine,* 24 (November): 63–74, 1996.

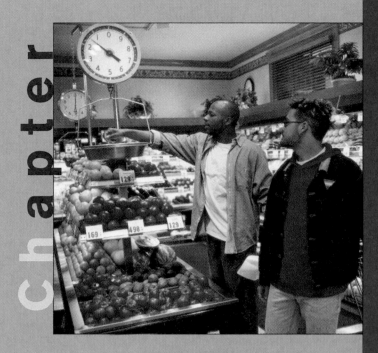

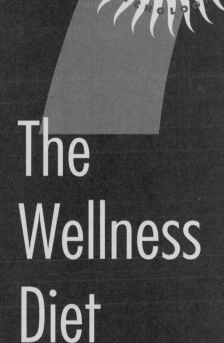

The Wellness Diet

One Student's View

In my pre-college days, my food intake was limited in variety by what my parents could afford to buy and what they wanted to eat. Now I live in the dorms and have access to an all-you-can-eat menu where I can choose to eat many more fruits, vegetables, and vegetarian meals than I ordinarily would be able to eat. I make the decisions of what I want to eat, so I choose healthy foods that I enjoy.

—Christopher John Voster

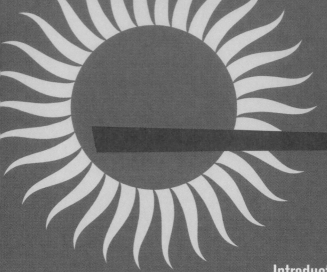

Introduction

The bell sounds. You rush off to the dorm before the cafeteria closes to grab a bite to eat before your next class. After an afternoon filled with lectures and labs, you manage to get a workout in before meeting friends for pizza. Across town, a classmate races home to pick up her kids so she can fix dinner for her family before returning to campus to study for midterms. The demands placed on college students today require that we juggle our basic need for food with the responsibilities of family, friends, athletics, school, and work. Although food provides the energy to perform our daily tasks and maintain our physical health, choosing healthy options is often difficult. Knowing what is a good choice requires that you know how to balance your diet and how to "eat healthy" even when the choices are limited. You need not despair of an occasional lapse in eating nutritiously, as long as your long-term eating habits are healthy. Understanding good nutrition can help you make dietary choices that contribute to wellness.

Objectives

After reading this chapter, you should be able to

- **Define the functions of the nutrients in our food**

- **Outline the recommendations for the amount of carbohydrate, protein, and fat in your diet that is conducive to wellness**

- **Describe the Food Guide Pyramid plan for a balanced diet**

- **Identify the special nutritional considerations for physically active people**

- **Evaluate your current diet and recommend changes to improve your overall nutrition**

Food: A Source of Energy

At the risk of trivializing its amazing complexity, the human body can be compared to an automobile engine. The engine is constructed so that when a spark is applied to a mixture of oxygen and gasoline, the resulting explosion moves the pistons in the cylinders, which, in turn, causes the wheels to rotate. The mixture of oxygen and fuel and the release of the spark are regulated by the engine's carburetor and distributor. Thus, the engine converts the potential (stored) energy in the fuel to the mechanical energy of the turning wheels.

The body is infinitely more complicated, but, like the engine, it has a distinct structure, it uses energy, and its processes are regulated. In the body, the muscles are probably the closest approximation to the engine. Here, oxygen and fuel are mixed and, in a reaction regulated by enzymes, the energy that is released powers muscular contractions. Whereas a machine is assembled from manufactured parts, the human body is synthesized from within itself, the raw materials being provided from the food we eat. Food contains **nutrients**—the specific substances the body requires for energy and for structural and regulatory purposes.

Although we commonly speak of the energy in food in terms of **calories,** the correct terminology is kilocalories. For ease of calculation, food energy is measured in kilocalories (abbreviated as kcalorie or kcal; also seen as Calorie). One kcal is equivalent to the amount of heat necessary to raise the temperature of 1 kilogram of water one degree centigrade. Therefore, we say that a bagel contains the energy equivalent of 250 kcals.

Foods high in complex carbohydrates, such as grains, beans, and vegetables, or those with naturally occurring sugars, such as fruits, are usually relatively low in calories and contain a wide variety of vitamins and minerals. Foods that contain few calories per unit of weight are said to have a **low caloric density.** Fruits, vegetables, beans, and grains are foods with low caloric density, because water and/or fiber, which are noncaloric, make up a significant portion of their weight. These foods also have **nutritional density,** which refers to foods that are a good source of vitamins and minerals relative to their caloric content. Some sources of carbohydrates, such as table sugar, are considered to be **empty calories,** which refers to foods that have a high sugar and fat content and lack any significant amount of vitamins and minerals. Examples of foods that are low in nutritional density would be soft drinks, candy, and certain snack foods. In some cases, foods that in their natural state are nutritionally dense become high-calorie foods when prepared with sugar and fats. For example, cakes and cookies are made from flour, which is ground wheat, but a considerable amount of sugar and fat is added when they are baked. You should check food labels when you buy canned fruit or fruit juices to be sure that they have not been sweetened with sugar, which can make them high-calorie foods.

Nutrients for a Healthy Body

Nutrients serve three functions in the body: structural, regulatory, and energy providing. There are six types of nutrients in food: water, carbohydrates, fats (lipids), proteins, vitamins, and minerals. Water, proteins, fats, and minerals are the nutrients that have structural roles in the building and repair of body tissues. Vitamins, minerals, and proteins have regulatory roles in energy-yielding

nutrients specific substances that the body requires for energy and for structural and regulatory purposes

calorie common term for kilocalorie; the amount of energy required to raise the temperature of one kilogram of water one degree centigrade

low caloric density refers to foods that contain few calories per unit of weight

nutritional density refers to foods that are good sources of vitamins and minerals relative to their caloric content

empty calories refers to foods that have a high sugar and fat content and lack any significant amount of vitamins and minerals

metabolic reactions and in the distribution of water throughout the body. Carbohydrates, fats, and, to a lesser extent, proteins serve as energy sources.

Water

You might be surprised to learn that you are made up mostly of water, but in fact water accounts for 50% to 60% of your total body weight. Most of this water is located within the cells of the body (intracellular), with the rest of it (approximately 40%) found in the blood and in the fluid occupying the small spaces between the blood vessels and the cells (the interstitial spaces). Water provides the medium for transporting substances throughout the body in the blood or out of the body in the urine. In addition, it provides the environment for the many reactions that take place in the cells and tissues of the body. The distribution of water throughout the body also helps control body temperature.

Water is an important dietary component because you need to replenish the water your body loses each day. A person maintains a **hydrated** condition when the daily water intake is equal to the daily water loss. For the most part, your need for water is well served by your sensation of thirst. However, this may not be the case if you sweat heavily during exercise, because the water you drink after a vigorous workout may satisfy your thirst before it replenishes the water lost from sweating. The total amount of water that is lost each day, excluding exercise-induced sweat loss, averages about 2 to 2.5 quarts (2 to 2.25 liters) (see Figure 7.1). This is the amount that needs to be replenished to avoid becoming dehydrated. Sweat loss increases considerably if you exercise, particularly if you exercise in the heat, as discussed later in this chapter.

Not surprisingly, one of the best ways to replenish the water lost is to drink beverages. Water is an excellent choice because it is rapidly absorbed into the bloodstream and contains no calories. Skim milk and unsweetened fruit juices are also good choices because they contain many important nutrients and are relatively low in calories. Although soft drinks are perhaps the most popular beverage in the United States, they have little or no nutritional

Figure 7.1

These values show daily water intake and loss for a moderately active adult. With intake and loss being equal, this person is well hydrated.
Source: From Hales, 1994.

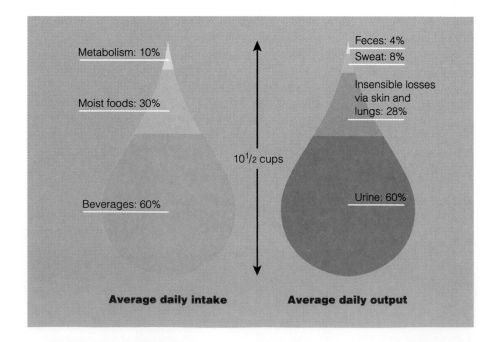

Metabolism: 10%

Feces: 4%
Sweat: 8%

Insensible losses via skin and lungs: 28%

Moist foods: 30%

10 1/2 cups

Beverages: 60%

Urine: 60%

Average daily intake   **Average daily output**

hydrated condition that exists when the daily body water losses are replenished by the daily water intake

value other than the water they contain. Soft drinks also can contain a large amount of sugar. Beer is another very popular beverage. However, as any beer drinker can tell you, alcohol is a diuretic—that is, it is a substance that stimulates urine production, thus contributing to fluid loss by the body. The nutrient content of beer is slight relative to the calories it contains: A 12-ounce can of light beer contains 100 kcal, while a can of regular beer has 145 kcal.

We also get significant amounts of water from solid food, particularly fruit and vegetables, which may be 80% to 90% water. Finally, we gain water through energy metabolism. When carbohydrates, fats, and proteins are aerobically metabolized to yield energy (as described in Chapter 2), an oxygen atom combines with two atoms of hydrogen (from the carbohydrate, fat, or protein) to form water.

Carbohydrates

Carbohydrates, a major source of energy in the diet, are almost exclusively of plant origin, occurring in grains (wheat, rice, corn), vegetables, fruits, and beans; they can also be found in an animal source—milk.

There are three types of carbohydrates: sugars, starches, and fiber. Sugars and starches, also known as simple and complex carbohydrates, respectively, are easily digestible sources of energy. Fiber, which is discussed later in this chapter, is indigestible and therefore does not provide energy to the body. However, fiber does provide an important function in health and wellness. A sample of foods that are good sources of carbohydrates is presented in Figure 7.2.

Americans typically get only 40% to 45% of their calories from carbohydrates, far short of the American Heart Association recommendation of 55% to 60%. If you are very physically active, you may need as much as 60% to 70% of your calories from carbohydrates to help replenish your muscle and liver carbohydrate stores (glycogen, see Chapter 2) between your exercise sessions. For a diet of 2,400 kcal each day, you would need to eat 360 grams (g) of carbohydrates to have 60% of your calories supplied by carbohydrates (1 g of carbohydrate contains 4 kcal). A diet with 60% of the calories from carbohydrate can be met by planning meals around grains, rice, pasta, fruits, and vegetables.

Fats

Fats (or lipids) are the most concentrated form of energy in the diet, containing 9 kcal/g. The major form of dietary fat is **triglyceride,** which is a collection of three fatty acids attached to a three-carbon carbohydrate called glycerol. **Fatty acids** are long chains of carbon atoms with hydrogen atoms attached; they come in three forms: saturated, monounsaturated, and polyunsaturated.

Saturated Versus Unsaturated Fatty Acids. If each carbon atom in a fatty acid is attached to as many hydrogen atoms as it can hold, which in most cases is two, it is termed a **saturated fatty acid.** In an **unsaturated fatty acid,** some of the carbon atoms do not bind with two hydrogen atoms, but instead form a double bond with a neighboring carbon atom. If there is one such double bond, the fatty acid is monounsaturated; if there is more than one double bond, the fatty acid is polyunsaturated. Figure 7.3 shows an example of a saturated, monounsaturated, and polyunsaturated fatty acid as part of a triglyceride.

carbohydrates major source of energy in the diet, in the form of sugars and starches found in grains, fruits, vegetables, and beans; also includes fiber, which is not digestible

fats most concentrated form of energy in the diet, containing 9 kilocalories per gram

triglyceride three fatty acids attached to a molecule of glycerol

fatty acids long chains of carbon atoms with hydrogen atoms attached that come in three forms: saturated, monounsaturated, and polyunsaturated

saturated fatty acid fatty acid in which each carbon atom is attached to as many hydrogen atoms as it can hold, which in most cases is two

unsaturated fatty acid fatty acid in which some of the carbon atoms do not bind with two hydrogen atoms, but instead form a double bond with a neighboring carbon atom

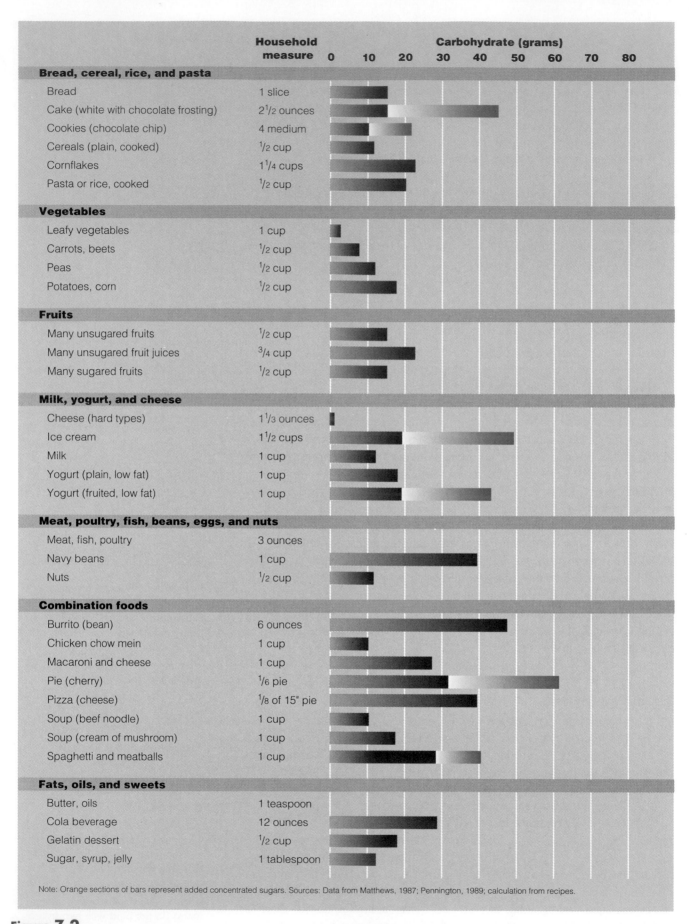

Figure 7.2

Note the wide disparity in the carbohydrate content of selected foods.

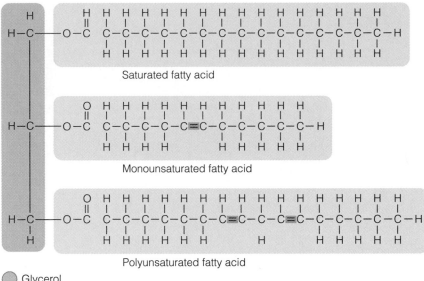

Saturated fatty acid

Monounsaturated fatty acid

Polyunsaturated fatty acid

● Glycerol
○ Fatty acid

Figure 7.3
The fatty acids attached to the glycerol backbone in this triglyceride are examples of each type of fatty acid: saturated, monounsaturated, and polyunsaturated.
Source: From Christian and Greger, 1994.

The distinction between saturated and unsaturated fats is important, because the consumption of saturated fats has been shown to elevate blood cholesterol levels, increasing the risk for coronary artery disease. In contrast, blood cholesterol levels are reduced when unsaturated fats replace saturated fats in the diet (see Chapter 13). Triglycerides with saturated fatty acids are usually of animal origin, such as beef fat and butter, and tend to be solid at room temperature. Unsaturated fatty acids usually come from plants and tend to be liquid at room temperature (oils). There are exceptions to these generalities, however. Coconut oil and palm oil, often referred to as tropical oils, are of plant origin, yet they contain predominantly saturated fatty acids. On the other hand, the oils found in fish contain many unsaturated fatty acids. Figure 7.4 compares several forms of fat for the proportion of saturated, monounsaturated, and polyunsaturated fat they contain.

The typical American diet is high in fat, with 35% to 40% of the calories supplied by this nutrient. The main dietary sources of fat are meat, fish and poultry, dairy products, and fats and oils. The last category represents fats that are added to other foods, such as salad dressings, baked goods, and fried foods. Because high-fat diets are associated with coronary artery disease, obesity, and cancers of the colon, breasts, and prostate, reducing fat consumption is strongly recommended. For example, the National Cholesterol Education Program and the American Heart Association recommend that fat should account for 30% or less of total daily calories, with saturated, monounsaturated, and polyunsaturated fat each contributing approximately one-third of this total. With a diet of 2,400 kcal each day, eating 80 g of fat would provide 30% of your total calories (since 1 g of fat contains 9 kcal).

One way to reduce the amount of fat in your diet is to increase your intake of carbohydrates. Grain and cereal products, beans, fruits, and vegetables contribute very little fat to your diet—unless you add fat in the form of butter or rich sauces.

To help you appreciate the variation in fat content among different foods, Table 7.1 presents some examples of foods and the amount of fat they contain. Keep in mind, however, that the goals for the amount of fat in your diet apply to the composition of foods you consume over several days, not necessarily to

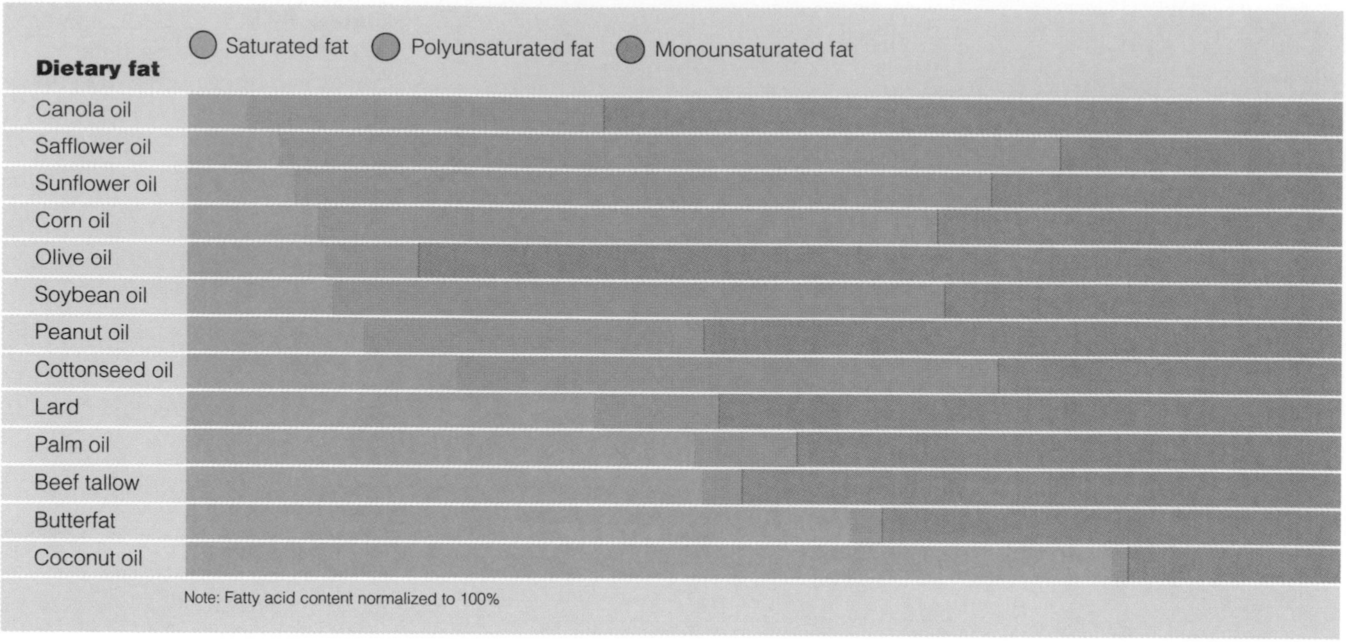

Dietary fat	◯ Saturated fat	◯ Polyunsaturated fat	◯ Monounsaturated fat
Canola oil			
Safflower oil			
Sunflower oil			
Corn oil			
Olive oil			
Soybean oil			
Peanut oil			
Cottonseed oil			
Lard			
Palm oil			
Beef tallow			
Butterfat			
Coconut oil			

Note: Fatty acid content normalized to 100%

Figure 7.4

Plant sources of oils are usually low in saturated fat, and animal sources of fat are usually high in saturated fat. Note, however, that coconut oil, a plant source, is high in saturated fat.

Source: From Christian and Greger, 1994.

cholesterol lipid of animal origin that is a factor in the development of heart disease

protein complex nutrient that is composed of combinations of amino acids and that serves all three functions of a nutrient: structural, regulatory, and energy-providing

amino acids building-block units of proteins, containing carbon, hydrogen, oxygen, nitrogen, and, in some cases, sulfur

each meal or each item of food. Note, too, that certain foods that may have more than 30% of their calories as fat, such as meat, cheese, and milk, can also be high-quality sources of protein, vitamins, and minerals. Selecting the low-fat form of these foods, such as skim milk or lean meats or poultry, will help you reduce your daily caloric intake and ensure that you do not exceed the recommended intake of fat (see Table 7.2).

Cholesterol. Another form of fat in the diet is **cholesterol,** a lipid of animal origin that is a factor in the development of heart disease. It is an important molecule, for it serves as a structural component of cell membranes, and it is the structure from which steroid hormones (such as estrogen and testosterone) and vitamin D are synthesized. Dietary cholesterol is found only in foods of animal origin such as red meat, whole milk, egg yolks, liver, and shellfish. Cholesterol is also synthesized in the body, primarily in the liver. The amount of cholesterol in a variety of foods is presented in Table 7.3. The National Cholesterol Education Program and the American Heart Association recommend that the daily intake of dietary cholesterol not exceed 300 milligrams (mg) per day.

Proteins

Protein is a complex nutrient composed of combinations of amino acids that serves all three functions of a nutrient: structural, regulatory, and energy providing. Like carbohydrates and fats, **amino acids,** the building-block units of proteins, contain carbon, hydrogen, and oxygen. The distinguishing feature of amino acids, and thus protein, is that they also contain nitrogen and, in some cases, sulfur. Different combinations of these elements produce the structure of the 20 amino acids that human cells use in the synthesis of proteins. Of the three functions that protein serves, the structural and regulatory are the most important. Not only is protein a structural component of all cells, but it also forms the enzymes that regulate cellular reactions. Carbohydrates and fats are the major sources of energy in human metabolism, but

TABLE 7.1

Fat Content of Selected Foods

ITEM	PORTION SIZE	TOTAL FAT CONTENT(G)	SATURATED FAT CONTENT(G)
Skim milk	1 cup	1	Less than 1
Dry cereal[a]	1 cup	Not more than 1	Less than 1
MacDonald's Quarter-Pounder hamburger	1 burger	20.7	8.1
Fruits[b]	1 whole or 1 cup	Less than 1	Less than 1

[a]Cheerios, Special K, Grape-Nuts, Corn Flakes, Frosted Flakes, Raisin Bran, or All-Bran
[b]bananas, apples, oranges, or strawberries

TABLE 7.2

U.S. Departments of Agriculture and Health and Human Services Guidelines for Reducing Dietary Fat

- Use fats and oils sparingly in cooking.
- Use small amounts of salad dressings and spreads, such as butter, margarine, and mayonnaise.
- Favor liquid vegetable oils because they are lower in saturated fat.
- Check labels on foods to see how much fat and saturated fat are in a serving.
- Have two or three servings each day, for a total of 6 ounces, from among the following: meat, poultry, fish, dry beans, and eggs.
- Trim fat from meat; remove skin from poultry.
- Substitute cooked dry beans and peas occasionally for meat.
- Moderate the use of egg yolks and organ meats (liver, kidneys).
- Have two or three servings of milk and milk products daily.
- Choose skim or low-fat milk and fat-free or low-fat yogurt and cheese most of the time.

proteins can also serve as a source of energy when, in the cell, the nitrogen has been removed from the amino acids.

Of about 20 amino acids used in the formation of proteins in your body, the **essential amino acids** are the 9 amino acids that cannot be synthesized by the body and thus must be obtained in the diet.

Essential Amino Acids	Nonessential Amino Acids
Histidine	Alanine
Isoleucine	Arginine
Leucine	Asparagine
Lysine	Aspartic Acid
Methionine	Cysteine
Phenylalanine	Glutamic Acid
Threonine	Glutamine
Tryptophan	Glycine
Valine	Proline
	Serine
	Tyrosine

essential amino acids nine amino acids that cannot be synthesized by the body and thus must be obtained in the diet

TABLE 7.3
The Cholesterol and Protein Content of Selected Foods

ITEM	PORTION SIZE	WEIGHT (G)	CHOLESTEROL (MG)	PROTEIN (G)
Beef—lean, composite of cuts	2 oz	57	51	14
Butter	1 pat (1 tsp)	5	11	0
Cheese				
American	1 oz	28	27	4
Cheddar	1 oz	28	30	7
Cottage, low-fat, 1%	1 cup	226	10	28
Swiss	1 oz	28	26	8
Chicken, roasted, no skin				
Dark meat	2 oz	57	54	16
Light meat	2 oz	57	48	16
Eggs, large	1 egg	50	213	6
Ice cream (about 10% fat)	1 cup	133	59	5
Margarine	1 tbsp	14	0	0
Milk				
Whole, 3.3% fat	1 cup	244	33	8
Low-fat, 2%	1 cup	244	18	8
Low-fat, 1%	1 cup	244	10	8
Skim	1 cup	244	5	8
Peanut butter	1 tbsp	16	0	4
Pizza with cheese[a]	1 slice	48	7	8

[a]Source of the cholesterol

Source: J. L. Christian and J. L. Greger, *Nutrition for Living*, 4th ed. (Redwood City, CA: Benjamin/Cummings, 1994), pp. 230, 253.

The other 11 amino acids are nonessential in the sense that the body can manufacture them from elements available in the cells. In special cases, some nonessential amino acids may become conditionally essential, as is the case with tyrosine in people with the inherited disorder phenylketonuria (PKU). Although most foods contain some protein, there is considerable variation in both the quantity (see Table 7.3) and the quality. The superior sources of protein contain the full complement of the essential amino acids in the proportions necessary to support protein synthesis in the cells of the body. Animal sources of protein are generally superior to plant sources. On a scale where eggs rate 100 as a protein source, cow's milk scores 93; fish,

76; beef, 74; the legumes soybeans, peas, and peanuts, 73, 64, and 53, respectively; and whole wheat, 65.

Individuals who refrain from eating meat but consume eggs and dairy products (the ovo-lacto vegetarians) will still have high-quality sources of protein in their diets. Those who abstain from all foods of animal origin (the vegans) must plan their diets to obtain the essential amino acids because most plant sources of protein lack one or more of these. **Complementary proteins** are proteins that do not contain all the essential amino acids but differ in the essential amino acids they lack, so that consuming them during the same day will provide all the essential amino acids and serve as a complete source of protein. For example, legumes (soybeans, peanuts, lentils, lima beans, peas) are complementary with grains (wheat, rice, corn) or nuts and seeds. For this reason, a peanut butter sandwich, a bean-and-rice casserole, a bean burrito, or hummus (ground chick peas and sesame seeds) each provides a high-quality protein meal.

The Recommended Dietary Allowances (RDA) for protein and certain vitamins and minerals have been established by the Food and Nutrition Board of the National Research Council/National Academy of Science. These recommendations reflect the consensus of the board for the amount of these nutrients that are adequate to meet the nutritional needs of practically all healthy people. The RDA for protein is 0.8 g per kilogram (kg) body weight, which translates to approximately 58 g to 63 g per day for males (weighing 160 to 173 pounds) and 46 g to 50 g per day for women (weighing 127 to 138 pounds).

The typical American diet provides sufficient protein, representing 12% to 15% of the total daily caloric intake. If protein intake exceeds the body's requirement, the excess will be used as an energy source (1 g of protein contains 4 kcal) or converted to fat and stored in the adipose tissue, because the body does not store protein. This being the case, and since protein sources of food tend to be expensive, there is no real benefit to making protein more than 15% of your total daily caloric intake. Therefore, if you eat an 8-ounce steak, three 8-ounce glasses of milk, and two eggs (a total of 100 g protein) in a day, it is likely the excess protein will be stored as fat!

Vitamins

Vitamins are complex organic compounds of widely varying structure and function that serve as regulators of the energy-yielding reactions of the cell (particularly the B vitamins) and also play a role in the structure or synthesis of body tissues. For example, vitamin D helps strengthen bones, vitamin C does the same for the connective tissues collagen and cartilage, vitamin K aids the clot-forming proteins in the blood, vitamin A helps form the visual pigment rhodopsin in the eye, and vitamins E, K, and C help to protect the integrity of cell membranes. Most foods contain vitamins; the major sources of each vitamin are listed in Table 7.4, which also summarizes the functions, symptoms of deficiency and excess, and RDA of each vitamin.

As shown in Table 7.4, consuming an excessive amount of several vitamins can produce serious side effects. Vitamins A, D, E, and K are fat-soluble vitamins, which means they can dissolve in fat and are usually obtained in dietary fat. Because they are stored in the fatty tissues of the body, an excess of these fat-soluble vitamins can accumulate with repeated high doses and lead to a risk of toxic effects from overconsumption, as can occur when taking a vitamin supplement. The B vitamins and vitamin C

complementary proteins
proteins that do not contain all the essential amino acids but differ in the essential amino acids they lack so that consuming them together in a meal will provide all the essential amino acids and serve as a complete source of protein

vitamins complex organic compounds of widely varying structure and function that serve as regulators of the energy-yielding reactions of the cell and also play a role in the structure or synthesis of body tissues

TABLE 7.4

Key Information About the Vitamins

VITAMIN	RDA FOR HEALTHY ADULTS AGES 19–50	MAJOR DIETARY SOURCES	MAJOR FUNCTIONS	SIGNS OF SEVERE, PROLONGED DEFICIENCY	SIGNS OF EXTREME EXCESS
Fat-Soluble					
A	Females: 800 RE[a] Males: 1000 RE[a]	Fat-containing and fortified dairy products, liver, provitamin carotene in orange and deep green fruits and vegetables	Vitamin A is a component of rhodopsin; carotenoids can serve as antioxidants; retinoic acid affects gene expression	Night blindness; damage to the cornea causing permanent blindness; dry, scaling skin; increased susceptibility to infection	Damage to liver, bone; headache, irritability; vomiting; hair loss; blurred vision; some fetal defects; yellowed skin
D	<25years: 10µg[b] >25 years: 5µg	Fortified and full-fat dairy products, egg yolk (diet often not as important as sunlight exposure)	Promotes absorption and use of calcium and phosphorus	Rickets (bone deformities) in children; osteomalacia (bone-softening) in adults	Calcium deposition in tissues leading to cerebral, cardiovascular, and kidney damage
E	Females: 8 α-tocopherol equivalents Males: 10 α-tocopherol equivalents	Vegetable oils and their products; nuts, seeds	Antioxidant to prevent cell membrane damage	Possible anemia and neurological effects	Generally nontoxic, but may worsen clotting defect in vitamin K deficiency
K	Females: <25: 60 µg >25: 65 µg Males: <25: 70 µg >25: 80 µg	Green vegetables, tea	Aids in formation of certain proteins, especially those for blood clotting	Defective blood coagulation causing severe bleeding on injury	Liver damage and anemia from high doses of the synthetic from menadione
Water-Soluble					
Thiamin (B$_1$)	Females: 1.1 mg[c] Males: 1.5 mg	Pork, legumes, peanuts, enriched or whole-grain products	Coenzyme used in energy metabolism	Nerve changes; edema; heart failure; beriberi	Generally nontoxic
Riboflavin (B$_2$)	Females: 1.3 mg Males: 1.7 mg	Dairy products, meats, eggs, enriched grain products, green leafy vegetables	Coenzyme used in energy metabolism	Skin lesions	Generally nontoxic

are water-soluble vitamins, which means they are distributed in the body fluids. The body cannot store these vitamins to any extent, so an excess is usually excreted in the urine. Thus, most of them do not have any toxic effects when taken in excess. Our requirement for energy and dietary protein can be met by consuming a limited selection of foods, but we would likely develop several vitamin deficiencies if we were to do so. Thus, a varied, well-balanced diet is important to ensure an adequate intake of vitamins and minerals. (See the Myths and Controversies box.)

TABLE 7.4 Continued

Key Information About the Vitamins

VITAMIN	RDA FOR HEALTHY ADULTS AGES 19–50	MAJOR DIETARY SOURCES	MAJOR FUNCTIONS	SIGNS OF SEVERE, PROLONGED DEFICIENCY	SIGNS OF EXTREME EXCESS
Niacin	Females: 15 niacin equivalents Males: 19 niacin equivalents	Nuts, meats; provitamin tryptophan in most proteins	Coenzyme used in energy metabolism	Pellagra (multiple vitamin deficiencies including niacin)	Flushing of face, neck, hands; potential liver damage
B₆	Females: 1.6 mg Males: 2.0 mg	High-protein foods in general	Coenzyme used in amino acid metabolism	Nervous, skin, and muscular disorders; anemia	Unstable gait, numb feet, poor coordination
Folic acid	Females: 180 μg Males: 200 μg	Green vegetables, orange juice, nuts, legumes, grain products	Coenzyme used in DNA and RNA metabolism; single carbon utilization	Megaloblastic anemia (large, immature red blood cells); GI disturbances	Masks vitamin B₁₂ deficiency; interferes with drugs to control epilepsy
B₁₂	2 μg	Animal products	Coenzyme used in DNA and RNA metabolism; single carbon utilization	Megaloblastic anemia; pernicious anemia; nervous system damage	Thought to be nontoxic
Pantothenic acid	4–7 mgᵃ	Animal products and whole grains; widely distributed in foods	Coenzyme used in energy metabolism	Fatigue, numbness, and tingling of hands and feet	Generally nontoxic; occasionally causes diarrhea
Biotin	30–100 μgᵃ	Widely distributed in foods	Coenzyme used in energy metabolism	Scaly dermatitis	Thought to be nontoxic
C (ascorbic acid)	60 mg	Fruits and vegetables, especially broccoli, cabbage, cantaloupe, cauliflower, citrus fruits, green pepper, kiwi fruit, strawberries	Functions in synthesis of collagen; is an antioxidant; aids in detoxification; improves iron absorption	Scurvy; weakness; delayed wound healing; impaired immune response	GI upsets

ᵃEstimated safe and adequate daily dietary intake in 1989 RDAs
ᵇμg = micrograms
ᶜml = milligrams
Source: From Shils and Young, 1988.

Minerals

Minerals are the inorganic chemical elements other than carbon, hydrogen, oxygen, and nitrogen that make up the body. Twenty to 22 of these elements are considered to be essential. The major minerals—those present in large quantities—include calcium and phosphorus (concentrated in bone), sulfur, potassium, sodium, chloride, and magnesium; the minerals present in only small amounts are referred to as trace minerals (see Table 7.5). As a nutrient, minerals are important in the structure of bone, teeth, connective tissue,

minerals inorganic chemical elements other than carbon, hydrogen, oxygen, and nitrogen

MYTHS & CONTROVERSIES

Controversy **Vitamin and mineral supplements are essential for today's active adults.** Currently, there is no evidence that physically active people or athletes require nutrients that cannot be provided by a well-balanced diet. Our food supply is rich in vitamins and minerals necessary for an active lifestyle. Many people view taking vitamin or mineral supplements as a nutritional insurance policy—a way of ensuring that they get enough of these nutrients. This practice often results in vitamin-enriched urine, because excessive amounts of the water-soluble vitamins are simply excreted.

In certain situations, a vitamin and mineral supplement may be necessary. Vitamin and mineral supplementation is needed when a person does not take in adequate calories or eat a well-balanced diet—when restricting food intake to lose weight, during illness, when under stress, when consuming a significant portion of calories as empty calories (soft drinks, sweets, snack foods), when following a vegetarian diet, or when undergoing chemotherapy, radiation therapy or surgery. People who have been diagnosed with nutritional deficiency conditions (such as low iron stores) require supplementation. Also, certain conditions increase the requirement for vitamins and minerals, such as pregnancy and lactation.

Vitamin and mineral supplements have been touted for increasing endurance, improving performance, and increasing muscle mass. There are few well-controlled studies that verify many of the proposed claims. Supplements such as blue-green algae, creatine, amino acid supplements and chromium picolinate are popular among athletes. Antioxidants, such as vitamin C, E, selenium, and beta-carotene, are currently under investigation for their protective effects on cells from environmental and metabolic oxidative damage. It is not yet clear, however, whether taking these vitamin supplements provides any assistance to the antioxidants that the body produces on its own to protect the integrity of the cells. Some studies show a lower incidence of certain cancers in people with higher intakes of the antioxidant vitamins, but more research is needed before recommendations can be made for supplementing your diet. Furthermore, excessive amounts of the fat-soluble vitamins (A, D, E, K) or such minerals as iron, calcium, iodine, or zinc can impair the absorption of other minerals and/or result in tissue damage or death. Unless you have been diagnosed as deficient in a particular fat-soluble vitamin or a mineral, you should be cautious about taking a supplement.

enzymes, hemoglobin, and myoglobin. They are also important in maintaining water balance, nerve function, and enzyme activity.

Calcium. All the minerals are important, but calcium, iron, and sodium have received special attention because of their relationship to osteoporosis, anemia, and high blood pressure, respectively. Osteoporosis is the demineralization and weakening of the bones, which makes them more susceptible to fractures. This disease, discussed at length in Chapter 13, is much more prevalent in women than men, especially in postmenopausal women. Inadequate calcium intake, low estrogen levels, and sedentary lifestyles are associated with low bone density in women.

For both women and men, it is important to establish strong bones as a young adult so that the inevitable loss of bone that occurs with aging will not result in critically low bone density and brittle bones. Sufficient intake of calcium, estrogen therapy (if medically necessary), and regular exercise have been shown to increase bone density in the young adult and to slow the rate of bone loss in the elderly. The RDA for calcium is 1,200 mg for men and women ages 19 to 24 and 800 mg for those 25 and older, although some experts feel that intakes up to 1,500 mg per day is more appropriate for women. In any case, few women consume adequate amounts of calcium; surveys show that their average daily calcium intake is less than 800 mg.

Dairy products are the best food sources of calcium, with an 8-ounce glass of milk providing 300 mg and an 8-ounce serving of yogurt providing

TABLE 7.5

Key Information About Many Essential Minerals

MINERAL	RDA FOR HEALTHY ADULTS AGES 19–50	MAJOR DIETARY SOURCES	MAJOR FUNCTIONS	SIGNS OF SEVERE, PROLONGED DEFICIENCY	SIGNS OF EXTREME EXCESS
Major Minerals					
Calcium	1,200 mg for ages 19–24; 800 mg for 25 and older	Milk, cheese, dark green vegetables, legumes	Bone and tooth formation; blood clotting; nerve transmission	Stunted growth; perhaps less bone mass	Depressed absorption of some other minerals; perhaps kidney damage
Phosphorus	1,200 mg for ages 19–24; 800 mg for 25 and older	Milk, cheese, meat, poultry, whole grains	Bone and tooth formation; acid-base balance; component of coenzymes	Weakness; demineralization of bone	Depressed absorption of some minerals
Magnesium	Females: 350mg Males: 350mg	Whole grains, green leafy vegetables	Component of enzymes	Neurological disturbances	Neurological disturbances
Sulfur	(Provided by sulfur amino acids)	Sulfur amino acids in dietary products	Component of cartilage, tendons, and proteins	(Related to protein deficiency)	Excess sulfur-containing amino acid intake leading to poor growth; liver damage
Sodium	a	Salt, soy sauce, cured meats, pickles, canned soups, processed cheese	Body water balance; nerve function	Muscle cramps; reduced appetite	High blood pressure in genetically predisposed individuals
Potassium	a	Meats, milk, many fruits and vegetables, whole grains	Body water balance; nerve function	Muscular weakness; paralysis	Muscular weakness; cardiac arrest
Chloride	a	Same as for sodium	Plays a role in acid-base balance; formation of gastric juice	Muscle cramps; reduced appetite; poor growth	High blood pressure in genetically predisposed individuals
Trace Minerals					
Iron	Females: 15 mg Males: 10 mg	Meats, eggs, legumes, whole grains, green leafy vegetables	Components of hemoglobin, myoglobin, and enzymes	Iron deficiency anemia; weakness; impaired immune function	Acute: shock; death Chronic: liver damage; cardiac failure
Iodine	0.15 mg	Marine fish and shellfish, dairy products, iodized salt, some breads	Component of thyroid hormones	Goiter (enlarged thyroid)	Iodide goiter
Fluoride	1.5–4.0 mg[b]	Drinking water, tea, seafood	Maintenance of tooth (and maybe bone) structure	Higher frequency of tooth decay	Acute: GI distress Chronic: mottling of teeth; skeletal deformation

(Continued on next page)

TABLE 7.5 Continued

Key Information About Many Essential Minerals

MINERAL	RDA FOR HEALTHY ADULTS AGES 19–50	MAJOR DIETARY SOURCES	MAJOR FUNCTIONS	SIGNS OF SEVERE, PROLONGED DEFICIENCY	SIGNS OF EXTREME EXCESS
Zinc	Females: 12 mg Males: 15 mg	Meats seafood, whole grains	Component of enzymes	Growth failure; scaly dermatitis; reproductive failure; impaired immune function	Acute: nausea; vomiting; diarrhea Chronic: adversely affects copper metabolism and immune function; anemia
Selenium	Females: 0.055 mg Males: 0.070 mg	Seafood, meats, whole grains	Component of enzymes; functions in close association with vitamin E	Muscle pain; maybe heart muscle deterioration	Nausea and vomiting; hair and nail loss
Copper	1.5–3.0 mg[b]	Seafood, nuts, legumes, organ meats	Component of enzymes	Anemia; bone and cardiovascular changes	Nausea; liver damage
Cobalt	(Required as vitamin B_{12})[a]	Animal products	Component of vitamin B_{12}	Not reported except as vitamin B_{12} deficiency	With alcohol: heart failure
Chromium	0.05–0.2 mg[b]	Brewer's yeast, liver, seafood, meat, some vegetables	Involved in glucose and energy metabolism	Impaired glucose metabolism	Lung and kidney damage (occupational exposures only)
Manganese	2.0–5.0 mg[b]	Nuts, whole grains, vegetables and fruits, tea	Component of enzymes	Abnormal bone and cartilage	Central nervous system damage (occupational exposures)
Molybdenum	0.075–0.25 mg[b]	Legumes, cereals, some vegetables	Component of enzymes	Disorder in nitrogen excretion	Inhibition of enzymes; adverse effect on copper metabolism

[a]No formal recommendation
[b]Estimated safe and adequate daily dietary intake
Source: Data from M. E. Shils, V. F. Fairbanks, E. Beutler, and N. W. Solomons in *Modern Nutrition in Health & Disease*, Philadelphia: Lea & Febiger, 1988; RDA Subcommittee, 1989; E. J. Underwood, *Trace Elements in Human and Animal Nutrition*, New York: Academic Press, 1977.

approximately 400 mg. Dark green, leafy vegetables, such as spinach and turnip greens, are good nondairy sources of calcium. Some foods, such as orange juice, are now available in a calcium-fortified form. You can also use calcium supplements if your food sources are inadequate.

Iron. Iron is an essential constituent of the oxygen-carrying molecules of hemoglobin (in the red blood cells) and myoglobin (in the muscle fibers). It is also a vital element in the structure of the mitochondria and plays an important role in the metabolic reactions that generate energy from the breakdown of carbohydrates, fat, and protein (see Chapter 2). When blood hemoglobin levels are low, the body's ability to transport oxygen to cells is impaired, and this condition reduces the person's capacity to exercise or to do work. **Anemia** refers to a deficiency in blood hemoglobin levels (less than 12 mg per 100 milliliter [ml] of blood for women and less than 13 mg per 100 ml of blood for men), and it is usually caused by an insufficiency in iron intake.

Because of the iron lost during menstruation, women have a greater need for dietary iron than men: 15 mg per day, as opposed to 10 mg per day for men. Animal sources of iron (heme iron) are absorbed more effectively than plant sources (nonheme iron), but the absorption of nonheme iron can be improved if it is consumed with sources of vitamin C, such as orange juice. Meat, fish, and poultry are the best sources of iron in the diet, but eggs, legumes, whole grains, and enriched cereals also contain appreciable amounts. In addition, cooking with cast-iron cookware will increase the iron content of foods.

Sodium. Sodium, potassium, and chloride are termed electrolytes because they dissolve into the body water and have an electrical charge (sodium and potassium have a positive charge; chloride has a negative charge). Electrolytes are involved in the transmission of nerve impulses and the contraction of muscle fibers. The concentration of these electrolytes influences the distribution of water in the body, which is an important factor in the regulation of blood pressure. For most people, the balance between sodium intake in the diet and sodium excretion by the kidneys is usually well maintained. For some "sodium sensitive" individuals, however, increased intake of sodium is not matched by increased sodium excretion, and high blood pressure results. High blood pressure, or **hypertension,** is a disorder that contributes to the incidence of heart disease, stroke, kidney damage, and eye problems.

Because most people consume more sodium than they need, and because some people (the "sodium sensitive") will experience a reduction in their blood pressure when they reduce their sodium intake, everyone is advised to moderate his or her consumption of sodium. Currently, Americans consume 4 to 6 g of sodium per day. There is no RDA for sodium, but the minimum requirement is considered to be 0.5 g (500mg). One teaspoon of salt contains 2g (2,000 mg) sodium. Experts agree that sodium intake should be limited, but they differ somewhat in setting the maximum amount. For example, the American Heart Association recommends that sodium intake not exceed 3 g (3,000 mg or 1½ teaspoons of salt) per day, whereas the National Academy of Sciences recommends an upper limit of 2.4 g (2,400 mg or approximately 1¼ teaspoons of salt) per day. The difference in the recommendations is probably not significant, from a health standpoint.

Table salt (40% sodium and 60% chloride) provides approximately one-third of our daily sodium intake, another third comes from the salt in processed foods (soups, processed cheeses, and processed luncheon meats, hot dogs, or bacon), and the final third occurs naturally in foods (see Table 7.6). Adding less salt to food and avoiding foods that already have salt added to them will greatly reduce your daily intake of sodium. Salt tablets, once recommended to replace the salt lost in sweat, are not recommended and may even be dangerous to your health.

anemia deficiency in blood hemoglobin levels (less than 12 mg per 100 ml of blood for women and less than 13 mg per 100 ml of blood for men)

hypertension high blood pressure, a disorder that contributes to the incidence of heart disease, stroke, kidney damage, and eye problems

TABLE 7.6

Sodium Content of Selected Foods[a]

ITEM	PORTION SIZE	SODIUM (MG)
Vegetables		
Beans, green, cooked without salt	½ cup	19
Beans, green, canned with salt	½ cup	170
Cucumber, chopped	½ cup	1
Dill pickle	1 medium	928
Potato, baked	1 average	16
Potato chips	1 oz (14 chips)	132
Milk, yogurt, cheese		
Milk, 2% fat	1 cup	122
Cheese, cheddar	1⅓ oz	235
Cheese, processed	2 oz	448
Yogurt, plain low-fat	1 cup	159
Meats, poultry, fish, eggs, beans, nuts		
Beans, refried	1 cup	1073
Beef, ground, cooked without salt	2 oz	33
Corned beef, canned	2 oz	553
Frankfurter	2 oz	638
Salmon, broiled	2 oz	33
Salmon, canned with salt	2 oz	310
Peanut butter, chunky style	¼ cup	313
Combination foods		
Bean, cheese burrito	1 oz	583
Cheese pizza	1 slice (4½ oz)	622
Chicken chow mein	1 cup	722
Spaghetti, canned entree with meat	1 cup	220
Fats, oils, sweets		
Beer	12 oz	8
Butter	1 tsp	39
Soy sauce	1 tbsp	1029
Sugar	1 tbsp	trace

[a]Estimated minimum requirement of healthy adults is 500 mg sodium.
Source: From Christian and Greger, 1994.

Balancing the Diet: The Food Guide Pyramid

Now that you know the functions and some of the dietary sources of the nutrients you require, you need to learn how to ensure that your diet provides them in adequate amounts. The most practical approach to dietary planning is to group foods into five categories: (1) fruits, (2) vegetables, (3) grain products, (4) milk and milk products, and (5) meats and meat alternatives. The various foods in each category have similar nutrient values. Thus, rather than analyze each item of food for its nutrient content, you can select the recommended amounts of food from each of the food groups on a daily basis and be confident that you are receiving an adequate supply of your RDA for water, carbohydrates, fat, protein, vitamins, and minerals. Table 7.7 presents examples from each food group and lists the major nutrients found in each group.

TABLE 7.7

The Five Food Groups and Their Major Nutrients

FOOD GROUP	EXAMPLES	MAJOR NUTRIENTS PROVIDED	REPRESENTATIVE SERVING SIZES
Fruits	Apples, oranges, bananas, berries, tomatoes, pears	Carbohydrate (and fiber[a]) Water Vitamins: A[a], C[a], folic acid[a] Minerals: iron[a], calcium[a]	Average piece of fruit ½ cup of fresh, frozen, or canned fruit ¼ cup dried fruit
Vegetables	Broccoli, lettuce, green beans, potatoes, cabbage	Carbohydrate (and fiber) Water Vitamins: A[a], C[a], folic acid[a] Minerals: iron[a], calcium[a]	½ cup of fresh, frozen, or canned vegetable 1 cup raw leafy vegetable ¼ cup dried vegetable
Bread, cereal, rice, and pasta	Breads, rolls, bagels; cereals, dry and cooked; pasta; rice, corn, and other grains; popcorn, crackers, pancakes, muffins, tortillas	Carbohydrate (and fiber[a]) Protein Vitamins: thiamin, niacin Minerals: iron[a], magnesium[a], selenium[a] Water[a]	Slice of bread 1 cup cereal 1 cup pasta 3 cups popped popcorn 6 saltines, snack crackers, or 3-ring pretzels 1 bagel, dinner roll, or English muffin
Milk, yogurt, and cheese	Milk, yogurt; cheese; ice cream, ice milk, frozen yogurt	Protein Carbohydrate[a] Fat[a] Vitamins: riboflavin, B$_{12}$, A[a], D[a] Minerals: calcium, phosphorus Water[a]	1 cup milk or yogurt 1½ slices cheese or 1⅓ oz hard cheese 1½ cups ice cream or ice milk 2 cups cottage cheese
Meats, poultry, fish, dry beans, eggs, and nuts	Meat, fish, poultry; eggs; seeds; nuts; soybeans, tofu; other legumes (peas and beans)	Protein Carbohydrate[a] (and fiber[a]) Fat[a] Vitamins: niacin, B$_6$, B$_{12}$[a], thiamin[a] Minerals: iron, zinc Water[a]	2–3 oz lean cooked meat, fish, or poultry 2 eggs 1 cup dried peas or beans 4 tbsp peanut butter 2 oz nuts or seeds

[a]Found in some, but not all, foods in this group
Source: Nutrition and Your Health: *Dietary Guidelines for Americans,* USDA and DHHS, 1980, 1985, 1990.

Figure 7.5

The Food Guide Pyramid was developed by the U.S. Department of Agriculture to convey their nutritional recommendations. With the lowest, widest levels of the pyramid being the bread, vegetable, and fruit groups, the pyramid emphasizes the role of high-carbohydrate, low-fat, and high-fiber foods.

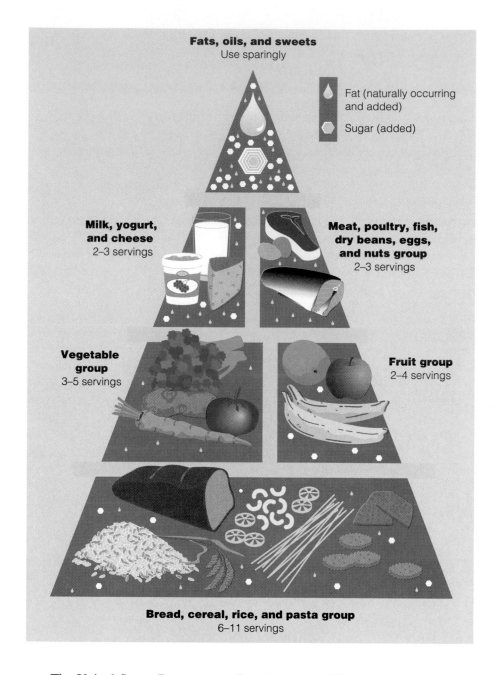

Fats, oils, and sweets
Use sparingly

Fat (naturally occurring and added)

Sugar (added)

Milk, yogurt, and cheese
2–3 servings

Meat, poultry, fish, dry beans, eggs, and nuts group
2–3 servings

Vegetable group
3–5 servings

Fruit group
2–4 servings

Bread, cereal, rice, and pasta group
6–11 servings

The United States Department of Agriculture (USDA) has recently developed a new design for illustrating the healthful diet: the Food Guide Pyramid (see Figure 7.5). The pyramid promotes the consumption of a diversity of foods while also limiting fats and sugars in the diet. To show that carbohydrates should constitute 55% to 60% of your total daily caloric intake, the first two levels of the pyramid are made up of the bread, cereal, rice, and pasta group (6–11 servings), the vegetable group (3–5 servings), and the fruit group (2–4 servings). The major sources of protein, which should constitute 12% to 15% of your total daily caloric intake, are on the third level of the tapering pyramid: the milk, yogurt, and cheese group (2–3 servings) and the meat, poultry, fish, dry beans, eggs, and nuts group (2–3 servings). Finally, the tip of the pyramid shows not a food group but rather the proportion of your daily calories contributed by the high-calorie, low-nutrient fats, oils, and sweets, which should be eaten only sparingly. By the use of a symbol representing the fat that has been added to or may already be a significant component of the original food item, the pyramid demonstrates that the dairy and meat groups can contain much of the fat in your diet. Thus, you should select the low-fat forms of these foods to limit fat to 20% to 30% of the calories you consume while still obtaining the protein, vitamins, and minerals they provide.

Following the Food Guide Pyramid is relatively simple and allows for differences in food preferences and for seasonal variation in food availability. As you plan your diet, keep these recommendations in mind:

1. *Choose a variety of foods.* Even though the foods in each food group are nutritionally similar, some will be a better source of a particular vitamin or mineral than others. For example, among the three fruits oranges, apricots, and bananas, apricots are the best source of vitamin A, oranges of vitamin C, and bananas of potassium. Choosing a variety of foods from a food group will make the nutritional strengths and weaknesses of the foods complement one another. By contrast, consuming only a narrow assortment of foods from a given group will eventually lead to nutritional deficiencies.

2. *Eat foods in moderation.* Even healthful foods may contain nutrients that should be restricted. Some foods, such as meat, can be an excellent source of high-quality protein and also be the major source of certain vitamins (for example, B_6 and B_{12}) or minerals (iron, zinc); at the same time, they are a source of fat and cholesterol.

3. *Choose wholesome foods.* As foods are processed, vitamins, minerals, and fiber are lost when parts of the food are removed (for example, the skin of the potato or apple, or the bran or germ of wheat) or as a result of cooking. Adding sugar, salt, and/or fat to the food may make it tastier, but these additives can contribute to the development of high blood pressure, obesity, and elevated blood cholesterol levels. For example, when a potato is processed into a potato chip, a wholesome, high-carbohydrate, low-fat food becomes a high-fat, high-sodium snack food. Similarly, orange juice gives you the natural sweetness, vitamins, and fiber (in the pulp) of an orange; orange drinks are diluted with water, sugar is added, and the pulp is removed. Again, a wholesome food has been turned into a high-calorie food with little nutritious value.

Adopting a healthier diet may be easier than you think. Start with the base of the Food Guide Pyramid by adding several bread items, cereal, pasta and/or rice to your meal. This could include oatmeal and a couple of pieces of toast for breakfast, a sandwich on whole grain bread for lunch or a pasta dish for dinner. Next, include vegetables in the meal, in the form of a stir-fry, a side dish, in a soup, or as a raw appetizer while you're preparing your meal. Fruits can be included as a juice with a meal, as a dessert, or even as a snack. Meats should be thought of as a side dish and not as the main focus of the meal. Add some meat to a stir-fry, to a pasta dish, or to a salad. Canned meats and ready-to-eat meats may work if you are in a hurry. Beans, fish, and poultry are also excellent sources of protein. Dairy products can be included on salad (cheese), as a topping for a baked potato (cottage cheese), as a beverage (milk), or as a dessert (frozen yogurt). All fats, no matter what type, should be used sparingly. Wherever possible, try to use only a small amount of salad dressing, margarine, and oils in cooking. This is not to say that "other foods" such as snack foods,

STATS-AT-A-GLANCE
Current Eating Patterns of Americans

■ % of American adults who eat breakfast: 75%

■ % of college students who call themselves vegetarians: 15%

■ # of times the average American eats out per year: 198

■ # of meals eaten out per week: 4

■ Average sugar consumption per year from all sources: 143 pounds

■ # of cups of coffee the average American consumes per day: 3.5 cups

■ # of servings of vegetables the average American eats per day: 2–3

(University of California at Berkeley Wellness Letter, Oct., 1996, Dec., 1995, April, 1996; *FoodService Director*, 10 (8), August 15, 1997, p.136)

fast foods, and dessert foods cannot be included. Keep in mind that it is your intake of foods and nutrients for the total day that is important. An occasional treat, as long as you are making healthy food choices on a daily basis, is all right.

The Modern Diet

American Eating Habits

Less time is spent today sitting down with our families for a traditional family meal than was the pattern 25 or 30 years ago. Mealtime is less formal today, with only 25% of American households having sit-down meals five nights per week. There is more snacking (or "grazing") that occurs between meals and even as meals are prepared. Take-out meals are more prevalent today, with pizza and Chinese food two of the more popular options. Prepared entrees, fast foods, and ready-made meals, all available at grocery stores, make planning of meals a thing of the past for many people. People plan meals more on a spur of the moment. These trends make it increasingly difficult to eat a low-fat, nutrient-dense diet rich in whole grains, fruits, and vegetables. The good news is that eating establishments have responded to people's desire to eat more healthfully. Increasingly, salad bars, low-fat entrees, and fresh fruits/vegetables are appearing on menus. Consumers are still ultimately in control of balancing their daily intake to include foods from the Food Guide Pyramid.

Fiber, Fruits, and Vegetables

Even though we cannot digest **dietary fiber** and it has no calories, fiber helps prevent constipation, may lower the risk of some cancers (such as colon cancer), and is generally underconsumed by people with a Western diet. The level of fiber recommended by the American Dietetic Association is 20 g to 35 g per day. By selecting whole grain breads and cereals and eating at least 5 servings of fruits and vegetables, especially green and yellow vegetables and citrus fruits, your fiber intake would be met. This recommendation has recently received strong reinforcement with the finding that broccoli and other cruciferous vegetables (cauliflower, cress, brussels sprouts, and cabbage) have a chemical, sulforaphane, that detoxifies carcinogens (agents that promote cancer development in cells). Unfortunately, surveys continue to show that most people (up to 77%) do not eat five or more servings of fruits and vegetables per day. The National Cancer Institute reports that Americans average between three and four servings per day. If you can develop the habit of thinking of fruits when you want a snack, you will be well on your way to a more healthful diet.

Dietary fiber occurs as the **insoluble,** fibrous form (found primarily in the cell walls of plants) or the **soluble,** nonfibrous form that dissolves in water to form a gel (such as the fiber found in oats, beans, and apples). Both forms cannot be broken down by human digestive enzymes. Insoluble fiber is responsible for helping to prevent certain types of cancers and for preventing constipation. Soluble fiber is credited with decreasing blood cholesterol levels.

dietary fiber complex carbohydrate substances in food that cannot be broken down by human digestive enzymes

insoluble fiber dietary fiber that does not dissolve in water, but "holds" water; typically found in plant cell walls

soluble fiber dietary fiber that dissolves in water to form a gel

A ◆ WELLNESS ◆ DIET

Do

▲ Keep your fat intake to less than 30% of your total daily calories.

▲ Learn which foods are high in fat and eat them only occasionally.

▲ Eat lots of carbohydrates—six to eleven servings per day.

▲ Keep fruits and vegetables on hand for snacks.

▲ Eat fresh or minimally processed foods as much as possible.

▲ Drink plenty of water.

▲ Learn to read food labels and look at them when you shop.

▲ Look for healthier options at fast-food restaurants, such as salads with low-fat dressings, baked potatoes, fruit juices, and burgers without cheese, mayonnaise, or bacon.

▲ Substitute fish, chicken, or meatless dishes for some red meat.

▲ Use skim or low-fat milk and milk products.

▲ Broil, bake, or boil foods instead of frying them in fat.

▲ Get curious about those unfamiliar things in the produce section. Try a new fruit or vegetable every week.

▲ Help children develop good eating habits that will stay with them for life.

Don't

▼ Eat fast food every day; save it for an occasional treat.

▼ Develop the snack food habit; try fruits and veggies instead of chips, cookies, and candy.

▼ Add salt to food without tasting it first.

▼ Get taken in by false nutritional claims. If a product promises results that seem too good to be true, they probably are.

Vegetarianism

There is no one vegetarian diet. Vegetarians range from those who avoid red meat, to those who exclude all foods from animal sources (meat, poultry, fish, eggs, milk). In our country, people are vegetarian for a variety of reasons.

There may be a lack of affordability or availability of animal products, a desire to avoid harm to animals, a religious belief that prohibits eating certain animal products, a desire to eat "low on the food chain," a desire to preserve the world's food supply, or a desire to avoid animal sources for health reasons. Vegetarianism is associated with a lower risk of developing obesity, heart disease, hypertension, diabetes, and colon cancer. The common types of vegetarianism include semi-vegetarians (or partial-vegetarians), who eat small amounts of poultry, fish, and seafood in addition to plant foods; **ovo-lacto-vegetarians,** who include eggs ("ovo") and dairy products ("lacto") in addition to plant foods; **lacto-vegetarians,** who include only dairy products and plant foods in their diet; and **vegans** (the strictest vegetarians) who eat only foods of plant origin. Just because a diet is vegetarian does not necessarily mean it is healthy. Careful diet planning to obtain all the essential nutrients becomes increasingly more difficult as the vegetarian diet becomes stricter or more restricted. A vegan must plan foods with adequate amounts of protein, riboflavin, vitamin D, vitamin B_{12}, calcium, iron, and zinc. Includ-

Sound Decision Making

RUNNING CLEAN ON BETTER FUEL

Eduardo grew up in a large, close-knit family in which holidays and special events were usually celebrated with a feast. Fried chicken, cake, pastries, chips—these foods still signal comfort and good times to him. And because Eduardo has never had a problem with his weight, he hasn't thought much about what he eats. Since he started running regularly last semester, however, his awareness of his body and its needs has increased, and Eduardo has started to think seriously about paying more attention to his diet. If running could make such a big difference in how he feels, maybe eating more healthfully would also be a change for the better.

Eduardo starts by keeping a food diary of everything he eats for three days. He also notes whom he is with at the time and how he feels. In analyzing the food diary, Eduardo notices that eating is often a social activity for him, and he eats most of his high-fat foods while watching sports on TV with his brothers or at fast-food restaurants with his friends. He also snacks a lot on candy and chips while he is at school or studying, and he rarely eats fresh vegetables. On the positive side, Eduardo usually has a healthy breakfast of cereal and fruit, and he eats lots of carbohydrates in the form of bread and pasta. Based on this information, Eduardo sets three goals for himself: he will limit fast food meals to once a week, he will substitute healthy snacks for chips and candy, and he will eat three servings of vegetables per day.

Limiting his trips to fast food places turns out to be very difficult for Eduardo because it means spending less time with his friends. So he revises his plan to allow him to go to the restaurants, but to eat baked potatoes and salads instead of burgers and fries. Changing his snacking habits means a certain amount of preparation every morning. He makes little bags of treats like fruit, carrots, and baked corn chips to take with him to school and while he studies. Eduardo finds he likes the sense of self-sufficiency he gets from preparing his own snacks. To add more vegetables to his diet, Eduardo starts out by cooking large portions of broccoli and squash to go with his dinner. This doesn't work out too well because he doesn't really like these vegetables, and for awhile he thinks there is no way for him to enjoy three servings of vegetables each day. But slowly he starts to add vegetables to other things: peppers and onions on pizza, tomato and cucumber on sandwiches, and an occasional baked potato for lunch. By eating this way, Eduardo is able to meet his goal to eat more vegetables.

Two months later Eduardo has ironed out most of the difficulties with his plan and eating more healthfully has become a habit instead of a chore. Eduardo does feel better about his body, and more in control of his lifestyle. As he runs each evening, he imagines that his body runs cleaner on vegetables than it did on fast-food burgers.

ing 11 servings from the grain group and 4 servings of legumes, nuts, and seeds per day will help meet the protein requirements. Tofu and soy milk also contribute protein as well as calcium. Our bodies can make vitamin D from a cholesterol precursor if we spend approximately one half-hour per day outside in the sun. If not, a supplement may be necessary. Vitamin B_{12}, found only in animal foods, occurs in foods fortified with B_{12}, such as yeast products, breakfast cereals, and soy milk. Otherwise, a vitamin B_{12} supplement may be necessary. Riboflavin is found in green leafy vegetables, whole grains, yeast, and legumes. Calcium is found in fortified tofu, green leafy vegetables, nuts, fortified orange juice, bread, and fortified soy milk. Again, supplements may be necessary to consume the recommended amount. Iron can be found in whole grains, fortified breakfast cereals, dried fruits, nuts, and legumes. And good sources of zinc include whole grains and legumes.

If you are a vegetarian, or planning on becoming one, take time to plan your diet to make sure you are consuming foods in the correct amounts with the nutrients you need. Eating a variety of foods is the key.

Food Irradiation

Food irradiation is already here. Many of us are not aware that we are eating food that has been irradiated. For example, potatoes are irradiated to inhibit sprouting, wheat is irradiated to eliminate insects, and spices are irradiated to destroy pathogenic microbes. Pork is irradiated to control trichinae worm infestations. In irradiation, a gamma ray (similar to those produced by microwaves or ultraviolet light) is passed through a food. The process controls pathogens. An irradiated food is no more dangerous than conventionally processed foods and contains compounds similar to those found in foods processed by older methods. Because food irradiation generates little heat and deactivates microbes that are deleterious to quality, irradiated food remains fresh longer, and nutrient losses are minimal. Food irradiation is a safer alternative in food preservation than the use of chemicals and fumigants to decrease microbial counts in spices.

Interpreting Food Labels

The healthy diet is high in carbohydrates; low in fat, sodium, cholesterol, and sugar; and adequate in protein, calcium, and other minerals and vitamins. One of the best ways to find out whether your diet meets these requirements is to read the nutritional labels on the foods you eat. (For foods without labels such as fruits, vegetables, fish, eggs, and meat, consult a food composition table to determine their nutritional content. Such a table is found in the Appendix of this text.) The Food and Drug Administration (FDA) implemented the following regulations to make food labels more user friendly and informative:

- The label prominently displays the fat, cholesterol, carbohydrate, sodium, and protein content of a serving and the number of calories it contains. It also lists the recommended levels of these items, except for protein, and the percentage each serving will provide. The format for food labels is depicted in Figure 7.6.

- The serving size listed is more realistic with regard to the customarily consumed portion. In the past, the serving size listed was often smaller

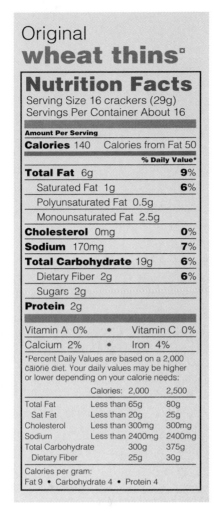

Figure 7.6

Food labels are a useful source of information if you know how to read them. The new food label is designed to be more user friendly than before.
Source: From Nabisco, Inc.

ovo-lacto-vegetarians vegetarians who eat eggs ("ovo") and dairy products ("lacto") in addition to plant foods

lacto-vegetarians vegetarians who eat only dairy products and plant foods in their diet

vegans vegetarians who eat only foods of plant origin.

than what people usually consumed; this measurement implied that the item contained fewer calories and that the package contained more servings than it actually did.

■ The use of descriptive terms has been limited and their meanings standardized. For example, "fat free" means less than 0.5 g of fat per serving, with no added ingredient that is fat or oil; "low fat" means 3 g or less of fat per serving and per 100 g of the food; and a claim of "no cholesterol" or "low cholesterol" cannot be made if the food contains more than 2 g of saturated fat per serving.

■ Health claims for foods can be made for the following nutrient-disease relationships:

cancer and fat

cancer and fiber-containing grain products, fruits, and vegetables

cancer and fruits and vegetables

cardiovascular disease and saturated fat and cholesterol

cardiovascular disease and fiber-containing grain products, fruits, and vegetables

osteoporosis and calcium

hypertension and sodium

■ When more than one sweetener is used in a food, all sweeteners are listed together in the ingredients, under the collective term *sweeteners,* and then listed individually. All ingredients in a product are listed in descending order of their predominance. Collecting all the sweeteners into one item shows their proportion in the food. If they were listed individually, the various sweeteners (sugar, corn syrup, fructose, and so on) would be distributed throughout the list, which could obscure the fact that, collectively, these sweeteners were the major ingredient in the food.

If you are to eat right, you must think of food labels as required reading. Spend a little time in the supermarket aisle looking them over as you choose the foods in your wellness diet.

Nutritional Needs of the Physically Active Person

This text strongly promotes a physically active lifestyle. People often wonder whether the increased expenditure of energy that comes with being physically active alters a person's nutritional needs. In general, it does not. The active person's need for vitamins and minerals is, for the most part, identical to that of the inactive person. However, a deficient state may become more apparent to a regular exerciser than to a sedentary person because the deficiency may cause an impairment in performance. For example, a man with anemia will notice a lack of energy for his exercise sessions because of the iron deficiency and resultant reduced capacity of his blood to transport oxygen to the exercising muscles. Likewise, a woman who is deficient in calcium may have weak bones regardless of whether she exercises, but the stresses applied to the skeleton during such exercises as running may result in a fracture that the inactive woman would not experience until a later point in life, when her bones became even more brittle.

One of the advantages of the physically active lifestyle is that the increased expenditure of energy makes it easier to maintain an energy balance. A **positive caloric balance** is achieved when the daily consumption of food energy exceeds the amount of energy expended, resulting in an increase in body fat. When you participate in regular exercise, you have a larger total energy expenditure than if you are sedentary, which means you can consume more food while still maintaining your body weight. By consuming more food, particularly nutritionally dense foods, you are more likely to be receiving your daily requirements in protein, vitamins, and minerals. Being physically active can also allow you to consume some empty calories, such as desserts or soft drinks, because the nutritionally sound diet can provide the nutrients you need in fewer calories than what is needed to balance the energy expended during the day. Of course, this should be done in moderation to avoid ingesting too much dietary fat or displacing more nutritious foods from your diet.

Water

When you exercise, your muscles generate heat. To avoid elevating your body temperature to dangerously high levels, this heat must be transmitted to the environment. The major mechanism for releasing heat when you exercise is the secretion of sweat from the sweat glands in the skin. The sweat absorbs heat from the skin and evaporates, cooling the skin and the blood beneath it, but the cooling effect of evaporation is at the expense of your body water supply. An exercise-trained person can lose up to 2 or 3 liters of body water in an hour of heavy exercise. The reduced blood volume that results from water loss will impair the transfer of heat from the muscles to the skin, and heat injury can occur (see Chapter 6). Thus, you need to maintain water levels while you exercise and to **rehydrate**—to replenish the water in the body, particularly following heavy sweat losses—afterward.

The main goal is to replenish your body water levels, so plain water would seem to be the best rehydrating drink. However, Ethan Nadel, an authority on the physiological responses to exercising in the heat, reports that rehydration occurs more rapidly and completely if the beverage consumed contains some sodium. Apparently, when you drink plain water, your blood becomes more dilute, which blunts your thirst and also stimulates urine production. With some sodium (50–100 mg per cup) in the drink, your thirst is maintained, so you consume more fluid and restore body water more effectively. And while sport drinks are often promoted as electrolyte replacement beverages (because sodium and potassium are lost in sweat), there is no special need to replace these minerals through the beverages you consume after exercise. The normal foods and fruit drinks in your diet will readily replace whatever electrolytes were lost in your sweat. The inclusion of electrolytes in sport drinks serves a more important purpose by enhancing the consumption of enough fluids to replenish the fluids lost during exercise.

To best maintain a hydrated state when exercising in the heat, follow these steps:

1. Weigh yourself before and after workouts, and replenish your fluid loss at the rate of 1 pint (16 fluid ounces) for every pound of weight lost.

2. Drink beverages containing sodium to enhance rehydration.

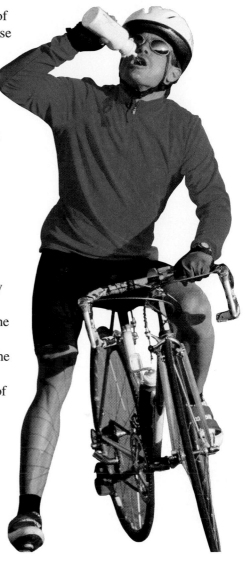

The water lost from sweating during exercise should be replenished to avoid the harmful effects of dehydration.

positive caloric balance condition in which the daily consumption of food energy exceeds the amount of energy expended during a day, resulting in an increase in body fat

rehydrate to replenish the water in the body, particularly following heavy sweat losses

3. Drink beverages that contain 6% to 8% carbohydrates (the sugars glucose and/or sucrose) to improve palatability.

4. Do not restrict fluids before or during exercise. If the exercise is quite prolonged (over an hour), drinking beverages containing carbohydrates during the exercise can help to maintain blood and muscle glucose levels.

Proteins

There is a common perception that your need for protein increases when you exercise regularly. Indeed, in reviewing the research on the topic, Lemon reports that strength-trained athletes and even endurance athletes (for example, runners) need more than the RDA of 0.8 g of protein per kg body weight. These studies indicate that strength and power athletes should consume 1.2 g to 1.7 g of protein per kg body weight and that endurance athletes should consume 1.2 g to 1.4 g of protein per kg body weight. Although these athletes need more than the RDA for protein, they do not need to increase the amount of protein in their diet. Rather, by following the recommendations to have 12% to 15% of their total daily caloric intake as protein, they will more than adequately meet their protein requirements. The typical American diet contains a sufficient amount of protein to support an active lifestyle.

Carbohydrates

Carbohydrates are an important source of energy during exercise, but the body's capacity to store carbohydrates as muscle and liver glycogen is rather limited. Thus, an extended bout of exercise can deplete the exercising muscles of virtually all their glycogen. Consecutive days of vigorous exercise combined with a diet that is low in carbohydrates will also result in muscle glycogen depletion. Insufficient carbohydrate in the diet is one cause of the chronic fatigue some athletes experience during periods of heavy training. Researchers have shown that a diet that was 70% carbohydrates was necessary to refill muscle glycogen stores between workouts when runners were performing 2-hour training sessions on consecutive days (Costill). When their diet was just 40% carbohydrates, similar to the typical American diet, they were unable to restore the glycogen that was used in their workouts, leaving many of them incapable of completing the third day's training session.

Recall that the recommended proportion of carbohydrates in your diet is 55% to 60%. The person actively engaged in a fitness program should be sure to follow that prescription. Such a diet reduces the amount of fat you consume, which is beneficial from a health standpoint, and it keeps your body's glycogen stores replenished. For the person in heavy exercise training, a diet with 60% to 70% of its calories in the form of carbohydrates may be necessary to refill glycogen stores. The complex carbohydrates found in cereals, grains, fruits, and vegetables are preferable to the refined carbohydrates found in sweets and soft drinks. Both types of carbohydrates can restore glycogen levels, but the refined carbohydrates have little other nutritional value. By contrast, the complex carbohydrates are also a good source of vitamins, minerals, and fiber.

The Pre-Exercise Meal

A special consideration for people who exercise is how to integrate their meals with their workouts. On a day-to-day basis, the main concern is to time your workouts with your meals so that you avoid the discomfort associ-

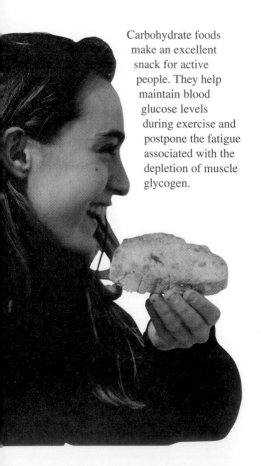

Carbohydrate foods make an excellent snack for active people. They help maintain blood glucose levels during exercise and postpone the fatigue associated with the depletion of muscle glycogen.

ated with exercising on a full stomach. It is generally best to allow 3 to 4 hours to pass between eating a meal and performing vigorous exercise. For light- or moderate-intensity activities, you can shorten the time period. In fact, most people do not encounter any problem going for a walk shortly after eating dinner. A little trial-and-error will show what works best for you. Experience will also teach you whether particular foods are not compatible with a workout several hours later. For example, starchy or spicy foods can give you heartburn or indigestion during a workout, whereas high-fiber foods might have you searching for a restroom during your afternoon run.

Meals that are high in carbohydrates make good pre-competition fare. An example would be a cereal (such as oatmeal) with skim milk; a bagel, toast, or English muffin with butter or jelly; orange juice; and, if you like, coffee. High-carbohydrate foods such as fruits, bagels, granola bars, and the like are good snacks or meals to pack for hikes or bike tours. They provide a readily available source of glucose for the muscles and help maintain your blood glucose levels.

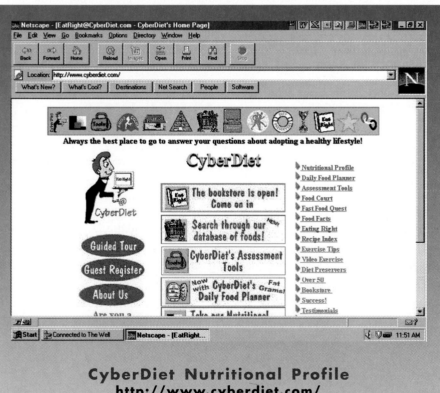

CyberDiet Nutritional Profile
http://www.cyberdiet.com/

This site allows you to calculate your calorie and nutrition needs based on your current or target body weight, and it creates a personalized nutrient profile for you. It also features a Daily Food Planner, a comparison of fast food meals, several nutritional assessments, a recipe index, and much more.

Critical thinking: Is using a computerized dietary assessment different for you from using a similar paper and pencil one like Laboratory 7.1? Does one have a greater impact on you? Why?
Source: From Gustafson, 1998.

Lifestyle Choices: Plan for Action

How does your current diet measure up to the principles and guidelines presented in this chapter? How might you adapt your lifestyle or change your eating habits to achieve a higher level of wellness? To evaluate your diet, refer to Section III of the Wellness Inventory in Chapter 1. If you scored below 42 points, you should consider making some changes in your diet. The lower your score, the more important it is for you to modify your diet.

Review your responses to the questions to identify which parts of your diet are most in need of change and make them your first targets for modification. Start the shift to a better diet by listing the foods that will be added to your diet and/or the foods or drinks that you will stop consuming to make this change. Consult the tables throughout the chapter to identify foods in the various food groups that are good sources of complex carbohydrates, protein, calcium, or iron that you may want to add to your diet, or to identify foods that are high in cholesterol, salt, fat, saturated fat, or sugar that you may need to reduce or eliminate from your diet. Also list any barriers to adopting a wellness diet.

POTENTIAL CHANGES **POTENTIAL BARRIERS**

_____ _____

_____ _____

_____ _____

Now set out the plan of action you have for the next month, listing the changes you will make each week. Make a contract with yourself by putting your intentions in writing and then signing it. This formality helps to move you from the thinking stage to the doing stage.

WEEK 1

This week I will make the following change in my diet:

_____

To do this, I will consume more of the following foods:

_____

and less of the following foods:

_____

WEEK 2

This week I will make the following change in my diet:

_____

To do this, I will consume more of the following foods:

_____

and less of the following foods:

_____

WEEK 3

This week I will make the following change in my diet:

_____

To do this, I will consume more of the following foods:

_____

and less of the following foods:

_____

WEEK 4

This week I will make the following change in my diet:

_____

To do this, I will consume more of the following foods:

_____

and less of the following foods:

_____

_____   _____

(signature)   *(date)*

At the end of the month, review your progress. How many of the changes
were you able to make? What turned out to be more difficult to change? If
you had some problems including more vegetables, fruits, cereals, rice,
breads, or pasta in your diet, keep trying! There are so many types of these
foods, you should be able to find some that you like and can add to your
meals. Have you been able to reduce the fat in your diet? Or the salt? Or
the cholesterol? Don't worry if it takes a while to modify your diet. Just
don't give up!

Summary

Making the correct choices in your diet will benefit you now and in the future. Eating right will give you the energy you need for the daily stresses of school or work and for your fitness program. Along with your daily physical activity, your diet determines whether you maintain your body weight or increase the amount of fat on your body.

Key concepts that you have learned in this chapter include these:

- Food contains the nutrients your body needs to build tissue, to regulate body functions, and to generate energy.

- The nutrients your body requires are water, carbohydrates, fats, proteins, vitamins, and minerals.

- Carbohydrates are the main dietary source of energy and come primarily from plant sources (fruits, vegetables, grains, and beans).

- Fats, the most concentrated form of energy, can be either saturated or unsaturated.

- Protein primarily serves as a structural component in cells and forms the enzymes that regulate cellular reactions.

- Vitamins regulate the energy-yielding reactions of cells and play a role in the structure or synthesis of body tissues.

- Calcium, iron, and sodium are key minerals because of their relationship to osteoporosis, anemia, and high blood pressure, respectively.

- The Food Guide Pyramid presents a strategy for dietary planning that ensures consumption of essential nutrients while limiting intake of foods that are high in sugar, fat, and sodium.

- Learning to read and interpret food labels is a key to achieving a wellness diet.

- The physically active person has essentially the same vitamin and mineral needs as the sedentary individual but may require more carbohydrates to ensure that muscle glycogen is replenished.

References

Applegate, E. A., and L. E. Grivetti. Search for the competitive edge: a history of dietary fads and supplements. *Journal of Nutrition,* 127 (5 Suppl): 869S–873S, 1997

Armstrong, L. E., and C. M. Maresh. Vitamin and mineral supplements as nutritional aides to exercise performance and health. *Nutrition Reviews,* 54(4 Pt.2): S149–S158, 1996.

Christian, J. L., and J. L. Greger. *Nutrition for Living,* 4th ed. Redwood City, CA: Benjamin/Cummings, 1994.

Clark, N. *Sports Nutrition Guidebook,* 2nd ed. Champaign, IL: Leisure Press, 1996.

Clarkson, P. M. Antioxidants and physical performance. *Critical Reviews of Food Science and Nutrition,* 35(1-2): 131–141, 1995.

Clarkson, P. M. Micronutrients and exercise: Anti-oxidants and minerals. *Journal of Sports Science,* 13 Spec. No. S11–S24, 1995.

Clarkson, P. M. Nutrition for improved sports performance. Current issues on ergogenic aids. *Sports Medicine,* 21(6): 393–401, 1996.

Clarkson, P. M. and E. M. Haymes. Trace mineral requirements for athletes. *International Journal of Sports Nutrition,* 4(2): 104–119, 1994.

Coleman, E. *The Ultimate Sports Nutrition Handbook.* Bull Publishers, Menlo Park, CA, 1996

Convertino, V. A., L. E. Armstrong, E. F. Coyle, G. W. Mack, M. N. Sawka, L. C. Senay, and W. M. Sherman. American College of Sports Medicine position stand. Exercise and fluid replacement. *Medicine and Science in Sports and Exercise,* 28(1): i–vii, 1996.

Costill, D. L. Carbohydrates for exercise: Dietary demands for optimal performance. *International Journal of Sports Medicine,* 9: 1–18, 1988.

Craig, W. J. Phytochemicals: Guardians of our health. *Journal of the American Dietetic Association.* 97(10 Suppl 2): S199–S204, 1997.

Dietary Guidelines for Americans, 4th ed. U.S. Department of Agriculture, U.S. Department of Health and Human Services, December, 1995, Home & Garden Bulletin No. 232.

Food and Nutrition Board. *Recommended Dietary Allowances,* 10th edition. Washington, DC: National Academy of Sciences, 1989.

The Food Guide Pyramid. U.S. Department of Agriculture, U.S. Department of Health and Human Services, 1992, Home & Garden Bulletin No. 252.

Glade, M. J. NIH workshop on the role of dietary supplements for physically active people. Bethesda, Maryland, June 3–4, 1996. *Nutrition,* 13(3): 257–262, 1997.

Hawley, J. A., E. J. Schabort, T. D. Noakes, and S. C. Dennis. Carbohydrate-loading and exercise performance. An update. *Sports Medicine,* 24(2): 73–81, 1997.

Holloszy, J. O., and W. M. Kohrt. Regulation of carbohydrate and fat metabolism during and after exercise. *Annual Review of Nutrition,* 16: 121–138, 1996.

Katch, F. L., and W. D. McArdle. *Introduction to Nutrition, Exercise and Health.* Philadelphia: Lea & Febiger, 1993.

Kennedy, E., L. Meyer, and W. Layden. The 1995 dietary guidelines for Americans: an overview. *Journal of the American Dietetic Association,* 96(3): 234–237, 1996.

Kreider, R. B., M. Ferreira, M. Wilson, P. Grindstaff, S. Plisk, J. Reinardy, E. Cantler, and A. L. Almada. Effects of creatine supplementation on body composition, strength, and sprint performance. *Medicine and Science in Sports and Exercise,* 30: 73–82, 1998.

Lappe, F. M. *Diet for a Small Planet.* New York: Ballantine Books, 1991.

Lemon, P.W.R. Effect of exercise on protein requirements. *Journal of Sports Sciences,* 9: 53–70, 1991.

Matthews, R. H., P. R. Pehrsson, and M. Farhat-Sabet. Sugar content of selected foods. Washington, DC: United States Department of Agriculture, 1987.

Maughan, R. J., and T. D. Noakes. Fluid replacement and exercise stress. A brief review of studies on fluid replacement and some guidelines for the athlete. *Sports Medicine,* 12(1): 16–31, 1991.

McArdle, W. D., F. I. Katch, and V. L. Katch. *Exercise Physiology: Energy, Nutrition and Human Performance.* Philadelphia: Lea & Fibiger, 1996.

National Cholesterol Education Program. Summary of the second report of the National Cholesterol Education Program (NCEP) expert panel on detection, evaluation, and treatment of high blood cholesterol in adults (Adult Treatment Panel II). *Journal of the American Medical Association,* 296: 3015–3023, 1993.

Pennington, J. A. *Food values of portions commonly used.* New York: Harper and Row, 1989.

Position of the American Dietetic Association: Food irradiation. *Journal of the American Dietetic Association,* 96(1): 69–72, 1996.

Position of the American Dietetic Association: Phytochemicals and functional foods. *Journal of the American Dietetic Association,* 95(4): 493–496, 1995.

Sizer, F., and E. Whitney. *Nutrition: Concepts and Controversies,* 7th ed. Belmont, CA: Wadsworth, 1997.

Volek, J. S., W. J. Draemer, J. A. Bush, M. Boetes, T. Incledon, K. L. Clark, and J. M. Lynch. Creatine supplementation enhances muscular performance during high intensity resistance exercise. *Journal of the American Dietetic Association* (H6F), 7: 765–770, 1997.

Williams, C. Macronutrients and performance. *Journal of Sports Science,* 13: S1–S10, 1995.

Analyzing Your Diet

Set aside one day to keep a diary of all of the foods you consume, noting the types and amounts of foods that make up each of your meals. (Use the Food Record form provided.) It is important that you also record any snacks and beverages that you consume between meals, because people are often unaware of the amount of calories they ingest outside of formal meal settings. The accuracy of this dietary analysis depends on several factors:

- How typical or representative the day you analyzed is of your regular diet.

- How thorough you were in recording everything you ate or drank.

- How accurately you quantified your portion sizes. To be precise, you need to weigh or measure each item you consume with a food scale or measuring cup. For the purposes of this lab, make your best judgment of portion sizes if you do not actually measure them. Refer to the labels on the foods you eat, especially if you eat something that has only one serving per container.

Once you have compiled an accurate list of your day's food intake, perform a careful analysis of each food. Use the food label to determine the caloric content, the amount of cholesterol and sodium, and the grams of carbohydrates, proteins, and fat in the food. A food composition table is provided as an Appendix in this text. Check with your instructor to see if you have access to diet analysis software; such a program can quickly give you a detailed analysis of your diet when you enter the types and amounts of foods you consume. This laboratory will make you more aware of what foods you eat and how your diet compares with the nutritional recommendations (55%–60% or more of your calories in the form of carbohydrates, 12%–15% in the form of proteins, and 30% or less in the form of fat).

Dietary Analysis Form

After you have recorded and analyzed each item of food in the Food Record, calculate the total number of kilocalories you consumed for the day. Also total the number of grams of carbohydrates, proteins, fat, saturated fat, monounsaturated fat, and polyunsaturated fat you consumed. With this information you will be able to calculate the percentage of your total caloric intake that is coming from the various sources of energy. The steps for these computations are outlined following.

Carbohydrates

_____ g of carbohydrate × 4 kcal/g =
_____ kcal from carbohydrate

_____ kcal carbohydrate

$$\frac{\text{\_\_\_\_\_ kcal carbohydrate}}{\text{\_\_\_\_\_ total kcal}} \times 100 =$$
_____ % kcal from carbohydrate

_____ total kcal

Proteins

_____ g of protein × 4 kcal/g = _____ kcal from protein

_____ kcal protein

$$\frac{\text{\_\_\_\_\_ kcal protein}}{\text{\_\_\_\_\_ total kcal}} \times 100 =$$
_____ % kcal from protein

_____ total kcal

Fat

_____ g of fat × 9 kcal/g = _____ kcal from fat

_____ kcal fat

$$\frac{\text{\_\_\_\_\_ kcal fat}}{\text{\_\_\_\_\_ total kcal}} \times 100 =$$
_____ % kcal from fat

_____ total kcal

Saturated Fat

_____ g of saturated fat × 9 kcal/g =
_____ kcal from saturated fat

_____ kcal saturated fat

$$\frac{\text{\_\_\_\_\_ kcal saturated fat}}{\text{\_\_\_\_\_ total kcal}} \times 100 =$$
_____ % kcal from saturated fat

_____ total kcal

Monounsaturated Fat

_____ g of monounsaturated fat × 9 kcal/g =
_____ kcal from monounsaturated fat

_____ kcal monounsaturated fat

$$\frac{\text{\_\_\_\_\_ kcal monounsaturated fat}}{\text{\_\_\_\_\_ total kcal}} \times 100 =$$
_____ % kcal from monounsaturated fat

_____ total kcal

Polyunsaturated Fat

_____ g of polyunsaturated fat × 9 kcal/g
= _____ kcal from polyunsaturated fat

_____ kcal polyunsaturated fat

$$\frac{\text{\_\_\_\_\_ kcal polyunsaturated fat}}{\text{\_\_\_\_\_ total kcal}} \times 100 =$$
_____ % kcal from polyunsaturated fat

_____ total kcal

Food Record

Day: S M T W T F S   Date: _____

Food or Beverage	Amount	Kilo-calories	Choles-terol (mg)	Sodium (mg)	Carbo-hydrate (g)	Protein (g)	Fat (g)	Saturated Fat (g)	Monoun-saturated Fat (g)	Polyunsat-urated Fat (g)

Total: _____   _____   _____   _____   _____   _____   _____   _____   _____

Is total cholesterol less than 300 mg? _____   Is total sodium less than 3,000 mg (3g)? _____

Dietary Analysis Using the Food Guide Pyramid

A simplified dietary analysis using the Food Guide Pyramid can give a quick and useful assessment of your diet. It begins with an estimate of your daily caloric requirement. The number of calories you should consume each day is determined by such factors as your age, sex, body size, and activity levels. The exact daily requirement of calories is different for each person, but some general guidelines from the USDA's Food Guide Pyramid may help you estimate the approximate value for you:

> 1600 kcal—many sedentary women, some older adults
>
> 2200 kcal—teenage girls, active women, many sedentary men
>
> 2800 kcal—teenage boys, many active men, some very active women

If you are in the lower range of total daily calories, then you should consume the lower number of servings given for the food groups in the Food Guide Pyramid (see Figure 7.6 on page 209). For example, you would have 6 servings from the bread group, 2 servings of fruit, 3 servings of vegetables, 2 servings from the milk group, and 2 servings from the meat group. If you are in the upper range of total daily calories, then you need to consume the higher numbers of servings from the food groups: 11 servings from the bread group, 4 servings of fruit, 5 servings of vegetables, 3 servings from the milk group, and 3 servings from the meat group.

Another consideration in dietary planning is to limit the amount of fat you consume so that it does not exceed 30% of the calories in your diet. This means that you should not exceed 53 g of fat in your diet if you consume 1600 kcal per day, 73 g of fat if you consume 2200 kcal per day, or 93 g of fat if you consume 2800 kcal per day.

Complete the following diet form to determine whether you are meeting the Food Guide Pyramid goals for the well-balanced, low-fat diet:

Step 1: Record everything you ate for meals and snacks during a typical day on the Food Record form in Laboratory 7.1. If you have already completed Laboratory 7.1, you can use the data you have compiled in this lab, too.

Step 2: Classify everything you ate into its food group. Did you have the number of servings from the five food groups that is appropriate for your caloric intake? Keep in mind that one food item may contain several servings from the food groups. For example, a sandwich will have two servings

from the bread group (two slices of bread) and, depending on what kind of sandwich it is, it may have one serving from the meat group, dairy group, and/or vegetable group. Use Table 7.7 on page 203 to determine serving sizes.

	Servings Right For You						Servings You Had
Bread group	6	7	8	9	10	11	_____
Vegetable group	3	4	5				_____
Fruit group	2	3	4				_____
Milk group	2	3					_____
Meat group	2	3					_____

Step 3: Determine the amount of fat in your diet. Use the food labels or a food composition table to determine the grams of fat in the foods you ate and enter the value in the "Grams of Fat" column of the food record. Add together all these values to determine the total number of grams of fat you ate. Enter that value below and compare it to the recommended number of grams to be no more than 30% of the calories of a diet of 1,600, 2,200, or 2,800 kcals.

	Grams Right For You			Grams You Had
Fat	53	73	93	_____

Step 4: Making changes in your diet. If you were eating fewer servings from some of the food groups, list some foods you can add to better balance your diet. If your diet has more than 30% of its calories from fat, list some low-fat foods you can add to your diet and the high-fat foods you will try to avoid.

Foods I Will Add To My Diet	Foods I Will Try To Avoid
_____	_____
_____	_____
_____	_____
_____	_____
_____	_____

Laboratory 7.3

Analyzing an Individual Item of Food

After you have completed your Food Record, analyze the label of several foods that you consume. To do so, select four food labels, one from each of the following types of food—significant protein source, carbohydrate source, fat source, and a mixed-food item (for example, macaroni and cheese, canned soup or stew, frozen dinner)—and complete the following analysis form for each. (You will need to make copies of the form to use with each food item.)

Food Label Analysis Form

Food: _____

Significant source of (check one):

❑ Carbohydrate (bread, cereal, pasta)

❑ Protein (some dairy products, meat)

❑ Fat (dessert, some dairy products)

❑ Mixed-food source (e.g., macaroni and cheese, packaged dinner)

Manufacturer: _____

Serving size: _____ grams / ounces
(circle the appropriate units or indicate other units)

Total calories (kcals) per serving: _____ kcals

Grams of carbohydrate per serving: _____ g

Grams of protein per serving: _____ g

Grams of fat per serving: _____ g

Carbohydrates

_____ g of carbohydrate × 4 kcal/g =
_____ kcal from carbohydrate

_____ kcal carbohydrate
―――――――――――――――――― × 100 =
_____ % kcal from carbohydrate

_____ total kcal/serving

Proteins

_____ g of protein × 4 kcal/g = _____ kcal from protein

_____ kcal protein
―――――――――――――――――― × 100 =
_____ % kcal from protein

_____ total kcal/serving

Fat

_____ g of fat × 9 kcal/g = _____ kcal from fat

_____ kcal fat
―――――――――――――――――― × 100 =
_____ % kcal from fat

_____ total kcal/serving

Examine the label, including the list of ingredients, and complete the following:

1. List any source(s) of added sugar.

2. List the cholesterol content per serving.
    Is it low in cholesterol (< 20 mg per serving)?

3. List the sodium content per serving.
    Is it low in sodium (< 140 mg per serving)?

4. List any added vitamins or minerals.

Chapter 8

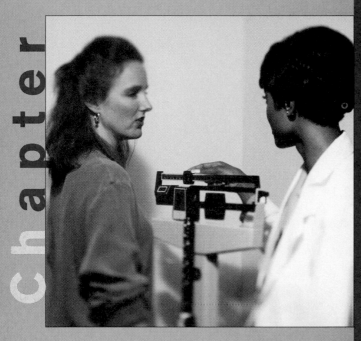

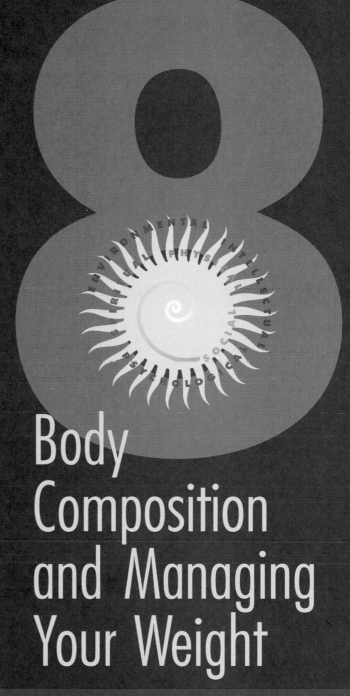

Body Composition and Managing Your Weight

One Student's View

I've found that eating three balanced meals a day and exercising regularly is the best way to maintain an appropriate level of body composition. My advice to someone who is trying to lose weight is to first set a reasonable goal. Second, concentrate on becoming active—don't initially focus on your food intake. Then, once you're exercising regularly, take a look at your diet and make sure you're eating a variety of foods.

—Kim Bentley

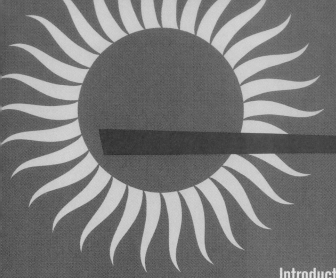

Introduction

Few of us are satisfied with the proportions of fat and muscle on our bodies. If we could turn wishes into reality, most of us would change something about our bodies: reduce the amount of fat on our abdomens, hips, or thighs, and maybe increase the muscular development of our chest, arms, or legs. Yet the trends in America lead to exactly the opposite result: People are consuming more high-calorie fast foods, and they are, for the most part, physically inactive. As an example, when the authors of this text, who are in their mid-forties, were in college, there was a phenomenon known as "the freshman 10," which referred to the almost inevitable 10 pounds of weight freshmen gained during the first year in college. Current freshmen speak of the same phenomenon, but it is now known as "the freshman 15."

The term *body composition* refers to the quantification of the amount of fat on your body. This physical characteristic is a wellness component because *obesity,* an excessive amount of body fat, is directly related to many health problems, including heart disease, gout, gall bladder disorders, diabetes, hypertension, osteoarthritis, and some forms of cancer. Body composition also influences body shape and appearance. The way you look can have a bearing on your self-image, which in turn can affect the psychological as well as the social aspects of wellness. By some estimates, the economic cost of obesity is over $39 billion each year.

The National Health and Nutrition Examination Survey (NHANES) has been tracking trends in the heights and weights of the American population since 1960. From 1960 through 1980, the prevalence of overweight among Americans was quite stable, ranging between 24.3% and 25.4%. However, when NHANES conducted an assessment of over 8,000 people between 1988 and 1991, they found that the prevalence of overweight had increased to 33.3%! In a 10-year interval, the incidence of overweight increased from 1 person in 4 to 1 person in 3. Figure 8.1, shows that the

Objectives

After reading this chapter, you should be able to

- **Define body composition and the fat and lean compartments of the body**

- **Describe the methods for determining body composition**

- **Describe the differences in body fat levels and distribution in males and females, and present the norms for body fat for each sex**

- **Identify the factors that determine the total daily energy expenditure**

- **Outline the unique contributions of exercise in a fat-reduction program**

- **Describe the exercise prescription for weight management**

incidence of overweight increases with age until people are in their 60s, and the incidence differs by race and by gender. Grouping all races together, approximately 20% of the men and women in their twenties are overweight, approximately 37% of the men and women in their forties, and 42% of the men and 52% of the women in their fifties. Grouping all ages together, 32% of white men and women are overweight; 31% and 49% of African-American men and women, respectively, are overweight; and 39% and 41% of Mexican-American men and women, respectively, are overweight (Kuczmarski et al.).

At any one time, approximately 50% of American women and 25% of American men are dieting to lose weight. Interestingly, more women are dieting than would be classified as overweight, whereas the reverse is true for men. This disparity is due largely to our society's strict and often unrealistic standards of physical appearance for women: We place a high value on the thin and youthful-looking body. If people in general, and the young adult female in particular, could be guided by standards of health only, far fewer of them would think they had a weight problem.

The amount of fat and muscle on your body is the result of your genetic inheritance interacting with your eating and exercise habits. The genetic factor accounts for 25% of the variability in percentage of body fat in the population (Bouchard). That leaves you a considerable amount of control over your body fat level. You decide what, when, and how much you eat. You decide how much exercise and physical activity you get. By following the advice for proper nutrition and exercise presented in the earlier chapters of this text and the advice concerning your personal health presented in the later chapters, your body will be as fit and healthy as it is capable of being.

In this chapter, you will learn how to establish a healthful and realistic expectation for your level of body fatness. You will also learn appropriate means of reducing body fat when reduction is called for. As we shall see, dieting is not necessarily the best approach. Physical activity has proven to be an essential part of successful interventions to prevent weight gain or to reduce body fat. With obesity, as with other health issues, prevention is preferable to cure.

Body Composition

Our bodies are composed of a variety of different tissues, which can be categorized as being part of either the lean or the fat compartment of the body.

The Lean and Fat Compartments

The **lean compartment** is composed primarily of the muscles, skeleton, and organs of the body; the **fat compartment** can be differentiated into the essential and storage fat in the body. The **essential fat** is fat that serves structural and functional roles in the body. For example, essential fat (lipid) is part of every cell membrane in the body, and it is a major constituent of certain specialized tissue, such as nerves and bone marrow. Although fat has a negative connotation for many people, it plays a key role in our healthful functioning—hence the term *essential*.

lean compartment muscles, skeleton, and organs in the body

fat compartment essential and storage fat in the body

essential fat fat that serves structural and functional roles in the body

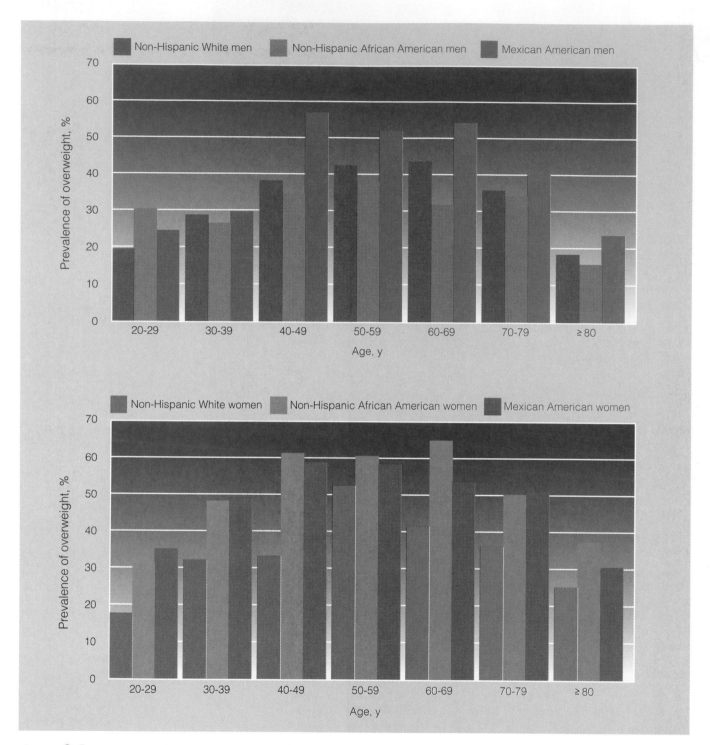

Figure 8.1

Prevalence of overweight in the United States by age and race/ethnicity for men and women. White women tend to have a lower incidence of overweight than African American and Mexican American women; the prevalence of overweight is similar among the race/ethnicity classifications of men, until after 40, when the Mexican American men have a higher incidence of overweight (Kuczmarski et al.).

The other form of fat, storage fat, is what many people perceive as being their nemesis. **Storage fat** is the fat that serves as the energy reservoir of the body and is just as necessary for life as the functions described for essential fat. Thus, it would be a mistake to try to achieve a fat-free body. Most storage fat is located in the **adipose tissue,** which is a collection of fat cells, each of which stores energy in the form of fat called triglyceride (see Chapter 7). When energy is required, as when you are exercising or when you have used up the ready energy from your last meal, triglyceride is split and released into the bloodstream, making the energy it contains available

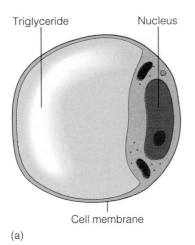

Triglyceride   Nucleus

Cell membrane

(a)

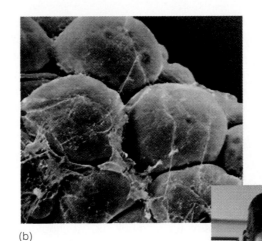

(b)

Figure 8.2
Human adipose tissue contains billions of fat cells. **(a)** Each cell is a sphere filled primarily with triglyceride. **(b)** A micrograph of human adipose tissue.
Source: From Christian and Greger, 1994.

throughout the body. Storage fat also serves to insulate and protect the body by virtue of its location just below the skin (subcutaneous) and surrounding the internal organs.

The Development of Body Fat

A unique characteristic of adipose tissue is its capacity to enlarge and store enormous quantities of energy if a person consistently ingests more energy than he or she expends in activity or exercise. For the most part, when adults experience changes in body weight, particularly weight gain, these are reflective of changes in their storage fat compartment.

Our adipose tissue contains many billions of fat cells (see Figure 8.2). A person with a normal amount of body fat may have 20 to 40 billion of them. Structurally, each fat cell is a sphere, with the majority of its volume filled with triglyceride. If triglyceride is added to or removed from the cell, the fat cell will increase or decrease in size accordingly. When this enlargement or reduction is occurring throughout the billions of fat cells we possess, an observable increase or decrease in our overall body fat level will result.

The amount of adipose tissue we have can be increased through the development of additional fat cells or the enlargement of the existing cells. As we grow up, the number of fat cells we have increases, particularly in the first few years of life and again during the adolescent growth spurt. When people develop obesity during childhood, an abnormally large increase in the number of their fat cells occurs. By the time these people become adults, they may have 70 to 100 billion fat cells and suffer from **hyperplastic obesity**—the obesity that results from an elevated number of fat cells.

With adult-onset obesity, the enlargement of the adipose mass is primarily the result of the enlargement of the individual fat cells, with little or no change in numbers of fat cells. **Hypertrophic obesity** is the obesity that results from having fat cells that are greatly enlarged although the number of fat cells is normal. This phenomenon has been referred to as *creeping obesity,* because it can be a process that slowly but steadily progresses until a person has amassed an excessive amount of body fat. As Figure 8.1 shows, most cases of obesity occur when people are beyond their early twenties. Thus, most Americans who are obese have hypertrophic obesity. When we

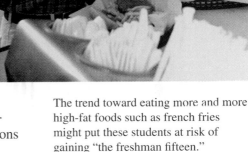

The trend toward eating more and more high-fat foods such as french fries might put these students at risk of gaining "the freshman fifteen."

storage fat fat that serves as the energy reservoir of the body

adipose tissue collection of fat cells, each of which stores energy in the form of triglyceride

hyperplastic obesity obesity that results from an elevated number of fat cells

hypertrophic obesity obesity that results from having fat cells that are greatly enlarged although the number of fat cells in the body is normal

reduce our levels of body fat, the fat cells become smaller. The triglyceride in the fat cells is broken down and released into the bloodstream, to be used as a source of energy for tissues throughout the body. Although we can reduce the *size* of our fat cells, we cannot reduce the *number*. Therefore, people with hyperplastic obesity will continue to have an excessive number of fat cells even when they reduce their levels of body fat. They will have to lose fat to the point of shrinking their fat cells to below-normal size to compensate for having so many of them.

The only way you can reduce the number of fat cells you have is by removing them surgically. **Liposuction** is the surgical removal, by a suctioning technique, of adipose tissue located in subcutaneous depots, such as the abdomen, hips, or thighs. Considering the societal emphasis on thinness and the desire for a "quick fix," it should come as no surprise that liposuction is the most commonly performed type of plastic surgery. Liposuction is not without its risks and discomforts, however. For example, it can cause numbness or pain that lasts for weeks, and several people have died from complications following the procedure. The amount of adipose tissue that can be safely removed is limited, so the operation is used for what plastic surgeons refer to as "body shaping" rather than as a cure for obesity. Again, prevention is preferable to cure. The principles outlined in this chapter will help you avoid creeping obesity.

Norms for Body Composition

Males and females differ in their body composition (see Table 8.1). For men, the average percentage of body fat is 15%, and levels above 23% are considered obese. For women, the average percentage of body fat is 23%, and levels above 32% are considered obese. Generally, males and females have similar levels of storage fat. Where they differ is in the amount of essential fat they carry. The additional fat associated with the female's reproductive capacity to support a pregnancy and lactation is considered part of the essential fat component of her body composition. The most important reference point in terms of body fat is the level that represents obesity, because various health problems (heart disease, diabetes, gout, hypertension) are associated with that degree of body fatness. Men above 23% and women above 32% body fat are advised to reduce their body fat.

Athletes often have below-average body fat levels, particularly those who engage in endurance events (runners, swimmers, cyclists, cross-country skiers), in sports that are divided into weight classifications (boxers, wrestlers, rowers), or in events in which appearance is a factor because performances are judged (gymnasts, figure skaters, divers). For many sports, body fat can be an impediment to high-level performance because it represents a weight that must be transported but does not actively contribute to running faster, throwing farther, or jumping higher. Even the lean male marathoner, who may have only 5% body fat, will not come close to depleting his storage fat during his 26.2-mile race. Marathon runners represent the extreme in low body fat (3% to 10% for males, 8% to 18% for females), and this is the result of their long hours of heavy training and the unique body type they inherited.

Athletes and, for that matter, fashion models are a very select and nonrepresentative portion of the wide array of body types that make up our general population. For this reason, they should not become the standard of body fat levels that all aspire to achieve. A positive outcome of the recent

---

liposuction surgical removal, by a suctioning technique, of adipose tissue located in subcutaneous depots

TABLE 8.1

Body Composition of an Average Young Adult Male and Female

	MALE	FEMALE
Height	170 cm (67 in)	163.8 cm (64.5 in)
Weight	70 kg (154 lb)	53.8 kg (118 lb)
Total fat	10.5 kg (15%)	12.4 kg (23%)
Storage fat	8.4 kg (12%)	5.9 kg (11%)
Essential fat	2.1 kg (3%)	6.5 kg (12%)
Lean mass	59.5 kg (85%)	41.4 kg (77%)
Muscle	31.3 kg (45%)	20.4 kg (38%)
Bone	10.6 kg (15%)	6.9 kg (13%)
Remainder	17.6 kg (25%)	14.1 kg (26%)

Note: Percentages given are percentage of total body weight.
Source: From McArdle, Katch, and Katch, 1991.

fitness orientation of our society has been the development of more functional standards of beauty—that is, the body that has developed endurance, strength, and flexibility through regular exercise is seen as being attractive. These are standards most of us can meet as our bodies are shaped by the specific type of exercise we perform.

People who are obese should undertake a prudent program of diet and exercise to reduce their body fat. The National Health and Nutrition Examination Survey (NHANES) report showed that most people in their twenties are not overweight and, thus, need not concern themselves with losing weight. However, having an acceptable and healthy body composition now is no guarantee that you will continue to have it when you are older. The average percentage of body fat of people in their fifties is higher than that of people in their twenties. This increase in body fatness is not a necessary biological consequence of aging, but rather the result of the reduction in physical activity that typically occurs as we age. For this reason, the body fat standards presented earlier are appropriate for older people, too, though some experts feel they can be relaxed slightly upward to reflect the increase in body fat most people experience as they age. With this adjustment, men and women over age 40 should keep their percentage of body fat below 26% and 35%, respectively.

Unhealthy Responses to Body Composition

People can make themselves unhealthy if they become obsessive about having low levels of body fat. For example, someone who has above-average body fat levels but is not obese should avoid becoming fatter, but this person does not necessarily have a health reason for reducing body fat levels. Nonetheless, many people in this situation think of themselves as too fat and feel they should lose weight. They believe this because our standards of

People who suffer from anorexia nervosa have a distorted body image, seeing themselves as too fat in spite of their obvious underweight.

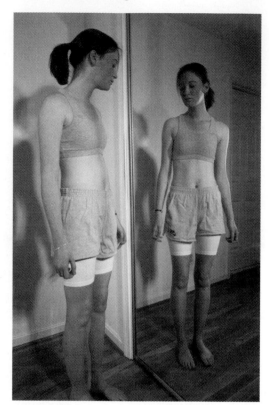

anorexia nervosa psychological disorder characterized by self-starvation, an intense fear of becoming fat, and a refusal to maintain a minimal normal weight

bulimia nervosa psychological disorder characterized by episodes of uncontrolled binge eating followed by purging behavior, such as self-induced vomiting, the use of diuretics or laxatives, strict dieting, or exercise to avoid weight gain from food consumed

android pattern accumulation of fat on the trunk, particularly the abdomen, which is typically found in males

gynoid pattern accumulation of fat on the limbs, particularly the hips and thighs, which is typically found in females

appearance are often a more powerful force in shaping our perceptions of acceptable levels of body fat than are health considerations.

Finding themselves in a society that worships thinness, a small percentage of women and an even smaller percentage of men have adopted abnormal eating practices in an attempt to control their body weight. Adolescent and young adult females are particularly vulnerable to eating disorders. A fear of fatness is instilled in them at a time when hormonal changes following puberty produce an increase in body fatness. The two most common eating disorders, anorexia nervosa and bulimia nervosa, have received increased attention during the past 20 years, although neither is a recent phenomenon. **Anorexia nervosa** is a psychological disorder characterized by self-starvation, an intense fear of becoming fat, and a refusal to maintain a minimal normal weight. Anorexics view themselves as fat in spite of their emaciated condition. It is estimated that approximately 1% of the population is anorexic, with the majority of the cases (over 90%) being female.

Bulimia nervosa is a psychological disorder characterized by episodes of uncontrolled binge eating followed by purging behavior such as self-induced vomiting, the use of diuretics or laxatives, strict dieting, or exercise to avoid weight gain from the food consumed. Unlike the anorexic, the bulimic is not necessarily below average in body weight. A survey of female students at the University of California at Los Angeles found that 2.1% were bulimic at the time of the survey, and 4.8% had been bulimic at some time during their lives (Kurtzman et al.). Like anorexia nervosa, bulimia nervosa is more prevalent among females than males.

Clearly, starvation or bingeing and purging are not healthy practices. The anorexic female will become malnourished, a condition that will cause a reduction in estrogen production, amenorrhea (cessation of menstruation), osteoporosis, abnormal heart function, and possibly death. A mortality rate of 5% to 18% for those with anorexia nervosa has been reported (Leon; Wilmore). The purging practices of the bulimic can result in mineral disturbances through losses in vomiting or the use of diuretics or laxatives. Excessive loss of potassium can lead to fatal disruptions in the contraction of the heart. Other side effects of bulimia include an erosion of the lining of the throat, dark eye circles, and chronic stomach pains.

Both conditions are serious psychological disorders that require professional diagnosis and treatment. If you suspect that you have an eating disorder, seek out professional help. If someone you know exhibits the behaviors associated with these eating disorders, encourage him or her to get counseling. Community and university hospitals and health clinics have physicians, nutritionists, and psychiatrists who are trained in identifying and treating eating disorders.

Body Fat Distribution

Characteristically, males and females differ in the distribution of fat on their bodies. Males are more likely to accumulate fat on the trunk, particularly the abdomen, and this has been termed the **android pattern** of fat distribution. Females are more likely to accumulate fat on the limbs, particularly the hips and thighs, and this is termed the **gynoid pattern** of fat distribution (see Figure 8.3). These patterns are not entirely sex-specific, however, as males can have the gynoid distribution and females can have the android distribution.

Where fat accumulates on the body has important health implications People, male or female, who carry an excessive amount of abdominal fat have a greater risk for the development of cardiovascular disease and diabetes. Obese individuals with the gynoid pattern of fat accumulation do not share this increased risk. Abdominal fat is more active in the flux of fat into and out of the bloodstream. This increased release of fat into the bloodstream influences blood levels of triglyceride, lipoproteins, glucose, and insulin, which may be the mechanism by which excessive amounts of abdominal fat contribute to hypertension, diabetes, and cardiovascular disease. Fat on the hips and thighs is not released as readily and thus shows a much lower association to these diseased states. (See the Myths and Controversies box.)

The waist-hip ratio is used to assess whether you have the android pattern of body fat distribution. The directions for making this measurement and the criteria for interpreting the results are presented in Laboratory 8.1.

Assessing Body Composition

Several different methods are used to quantify body composition, ranging from the traditional height-weight tables and body mass indexes to the laboratory measures that involve underwater weighing, skinfold measurements, and bioelectrical impedance analysis.

Height-Weight Tables

The Metropolitan Life Insurance Company has developed tables listing desirable weights for height based on large-scale studies conducted on the American population (see Table 8.2). Height-weight tables are widely used by health professionals for two reasons: (1) Height and weight are very easy and straightforward measurements to obtain, and (2) a considerable amount of research has been conducted with height-weight data as the sole indicator of body composition. Based on the relationship between weight-for-height and health problems, it has become accepted that being 20% or more above

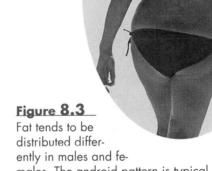

Figure 8.3

Fat tends to be distributed differently in males and females. The android pattern is typical in males (left); the gynoid pattern is typical in females (right).

MYTHS & CONTROVERSIES

Myth   **Cellulite is a distinct form of adipose tissue.** *Cellulite* is a nonscientific term used to describe the accumulation of fat on the thighs, which can be distinguished from normal adipose tissue by its dimpled, "cottage cheese"-like appearance. Supposedly, cellulite is especially difficult to lose. For this reason, a multitude of creams, rubs, special exercises, and equipment are advertised in women's magazines that claim to facilitate cellulite reduction.

The truth is that cellulite, as a distinct type of adipose tissue, does not exist. The adipose tissue on the thighs is no different from the adipose tissue elsewhere in the body. The way an accumulation of fat on the thighs distributes when weight is placed on it during sitting can give it a lumpy and dimpled appearance. Commercially available creams or special massages will not help reduce the amount of fat on the thighs or anywhere else on the body. Adipose tissue is reduced when the individual fat cells become smaller, and the only sure way for that to happen is for the cells to release the stored fat they contain into the bloodstream to be used as a source of energy for the body.

TABLE 8.2

The 1959 Metropolitan Life Height-Weight Tables

MEN				WOMEN			
HEIGHT (FT/IN)	**WEIGHT (LBS)**			**HEIGHT (FT/IN)**	**WEIGHT (LBS)**		
	SMALL FRAME	**MEDIUM FRAME**	**LARGE FRAME**		**SMALL FRAME**	**MEDIUM FRAME**	**LARGE FRAME**
5'2"	112–120	118–129	126–141	4'10"	92–98	96–107	104–119
5'3"	115–123	121–133	129–144	4'11"	94–101	98–110	106–122
5'4"	118–126	124–136	132–148	5'0"	96–104	101–113	109–125
5'5"	121–129	127–139	135–152	5'1"	99–107	104–116	112–128
5'6"	124–133	130–143	138–156	5'2"	102–110	107–119	115–131
5'7"	128–137	134–147	142–161	5'3"	105–113	110–122	118–134
5'8"	132–141	138–152	147–166	5'4"	108–116	113–126	121–138
5'9"	136–145	142–156	151–170	5'5"	111–119	116–130	125–142
5'10"	140–150	146–160	155–174	5'6"	114–123	120–135	129–146
5'11"	144–154	150–165	159–179	5'7"	118–127	124–139	133–150
6'0"	148–158	154–170	164–184	5'8"	122–131	128–143	137–154
6'1"	152–162	158–175	168–189	5'9"	126–135	132–147	141–158
6'2"	156–167	162–180	173–194	5'10"	130–140	136–151	145–163
6'3"	160–171	167–185	178–199	5'11"	134–144	140–155	149–168
6'4"	164–175	172–190	182–204	6'0"	138–148	144–159	153–173

Note: Men's height assumes shoes with 1-in heels; women's assumes 2-in heels. Weight for both sexes includes indoor clothing. For nude weight for men, deduct 5–7 lbs; for women, deduct 2–4 lbs.
Source: From Metropolitan Life Insurance Co., 1959.

your ideal weight (as determined from the height-weight tables) places you at a health risk and classifies you as being overweight.

When you use height-weight tables, however, be aware of this: A scale can very accurately measure your weight, but it is incapable of determining how much of that weight is lean tissue and how much is fat. Thus, it is necessary to distinguish between the terms *overweight* and *overfat*, because a person can be one without being the other. Being overweight means weighing more than the norm for one's height. This is not synonymous with being overfat, because a person can be overweight by virtue of having a large lean body mass while being low or average in body fatness. One can also be overfat without being overweight if a below-average lean body mass coincides with an excessive amount of body fat. Thus, keep in mind that the height-weight tables can be misleading in suggesting that all cases of being overweight are due to an excessive amount of body fat and suggesting that all cases within the normal range of body weight are incapable of being overfat. Therefore, the term *overweight* is used instead of *obese* if the determination is based on height-weight data, such as with the height-weight tables or by the body mass index (described below). When there is a quantification of the fat component of a person's body weight, as with the underwater weighing, skinfold, or bioelectrical impedance methods, then it is appropriate to use the term *obese.*

The most recent version of the height-weight tables was published in 1983. Objecting to the higher weights allowed for the various heights, many health professionals have continued to use the 1959 version (the one presented in Table 8.2). Note that the heights and weights are based on individuals wearing shoes and wearing indoor clothing, respectively. For each height, a range of ideal body weights is given for people with small, medium, or large frame sizes. Table 8.3 enables you to derive a determination of your frame size based on the width of your elbow.

Body Mass Index

Another tool used to relate height and weight is the **body mass index (BMI),** which is your weight (in kilograms) divided by the square of your height (in meters):

$$BMI = \frac{Weight\ (kg)}{[Height\ (m)]^2}$$

The advantage of using BMI is that you do not need to refer to a table to determine what is normal and what is obese. According to the most

---

TABLE 8.3

Determining Frame Size Based on Elbow Width

These tables list the elbow measurements[a] for medium-frame men and women of various heights. Measurements lower than those listed indicate that you have a small frame, and higher measurements indicate a large frame.

MEDIUM-FRAME MEN

HEIGHT (FT/IN)	ELBOW BREADTH (in INCHES)	ELBOW BREADTH (in CM)
5'1"–5'2"	2½"–2⅞"	6.35–7.30
5'3"–5'6"	2⅝"–2⅞"	6.67–7.30
5'7"–5'10"	2¾"–3"	7.00–7.62
5'11"–6'2"	2¾"–3⅛"	7.00–7.94
6'3"	2⅞"–3¼"	7.30–8.26

MEDIUM-FRAME WOMEN

HEIGHT (FT/IN)	ELBOW BREADTH (in INCHES)	ELBOW BREADTH (in CM)
4'9"–4'10"	2¼"–2½"	5.72–6.35
4'11"–5'2"	2¼"–2½"	5.72–6.35
5'3"–5'6"	2⅜"–2⅝"	6.03–6.67
5'7"–5'10"	2⅜"–2⅝"	6.03–6.67
5'11"	2½"–2¾"	6.35–7.00

[a]For the most accurate measurement, measure your elbow breadth with a caliper.
Source: From Metropolitan Life Insurance Company, 1983.

---

body mass index (BMI) weight (in kilograms) divided by the square of height (in meters)

recently published guidelines of the National Institutes of Health, the accepted range of healthy for BMI is below 25, values from 25 to 29.9 are considered overweight, and values of 30 or greater are considered indicative of obesity. Because BMI is computed from height and weight data, it suffers from the same limitation as height-weight tables—that is, its inability to differentiate fat weight from lean weight. Calculation Box 8.1 shows how to compute a sample BMI.

Underwater Weighing

The laboratory standard for determining body composition is underwater weighing (see Figure 8.4). The underwater weighing procedure is an application of Archimedes' principle, which states that an object submerged in water will displace a volume of water equal to the volume of the object. Once your body volume is determined, it is possible to compute your body density (body density equals body weight divided by body volume). Fat has a low density; lean tissue has a high density. If your body density is relatively low, then fat makes up a high proportion of your total body weight. If your body density is relatively high, then fat makes up a small proportion of your total body weight. Refer to Calculation Box 8.2 to see the formulas for computing the percent body fat from underwater weighing data. When you know your percent body fat, you can calculate your fat weight, your lean body weight, and a target body weight for yourself. These computations are described in Laboratory 8.1.

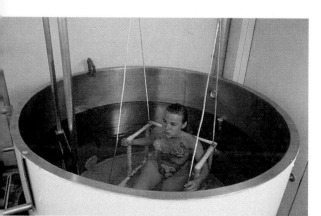

Figure 8.4

The fat and lean components of the body can be determined by underwater weighing.

Although underwater weighing gives a reasonably accurate measure of the percent body fat, it is not an absolutely precise procedure. For one thing, there is the possibility of inaccuracies in collecting the underwater weighing data. For another, the equation that converts body density into a percent body fat value makes assumptions about the densities of the tissues of the body that do not apply to everyone. Body fat determination by underwater weighing has an estimated accuracy of ±2.5%, which means that if underwater weighing yields a figure of 20% body fat, the true figure is likely between 17.5% and 22.5% body fat.

Skinfold Measurements

When underwater weighing is either unavailable or inconvenient, a common alternative is to predict the percent body fat from measurement of skinfold fat thicknesses. Because much of our adipose tissue is distributed in subcuta-

---

CALCULATION BOX 8.1

Body Mass Index

Consider a person who weighs 160 pounds and is 6 feet 1 inch tall. To convert these values into metric units, we divide 160 pounds by 2.2 pounds/kilogram to get 72.73 kg, and we divide 73 inches by 39.37 inches/meter to get 1.85 m. Now we can compute the BMI:

$$\text{BMI} = \frac{72.73 \text{ kg}}{(1.85 \text{ m})^2}$$

$$= \frac{72.73 \text{ kg}}{3.44 \text{ m}^2}$$

$$= 21.2 \text{ kg/m}^2$$

CALCULATION BOX 8.2

Computing Percent Body Fat

The purpose of underwater weighing is to determine a person's body volume, which, when corrected for the density of water and the air in the lungs, becomes the denominator in the equation for body density. The formulas for these calculations are shown below:

$$\text{Density} = \frac{\text{Mass}}{\text{Volume}}$$

$$\frac{\text{Body}}{\text{density}} = \frac{\text{Body mass}}{\text{Body volume}} = \frac{\text{Wt}_{air}}{\dfrac{\text{Wt}_{air} - \text{Wt}_{H_2O}}{\text{Density of } H_2O} - \text{RV}}$$

- Wt_{air} = weight on a scale on land, in kg
- Wt_{H_2O} = underwater weight, in kg

- Density of H_2O = the density of water is 1.0 g/cc (or 1.0 kg/l) at 4° C. Underwater weighing is conducted in water that is near body temperature (37° C), and a table must be consulted to obtain the water density at that temperature.

- RV = the residual lung volume, in liters, is the volume of air remaining in the lungs at the end of a maximal exhale. This must be determined or predicted to correct the body volume for the air in the lungs at the time of underwater weighing.

The body density value derived from the above equation is inserted into the following equation to convert it into a percent body fat value:

$$\% \text{ Body fat} = \frac{495}{\text{Body Density}} - 450$$

neous locations around the body, measuring the thicknesses of these sites with skinfold calipers can be used to derive a useful estimate of total body fat.

The most common locations on the body for skinfold assessment are the chest (along the pectoral muscle), axilla (under the arm, on the side of the ribs), triceps (at the back of the upper arm), subscapula (below the lower edge of the shoulder blade), suprailiac (at the hip, just above the iliac crest), abdomen (next to the navel), and thigh (at the front of the upper leg) (see Figure 8.5). Most prediction equations will use at least three of these sites. The skinfold caliper is a precision instrument that will measure a skinfold to the nearest 0.1 or 0.5 mm (depending on the model).

The accuracy of the skinfold technique depends on the skill of the person doing the measuring. A technician experienced in skinfold measurements has developed consistency in the way he or she takes the skinfold reading

Figure 8.5

Skinfold measurements are commonly taken from the following seven sites: chest, axilla, triceps, subscapular, suprailiac, abdomen, and thigh. Note that some of the skinfolds are taken with a vertical orientation and others with a diagonal orientation. The measurements are taken on the right side of the body.

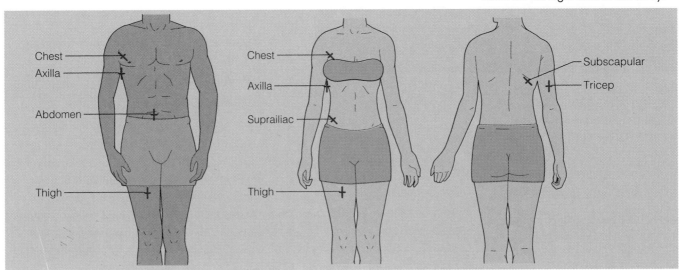

and has expertise in measuring the skinfold at the defined body locations. The choice of the equation used to convert the skinfold data into a percent body fat value is also very important because there are literally hundreds of equations to choose from. The skinfold equations that have been selected for use in Laboratory 8.1 are among those most consistently accurate for estimating percent body fat.

Because underwater weighing is used as the standard of accuracy in the development of the skinfold equations, body fat determinations from skinfold measures cannot be more accurate than those obtained from underwater weighing. The prediction equations used in Laboratory 8.1 are within ± 3.5% to 3.8% of the percent body fat determined from underwater weighing. This disparity between the two methods is due partly to the different patterns of fat distribution on the body. Some people may have a relatively large amount of fat in a subcutaneous site that was not measured for the prediction, or they may have more of their fat located in deep, internal deposits. However, for most people the accuracy of skinfold equations is reasonably good, which makes this measure a useful means of assessing percent body fat.

Bioelectrical Impedance Analysis

A recent innovation in the measurement of body composition is the bioelectrical impedance analysis (BIA) technique (see Figure 8.6). The BIA procedure takes only a few minutes, and the measurement can be made while you are in your street clothes. You lie down on a table, and small adhesive electrodes are placed on your wrist, on the back of your hand, on your ankle, and on the top of your foot. A very mild current of electricity, which is entirely safe and imperceptible, is sent through your body, and the resistance to its passage is measured by the instrument. The current flows most readily through your lean tissue, which has a high water content, and encounters more resistance in your adipose tissue, which contains very little water. The BIA computer combines the body resistance measurement with data such as your height, weight, age, and sex and calculates your percent body fat.

The simplicity of the technique is appealing, and many fitness clubs and clinics have purchased the instrument and offer the assessment to their members and clients. However, BIA determinations of percent body fat have not proven to be as accurate as those by the skinfold equations presented in Laboratory 8.1. Predictions of percent body fat by BIA have an error of ±5% to 6% compared to the determination made by underwater weighing. The inaccuracy is due, in large part, to variations in your state of hydration (your body water level). The amount of water in your body affects the passage of the electrical current. Therefore, variables that change your hydration level, such as recently consumed food or beverages, caffeine, alcohol, drugs, exercise, or, for women, hormonal changes during the menstrual cycle, will weaken the relationship between electrical impedance and your percent body fat.

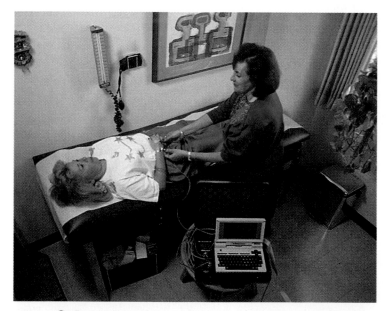

Figure 8.6

Bioelectrical impedance analysis (BIA) is a new technique for measuring body composition, but it may not be as accurate as calculations from measuring skinfold fat.

metabolic rate sum total of all the energy-utilizing reactions occurring throughout the body at any particular time

Weight Management

Without our being very conscious of it, our bodies are performing a daily balancing act in energy management. On the one hand, our bodies are constantly using energy. Our **metabolic rate** is the sum total of all the energy-utilizing reactions occurring throughout the body at any particular time. The metabolic rate ranges from the very low rate of energy expenditure associated with sleep to the very high rate of energy expenditure occurring when we exercise at our maximal capacity. Most of our time is spent somewhere between these two metabolic extremes, usually much closer to the sleep end than the heavy-exercise end (Figure 8.7).

On the other hand, our bodies are constantly providing a supply of fuel as a source of energy. The cells have energy-yielding pathways where carbohydrates, fats, and proteins are broken down and the energy they contain is released and converted into the form the cells can use: ATP (see Chapter 2). Our energy supply is maintained by the foods we consume. On a daily basis, then, energy is introduced into our bodies in the food we eat, and energy is expended in all the metabolic reactions occurring throughout our bodies.

Like everything else in the universe, our bodies abide by the First Law of Thermodynamics, which states that energy is neither created nor destroyed. Therefore, the relationship between the quantity of energy ingested and the quantity of energy expended will ultimately control our body weight. Because energy cannot be created, it must be provided to the cells when they need it. If our diet does not contain sufficient energy to meet the body's metabolic requirements, then our adipose tissue will make its stores of energy available to the tissues. If this situation persists, we will reduce our body fat levels. And because energy cannot be destroyed, once food energy is introduced into the body it must be either used to do work, converted into heat energy, or placed in storage. If our diet provides more energy than the body requires,

Figure 8.7

The energy expenditure spectrum encompasses a wide range in metabolic rates.

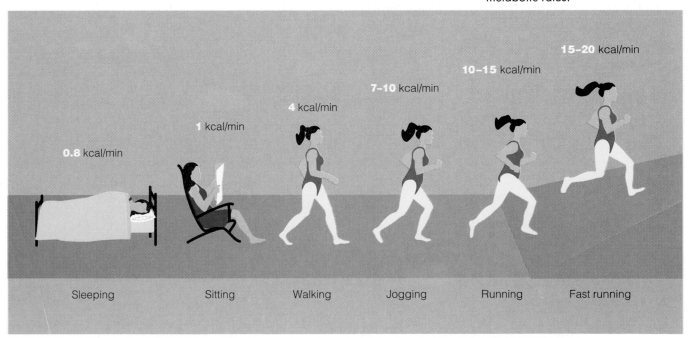

| 0.8 kcal/min | 1 kcal/min | 4 kcal/min | 7–10 kcal/min | 10–15 kcal/min | 15–20 kcal/min |
| Sleeping | Sitting | Walking | Jogging | Running | Fast running |

the excess will be converted to fat and stored in our adipose tissue. Over time, this situation will increase the amount of fat on our body.

Energy intake can relate to energy expenditure in one of three ways:

■ *Caloric (energy) balance: energy intake = energy expenditure.* We maintain a stable body weight when we are in energy balance. There is no excess energy to be stored as fat and no shortfall in energy intake, which would reduce the fat stores.

■ *Positive caloric balance: energy intake > energy expenditure.* We gain weight when we are in a positive caloric balance. Because more energy is being consumed than is being utilized, the excess will be stored as triglyceride in our adipose tissue.

■ *Negative caloric balance: energy intake < energy expenditure.* We lose body fat when we are in a negative caloric balance. Because more energy is being used than is being consumed, we must draw from our energy reserves in the adipose tissue to supplement the diet in meeting our body's metabolic requirements. (See Figure 8.8).

Figure 8.8

Energy intake can relate to energy expenditure in one of three ways: caloric (energy) balance, positive caloric balance, and negative caloric balance.

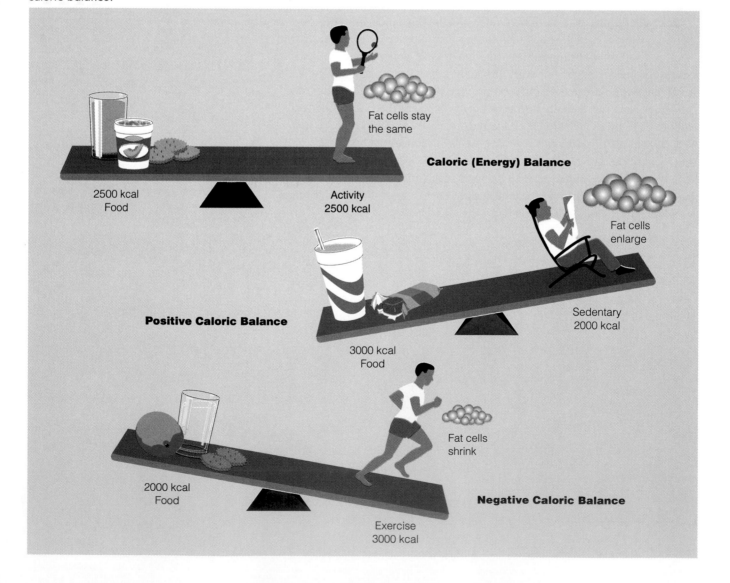

Fat cells stay the same

Caloric (Energy) Balance

2500 kcal Food

Activity 2500 kcal

Fat cells enlarge

Positive Caloric Balance

3000 kcal Food

Sedentary 2000 kcal

Fat cells shrink

2000 kcal Food

Negative Caloric Balance

Exercise 3000 kcal

Elements of the Energy Balance

The energy intake side of energy balance is easy to understand: It is merely the energy contained in the food we consume. As you discovered when you completed the diet analysis laboratory in Chapter 7, determining the total number of kilocalories you consume in a day requires a detailed record of everything you eat plus the size of the portions. Energy expenditure is more complicated than energy intake, for several factors contribute to the total amount of energy the body uses during a day, including basal metabolic rate, physical activity, and thermic effects.

Basal Metabolic Rate

The first factor in your daily energy expenditure is the **basal metabolic rate (BMR),** which is the amount of energy used by the body while awake and in a state of complete rest. The BMR is the starting point in your daily energy expenditure. Even if you did nothing but lie down all day, your total caloric expenditure would be substantial. Your BMR itself is a low level of energy expenditure, but it adds up over a 24-hour period. This basal, or minimal, rate of energy utilization is determined under a very prescribed set of conditions: lying down (sitting up requires more energy than lying down), 12 hours after consuming a meal (eating a meal stimulates the metabolism), and in a room at a comfortable temperature (heat stimulates metabolism while cold stimulates heat-generating reactions to maintain body temperature). The **resting metabolic rate**—the amount of energy used by the body at rest but sitting up, only several hours since the last meal—is slightly greater than the BMR.

Although a precise measurement of your BMR can be achieved only in human performance laboratories and hospitals, you can compute a prediction of your BMR using the following equations:

Males: 1.0 kcal/hr/kg × body wt (kg) × 24 hr/day = kcal/day

Females: 0.9 kcal/hr/kg × body wt (kg) × 24 hr/day = kcal/day

For example, the predicted BMR of a female who weighs 135 pounds (61.4 kg) is 1,326 kcal/day (0.9 kcal/hr/kg × 61.4 kg × 24 hr/day = 1,326 kcal/day).

The prediction is only a rough estimate because there is considerable variation in BMR among normal individuals. Some people have a fast metabolism whereas others have a slow metabolism. People with a higher BMR are like a car with a fast idle: They use more energy even when they are not doing anything. Although fuel efficiency is desirable in a car, in the human, fuel efficiency can lead to weight gain. The person with a lower BMR, or a slow idle, will be using less energy and so may more easily fall into a positive caloric balance. The food energy not being used in the BMR will be stored as fat in the adipose tissue unless the person engages in sufficient physical activity to expend it.

BMR tends to be higher in men than women because of differences in body composition between the sexes (see Figure 8.9). Men have more lean tissue than women, and lean tissue has a higher metabolic rate than adipose tissue. For both men and women, BMR declines by about 2% to 3% per

basal metabolic rate (BMR) amount of energy used by the body while awake and in a state of complete rest

resting metabolic rate amount of energy used by the body at rest but while sitting up, only several hours since the last meal; slightly greater than the BMR

Figure 8.9

The basal metabolic rate (expressed relative to body surface area) is slightly higher in males than in females, but both males and females experience a decline in BMR as they age.
Source: From Christian and Greger, 1994.

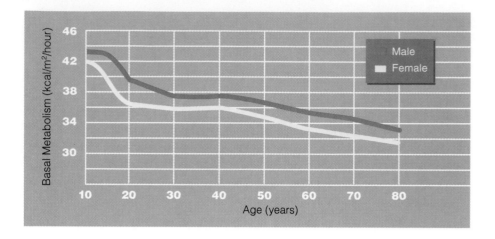

decade after age 25. The loss of lean tissue that often accompanies aging causes a reduction in the BMR, and this reduction in energy expenditure contributes to a gradual increase in body fat. A regular exercise program throughout your lifetime will help prevent a decline in both your lean body mass and your BMR as you age.

Physical Activity

With the BMR establishing the baseline, anything you do above basal conditions will add to your total daily caloric expenditure. Sitting up, walking around, climbing stairs, doing chores, and working in the yard all increase your rate of metabolism. Exercise is a very concentrated form of physical activity and has a very potent stimulating effect on your metabolism. For example, your BMR may be in the neighborhood of 1 kcal/min. By comparison, jogging at 6 mph will cause you to expend energy at a rate of approximately 10 kcal/min. Highly trained athletes can exercise at intensities in which they are expending 20 kcal/min or more. (See Figure 8.7.) A consistent program of regular exercise can elevate your total daily energy expenditure to a level that prevents you from gaining weight or, if necessary, helps you lose weight. The need to rely on exercise to maintain a caloric balance would be lessened if you also incorporated other forms of physical activity into your daily routine. For example, you could walk or ride a bike rather than using your car; you could take the stairs rather than the elevator; and you could engage in such activities as gardening, yard work, house-cleaning, and so on.

Thermic Effects

thermic effect of food increase in metabolism that occurs as a meal is digested, absorbed, and stored

adaptive thermogenesis energy expended to maintain body temperature

The BMR and physical activity are the major factors determining your daily energy expenditure. Two other metabolic processes play a lesser role: the thermic effect of food and adaptive thermogenesis. The **thermic effect of food** is the increase in metabolism that occurs as a meal is digested, absorbed, and stored. Your resting metabolism can be increased by 7% to 10% after consuming a meal. **Adaptive thermogenesis** refers to the energy expended to maintain body temperature. Although the two factors are not the major contributors to the total daily energy expenditure, they are thought to play a role in the development of obesity. Some studies have reported a smaller thermic effect of food and a reduced adaptive thermogenesis in obese individuals. Researchers do not know whether this is a cause or a consequence of obesity, but it definitely makes achieving the caloric deficit necessary to lose weight more difficult.

MANAGING ◆ YOUR ◆ WEIGHT

Do

▲ Manage your weight by eating well and exercising regularly.

▲ Eat slowly and really notice the flavor of what you eat.

▲ Clear your kitchen of high-calorie food and snacks.

▲ Limit your intake of ice cream, candy, sweets, cheese, salad dressing, butter, and other high-fat foods.

▲ Keep a supply of healthful snacks on hand, like fruit, veggies, plain popcorn, and nonfat yogurt.

▲ Bake, broil, boil, or poach foods instead of frying.

▲ Switch to skim or low-fat milk and milk products.

▲ Find an exercise you truly enjoy and will stick with for the long run.

▲ Stay away from situations where you know you will be tempted with high-fat foods.

▲ Consider joining a support group if weight is a major issue for you.

▲ Seek help if you think you may have an eating disorder.

Don't

▼ Rely on crash or fad diets to lose weight.

▼ "Diet" if you are not seriously overweight; try improving your diet and exercising more instead.

▼ Compare your body to those of models, movie stars, or athletes.

▼ Feel that you must be thin to be happy and successful.

▼ Try to lose weight just to please someone else.

▼ Rely on drugs or pills to lose weight.

▼ Resort to fasting or bingeing and purging to lose weight.

Achieving a Negative Caloric Balance

The comparison of your energy intake with your energy expenditure cannot be made on a minute-by-minute or hour-by-hour basis; although your body is constantly using energy, the periods of energy intake are usually separated by several hours. Thus, your energy balance is usually assessed over a 24-hour period of time, with the total number of calories you consume during a day being compared to the total number calories you expend during that same day. This assessment is only a "snapshot" of your energy balance, as it represents just one day of food intake and energy expenditure, both of which will vary from day to day. Whether you maintain a stable weight, gain body fat, or lose body fat is the cumulative result of how your energy intake and expenditure compare with each other over time.

Options for Creating the Negative Caloric Balance

By completing Laboratory 8.1, you can determine whether your percent body fat is appropriate or if it is excessive. If you have a satisfactory level of body fat, then you should try to maintain a caloric balance. If you find that you have more fat than is healthy for you, then you should try to reduce your level of body fat. To do so, you must create a negative caloric balance. This can be achieved three ways:

■ *Diet.* By restricting your food consumption, you can reduce your energy intake to a level that is below your energy expenditure.

■ *Exercise.* By increasing your physical activity, you can elevate your energy expenditure to a level that exceeds your energy intake.

■ *Diet plus exercise.* By doing both, you can manipulate both sides of the energy balance, giving yourself more leverage in creating the caloric imbalance. Energy expenditure can more readily exceed energy intake if intake is being reduced at the same time expenditure is being elevated.

Although all three options can create a negative caloric balance, diet plus exercise is the most effective method. Moderate changes in your food intake and level of physical activity will create a caloric deficit that would require more drastic changes if it were to be created by diet or exercise alone. Long-term success in weight control requires a modification in your lifestyle whereby the behaviors necessary to lose the fat and keep it off become lifelong habits. Diets are usually temporary conditions. When they are over, you may be tempted to return to your previous eating habits and you are likely to regain the weight you lost. If exercise is the sole means by which fat is reduced, you may have to commit a considerable amount of time to it each week to ensure that your energy expenditure exceeds your intake.

To put the discussion of caloric deficits in more concrete terms, a pound of fat contains approximately 3,500 kcal. This means that a negative caloric balance of 3,500 kcal must be created to lose a pound of fat. Fat is a very concentrated form of energy, with many calories contained in a relatively small unit of weight that is an advantage for us as mobile beings: We can carry a large energy reserve in just a few pounds of body fat. The fat concentration can seem to be a disadvantage, though, if you are trying to lose a few pounds of fat, for it means that you have to expend thousands of calories to do so. This reality underscores the need to take the long view in fat reduction. Establish a reasonable caloric deficit on a daily basis and allow it to accumulate over time. Slowly but surely, you will lose fat.

Diet Versus Exercise

There is a common perception that people who are obese eat more food than those who are not obese. However, numerous studies have failed to bear this out. In fact, some studies report that it is not uncommon for the obese to eat *less* food than the nonobese. Overeating is a relative term, and relative to others, most obese people are not overeaters. However, anyone who is gaining in body fat is eating more than he or she is expending; thus, relative to their energy expenditure, the obese can be said to be overeaters. When people eating normal amounts of food gain weight, their energy expenditure is too low. It is very easy to fall into a positive caloric balance, and thereby increase body fatness, when you lead a sedentary life.

The Pitfalls of Dieting. People often turn to diets to lose weight when it is the energy expenditure side of the energy balance that is creating the problem. It is very difficult to create a negative caloric balance by dieting when the total daily energy expenditure is low. To do so, you must restrict caloric intake to very low levels, which can leave you in a constant state of hunger. In the long run, this approach is destined to fail. It can also create some serious nutritional deficiencies. Very low calorie diets (less than 1,000 kcal per day) are appropriate only for severe cases of obesity and should be followed only under medical supervision.

Weight-loss diets are notorious for their failure rates. When weight reduction is achieved, most people are not able to maintain the lower weight and eventually regain most, if not all, of the weight they lost. Later, they may go on another diet, lose some weight, but again gradually regain it. This pattern of weight loss and subsequent regain is termed **weight cycling** but is more commonly known as *yo-yo dieting*.

One can easily imagine the frustration of people caught in these futile cycles. In addition, yo-yo diets can lead to a reduction in the resting metabolic rate, making weight loss more difficult and weight regain more likely. Not only is it discouraging to be trapped on a body weight roller coaster, but weight cycling apparently takes a health toll as well. Analysis of the data from the famous Framingham Heart Study shows that weight cycling is associated with an increased risk of coronary heart disease, death from coronary heart disease, and death from all causes in both men and women. The youngest age group studied (ages 30–44), the ones most likely to be dieting, demonstrated the strongest association between weight cycling and the adverse health outcomes. The study reported that the relative risks of weight cycling are comparable to the relative risks attributed to obesity itself (Lissner et al.). However, researchers have not yet discovered what it is about weight cycling that increases the risk of heart disease and death.

You might conclude from this that you would be better off not trying to lose weight than running the risk of slowing your metabolism through dieting and increasing your risk for heart disease by weight cycling. These studies actually emphasize the importance of committing to a prudent and

weight cycling pattern of weight loss and subsequent regain

realistic weight-loss program. The healthiest situation is to achieve and then maintain your proper body weight.

The Importance of Exercising. Physical activity is an essential part of every fat-reducing program for several reasons:

■ *A low level of energy expenditure is a primary cause of weight gain.* Physical activity is the component of energy expenditure that we can control, and increasing it directly addresses the source of the problem.

■ *Exercise stimulates metabolism.* Low-calorie diets can cause a slowing in the basal metabolic rate. In effect, the body reduces its use of energy during this period of energy deprivation. This response is counterproductive to the goal of creating a negative caloric balance. When the BMR slows, the gap between caloric expenditure and caloric intake is lessened (see Figure 8.10). The decreased BMR makes weight loss more difficult and weight gain more likely. Exercise, on the other hand, greatly elevates the metabolic rate during the time it is being performed, and it remains somewhat elevated for a limited time once the workout is over. The diet-induced slowing of the BMR can be avoided if exercise is carried out along with the dieting.

■ *Exercise relies heavily on fat as its source of energy.* As your aerobic fitness increases, so, too, does your ability to use fat as your energy source. This makes your negative caloric balance more likely to be drawn from the fat in your adipose tissue than from the carbohydrates and proteins in your lean tissue. With dieting, some of the weight loss will be from the lean compartment, whereas exercise has repeatedly been shown to preserve or increase lean body mass.

■ *Exercise is a positive approach with a healthy outcome.* Losing weight, however it is achieved, is an act of willpower. Many people find it easier to gather up the willpower necessary to take the active role of exercising than to exert the willpower necessary to deprive themselves of food. It is difficult to ignore your hunger pangs, whereas you can eat enough food to keep from feeling hungry as long as you exercise enough to work it off. Regardless of the amount of weight you lose, a regular program of aerobic exercise will confer many health benefits, such as reducing your risk of developing heart disease, cancer, diabetes, hypertension, and hyperlipidemia.

Figure 8.10

The decline in the basal metabolic rate during a low-calorie diet decreases the caloric expenditure, which, in turn, reduces the caloric deficit. When this happens, the diet is less effective in causing fat reduction.

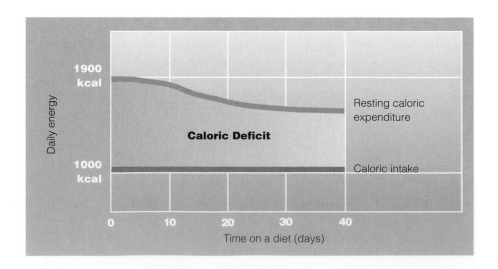

In spite of the advantages just listed, exercise has been underutilized as a tool in reducing body fat. For too long, many people have relied on diets to lose weight, even though research has shown that maintaining weight loss is more successfully accomplished when exercise is part of the program.

Exercise and Appetite

One of the reservations people have about using exercise to lose weight is the belief that exercise increases the appetite. If this were true, exercise would not be an effective way to create a negative caloric balance, for the additional food consumed would offset the energy expended in the exercise. The large quantities of food consumed by some endurance athletes or people engaged in heavy physical labor is taken as evidence to support this view.

The relationship between exercise and appetite has long intrigued scientists, but it has been very difficult to study. The careful food records necessary to quantify energy intake make its measurement very challenging. Quantifying energy expenditure is much more difficult, for it would require measuring oxygen consumption throughout the whole day! For this reason, much of the research on the topic has been conducted with animals because the food they eat can be easily measured and their level of daily physical activity controlled. The animal studies generally report a reduction or no difference in food intake when exercising animals are compared to sedentary animals.

The research with humans is inconclusive. One study reports a reduction or no change in food intake when an exercise program is undertaken (King and

"SLOW AND STEADY" WORKS

Sound Decision Making

Julie was chubby even as a child, but it didn't bother her until she started junior high school. There, the "fat kids" were often cruelly taunted, and suddenly it seemed very important to have a slim figure. Over the next several years, Julie tried every diet in the book, and she'd often lose ten or twenty pounds, only to gain it all back plus a bit more after she went off the diet. As she enters college, Julie wants to make a fresh start in her weight-loss efforts. She enrolls in a wellness class hoping to learn some weight-loss secrets.

Julie doesn't learn any secrets, but she does learn a lot about nutrition and fitness. Julie is currently 30% body fat and she decides she would like to reduce that to 25% by the end of the school year. Her short-term goal is to achieve a negative calorie balance of 500 calories. Julie enlists the support of her roommate and her sister, who will provide encouragement.

To meet her short-term goal, Julie starts a program of walking 3 miles per day, and reduces her caloric intake by 300 calories. She finds she can reduce her calories by this much with some fairly simple and relatively painless substitutions. She drinks water or tea instead of soda, and snacks on fruit or popcorn instead of chips and candy. After her first two weeks on her weight-loss program, Julie is a little disappointed that she has lost only three pounds. But she does not feel deprived like she always did on those diets; actually, she feels more energetic than she has in quite a while.

Six weeks into what she calls her "slow and steady" weight-loss plan, Julie is looking noticeably slimmer. She has made friends with a group of women from her wellness class, and they have started race-walking together three times per week. She even finds that she enjoys her new healthier eating habits, and has found a new joy in cooking from some low-fat cookbooks her sister gave her for her birthday. The best thing about it is that Julie knows that this is a lifestyle she can stick with to get down to a healthy weight and maintain it.

Tribble); others, however, have found exercisers to consume more food than nonexercisers. In spite of this, the exercisers were leaner than the nonexercisers. A study of formerly sedentary adults who completed a 2-year jogging program found a significant reduction in percent body fat even though food intake increased by approximately 300 kcal per day (Blair et al.). This finding indicates that the increase in energy intake was less than the increase in energy expenditure. Additional research is needed to give us a better understanding of the interaction between exercise and appetite, but for now we can accept that the increase in energy expenditure brought about by exercise is not undone by subsequent eating behavior.

Designing an Exercise Program for Weight Loss

The principle for weight loss is simple and unavoidable: Eat less and exercise more. The chances for long-term success are greater when new habits have replaced the lifestyle behaviors that led to weight gain. Rapid rates of weight loss are usually the result of changes in eating or exercise practices that are too drastic to become habits and are very likely to lead to the yo-yo pattern of weight loss and regain. The slow-but-steady approach to weight loss has a better track record.

Exercise is probably the most effective means you have to reduce the amount of fat on your body. To tailor your use of exercise for the purpose of losing weight, follow these steps:

1. *Assess your body composition.* You may be thinking that you should lose weight based on the height-weight tables or simply based on how you look in the mirror. Whether you truly need to lose weight is a matter of the amount of body fat you have. Complete Laboratory 8.1, or assess your percent body fat by underwater weighing. With this information, you can determine whether you need to lower your percent body fat and, if so, what your target body weight should be.

2. *Set realistic goals.* Your target body weight must be based on your body composition assessment. Too often people arbitrarily determine that they should lose 5, 10, or 15 pounds without knowing whether they even have that much extra fat to lose. Thus, you need to set realistic goals for the rate of fat reduction. People trying to lose body fat are advised to establish a steady rate of 1–2 pounds of weight loss per week. This may seem to be a modest goal, but it is achievable with modifications in diet and exercise that can be sustained indefinitely.

3. *Design your exercise program.* The exercise prescription for fat reduction is the same as the one described in Chapter 3 for developing cardiorespiratory fitness, because aerobic activity benefits both the cardiorespiratory system and body composition. Like the prescription given in Chapter 3, you need to make decisions concerning the mode of exercise and exercise intensity, duration, and frequency. You may find it helpful to keep a record of your physical activity or exercise sessions by jotting on your calendar the length of time you walked, worked out, and so on. This will allow you to chart your exercise frequency and duration and will serve as a guard against your doing too much or letting your program slip with too many days without significant physical activity.

4. *Evaluate your progress.* Weigh yourself once a week, under similar circumstances (for example, in the morning, after going to the bathroom). Remember, fat loss and weight loss are not synonymous. When you exercise, you will likely experience a gain in lean body weight, which will offset some of the weight loss due to fat reduction. A more accurate and direct assessment of your progress would be to repeat the measurement of your body composition (underwater weighing, skinfold, or BIA) every three months. If you are not satisfied with the rate of fat reduction, you should increase the amount of exercise you are doing and/or further reduce your food intake. Again, make sensible and gradual changes in your lifestyle, and be patient.

Choice of Exercise

Any form of aerobic exercise is appropriate. Weight-bearing activities such as walking or jogging are effective for ensuring a substantial caloric expenditure. In activities in which your body weight is supported, such as in cycling or swimming, your caloric expenditure will vary depending on whether you are exercising vigorously or are gliding or floating. The advantage of the weight-supported exercises is that there is less impact on your muscles, joints, and bones, and avoiding injury is an important factor in determining how often you can exercise. Ultimately, it's the regularity of your exercise sessions that will work off the pounds.

Intensity

When the object of the exercise program is to expend energy, there is no virtue in being energy efficient. For this reason, people often carry hand weights and/or move their arms in an exaggerated fashion as they walk or jog, which increases the caloric cost of the activity. Because the energy cost of walking or jogging is determined by the weight you are transporting and the distance you cover, you will expend fewer calories per mile when you lose weight. However, the training that resulted in your weight loss will also develop your aerobic fitness, so you will be able to walk or jog for a greater distance.

Recall from Chapter 2 that fat utilization during exercise is influenced by the intensity of the exercise. Fat contributes a larger proportion of the energy utilized during exercise at lower intensities. At higher intensities, the proportion of energy derived from fat decreases and the proportion derived from carbohydrates increases. For this reason, some people in the fitness field have asserted that low-intensity exercise is preferable for fat reduction. Such advice fails to recognize that the bottom line in fat reduction is how many calories are expended each day, not whether the calories expended in the exercise session came from fat or carbohydrates. Although fat may provide the greater proportion of kilocalories used during a low-intensity workout, more kilocalories are expended per minute in exercise at higher intensities. Unless you continue the low-intensity exercise long enough to equal or exceed the energy expended in a moderate- or high-intensity workout, the low-intensity workout will be less effective for fat reduction. This is not to say that you should push yourself hard in your workouts, because that may lead to burnout or injury. Rather, you should exercise at the intensity most comfortable to you without thinking you should lower it in the belief that "less is more."

Frequency and Duration

More exercise is generally required to reduce body fat than to achieve cardiorespiratory fitness. Numerous studies have demonstrated that three sessions per week of aerobic exercise that expends 300 to 500 kcal per workout will develop cardiorespiratory fitness over a 10- to 15-week period. This exercise regimen adds up to a 900- to 1,500-kcal expenditure per week. You can reduce body fat with that amount of exercise per week, but if the exercise represents the caloric imbalance, it will take 2 to 4 weeks to lose a pound of fat (3,500 kcal/pound fat divided by 900 kcal expended in exercise per week gives 3.9 weeks to lose a pound of fat; dividing 3,500 kcal/pound fat by 1,500 kcal/week gives 2.3 weeks/lb fat).

To be most effective, exercise programs for fat reduction must emphasize caloric expenditure. This can be done by gradually extending the length of the individual exercise sessions and/or increasing exercise frequency to 5 to 7 days per week. As always, increasing either of these aspects of an exercise program should be done gradually to ensure development of the fitness necessary to tolerate the increased exercise and to reduce the risk of injury.

Become a calorie burner. The following section gives you specifics on the number of calories you expend in a variety of exercises. The key is to be consistent and to be realistic. Most of all, do not become impatient. It took time for you to accumulate the 3,500 kcal in each pound of fat you gained, and it will take time for you to create the deficit that will whittle them away. Stick with it!

The Caloric Cost of Exercise

The key to success in losing weight and keeping it off is to establish a consistent habit of exercising. This will happen only if you enjoy your workouts. Staking your hopes for weight loss on a high-calorie-burning exercise such as running when you do not like to run sets you up for failure. If you like the activity, you are more likely to stick with it. A low- or moderate-calorie-burning activity that you do with regularity uses far more calories than a high-calorie-burning activity that you will not do. Table 8.4 shows you the caloric expenditure of many different physical activities.

Currently, many people vary their workouts within a week to exercise different parts of the body or to avoid the repetition of doing the same thing each workout. And the sport of triathlon, in which you consecutively swim, cycle, and run, has become very popular. Triathletes routinely rotate their workouts among running, swimming, and cycling—even within the same day! The question will arise, How can you compare a workout doing one of these activities with a workout doing another? The answer: by comparing the number of calories expended in each workout. The training benefits of two different forms of aerobic exercise (for example, cycling and running) are comparable if a similar number of kilocalories is expended in each.

The following will provide you with an approximate but useful estimate of the caloric costs of running, swimming, and cycling. First, an estimate of the kilocalories expended when running is

$$\text{kcal/mile run} = 0.74 \text{ kcal/lb/mile} \times \text{body wt (lb)}$$

Table 8.4

Caloric Expenditures During Selected Physical Activities

ACTIVITY	KCAL/KG/MINUTE	ACTIVITY	KCAL/KG/MINUTE
Bicycling (racing)	0.127	Piano-playing	0.018
Bicycling (leisurely)	0.042	Rowing in a race	0.267
Canoeing (leisurely)	0.024	Running (5½ min/mile)	0.269
Carpentry	0.045	Running (7 min/mile)	0.208
Cleaning (light)	0.030	Running (9 min/mile)	0.173
Cooking	0.015	Sewing (hand or machine)	0.007
Dancing (fast)	0.148	Singing (loud)	0.013
Dancing (slowly)	0.050	Sitting (writing)	0.007
Dishwashing	0.017	Skating	0.058
Dressing, personal care	0.025	Skiing	
Driving a car	0.015	(cross-country, level)	0.099
Eating	0.007	Skiing	
Field hockey	0.114	(cross-country, uphill)	0.254
Grocery shopping	0.040	Squash	0.192
Football	0.112	Standing (relaxed)	0.008
Garage work (repairs)	0.046	Stock-clerking	0.034
Golf	0.065	Swimming (2 mph)	0.132
Gymnastics	0.046	Tennis	0.089
Horseback riding (walk)	0.023	Violin playing	0.010
Horseback riding (gallop)	0.112	Volleyball	0.030
Judo	0.175	Walking (3 mph)	0.039
Knitting	0.012	Walking (4 mph)	0.057
Laboratory work	0.018	Walking downstairs	
Laundry (light)	0.022	(kcal/flight)	0.012
Painting inside	0.014	Walking upstairs	
Painting outside	0.057	(kcal/flight)	0.036
Playing Ping-Pong	0.073		

Note: Values have been modified to eliminate energy expended for BMR and the thermic effect of food. As values for the same activity vary from one source to another, these values are unavoidably less precise than they appear.

Source: Data from C. M. Taylor and G. McLeod, *Rose's Laboratory Handbook for Dietetics,* 5th ed. (New York: Macmillan: 1949), p. 18; J. V. G. A. Durnin and R. Passmore, "Energy, work and leisure," *Energy and Protein Requirements,* FAO/WHO, 1967; W. D. McArdle, F. I. Katch, and V. I. Katch, *Exercise Physiology: Energy, Nutrition, and Human Performance,* 4th ed. (Philadelphia: Lea & Febiger, 1996); R. Passmore and J. V. G. A. Durnin, "Human energy expenditure," *Physiological Reviews,* 35: 801–840, 1955.

For example, if you weigh 140 lbs, you will expend approximately 104 kcal to run or jog a mile (0.74 kcal/lb/mile × 140 lb = 103.6 kcal/mile). Notice that this equation gives you the number of kilocalories expended per mile. As long as you are running or jogging, it does not matter what speed you are going— you expend virtually the same number of kilocalories per mile run. Obviously, when you are running faster, you cover the mile in a shorter period of time and so can run a greater distance within a 30- or 60-minute time interval.

With the caloric cost of running as our basis of comparison, it requires three to four times as many kilocalories to swim a mile as it does to run a mile. Water offers far more resistance to movement than does air, so there is a considerably greater energy cost when traveling through it. The inefficient swimmer can expend a large amount of energy flailing about in the water without producing much forward motion. The average swimmer may have a 4-to-1 ratio between energy expended swimming a mile compared to energy expended running a mile. For the poor swimmer, the ratio might be 5-to-1. For the good swimmer, the ratio may be 3-to-1, which means swimming 1 mile is equivalent to running 3 miles. As it turns out, it takes approximately three to four times as long to swim a mile as to run a mile, so these activities are comparable in the number of calories expended per minute.

Cycling is more efficient than running. Cycling a mile will require approximately half the energy of running a mile. Thus, cycling 2 miles is roughly equal to running 1 mile. This relationship holds for level cycling, as opposed to uphill or downhill cycling, and varies somewhat with the aerodynamic and technological sophistication of the bicycle.

To illustrate: A 140-lb woman runs 4 miles per day and wants to calculate its equivalent in swimming and cycling. The energy cost of her workouts is 0.74 kcal/lb/mile × 140 lb × 4 miles = 414 kcal. To expend this energy in a swim workout would require 1 mile of swimming (4 miles running divided by 4 miles running/mile swimming). She would need to cycle 8 miles to get a comparable workout (4 miles running × 2 miles cycling/mile running).

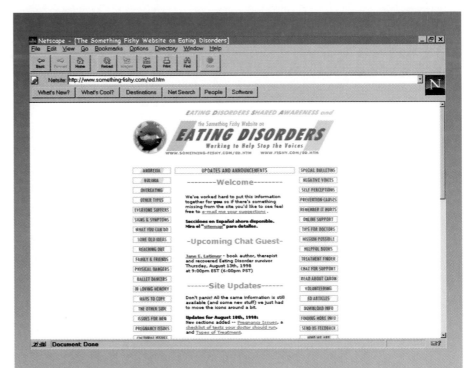

The Something Fishy Website on Eating Disorders
http://www.something-fishy.com/ed.htm

This excellent site provides lots of information on eating disorders, including anorexia nervosa, bulimia nervosa, and compulsive eating. It addresses some causes, symptoms, associated problems, physical consequences, and prevention methods. There is also information on what you can do if you are concerned about a loved one, resources for help, and treatment options.

Critical thinking: Eating disorders are particularly prevalent among college women. What is your school doing to reduce the incidence of eating disorders on campus? What more could it do?

Source: From Something Fishy Music & Publishing, 1996–1998.

Remember that exercise is the most potent means of increasing the number of calories you expend. For this reason, it is your best insurance against falling victim to creeping obesity as you age. Should obesity develop, exercise is an effective treatment in the weight-loss program. Choose the activity you enjoy and do it regularly. At the same time, follow the nutritional recommendations in Chapter 7: Restrict your consumption of desserts, cookies, pastries, potato chips, soft drinks, ice cream, butter and margarine, and high-fat varieties of meats, cheeses, and dairy products. Eat the recommended number of servings of the foods from the Food Guide Pyramid. When your diet comprises foods from the cereal, bread, and grain and the fruit and vegetable food groups, and when you choose the low-fat options from the dairy and the meat groups, you maximize the nutritional content of the calories you consume. At the same time, you make it less likely that you will create a positive caloric balance.

Your body composition is determined by your genetic inheritance, your diet, and your exercise and physical activity habits. As stated at the start of this chapter, your body composition influences your predilection for a number of chronic diseases, your ability to be vigorous in your daily activities, and your self-image. Modest increases in physical activity coupled with a diet that accentuates the food groups that make up the lower part of the Food Guide Pyramid will produce improvements in your health and fitness relatively quickly. It will take somewhat longer for the improvements in body composition to become evident, but that, too, will follow.

Lifestyle Choices: Plan for Action

Now that you are familiar with the principles of body composition and weight management, you are in a position to make the necessary lifestyle changes to ensure that you manage your personal energy reserves to achieve a high degree of wellness. Begin by reviewing your responses to the Body Composition and Weight-Control Checklist in Laboratory 1.1.

If you scored below 35 points, you should try to make some changes in your lifestyle. The lower your score, the more important it is for you to improve your exercise habits and perhaps modify your eating habits. Review your responses to the questions to identify which factors relating to body composition are most in need of change and make them your first targets for modification. Start by listing the potential benefits and barriers to your adopting the wellness lifestyle for weight control.

POTENTIAL BENEFITS   **POTENTIAL BARRIERS**

_____   _____

_____   _____

_____   _____

_____   _____

_____   _____

It may be helpful to develop your action plan for lifestyle changes in terms of a caloric adjustment achieved through increasing your level of physical activity and/or reducing your food or beverage consumption. For example, your first week's goal might be to change your daily caloric balance by 100 kcal by walking an additional mile each day. For the second week, you can build this up to 200 kcal each day by extending your walk to 2 miles. Then, for the third week, you can maintain your 2-mile daily walks and also give up that 300-kcal 24-ounce soft drink. Your daily caloric imbalance would now be up to 500 kcal. And so on. By relatively minor lifestyle modifications, you can create a caloric deficit that, with time, will really change your body composition.

Set out your plan of action for the next month, listing the changes you will make each week. Keep in mind that you do not need to implement a new change every week. You may want to continue with the changes made in the previous week and increase the caloric adjustment only at 2-week intervals. Do whatever works best for you. Make a contract with yourself by putting your intention in writing and then signing it. This formality helps to move you from the thinking stage to the doing stage.

WEEK 1

This week I will make the following caloric adjustment in my lifestyle:

_____

To do this, I will make the following modifications in my activity and/or eating behaviors:

_____

_____

_____

WEEK 2

This week I will make the following caloric adjustment in my lifestyle:

_____

To do this, I will make the following modifications in my activity and/or eating behaviors:

_____

_____

_____

WEEK 3

This week I will make the following caloric adjustment in my lifestyle:

_____

To do this, I will make the following modifications in my activity and/or eating behaviors:

_____

_____

_____

WEEK 4

This week I will make the following caloric adjustment in my lifestyle:

_____

To do this, I will make the following modifications in my activity and/or eating behaviors:

_____

_____

_____

_____   _____
(signature)   *(date)*

At the end of the month, review your progress. How many of the changes were you able to make? What turned out to be more difficult to change, your activity or eating behaviors? If you were unable to reach your daily goal consistently in one week, continue with that goal during the next week. Don't let yourself become discouraged and don't expect rapid results. Remember, consistency is the key for long-term success.

Summary

Although most college students are not obese, the incidence of obesity increases steadily with older age groups, so younger men and women need to be aware of how to avoid developing creeping obesity or how to correct it if it occurs. The exercise prescription for cardiorespiratory fitness, described in Chapter 3, is appropriate for fat reduction. A regular program of exercise combined with a nutritious diet that avoids empty calories and limits fat intake is the lifelong habit that will keep body fat at healthful levels.

Key concepts that you have learned in this chapter include these:

- Obesity is a condition of excessive body fat that places a person at risk for heart disease, diabetes, hypertension, and other health problems.

- The human body is made up of lean tissue (muscles, skeleton, and organs) and fat tissue (essential and storage).

- Essential fat serves structural and functional roles; storage fat serves as the body's energy reservoir.

- The average amount of body fat for men is 15% and for women is 23%; men over 23% body fat are considered obese, as are women over 32%.

- The male (android) pattern of body fat distribution refers to fat accumulation on the abdomen; the female (gynoid) pattern refers to accumulation mainly on the hips and thighs.

- The height-weight tables provide limited information on body composition because of their inability to make a distinction between being overweight and being overfat.

- Underwater weighing is the best laboratory technique for assessing percent body fat, but skinfold equations to predict percent body fat are reasonably accurate and can give a useful estimate of body composition.

- A person gains body fat when the number of calories ingested as food exceeds the number of calories expended in physical activity (positive caloric balance); a person loses body fat when caloric expenditure exceeds caloric intake (negative caloric balance).

- Energy expenditure is the sum of the calories expended as the basal metabolic rate, physical activity, and thermic effects.

- The exercise prescription for fat reduction accentuates caloric expenditure through weight-bearing activities (walking, jogging), 3 to 7 days per week, for 20 or more minutes per session.

- Commitment to a lifestyle of exercise and moderate food intake is necessary for long-term success in losing fat and keeping it off.

References

Andersson, B., et al. The effects of exercise training on body composition and metabolism in men and women. *International Journal of Obesity,* 15: 75–81, 1991.

Baumgartner, R. N. Electrical impedance and total body electrical conductivity. In A. F. Roche, S. B. Heymsfield, and T. G. Lohman, eds., *Human Body Composition.* Champaign, IL: Human Kinetics, 1996, 79–107.

Bjorntorp, P. The role of adipose tissue in human obesity. In M. R. C. Greenwood, ed., *Obesity.* New York: Churchill Livingstone, 1983, 17–24.

Blair, S. N., et al. Comparison of nutrient intake in middle-aged men and women runners and controls. *Medicine and Science in Sports and Exercise,* 13: 310–315, 1981.

Bonge, D., and J. E. Donnelly. Trials to criteria for hydrostatic weighing at residual volume. *Research Quarterly for Exercise and Sport,* 60: 176–179, 1989.

Bouchard, C. Discussion: Heredity, fitness, and health. In C. Bouchard et al., eds., *Exercise, Fitness, and Health.* Champaign, IL: Human Kinetics, 1990, 147–153.

Bray, G. A. Controls of food intake and energy expenditure. In G. A. Bray et al., eds., *Diet and Obesity.* Tokyo: Japan Scientific Societies Press, 1988, 17–36.

Chatard, J. C., J. M. Lavoie, and J. R. Lacour. Energy cost of front-crawl swimming in women. *European Journal of Applied Physiology,* 63: 12–16, 1991.

Despres, J.-P., et al. Regional distribution of body fat, plasma lipoproteins, and cardiovascular disease. *Arteriosclerosis,* 10: 497–511, 1990.

DiCarlo, L. J., et al. Peak heart rates during maximal running and swimming: Implications for exercise prescription. *International Journal of Sports Medicine,* 12: 309–312, 1991.

Forbes, G. B. The abdomen:hip ratio: Normative data and observations on selected patients. *International Journal of Obesity,* 14: 149–157, 1990.

Frankle, R. T. Weight control for the adult and the elderly. In R. T. Frankle and M. U. Yang, eds., *Obesity and Weight Control.* Rockville, MD: Aspen, 1988, 363–390.

Frey-Hewitt, B., et al. The effect of weight loss by dieting or exercise on resting metabolic rate in overweight men. *International Journal of Obesity,* 14: 327–334, 1990.

Gaesser, G. A. *Big Fat Lies.* New York: Fawcett Columbine, 1996.

Heyward, V. H., and L. M. Stolarczyk. *Applied Body Composition.* Champaign, IL: Human Kinetics, 1996.

Jackson, A. S., and M. L. Pollock. Generalized equations for predicting body density of men. *British Journal of Nutrition,* 40: 497–504, 1978.

Jackson, A. S., M. L. Pollock, and A. Ward. Generalized equations for predicting body density of women. *Medicine and Science in Sports and Exercise,* 12: 175–182, 1980.

Jackson, A. S., et al. Reliability and validity of bioelectrical impedance in determining body composition. *Journal of Applied Physiology,* 64: 529–534, 1988.

King, A. C., and D. L. Tribble. The role of exercise in weight regulation in nonathletes, *Sports Medicine,* 11: 331–349, 1991.

Kuczmarski, R. J., et al. Increasing prevalence of overweight among U.S. Adults; The National Health and Nutrition Examination Surveys, 1960–1991. *Journal of the American Medical Association,* 272: 205–211, 1994.

Kurtzman, F. D., et al. Eating disorders among selected female student populations at UCLA. *Journal of the American Dietetic Association,* 89: 45–53, 1989.

LeBlanc, J. Exercise training and energy expenditure. In G. A. Bray et al., eds., *Diet and Obesity.* Tokyo: Japan Scientific Societies Press, 1988, 181–190.

Leon, G. R. Eating disorders in female athletes. *Sports Medicine,* 12: 219–227, 1991.

Lissner, L., et al. Variability of body weight and health outcomes in the Framingham population. *New England Journal of Medicine,* 324: 1839–1844, 1991.

Lohman, T. G. *Advances in Body Composition Assessment.* Champaign, IL: Human Kinetics, 1992.

Martin, A. D., and D. T. Drinkwater. Variability in the measures of body fat. *Sports Medicine,* 11: 277–288, 1991.

McArdle, W. D., F. L. Katch, and V. L. Katch. *Exercise Physiology: Energy, Nutrition, and Human Performance.* Philadelphia: Lea & Febiger, 1996.

Pi-Sunyer, F. X. Exercise in the treatment of obesity. In R. T. Frankle and M. U. Yang, eds., *Obesity and Weight Control.* Rockville, MD: Aspen, 1988, 241–256.

Pollock, M. L., and A. S. Jackson. Research progress in validation of clinical methods of assessing body composition. *Medicine and Science and Exercise,* 16: 606–613, 1984

Pollock, M. L., and J. H. Wilmore. *Exercise in Health and Disease.* Philadelphia: Saunders, 1990.

Rodin, J., et al. Weight cycling and fat distribution. *International Journal of Obesity,* 14: 303–310, 1990.

Stern, J. S. Adipose tissue cellularity and function and food intake regulation. In G. A. Bray et al., eds., *Diet and Obesity.* Tokyo: Japan Scientific Societies Press, 1988, 175–180

Stern, J. S. Diet and exercise. In M. R. C. Greenwood, ed., *Obesity.* New York: Churchill Livingstone, 1983, 65–84.

Wilmore, J. H. Eating and weight disorders in the female athlete. *International Journal of Sport Nutrition,* 1: 104–117, 1991.

Wilmore, J. H. Body composition in sport and exercise. Directions for future research. *Medicine and Science and Exercise,* 15: 21–31, 1983.

Yang, M. U. Composition and resting metabolic rate in obesity. In R. T. Frankle and M. U. Yang, eds., *Obesity and Weight Control.* Rockville, MD: Aspen, 1988, 71–96.

Laboratory 8.1

Assessing Body Composition

The most accurate determination of the relative proportions of fat and lean tissue in the human body is through underwater weighing and the computation of body density. However, access to laboratories that perform underwater weighing is limited, so other techniques have been developed to evaluate body composition. Although less accurate, they provide information that can be useful in fitness, weight management, or athletic training programs. In this laboratory, you will collect data that allow you to calculate your percent body fat based on skinfold thicknesses, to compute your waist:hip ratio, to compute your body mass index, and to utilize the height-weight tables.

Skinfold Measurements

Three skinfold measurements will be taken to derive an estimate of your percent body fat. By convention, all skinfold measures are taken on the right side of the body. Skinfold measures should not be taken through clothing, so you will need to be wearing shorts for the thigh skinfold to be measured. The location of the skinfold sites are illustrated in Figure 8.5.

For men, the following skinfold sites are used:

Chest: a diagonal skinfold taken along the pectoral (chest) muscle, halfway between the front fold of the armpit and the nipple

Abdomen: a vertical skinfold taken 2 cm (approximately 0.75 in) to the side of the navel

Thigh: a vertical skinfold taken on the front of the thigh, halfway between the crease made where the leg joins at the hip and the upper edge of the kneecap

For women, these skinfold sites are used:

Tricep: a vertical skinfold taken at the back of the upper arm, halfway between the top edge of the shoulder and the bony prominence of the elbow, with the arm straight and relaxed

Suprailiac: a diagonal skinfold taken above the upper edge of the hip bone at a point directly below an imaginary line straight down from the front fold of the armpit

Thigh: a vertical skinfold taken on the front of the thigh, halfway between the crease made where the leg joins at the hip and the upper edge of the kneecap

Your lab instructor will be trained in the use of the skinfold calipers and the technique of skinfold measures. Record the measurements on the lab data form and follow the instructions there for determining your percent body fat.

Waist:Hip Ratio

A comparison of your waist circumference to your hip circumference will give you an indication of whether you have the android (abdominal) pattern of fat accumulation. To compute this ratio, use a measuring tape to measure your waist at the level of your navel and your hips at the level of the maximal protrusion of the buttocks. Record these values on the data form and follow the instructions there for computing your waist:hip ratio to determine whether you have an android pattern of fat deposition.

Keep in mind that these circumference measures, while easily obtained, are not the best indicators of the extent of abdominal fat accumulation. For this reason, these ratios should be interpreted with caution. For example, two people with the same waist circumference can have very different waist:hip ratios if one has a small hip circumference and the other has a large hip circumference.

Body Mass Index (BMI)

BMI is an expression of your weight (in kilograms) over the square of your height (in meters). The National Institutes of Health have recently set stricter BMI guidelines for men and women: a value of 25–29.9 is considered overweight, and a value of 30 or greater is considered obese. In the NHANES study, which reported that 33% of U.S. adults are overweight, the criteria for determining overweight were BMI values greater than 27.8 for men and 27.3 for women. You are reminded that the BMI and height-weight tables cannot distinguish how much fat weight contributes to your total weight. This means that it is possible for you to be overweight without being overfat.

Follow the instructions on the data form to determine your BMI.

Height-Weight Tables

You will notice that Table 8.2, which contains the height-weight tables, presents the recommended weights for each height in groupings by frame size. To determine your frame size, use a caliper to measure the width of your elbow and refer to Table 8.3 to classify your frame size. During the measurement you should hold your upper arm in a horizontal position with your lower arm at a right-angle to the upper arm with your palm facing you. If you do not have access to a caliper, have someone use a ruler to sight the width of your elbow as accurately as possible. (When referring to the height-weight tables, notice that the measures were made of subjects wearing indoor clothing and shoes.) Follow the steps in the lab to determine whether you are overweight by height-weight standards.

Keep in mind that all these assessments are indirect indicators of your level of body fat. Of the four methods, the skinfold assessment is a more direct measure of body fat than the others, but it has a precision of only 3.5% to 4%. If you find that you are overweight based on the height-weight table and BMI, but are average in percent body fat as determined from the skinfold measures, then you may be overweight, but you are not overfat.

Body Composition Assessment Form

Name

Age _____ Sex: M _____ F _____

Weight: _____ lb × 0.455 kg/lb = _____ kg

Height: _____ in × 0.0254 m/in = _____ m

Skinfold Assessment

Males (mm)	Females (mm)
Chest _____	Tricep _____
Abdomen _____	Suprailiac _____
Thigh _____	Thigh _____
Sum _____	Sum _____

Consult Table 8.5 to derive a prediction of your percent body fat using the sum of the three skinfolds and your age. Record that value here:

% body fat _____ %

Use Table 8.6 on page 260 to evaluate your body composition.

Calculating Target Body Weight

1. Fat weight = Total weight (lb) $\times \dfrac{\% \text{ body fat}}{100}$ = _____ lb

   (By dividing % body fat and target % lean [see step 5] by 100, you are converting the percentile value into decimal format, which needs to be done prior to multiplying or dividing with these numbers. For example, 15% means 15/100 or 0.15.)

2. Lean body weight = Total weight (lb) − Fat weight (lb)
   = _____ lb

3. Your target % body fat = _____ %
   (using your educated judgment of what is appropriate for you)

4. Target % lean = 100% − Target % body fat
   = _____ %

5. Target body weight = $\dfrac{\text{Lean body weight}}{(\text{Target \% lean}/100)}$
   = _____ = _____ lb

Waist:Hip Ratio

Waist circumference _____ in

Hip circumference _____ in

Waist:hip ratio = $\dfrac{\text{Waist circumference}}{\text{Hip Circumference}}$
= _____ = _____

Use Table 8.7 on page 260 to determine whether you have an android pattern of fat deposition.

Body Mass Index

BMI = $\dfrac{\text{Weight (kg)}}{\text{Height (m)}^2}$ = _____ = _____

Use Table 8.8 on page 260 to determine whether your BMI is healthy, overweight, or obese.

Height-Weight Tables

1. Elbow width _____ in or cm

2. Frame size (from Table 8.3): small _____ medium _____ large _____

3. Your weight: _____ lb   Your height: _____ in

4. Weight range for your height and frame size (from Table 8.2): _____ lb

5. The weight that is considered overweight for your height and frame size:

   Midpoint of the weight range _____ lb × 1.2 lb = _____

6. Does your weight exceed the value that is 20% greater than the midpoint of your weight range (determined in step 5)? _____ yes _____ no

Summary of the Assessments

Method	Value	Interpretation (Check One)	
% Body fat by skinfolds	_____ %	☐ not obese	☐ obese
Waist:hip ratio		☐ not obese	☐ android obesity
BMI		☐ healthy	☐ overweight
		☐ obese	
Height-weight table	_____ lb	☐ not overweight	☐ overweight

TABLE 8.5

Percent Body Fat Values Based on Skinfold Measurements

Women: Percent Body Fat Values Based on the Sum of Three Skinfolds (tricep, suprailiac, and thigh) and Age

SUM OF SKINFOLDS (mm)	UNDER 22	23–27	28–32	33–37	38–42	43–47	48–52	53–57	OVER 58
23–25	9.7	9.9	10.2	10.4	10.7	10.9	11.2	11.4	11.7
26–28	11.0	11.2	11.5	11.7	12.0	12.3	12.5	12.7	13.0
29–31	12.3	12.5	12.8	13.0	13.3	13.5	13.8	14.0	14.3
32–34	13.6	13.8	14.0	14.3	14.5	14.8	15.0	15.3	15.5
35–37	14.8	15.0	15.3	15.5	15.8	16.0	16.3	16.5	16.8
38–40	16.0	16.3	16.5	16.7	17.0	17.2	17.5	17.7	18.0
41–43	17.2	17.4	17.7	17.9	18.2	18.4	18.7	18.9	19.2
44–46	18.3	18.6	18.8	19.1	19.3	19.6	19.8	20.1	20.3
47–49	19.5	19.7	20.0	20.2	20.5	20.7	21.0	21.2	21.5
50–52	20.6	20.8	21.1	21.3	21.6	21.8	22.1	22.3	22.6
53–55	21.7	21.9	22.1	22.4	22.6	22.9	23.1	23.4	23.6
56–58	22.7	23.0	23.2	23.4	23.7	23.9	24.2	24.4	24.7
59–61	23.7	24.0	24.2	24.5	24.7	25.0	25.2	25.5	25.7
62–64	24.7	25.0	25.2	25.5	25.7	26.0	26.7	26.4	26.7
65–67	25.7	25.9	26.2	26.4	26.7	26.9	27.2	27.4	27.7
68–70	26.6	26.9	27.1	27.4	27.6	27.9	28.1	28.4	28.6
71–73	27.5	27.8	28.0	28.3	28.5	28.8	28.0	29.3	29.5
74–76	28.4	28.7	28.9	29.2	29.4	29.7	29.9	30.2	30.4
77–79	29.3	29.5	29.8	30.0	30.3	30.5	30.8	31.0	31.3
80–82	30.1	30.4	30.6	30.9	31.1	31.4	31.6	31.9	32.1
83–85	30.9	31.2	31.4	31.7	31.9	32.2	32.4	32.7	32.9
86–88	31.7	32.0	32.2	32.5	32.7	32.9	33.2	33.4	33.7
89–91	32.5	32.7	33.0	33.2	33.5	33.7	33.9	34.2	34.4
92–94	33.2	33.4	33.7	33.9	34.2	34.4	34.7	34.9	35.2
95–97	33.9	34.1	34.4	34.6	34.9	35.1	35.4	35.6	35.9
98–100	34.6	34.8	35.1	35.3	35.5	35.8	36.0	36.3	36.5
101–103	35.3	35.4	35.7	35.9	36.2	36.4	36.7	36.9	37.2
104–106	35.8	36.1	36.3	36.6	36.8	37.1	37.3	37.5	37.8
107–109	36.4	36.7	36.9	37.1	37.4	37.6	37.9	38.1	38.4
110–112	37.0	37.2	37.5	37.7	38.0	38.2	38.5	38.7	38.9
113–115	37.5	37.8	38.0	38.2	38.5	38.7	39.0	39.2	39.5
116–118	38.0	38.3	38.5	38.8	39.0	39.3	39.5	39.7	40.0
119–121	38.5	38.7	39.0	39.2	39.5	39.7	40.0	40.2	40.5
122–124	39.0	39.2	39.4	39.7	39.9	40.2	40.4	40.7	40.9
125–127	39.4	39.6	39.9	40.1	40.4	40.6	40.9	41.1	41.4
128–130	39.8	40.0	40.3	40.5	40.8	41.0	41.3	41.5	41.8

TABLE 8.5 Continued

Percent Body Fat Values Based on Skinfold Measurements

Men: Percent Body Fat Values Based on the Sum of Three Skinfolds (chest, abdomen, and thigh) and Age

SUM OF	AGE								
SKINFOLDS (mm)	UNDER 22	23–27	28–32	33–37	38–42	43–47	48–52	53–57	OVER 58
8–10	1.3	1.8	2.3	2.9	3.4	3.9	4.5	5.0	5.5
11–13	2.2	2.8	3.3	3.9	4.4	4.9	5.5	6.0	6.5
14–16	3.2	3.8	4.3	4.8	5.4	5.9	6.4	7.0	7.5
17–19	4.2	4.7	5.3	5.8	6.3	6.9	7.4	8.0	8.5
20–22	5.1	5.7	6.2	6.8	7.3	7.9	8.4	8.9	9.5
23–25	6.1	6.6	7.2	7.7	8.3	8.8	9.4	9.9	10.5
26–28	7.0	7.6	8.1	8.7	9.2	9.8	10.3	10.9	11.4
29–31	8.0	8.5	9.1	9.6	10.2	10.7	11.3	11.8	12.4
32–34	8.9	9.4	10.0	10.5	11.1	11.6	12.2	12.8	13.3
35–37	9.8	10.4	10.9	11.5	12.0	12.6	13.1	13.7	14.3
38–40	10.7	11.3	11.8	12.4	12.9	13.5	14.1	14.6	15.2
41–43	11.6	12.2	12.7	13.3	13.8	14.4	15.0	15.5	16.1
44–46	12.5	13.1	13.6	14.2	14.7	15.3	15.9	16.4	17.0
47–49	13.4	13.9	14.5	15.1	15.6	16.2	16.8	17.3	17.9
50–52	14.3	14.8	15.4	15.9	16.5	17.1	17.6	18.2	18.8
53–55	15.1	15.7	16.2	16.8	17.4	17.9	18.5	19.1	19.7
56–58	16.0	16.5	17.1	17.7	18.2	18.8	19.4	20.0	20.5
59–61	16.9	17.4	17.9	18.5	19.1	19.7	20.2	20.8	21.4
62–64	17.6	18.2	18.8	19.4	19.9	20.5	21.1	21.7	22.2
65–67	18.5	19.0	19.6	20.2	20.8	21.3	21.9	22.5	23.1
68–70	19.3	19.9	20.4	21.0	21.6	22.2	22.7	23.3	23.9
71–73	20.1	20.7	21.2	21.8	22.4	23.0	23.6	24.1	24.7
74–76	20.9	21.5	22.0	22.6	23.2	23.8	24.4	25.0	25.5
77–79	21.7	22.2	22.8	23.4	24.0	24.6	25.2	25.8	26.3
80–82	22.4	23.0	23.6	24.2	24.8	25.4	25.9	26.5	27.1
93–85	23.2	23.8	24.4	25.0	25.5	26.1	26.7	27.3	27.9
86–88	24.0	24.5	25.1	25.7	26.3	26.9	27.5	28.1	28.7
89–91	24.7	25.3	25.9	26.5	27.1	27.6	28.2	28.8	29.4
92–94	25.4	26.0	26.6	27.2	27.8	28.4	29.0	29.6	30.2
95–97	26.1	26.7	27.3	27.9	28.5	29.1	29.7	30.3	30.9
98–100	26.9	27.4	28.0	28.6	29.2	29.8	30.4	31.0	31.6
101–103	27.5	28.1	28.7	29.3	29.9	30.5	31.1	31.7	32.3
104–106	28.2	28.8	29.4	30.0	30.6	31.2	31.8	32.4	33.0
107–109	28.9	29.5	30.1	30.7	31.3	31.9	32.5	33.1	33.7
110–112	29.6	30.2	30.8	31.4	32.0	32.6	33.2	33.8	34.4

(Continued on next page)

TABLE 8.5 Continued

Percent Body Fat Values Based on Skinfold Measurements

Men: Percent Body Fat Values Based on the Sum of Three Skinfolds (chest, abdomen, and thigh) and Age

SUM OF SKINFOLDS (mm)	AGE								
	UNDER 22	23–27	28–32	33–37	38–42	43–47	48–52	53–57	OVER 58
113–115	30.2	30.8	31.4	32.0	32.6	33.2	33.8	34.5	35.1
116–118	30.9	31.5	32.1	32.7	33.3	33.9	34.5	35.1	35.7
119–121	31.5	32.1	32.7	33.3	33.9	34.5	35.1	35.7	36.4
122–124	32.1	32.7	33.3	33.9	34.5	35.1	35.8	36.4	37.0
125–127	32.7	33.3	33.9	34.5	35.1	35.8	36.4	37.0	37.6

Source: From Pollack and Wilmore, 1990.

TABLE 8.6

Classification of Body Composition Values

	AVERAGE % BODY FAT	OBESE LEVELS % BODY FAT
Males	15%	> 25%
Females	23%	> 32%

TABLE 8.8

NIH Guidelines for BMI

HEALTHY	OVERWEIGHT	OBESE
< 25	25–29.9	> 30

TABLE 8.7

Waist:Hip Ratio and Android Obesity

	AVERAGE WAIST:HIP RATIO	RATIOS INDICATING ANDROID OBESITY
Males		
Under age 30	0.84	> 0.90
Ages 30–40	0.88	> 0.93
Age 40 and over	0.91	> 0.97
Females		
Under age 30	0.75	> 0.80
Ages 30–40	0.76	> 0.82
Age 40 and over	0.80	> 0.87

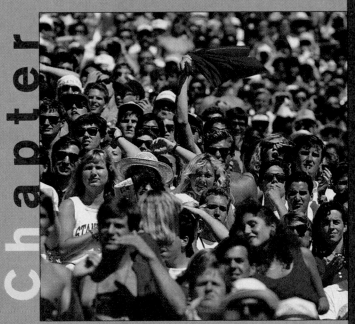

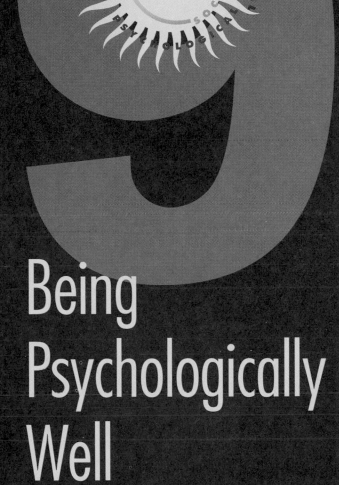

chapter

Being Psychologically Well

One Student's View

To me, wellness means being satisfied with my life and who I am. It means allowing myself to express all my emotions without bottling up my feelings. It means accomplishing my goals and being satisfied because I know that I did my best. It doesn't mean that I have to be happy all the time. It just means being able to smile and enjoy living my life.

—Shannon Ishikawa

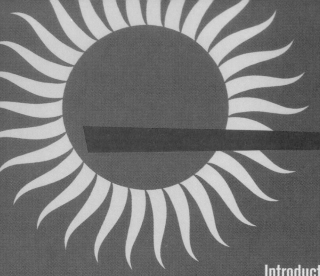

Introduction

If you are like most people, at some point you have probably responded to your alarm clock by covering your head with your pillow in dread of the day that faced you. Perhaps you lacked the energy to go to class, or the thought of getting started on that paper or studying for that exam was more than you could handle. In some cases, you may have dreaded running into someone or having to deal with interpersonal problems.

What did you do in this situation? Did you decide to "bag" the day and crawl back under the covers, or did you get up, pull yourself together, and get on with your day, functioning at a reasonable level of activity or at least in such a way that no one suspected that you were having problems? Chances are, you were able to drag yourself out of bed and face whatever real or imaginary adversary awaited you. Your family and/or friends probably would have supported you as you let the "blahs" pass, sorted through your problem, and regained a sense of control. Most of the time, when we are feeling "down," it is only temporary. We are able to find enough strength to respond in a fairly positive way, functioning normally in our social interactions, at school and at work. This type of *psychological resilience,* or ability to bounce back from life's crises, is a sign of psychological well-being. However, in increasing numbers, young adults are finding that they can't seem to get it together emotionally. For them, life may often seem like a pretty nasty place, complete with frustration, anxiety, boredom, and a general lack of zest for living. Their "funks" or "black holes" may seem impossible to crawl out of and lead to a spiraling downward crisis of depression, sleep disorders, eating disorders, and other problems. Why are so many people who should have so much to

Objectives

After reading this chapter, you should be able to

- Define mental, emotional, spiritual, and social health and understand why each of these dimensions of health is so important to your overall psychological well-being

- Describe the characteristics of psychological well-being

- List common psychological disorders experienced by college students and identify possible reasons to explain why college students may have unique risks for such problems

- Identify internal as well as external factors that predispose an individual to psychological wellness or disorder

- Define and distinguish between self-concept, self-esteem, self-efficacy, and locus of control, indicating the importance of each in individual psychosocial health

- Describe steps for enhancing psychological well-being and achieving optimal levels of wellness throughout the life span

look forward to in life in such bad places psychologically? Why are others able to face a seemingly constant barrage of adversity, yet come back ready for more? What elements seem to be most predictive of positive reactions to life's crises? What factors seem to be preludes to psychological and social problems?

Before we examine these important questions, we must explore what it really means to be psychologically well. The psychological dimension of wellness is closely linked to the other dimensions of wellness. Suppose you are really down about things in your life. You don't want to be around others, your bed is your refuge, you lack the energy to do much more than get a soda from the refrigerator or turn the channel on your television's remote control. Are you going to feel like getting up to go to the local gym or to go for a run? Probably not. Most likely, you aren't sleeping well, your diet is in a shambles, and your negative attitudes and comments have turned off enough of your friends that your isolation is chronic. Also, you might not be interacting with or noticing the beauty of nature or things in your immediate environment and your self-absorption may be extremely destructive. Thus, psychological problems may cause spiritual, physical, and social health to spiral out of control.

In this chapter, you will learn about many of the key aspects of psychological wellness and the factors that influence your psychological health. You will also begin to develop an appreciation for the complex interaction between psychological wellness and the other dimensions of wellness and how even slight imbalances in one aspect of your life can have profound effects on others. In addition, you will become familiar with some of the most common psychological health problems that face college students and where you or friends who may be experiencing problems can go to get help on most college campuses. Finally, you will learn how to use this information to recognize warning signs early and take positive actions to enhance your own well-being.

Defining Psychological Well-Being

As indicated above, some people have a seemingly endless capacity for dealing with life's ups and downs. They are able to respond to both the good and the bad by drawing on personal resources acquired through years of experiences. They have a high level of **psychological well-being**—the ability to respond in a positive, healthy manner to life's challenges using personal, social, spiritual, environmental, and physical resources.

If you are psychologically resilient, you may actually find that you are able to grow from each experience. For example, being "dumped" in a serious relationship may cause you great pain and emotional suffering. However, if you have a close network of friends, a realistic perspective on the significance of the situation, and a reasonably good opinion of yourself, you will eventually rebound and be ready for the next relationship. And if you are able to learn from the experience, you may be less likely to make similar mistakes the next time.

Less psychologically resilient individuals are easily devastated by even the smallest crises. For them, getting out of bed after a traumatic event, socializing with others, going to classes, studying, or performing other daily

psychological well-being
ability to respond in a positive, healthy manner to life's challenges using personal, social, environmental, and physical resources

activities may become impossible. They may become riddled with self-doubts and find it difficult to pull themselves together and get back on track again. Some may actually find that they lose the will to live and attempt suicide after excessive turmoil or adversity in their lives. Drug abuse, severe bouts of depression, dysfunctional relationships, and many other negative reactions to crisis reflect low levels of psychological well-being.

Why is one person able to respond positively and recover quickly from a major disappointment whereas another becomes socially isolated, angry, violent, or even suicidal? This question has been the basis of a great deal of research. Although much is known about the reasons some people respond in seemingly healthy ways and others respond in an unhealthy manner, many questions remain unanswered. Several factors appear to predispose individuals to varying degrees of psychological wellness.

Keys to Psychological Wellness

Being well psychologically is not something that just happens. The seeds of psychological wellness are planted when we are very young and then are either nurtured or ignored. Psychological wellness is the result of a complex interaction among several factors. Often, your conscious and unconscious thoughts about yourself, and your interpretation of events based on your history with such situations, may influence your emotional reactions. For example, if your last two partners have cheated on you with others, you might tend to be suspicious and anxious about your current partner. You are a product of your history and experiences in so many ways. The way you were raised by your parents; your interactions with young relatives and friends; your successes in school, athletics, music, and other areas all make you a very special and unique individual. That unique person you are will respond in a manner that has "worked" for you previously and you will repeat many behaviors based on past behaviors.

Thus, understanding how your thoughts and emotions influence you on a daily basis is an important first step in achieving psychological wellness.

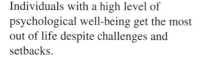

Individuals with a high level of psychological well-being get the most out of life despite challenges and setbacks.

Mental and Emotional Health

Two of the main aspects of psychological wellness are mental and emotional health. The term **mental health** is often used to describe the "thinking" or rational aspect of psychological wellness—that is, the way we think about or perceive reality. A mentally healthy person typically has a realistic view of life, free of most personal distortions. Such a person is able to make rational and effective choices even in confusing or difficult situations.

Emotional health generally refers to the "feeling" or subjective aspect of psychological wellness. An emotionally healthy person is aware of his or her feelings and is able to express them in an appropriate manner. Although the terms *emotion* and *feeling* are often used interchangeably, it would be more accurate to say that **emotions** are complex patterns of feelings such as anger, joy, love, and fear. Usually, emotions result in some type of physiological arousal that is expressed through feelings. For example, even an emotionally healthy person might respond with frustration and a bit of irritation at being cut off in traffic, particularly if the incident almost results in an accident and causes a rush of adrenaline. However, an emotionally healthy person would quickly control this burst of emotion. In contrast, an emotionally unhealthy person may experience what is aptly labeled *road rage,* chasing the driver who cut him or her off, banging into the offending car or even shooting the offending person. (Bowers, Fergeson, Alder)

Kleinginna and Kleinginna describe emotions as the interplay of four components: *physiological arousal, feelings, cognitive (thought) processes,* and *behavioral reactions.* For example, suppose your friend says to you, "I have something to tell you. I know you don't want to hear this but I can't hold off any longer. I have to tell you now." Instantly you break into a sweat and your heart starts to pound (physiological arousal). You are apprehensive/fearful and uncertain (feelings) and you think to yourself, "What is he going to say? What is wrong? This sounds important; I hope we can talk it out together and remain friends" (cognitive processes). You take a deep breath, sit down, and say to your friend, "Tell me what's on your mind" (behavioral reaction).

Often you can get an idea of someone's psychological health by looking at their outward appearance. However, external appearance does not always indicate that a person is emotionally well (or vice versa).

From this description of emotions, you can see that mental and emotional health are, in fact, very closely related. People who are psychologically healthy use their strengths in both these areas to respond in a positive way when things in life do not go as they would like. For example, a psychologically healthy student might be disappointed to receive a C− on a biology exam. However, he or she would typically maintain a sense of self-confidence despite the low grade, vow to do better the next time, and actually develop a plan of action for improving his or her study habits. By contrast, a psychologically unhealthy individual might conclude that the instructor did not like him or her, feel incapable of doing better, and spend the next few days getting drunk or running around doing anything *but* schoolwork.

Social Health

Another related aspect of our psychological health is our **social health,** or how we relate to others. A socially healthy person gets along well with others, takes their needs and perspectives into consideration, and is able to form meaningful, intimate relationships. Such a person is also able to maintain a healthy degree of independence, balancing time spent with others and time spent alone.

mental health "thinking" or rational aspect of psychological wellness

emotional health "feeling" or subjective aspect of psychological wellness

emotions complex patterns of feelings such as anger, joy, love, and fear

social health how we relate to others

Some psychologists measure sociability levels in terms of *introversion* and *extroversion*. Introverted people tend to direct their energies and emotions inward, enjoying their time alone. In extreme cases, they may become loners. Extroverted people prefer to seek out others and derive more pleasure from social activities.

Often, people who have psychological difficulties also experience problems in their social relations. They may develop distorted perceptions of others, become highly distrustful, or choose to avoid others. If they behave in unkind or antisocial ways, their friends may also choose to avoid them. In fact, they may become isolated at just the time when social support and a close-knit group of loved ones would be most needed.

Spiritual Health and Wellness

Although often given little attention in texts such as this, **spiritual health,** the process of creating and discovering meaning and purpose in life and demonstrating values through behaviors, is an essential part of your overall health/wellness profile. Perhaps because spiritual health is not as easily measured as blood pressure and other physical conditions, many assume that it can't really be assessed, and thus, probably can't be improved. Also, many wrongly assume that spirituality is synonymous with organized religion and tend to avoid discussions of anything spiritual in classes.

Many people do find their meaning and purpose in life and a sense of belonging through religion; many others, however, are spiritual individuals who are not religious. It is also quite possible to appear to be religious and yet not be spiritual. Spirituality can evolve through many different avenues. Religion may instill a sense of values and respect for others and for your own "place" in the universe. However, a sense of spirituality often develops through the values and beliefs of those people we surround ourselves with throughout our lives, through customs, through the education we receive, and through our sense of the "rightness" and "wrongness" of various social and environmental threats.

People who value life, value the lives of all living things, and work each day to make the world a healthier place for all living things may be said to be spiritual. Persons of a particular religious belief who revere certain objects, practices, or beliefs may be said to be spiritual. Spiritual leaders may be found among those who direct self-improvement/awareness seminars. A spiritual experience may be as simple as watching a beautiful sunset on a lake in Northern Wisconsin, with the call of the wild loon in the background, or watching a double rainbow form after a storm. By thinking about how you felt during one of those moments when you really observed something beautiful in nature or in life, and trying to re-create that moment in your everyday life, you may enhance the spiritual side of yourself. Taking time to "smell the roses" and realizing that you and the rose are both important in the greater scheme of life is an important part of spiritual wellness.

spiritual health process of creating and discovering meaning and purpose in life and demonstrating values through behaviors

Psychological Wellness Versus Illness

Psychologists have developed a variety of ways to recognize psychological well-being. Although at times they may respond emotionally, psychologically healthy individuals on the whole tend to behave more consistently and are less likely to demonstrate extreme emotional swings than less healthy people. They often are less impulsive and try to think through what is happening and how to respond rather than responding solely from "gut feelings." They tend to be more predictable and act more appropriately in times of extreme uncertainty or stress. Rather than lashing out physically at someone who makes them angry, they may try to reason with that person, ignore the problem because it isn't worth worrying about, or cope with the problem in any number of ways. For a summary of some typical characteristics of psychologically healthy and unhealthy people, see Table 9.1.

TABLE 9.1

Signs and Symptoms of Psychological Wellness and Illness

A PSYCHOLOGICALLY WELL PERSON	A PSYCHOLOGICALLY UNWELL PERSON
Has self-confidence	Lacks self-confidence and self-esteem, and has a low self-concept
Finds meaning and purpose in life	Finds little meaning and purpose in life
Cultivates his or her spiritual side	Ignores the spiritual side of life
Makes healthy choices	Makes poor health decisions
Is flexible and can adapt to situations	Is rigid and resistant to change
Feels comfortable with others	Is uncomfortable with others or uncomfortable alone
Accepts others for who they are	Has racist, ethnic, sexist, ageist, homophobic, or cultural biases
Is able to give and receive love	Finds it difficult to relate to others or to love and be loved
Accepts responsibility for his or her actions	Is often immature and irresponsible
Does not make excuses for personal mistakes/problems	Blames others for his or her mistakes
Responds in a positive way to life's problems	Fails to plan for the future
Plans ahead and establishes realistic goals	Acts without thinking and responds volatilely
Thinks before responding to emotions	Fails to manage emotions; lacks control
Handles stress effectively	Has poor stress-management skills
Respects others and acts to preserve nature	Lacks respect for others and nature
Is unselfish	Thinks only of self; is egocentric
Is always striving to improve	Is static, reluctant to change, or resists change

STATS-AT-A-GLANCE
Depression

Depression and a host of related problems continue to contribute to significant psychological problems in the world today. Although actual statistics may reflect only the "tip of the iceberg" of our U.S. problem, several key indicators point to a dramatic drain on our nation's population. Consider the following:

- Depression strikes over 17 million Americans each year, with less than half of those who suffer from it receiving the treatment that they need.

- More than 80% of people with depression can be treated successfully with medication, psychotherapy, or a combination of both.

- Over 16% of all Americans have sought help from mental health professionals in the last year, often for depression-related problems.

- The risk of depression increases if you have a parent or sibling who became depressed before age 30.

- Suicide is one of the leading causes of death in America today, and over 40,000 depressed people in the United States kill themselves every year.

- The known suicide rate among 15- to 19-year-olds has more than doubled since 1950. In the United States, suicide rates are higher among whites than blacks, and higher among males than females. Rates on college campuses have increased dramatically, forcing colleges and universities to reexamine their mental health policies and services.

Sources: U.S. Bureau of the Census, 1995; Health U.S.—1995; Clements, M., and D. Hales. 1997. How healthy are we? *Parade Magazine*, September 7, 1997, pp. 4–7.

Influences on Psychological Wellness

Many factors contribute to psychological wellness. Some of these influences are changeable, which means you can take specific actions to improve your wellness levels. Other influences are more ingrained and may be difficult or even impossible to change.

Internal Influences

Internal factors that have the greatest impact on psychological wellness include your heredity, physical health, and neurological and hormonal functioning. If any or all of these factors are malfunctioning, overall psychological wellness begins to decline.

Physical Health. One of the most important internal factors influencing your overall psychological well-being is your physical health. If you are ill, in pain, or worried about a mysterious lump that has appeared in your breast or elsewhere on your body, you may find it difficult to cope with other problems. Your energy level may be sapped from sleepless nights, poor eating habits, or other worries, and you may become easily depressed or distraught. You may react to adverse events without thinking or with an uncharacteristic emotional outburst. Conversely, if you are in good health and are physically fit, your energy level is likely to be much higher and you will be better able to cope with life's crises. In fact, exercise is believed to stimulate production of natural substances in the brain called *endorphins,* which may actually calm an overly anxious, stress-prone individual. See Chapter 10 for a more complete discussion of this.

In short, your physical condition can have a tremendous influence on your psychological health. Similarly, emotions can have a dramatic effect on physiological functioning. For example, extreme fright or anger may trigger increases in heart rate and blood pressure as well as changes in posture and facial expressions. Over time, negative emotions like excessive anger or frustration can contribute to high levels of stress, which can have a devastating effect on the body systems. (Chapter 10 discusses stress in detail.) Extreme unhappiness, loneliness, and depression can also affect physical health indirectly by causing people to attempt suicide or abuse their bodies in other ways, such as through drug or alcohol abuse, lack of sleep, or dietary extremes. (See the Myths and Controversies box.)

The Brain. Just as the brain functions to control physical bodily processes, it also has specialized centers for responding to psychological influences. Several areas within the brain, particularly the *cerebral cortex* and the limbic system, function to influence your emotions as well as serving many other vital tasks. The cerebral cortex is a major center for receiving and assessing sensory input, forming the basis of our perceptions. Perceptions are often the basis for an emotional reaction to a wide range of stimuli in the environment. The limbic system contains the *amygdala,* a small, bulblike organ that has been shown to be highly sensitive to external sensory stimulation. For example, when this area is stimulated in cats, they will arch their backs, hiss, and prepare to fight a would-be attacker. Evidence of such violent behavior has also been noted in humans who have tumors or

MYTHS & CONTROVERSIES

Controversy **What we eat can affect our behavior.** According to some current research by the Center for Science in the Public Interest, many food constituents including amino acids (the building blocks of protein), choline, and even carbohydrates can actually influence the chemical composition of the brain and thus our actions. For example, carbohydrates cause the pancreas to release insulin into the bloodstream that lowers the blood levels of all amino acids except tryptophan. The end result of increased levels of tryptophan passing into the brain is sleepiness and reduced appetite and pain levels. Furthermore, a high-carbohydrate lunch can make you sluggish, whereas the same dinner will relax you. Finally, the amino acid tyrosine has antistress effects and can enhance performance test scores. Although there is much speculation about foods such as turkey and other food products and their role in mood, there is also much room for additional research into this relatively unexplored area.

other pressures on the amygdala. In addition, tumors or abnormalities in blood flow to the brain can impair a person's ability to think or remember, as well as cause mood swings, erratic behaviors, and other aberrant actions.

Hormones. The **endocrine glands** secrete numerous hormones that are important for various bodily functions and that have a dramatic effect on emotions like fear, love, hate, anger, frustration, and the like. Hormone levels in the blood and urine have been shown to rise during times of emotional stress. (Hormones specific to the stress response are discussed in Chapter 10.)

Two of the major hormones related to emotions are the "sex" hormones —the androgens and the estrogens. Men produce large amounts of androgen and little estrogen; women produce large amounts of estrogen and little androgen. These secretory patterns have been associated, albeit inconclusively, with different emotional responses in men and women. For example, some researchers have demonstrated a link between an apparent male pattern of aggression and violence and variations in levels of *testosterone* (a type of androgen) (Rosenberg and Fenley). Variations in women's levels of estrogen during the menstrual cycle have led others to explore associations between low levels of estrogen just before or during the menstrual cycle and dramatic swings in mood, tension, and anxiety (Mednick et al.). Although the controversy surrounding this particular estrogen-related mood fluctuation continues, the syndrome of combined psychological and physiological symptoms during or prior to the menstrual cycle has been labeled **premenstrual syndrome (PMS)** by health professionals.

Other hormones secreted by the endocrine glands include the thyroid hormones, which are active in the metabolic process. Certain diseases as well as high levels of emotional stress can cause serious imbalances in the thyroid hormones. These imbalances can trigger a thyroid crisis resulting in emotional responses characterized by sudden, violent mood swings, hyperactivity, and depression.

Heredity. Although research in this area is inconclusive, an increasing number of theorists believe that we actually inherit genes that make us more likely to be either even tempered or hot headed, just as animals are bred for disposition and temperament. Thus, people inadvertently may be products of good or bad temperament lines. For example, some experts believe that we have an inherited "reaction range" for our emotional responses. Included within this reaction range are (1) *arousability*, measured by the amount of time that elapses before we respond to emotional stimuli; (2) *excitability*, measured by

endocrine glands glands that secrete numerous hormones important for various bodily functions and having a dramatic effect on emotions

premenstrual syndrome (PMS) syndrome of combined psychological and physiological symptoms that occur during or prior to the menstrual cycle

the amount of energy we can summon in response to emotional stimuli; and (3) *tempo,* measured by the rapidity of our emotional response. The shorter the inherited reaction range, the more volatile and emotional the individual is likely to be (Baranowski and Nader). Several recent studies of twins raised in very different environments provide indications that much of our temperament and our predisposition toward certain emotional responses and behaviors may be a product of our genetic make-up. Because depression tends to run in families, hereditary predisposition to this illness may be as much a cause of depression as a person's environment factors. Much is unknown about the complex associations between your genes and your propensity toward psychological wellness or illness. Someday we may be able to predict who will have difficulties with mental health problems merely by examining their family history. In the meantime, exploring the role that people's environment has on their psychological health may help us find clues to the mysteries of the mind.

External Influences

We are all born with the capacity to feel various emotions. Although some of us have a predisposition toward greater emotionality than others, our interpretations of and responses to events are largely the result of social and cultural influences. These learned behaviors may sabotage even the strongest genetic, hormonal, neurological, or other physiological factors.

How you are treated in the womb, as an infant and child, and later as an adult by your family, your friends, and the people around you are major influences on what you become. Socioeconomic status, education, culture, religion, and various environmental factors all have a profound role in making you who you are. Just as no two people experience the exact same set of social and environmental conditions during their formative years, no two people are identical from a psychological wellness perspective. For instance, the youngest child may have the same parents as older siblings but grow up to have completely different values, attitudes, and behaviors. One child may turn out completely normal by societal standards whereas another becomes a deviant. What could make these children—who have the same parents, who went to the same schools, and who had the same socioeconomic backgrounds—turn out so differently?

Early Environmental Influences. From its first months in the womb, a fetus apparently reacts to warmth, adequate nutrition, soothing sounds, and general healthy maternal status with displays of physiological contentment and relaxation. In such an environment, the baby's heart rate, blood pressure, and activity levels remain in a resting state, and normal bodily functions work as expected. However, maternal stress or abuse, dietary deprivation, chemical stimulation through drugs (such as alcohol or crack cocaine), and even yelling can cause serious disruptions. For example, fetuses who develop in disturbed environments may demonstrate erratic heart rate and blood pressure, jerky reflex movements, and continual fidgeting indicative of nervous stimulation. Some of these babies, particularly those born to cocaine-addicted mothers, may have a low birth weight, cry incessantly after birth, demonstrate frenzied movements, be unresponsive to external stimuli, and fail to develop normally. Today, many states have actually imposed legal sanctions against mothers who knowingly put their unborn baby's health in jeopardy.

In the first months of life, the newborn begins to develop an even more intricate set of psychological responses to life. Several experts in child development have shown that infants who are held, touched, talked to, fed, and cared for at regular intervals and who are in peaceful, safe environments gain weight more quickly, develop more fully, and appear to feel more content and secure once these basic human needs for love, warmth, food, and security are met (Buechler and Izard; Burgess and Draper).

Childhood and Young Adulthood. As we progress through childhood and into the teen years, we are continually shaped by various environmental forces. Influences outside the home take on an increasingly significant role. For example, children whose families do not have the money to buy them the latest fashions or the newest bicycle may feel insecure or inadequate at school. In adolescence and young adulthood, youths may come into contact with peers who pressure them to take drugs, have sexual relations, or engage in other high-risk activities that may cause guilt, anxiety, and other psychological problems.

Children who come from **dysfunctional families**—families that lack adequate levels of love, security, and trust, and that are often characterized by alcohol abuse, violence, and instability—are more likely than those from healthy families to succumb to peer pressures. Individuals who have been sexually, physically, and/or emotionally abused by a parent or sibling may bring deep emotional scars to their interactions outside the home. Some research suggests that people raised in dysfunctional family environments have an increased risk of engaging in physically or emotionally abusive behaviors (Hayes, Ackerman). Also, such persons are significantly more likely to marry an abuser (Woititz).

In striking contrast to persons who experienced strife-torn early years are those raised in relatively secure, healthy family environments in which they felt loved, nurtured, and valued. The more positive the influences during your formative years, the more likely you are to develop positive psychological responses. Remember, however, that not everyone brought up in an unhealthy environment develops into a psychologically unhealthy adult. Likewise, not all children who have been raised in a healthy environment become healthy adults. Understanding why one person experiences unspeakable childhood trauma but has the resilience to succeed in life is the basis for much research. For example, certain protective factors, such as having a positive role model in the midst of chaos and having a positive family, may help even the child with the greatest risk of psychological disorder remain healthy and well adjusted (Werner).

The Later Years. As an adult, you continue to carry much of the "baggage" of your formative years. Your successes and failures in school, with friends, in intimate relationships, in athletics, in your jobs, and in every aspect of life subtly shape your **psychosocial development,** or the way you view the world and respond to it.

By the time you reach adulthood, your personality, that unique mix of characteristic patterns of behavior that distinguishes you from others, typically has been fully established. Your personality determines how you adapt to the various situations that arise in your life and reflects the hereditary, environmental, cultural, and experiential factors that have influenced you along the way. A healthy personality is important for psychological wellbeing. Individuals with

dysfunctional family family that lacks adequate levels of love, security, and trust, and that is often characterized by alcohol abuse, violence, and instability

psychosocial development way you view the world and respond to it

healthy personalities demonstrate appropriate levels of emotionality, sociability, and impulsiveness. And, in their later years, they generally feel a sense of satisfaction and fulfillment over what they've accomplished.

Indicators of Psychological Wellness

People who are psychologically healthy tend to focus on those things they can change in their immediate environment to keep themselves on the positive side of the wellness continuum (see Figure 9.1). They are able to do this because they have a positive self-concept and demonstrate high levels of self-esteem, self-efficacy, and personal control—key indicators of psychological wellness.

Self-Concept and Self-Esteem

In broad terms **self-concept** is one's view of oneself, physically, mentally, emotionally, and socially. It is both the mirror you hold up to yourself and the reflection you see. Generally, it refers to all the thoughts and feelings that we have in response to the question, "Who am I?"

If you like what you see in your internal mirror and believe that you measure up well to others around you, your self-esteem is considered to be high, or positive. **Self-esteem** reflects one's evaluation of oneself—that is, one's sense of self-regard or feeling good or not so good about oneself, or self-worth. Because they are closely related, self-esteem is sometimes confused with self-concept in discussions of psychological wellness.

Self-esteem is not innate; it is something we develop, starting at an early age. Growing up in a nurturing, supportive environment helps to build a sense of accomplishment and self-worth. Among high school students, self-esteem has been linked to both psychological factors (self-regard, social confidence, and intelligence) and physical factors (appearance and ability) (Fleming and Courtney). The development of low self-esteem has also been linked with a history of childhood abuse, psychological disorders, poor physical health, alcoholism, and drug use (Robson).

Clearly, not only disruptive life events or conditions but simply feeling bad about yourself can lead to low self-esteem. In general, if you have a positive sense of self-worth, you will be more likely to take care of yourself and have a high regard for others. If you are dissatisfied with yourself and have low self-esteem, you may take out your negative feelings on yourself and others in destructive ways. Behaviors such as drinking excessively, disregarding personal hygiene, and isolating oneself socially can indicate low self-esteem.

Improving and Maintaining Self-Esteem Levels. If you do have a poor image of yourself, how can you go about improving it? Bolstering self-esteem can be a difficult task, particularly in adults, because patterns of long-term self-deprecation are difficult to break. If you have always felt you were worthless, you may find it difficult to convince yourself overnight that you are a worthwhile, valuable person. Changing how you feel about yourself is particularly difficult if you have never been able to meet your own self-imposed criteria for personal worth. Also, let's face it. There are always people who seem to take pleasure in being critical of others as a means of making up for their own deficits in self-esteem. If you happen to

self-concept broad term that indicates how one views oneself from the physical, mental, social, and emotional perspective

self-esteem one's evaluation of oneself or one's sense of self regard or feeling good or bad about oneself

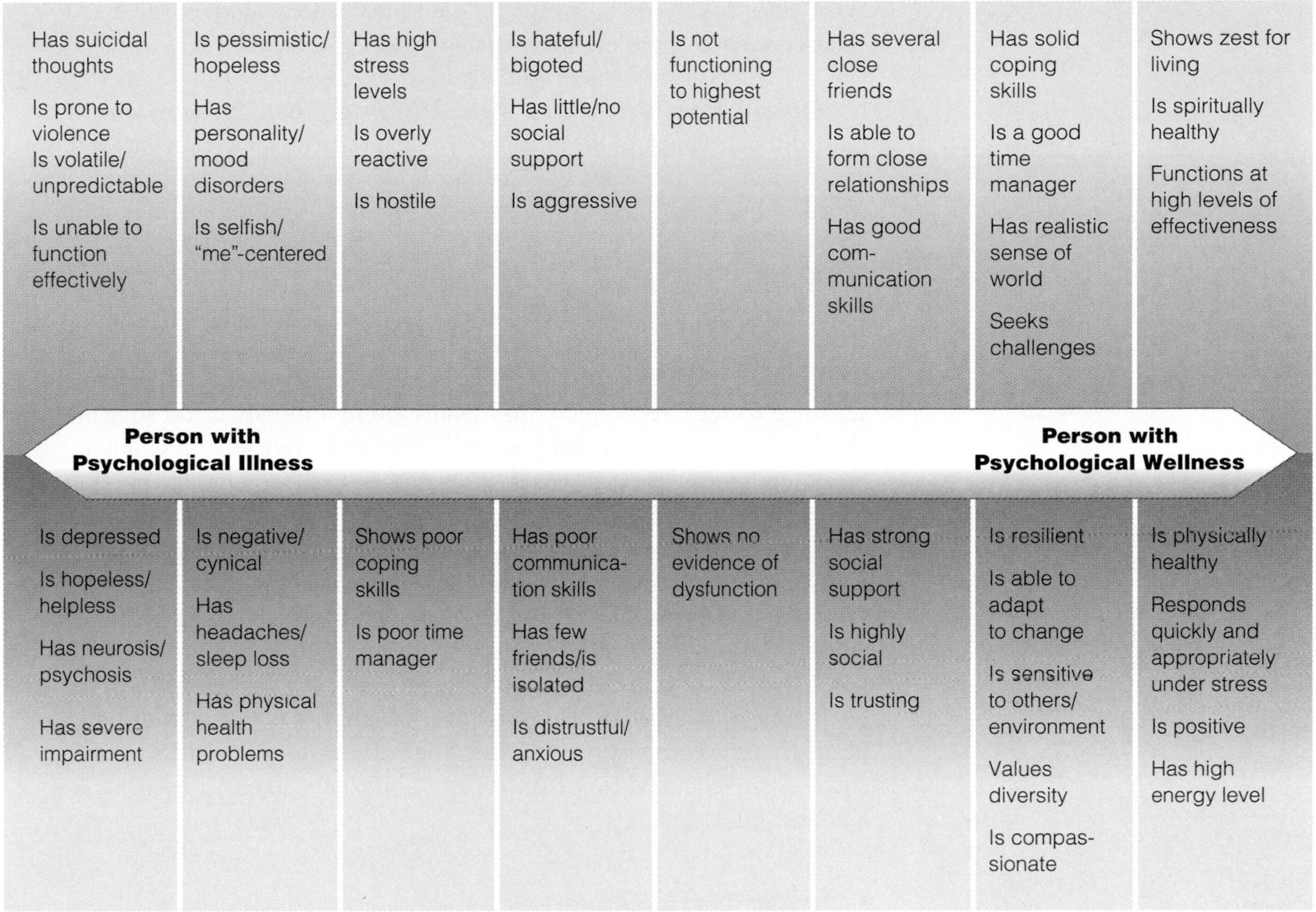

Has suicidal thoughts	Is pessimistic/ hopeless	Has high stress levels	Is hateful/ bigoted	Is not functioning to highest potential	Has several close friends	Has solid coping skills	Shows zest for living
Is prone to violence Is volatile/ unpredictable	Has personality/ mood disorders	Is overly reactive	Has little/no social support		Is able to form close relationships	Is a good time manager	Is spiritually healthy
Is unable to function effectively	Is selfish/ "me"-centered	Is hostile	Is aggressive		Has good communication skills	Has realistic sense of world Seeks challenges	Functions at high levels of effectiveness

Person with Psychological Illness ◁═══════════════════════════════▷ **Person with Psychological Wellness**

Is depressed Is hopeless/ helpless Has neurosis/ psychosis Has severe impairment	Is negative/ cynical Has headaches/ sleep loss Has physical health problems	Shows poor coping skills Is poor time manager	Has poor communica- tion skills Has few friends/is isolated Is distrustful/ anxious	Shows no evidence of dysfunction	Has strong social support Is highly social Is trusting	Is resilient Is able to adapt to change Is sensitive to others/ environment Values diversity Is compas- sionate	Is physically healthy Responds quickly and appropriately under stress Is positive Has high energy level

Figure 9.1
Psychological wellness and illness may be viewed on a continuum.

be around these self-appointed critics or if you are particularly sensitive to their attacks, you might find that your self-esteem is constantly being battered.

One of the most important ways to maintain or enhance self-esteem is by establishing a solid support system, particularly one made up of people who are willing to accept you for who you are and whatever flaws you may have. By building you up, and bolstering your self-regard, they may help you ward off problems when you are in a vulnerable state. In all stages of life, we need peers and/or family members who share our values, nurture us, and help validate our feelings rather than cause us to have self-doubt or place us under undue pressure. For some people with low self-esteem who also tend to isolate themselves, attempting to build a support group may mean taking the risk, perhaps for the first time, of reaching out to others. Participating in group therapy or a self-help support group can make this step easier.

Self-esteem can also be bolstered by making a conscious effort to prepare yourself to meet life's challenges. For example, if you schedule adequate time to study for a big exam, you can avoid potential failure due to self-defeating, last-minute cramming. This approach can also give you a realistic basis for anticipating the test results. By contrast, if you expect a top grade but have not invested the energy in studying, your unrealistic expectations may cause you to question your abilities when the test results are poor. Think about the things you do each day that tend to detract from your overall level of effec- tiveness in classes, in interpersonal interactions, and in your daily activities.

What steps might you take to make your own actions more positive and enhance your chances of strengthening your self-esteem?

Respecting Who You Are: Valuing You. Probably one of the most difficult things to do in American culture is to show by your own actions that you like yourself. The threat of seeming vain, egocentric, conceited, selfish, and a host of other "worries about what others may think" often compel us to think of ourselves *last* rather than first and to be our own worst critics. Taking time out for yourself and carefully protecting that time is an important aspect of maintaining and improving self-esteem. If you are worth something, you owe it to yourself to make your own needs and wants a priority in your life—and to set aside the necessary time. Allowing yourself time to read, relax, hike, play tennis, go to a movie, or do something else you enjoy is a sign that you are important to yourself. In addition, maintaining your physical health through diet, exercise, and attention to your body's signals of illness indicates that you value yourself. Feeling healthy and physically fit can increase your energy level and your overall sense of well-being. Sticking up for yourself and defending your point of view, acting to protect the environment that you care about, assessing what matters to you and what doesn't matter, and other self-protective behaviors indicate that you like yourself and value how you treat yourself as much as how you treat others. In short, whether you focus on your physical, social, or personal health or on a combination of these, your own actions designed to demonstrate self-respect and love of self can significantly improve even the lowest level of self-esteem.

Self-Efficacy

Albert Bandura, a well-known psychologist, defined **self-efficacy** as the perceptions or beliefs a person holds about his or her own competency that allow that person to act appropriately and successfully. That is, believing that we have the necessary personal skills and abilities is what enables us to succeed in a given situation. For example, if you were always the first one chosen for sporting events in your younger years and were generally good at whatever sports you played, you are likely to believe you can perform effectively in physical activities in later life. But if you were always the last one chosen for teams or fared poorly in measures of physical performance, you might see yourself as a "klutz," incapable of doing well in any type of physical activity.

Attribution styles, or how people explain the events in their lives and account for successes and failures, influence their levels of self-confidence and self-efficacy. If you expect to succeed, you will be more likely to do so; if you expect to fail, you are more likely to engage in less self-efficacious behavior and to meet with failure. Other researchers have theorized that people who continually fail actually learn to feel helpless and unable to respond (Seligman, 1975). Thus, **learned helplessness** reflects a pattern of failure that causes a person to feel incapable of acting to change a given situation, thus leading to continued failure. Often, this helplessness indicates deeper psychological disturbances.

In more recent studies, researchers have found that the key to choosing success over failure rests with our degree of optimism or pessimism. Optimists, whose attribution style leads them to expect the best in any situation,

self-efficacy perceptions or beliefs one holds about one's competency that allow one to act appropriately and successfully

attribution styles how one explains the events in one's life

learned helplessness pattern of failure that causes a person to feel incapable of acting to change a given situation, thus leading to continued failure

have been shown to be healthier both physically and psychologically. By contrast, pessimists, whose attribution style leads them to expect the worst, run an increased risk of psychological disorders (especially depression), have inferior physical health, visit the doctor more often, and are less likely to do well in school or on the job (Seligman, 1991).

Locus of Control

Another important aspect of psychological well-being that also involves our attributions is known as locus of control (locus meaning "place" or "source"). **Locus of control** refers to the belief that the outcome of your actions is either dependent on you (internal control) or dependent on events outside your control (external control). Feeling that external forces are in control of your life can lead you to blame others when things go wrong as well as create an expectation that negative outcomes are bound to occur. Having an internal control orientation, however, gives you a feeling of greater control over your destiny and is associated with psychological wellness. Psychologically healthy individuals have a strong appreciation for their own thoughts and motivations, but they also consider the needs and opinions of others.

How does locus of control apply to health-related behaviors? Actually, the answer to this is quite complex. We are all motivated by varying degrees of external and internal influences, depending on the particular situation, the value we place on the opinion of those involved, the possible consequences of our actions, and a host of other variables. Simply saying that you are motivated by internal factors or by external factors is an oversimplification of the locus of control concept. Perhaps the most important thing to consider here is *why* you might be acting in a particular way. Are you doing something because you staunchly believe it is the thing to do or because someone you want to impress is watching? What do you expect to *get* out of your actions? Determining why you are doing or *not* doing something may be one of the first steps in getting you on the right track. Individuals with an internal locus often are motivated by intrinsic rewards—feeling good, looking good, and so on. Externally motivated people are more likely to be motivated by praise from others, incentives, and external indicators of success. However, each of us may fluctuate in what motivates us on any given day or in any given circumstance, and that is actually quite normal. When a person is totally motivated by either internal or external factors and there is no balance between the two extremes, illness and/or dysfunctional behavior is often the result.

When Psychological Problems Begin

When the mental, emotional, and social aspects of psychological health deteriorate, people may experience sharp declines in rational thinking, a condition that can lead to a distorted perception of reality. They may become extremely cynical, distrustful, and/or emotional; experience volatile mood swings; or become unusually quiet and tend to isolate themselves from others. For individuals suffering from such **psychological disorders,** these negative mental reactions may threaten their life and health or the life and health of others around them. However, remember that most psychological disorders do not happen suddenly. They may be a reflection of how you were treated as a child, your experiences growing up, the behaviors you

locus of control belief that the outcome of one's actions is either up to oneself (internal control) or up to events outside one's control (external control)

psychological disorders negative mental reactions that may threaten the life and health of the individual or others around the individual

have learned, your reactions to life, and your current circumstances. Often, a person experiences psychological problems gradually; sometimes imperceptibly. Table 9.2 lists some common types of psychological disorders; some of these disorders are discussed in detail later in this chapter.

Whether they have actually been diagnosed with a psychological disorder, people who are emotionally unstable may have violent emotional outbursts or respond in inappropriate, sometimes frightening ways. They also may be extremely quiet and tend to shy away from others, or they may not act in any kind of way that might signal a problem until they have a major crisis and "act out" in some bizarre way, harming themselves or others. If you are in their way, they may harm you physically or attack your own psychological health, causing you significant problems

Psychological Problems Common to College Students

Although many of you will look back on the college years as carefree, fun, and free of major life difficulties, when you are actually experiencing

TABLE 9.2

Types of Psychological Disorders

TYPE	CHARACTERISTICS
A. Personality disorders	Chronic dysfunctional pattern of thinking, perceiving the world, and reacting
1. Dissociative disorders	Disturbance of memory or identity
a. Psychogenic amnesia	Forgetting personal experience (for psychological reasons)
b. Multiple personality	Two or more distinct personalities in one person
2. Anxiety disorders	Fear without apparent reason
a. Generalized anxiety	Chronic anxiety
b. Panic attacks	Brief, unexpected attacks of anxiety
c. Phobia	Fear of a specific object or situation (such as *agoraphobia*, fear of public places)
d. Obsessive-compulsive disorder	Anxiety caused by the need to perform compulsive behaviors (such as washing one's hands)
3. Affective disorders	Mood disturbances
a. Bipolar disorder	Alternation between elation and depression
b. Unipolar depression	Depression without episodes of elation
B. Schizophrenic disorders	Personality disintegration
1. Disorganized	Inappropriate behavior; incoherence
2. Catatonic	Frozen; no reaction to the environment
3. Paranoid	Delusions of persecution; hallucinations

them, they may seem far from idyllic. Adjusting to new academic surroundings; trying to live with a group of strangers who were raised differently from you and have very different ideas of cleanliness and order; being thrown into social situations where you feel constantly judged by others; worrying over grades, relationships, money, and the push and pull of home and family versus independence and self-discovery—all these can be difficult. Many people thrive in environments that are new and exciting; others have major problems and crises. Those who bring good coping skills, a strong sense of self, healthy self-esteem, and reliable social support from family and friends will usually have an easier time in adjusting and adapting. Those who relied too heavily on the support of past friends, the social acceptance of high school, and past successes and those who have low or variable levels of self-efficacy and self esteem may find that their past difficulties come with them to college. They may have been able to get by and handle things in their home towns, but an ever-changing and impersonal college campus may be the the catalyst for problems.

Some of the more typical problems affecting young, college-age people include depression, suicidal tendencies, and anxiety disorders. They may lead to difficulties in classes, failing grades, substance abuse, eating disorders, violent and erratic behaviors, and a host of other negative situations for students and those around them. Each of these problems may be prevented or at least reduced in severity through a better understanding of the nature and extent of the problem and fundamental causes, the ability to recognize early symptoms, and concerted campus efforts to promote positive health and psychological wellness among students before difficulties arise. One of the more insidious problems affecting today's students (as well as large segments of the general population) is depression.

Depression: A Common Threat

Psychological depression has been referred to as the "common cold" of psychological disorders because of its prevalence in the general population. Not to be confused with the "I'm bummed out" feelings you might have when someone close to you is ill, you do poorly in classes, or a relationship ends, depression is described as a "full-scale tumble into a void" (Rosenham and Seligman). In more clinical terms **depression** is a disturbance in mood or a prolonged emotional state characterized by feelings of hopelessness, helplessness, lethargy, and mental exhaustion. That exhaustion may make you so tired of life that death/suicide seems like a welcome relief from a seemingly unbearable existence.

Feelings of depression may progress gradually or come on suddenly. Regardless of the time it takes to develop full-blown symptoms, symptoms typically continue for weeks or even months. People who experience true depression may find it difficult to get out of bed in the morning, dress themselves, eat, or even motivate themselves to get to the bathroom on time. They may feel thoroughly empty emotionally and ready to cry over the smallest crisis or setback. They may suffer from lingering sadness, unexplainable fatigue, sleep disorders, increased or decreased appetite, loss of interest in work, loss of sex drive, withdrawal from friends and family, and feelings of worthlessness. They usually suffer from low self-esteem and tend to feel alienated from others. Often, they are just too tired to put on a happy face and be around friends. They may spend long periods of the day in bed

depression disturbance in mood or a prolonged emotional state characterized by feelings of hopelessness, helplessness, and mental exhaustion

or lounging around watching television. Determining when someone is just "down in the dumps" (such as after a sad event) or experiencing a major depressive event or series of events, (often manifested in true physiological/ biochemical disturbances) is difficult. In fact, many experts describe feelings of joy, contentment, sadness, and black despair as being different points on a continuum. Each of us is said to fluctuate on that continuum on a fairly regular basis, In fact, experiencing painful events such as the loss of a loved one and going through a grieving process is quite normal. However, if you have experienced pain and/or crisis in your life and have difficulty resuming your life over a period of time, you may be closer to experiencing true depression. Some have compared being in a blue mood after bad news or events and being truly depressed as the difference between gasping for breath after exercising and being chronically short of breath.

So, if you are down 1 to 2 hours a day, 1 to 2 days a week, only occasionally, regularly, or in some other pattern, are you actually depressed? How can you really tell whether your friend is in trouble from depression or just having a bit of a slump? Only a competent, highly skilled mental health professional can really make that assessment. There are no magic numbers and no exact science with depression. With careful physical examination, careful psychological examination, and a weighing of circumstances and situations, a trained mental health specialist can usually diagnose depression with fairly reliable accuracy using criteria established through the *Diagnostic and Statistical Manual of Mental Disorders* (DSM-IV; American Psychiatric Association).

Psychologists sometimes distinguish between two major types of depression, each of which requires its own form of treatment. **Endogenous depression** is biochemically derived and occurs when neurotransmitters in the brain become unbalanced or dysfunctional. Seligman suggests that this imbalance may be genetically caused, accounting for the large numbers of depressed individuals within certain families. Mitchell and colleagues theorize that factors in the family environment cause a person to learn specific coping styles, thereby increasing the risk of depression. Treatment of endogenous depression typically combines psychotherapeutic and pharmacological approaches. Psychotherapy is focused on emotional and social issues while drugs work chemically to relieve symptoms such as sleeplessness. The most commonly used drugs are *antidepressants,* which help restore biochemical balances and elevate mood. Prozac, Zoloft, and other antidepressant medications have been shown to be quite helpful when used under close supervision of a trained therapist and regular counseling sessions to help individuals work through chronic difficulties.

Exogenous depression is typically caused by an external event such as the loss of someone or something that has great personal significance. Persons suffering from exogenous depression can slip into endogenous depression if their condition becomes chronic. Symptoms of exogenous depression are similar to those experienced with endogenous depression, but treatment tends to focus more on psychological solutions, especially during early stages of the disorder. If symptoms do not begin to disappear with the help of professional therapists and/or mental health counselors or if suicide is a possibility, antidepressant therapy may be prescribed.

Hope for Depression? For many people, major depression resolves itself without professional help in less than 3 months, particularly for exogenous depression sufferers. Others need therapy, antidepressant drugs, or some

endogenous depression form of depression that is biochemically derived and occurs when neurotransmitters in the brain become unbalanced or dysfunctional

exogenous depression form of depression caused by an external event such as the loss of someone or something that has great personal significance

PSYCHOLOGICAL ◆ WELLNESS

Do

▲ Talk honestly about your problems with someone you trust.

▲ Focus on your strengths instead of on your weaknesses.

▲ Volunteer your time; helping others is a great way to feel better yourself.

▲ Set aside time each day to do something you really enjoy.

▲ Learn communication skills such as assertiveness and reflective listening.

▲ Keep a sense of humor about yourself and the world.

▲ Examine your assumptions about what you "need" to be happy.

▲ Face your problems squarely instead of just hoping they will go away.

▲ Seek professional help if you have a problem you can't solve on your own.

▲ Maintain a strong system of social support.

Don't

▼ Be a perfectionist; no one can measure up to standards of perfection.

▼ Rely on alcohol or drugs to deal with difficult feelings.

▼ Be too critical or negative about yourself or others.

▼ Feel that you have to live up to other people's expectations.

▼ Put up with violence of any kind; do what it takes to get out of an abusive relationship.

▼ Ignore a friend's talk of suicide; take it seriously and get help.

▼ Be afraid of getting professional help when a problem seems overwhelming.

combination of these two approaches to keep them functioning and to reduce their suicidal risks. Although these are all good treatment approaches, they do little to help prevent or intervene in the tremendous societal problems that we have with depression today. Why are so many people in the most affluent country in the world depressed beyond belief? Why are increasing numbers of children in grades 1 to 5 indicating that they are depressed? Although there are many possible explanations, much of the problem seems rooted in our society as a whole. Problems with self-worth, self-esteem, connectedness to others, a spiritual connection with other living things, and a social system that seems increasingly supportive of the rich and affluent members of society may predispose large numbers of people to feel rejected, dejected, and hopeless. Family values and other highly touted recipes for improving society and the problems that people have trying to cope have gained in popularity, but much could be gained by instilling in the whole of society values of self-worth, self-esteem, self-respect, respect for others, and a feeling of the value of life, regardless of a person's position or financial worth.

Currently, young and old, rich and poor, male and female all experience depression and related problems. Women tend to be more vulnerable to depression throughout their life span and they tend to experience more passive forms of depression, involving anxiety, sleep problems, and inhibited sexual desire. Men who experience depression tend to be more active in their responses, engaging in more alcohol abuse, antisocial behavior, and violent acts. It is interesting that college men and women appear to be equally vulnerable to depression episodes, a statistical phenomenon that is quite different from that of the general population and which has researchers puzzled. For an indicator of the nature and extent of depression-related problems in the United States, see the Stats-at-a-Glance section of this chapter.

Suicide

One of the leading causes of death and disability for Americans ages 15 to 24 is suicide: Over 26,000 annually decide that life is not worth living (Anderson et al.). Although this problem knows no social, economic, or cultural boundaries, certain risk factors have been established. These include a personal or family history of suicide threats or attempts; a history of severe emotional problems, drug abuse, major depression, or marital or relationship problems; chronic pain and illness; and a high level of chronic stress. Suicide rates are also high among certain minority groups, among victims of violent crimes or abuse, and among individuals who feel trapped in a bad situation.

People who drink heavily and who are also depressed are particularly vulnerable to suicide. College students who find the break from family and hometown friends unbearable may also be at high risk. They may feel emotionally, socially, and financially isolated. They may find themselves simultaneously facing pressure to succeed academically, gain social acceptance, and function independently without the level of social support to which they were accustomed. Ultimately, they may escape by taking their own lives. However, being psychologically healthy to begin with—having a reasonable level of self-esteem, adequate ways of coping, good communication skills, and a support network—makes a person less likely to think of ending it all when times get rough.

Although suicide is a crisis, it is not usually something that comes out of nowhere. Rather, it is often the result of a lifelong path of poor psychological health and is often triggered by a traumatic event. Obtaining immediate professional help for suicidal tendencies and/or threats and taking preventive actions designed to increase psychological wellness are important steps in suicide prevention.

Anxiety Disorders

You have most likely experienced some degree of fear or anxiety as part of the normal course of life. Perhaps you were anxious when you had to give a presentation for which you were not fully prepared or when a family member was going through a medical crisis. These feelings might have been unpleasant at the time, but they probably disappeared as soon as the immediate situation was resolved. For some people who suffer from an anxiety disorder, however, the feelings of anxiety become so severe and persistent that they interfere with normal functioning.

An **anxiety disorder** is a psychological problem, such as *claustrophobia* or *panic attacks*, characterized by persistent, vague feelings of fear, tension, or impending doom. Symptoms may include an accelerated heartbeat, sweating, unusual fatigue, headache, muscle tension, and general aches and pains. The symptoms may be more or less severe, depending on the particular disorder.

In a generalized anxiety disorder, a person experiences anxiety symptoms that are persistent but that are not necessarily tied to any recognizable object of fear. A *phobia*, on the other hand, is a deep-seated dread of specific objects, activities, or situations. For example, one common type of phobia is *claustrophobia* in which someone in a confined space may begin to squirm, sweat, or become nauseated or dizzy. While such an attack might not be life threatening, if it curtails your activities it could have a significant impact on your job or your social life. Other common phobias include fear of heights (acrophobia), fear of spiders (arachnophobia), and fear of crowds (agoraphobia). A *panic attack* is a sudden, extreme anxiety reaction in which an individual experiences rapid, disabling fits of terror. Symptoms of a panic attack may include shortness of breath, shaking, choking, convulsions, and other signs of acute fear.

Treatment of all forms of anxiety disorders usually involves a thorough physical examination to detect potential organic origins. Once physical causes are ruled out, therapy may focus on identifying the underlying psychological cause of the anxiety or may be directed primarily toward desensitizing the person toward the feared object or situation. Anti-anxiety drugs may also be prescribed.

Achieving Psychological Wellness

You are a complex product of your heredity, experiences, and environment. When psychological problems occur, there is typically no "quick fix" for undoing the negative emotional and behavioral patterns you have learned over many years. One-day workshops designed to enhance self-esteem may increase your awareness, but the emotional lift you get from such an event will not necessarily have a lasting impact on your well-being or help carry you through the difficult times ahead. Any long-term improvement in self-esteem, self-efficacy, or other measures of psychological wellness can only be achieved through hard work and a willingness to commit to taking small, slow, and even painful steps toward undoing the old, destructive patterns.

Each year, many of us make New Year's resolutions about how we are going to improve our health, yet most of these resolutions focus on the physical part of our bodies: losing weight, gaining muscular strength, losing

anxiety disorder psychological problem, such as claustrophobia or panic attacks, characterized by persistent vague feelings of fear, tension, or impending doom

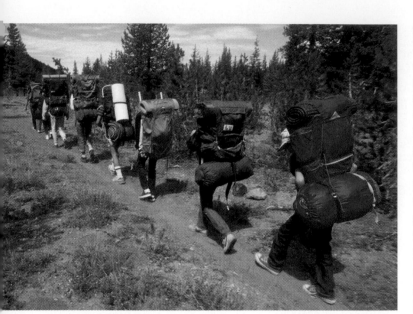

Taking time to enjoy nature, relax, refocus, and reenergize is often neglected by people who are too busy or burned out or who fail to recognize the importance of maintaining their psychological health.

inches, improving cardiovascular endurance. Few of us resolve to work consciously on our self-esteem, examine our self-doubts, take time to focus on our spiritual side, or dedicate ourselves to our psychosocial health. Perhaps one of the first steps to true wellness is to try to achieve a balance in the amount of effort we put on improving our "heads" and our relationships with others and the environment, and the time we spend on our physical appearance and physical functioning (Rowe and Kahn). Knowing where to get help and utilizing the resources available on campus and in the community are important first steps in psychological health. Acknowledging that everyone goes through challenging times in life and that it is all right to seek professional help for such problems is yet another marker of a wellness lifestyle.

Self-Help

Often we can do a lot ourselves to improve our psychological well-being, whether it be talking to a friend, joining a self-help support group, reading a self-help book, or simply making the time to do something for ourselves. Begin by considering what your major problems are, why you might have these problems, and what realistically you can do to change any negative patterns. Be sure to take careful stock of your positive attributes as you develop a plan for building on your best qualities. Avoid negative "self-talk"—self-deprecating thoughts about yourself—and try to focus on the things that you like best about yourself. Often we spend inordinate amounts of time focusing on the negative things about ourselves that we find troubling and/or disappointing while ignoring our good qualities. This negativity can become so habitual that we become our own worst enemies rather than our own biggest source of strength. Psychologically well individuals have little time for personal put-downs. Instead, they readily reaffirm that they are competent, worthy individuals who deserve to be treated with respect and care. If you find that you are continually berating yourself and/or focusing on the negative side of things, try to focus consciously on the more positive aspects. Practice saying good things about yourself to yourself and you may find that your overall outlook changes (see Table 9.3). Most important, do not try to change everything about yourself overnight.

If you are interested in finding a support group, you may want to consider a specialized group that focuses on your particular needs and issues. For example, Alcoholics Anonymous offers support in dealing with alcoholism; other groups focus on issues such as sexual abuse, overeating, or grief over the loss of a loved one. You can obtain phone numbers for these groups through your local community health center.

Professional Help

If you have exhausted your available self-help resources but still feel a need for change or more support from others, a trained professional can help. Seeking professional help is not an admission of failure or an indication that you are "crazy." Often people are willing to consult a physician for physical problems

TABLE 9.3

Negative Versus Positive Self-Talk

NEGATIVE/SELF-DEFEATING SELF-TALK	POSITIVE/CONSTRUCTIVE SELF-TALK
I'm really ugly. Nobody will find me attractive.	I have really nice eyes. My personality is great. Anyone who takes the time to get to know me will find this out.
I'm too busy to exercise. It would be embarrassing if anyone saw me in shorts.	I will find at least 15 minutes every day just to exercise. It doesn't matter what anyone else thinks about how I look.
I'll never understand how to do this. I might as well forget it.	I'm going to break this down into pieces and work on it until I get it. I know I can figure it out.
I'm addicted to eating chocolate. I can't stop.	I need to eat less chocolate. Starting today, I'm going to cut down gradually.
They really hate me. I can't trust any one.	They really seem to have a problem with me. They must be having a bad day for some reason.
It's impossible for me to be happy. Life is a bummer.	I'm going to try to focus on something pleasant and block out any negative thoughts.

but not a therapist for psychological problems. Fortunately, this attitude has changed substantially in recent years; in fact, record numbers of Americans are obtaining professional help for a variety of psychological ailments. In addition, many employers have staff counselors to deal with employee problems, and college and university health centers typically offer services to help students deal with many emotional problems.

If you decide that you need professional help to improve your psychological health, you should consider a variety of factors. Doing your homework at the outset may save you time, money, and effort down the road and help you avoid an unproductive experience. First, you should consider the type of mental health professional you want to see. These professionals may vary considerably in terms of their credentials, their fees, and their ability to treat your specific problem (see Table 9.4). In selecting a therapist, it is helpful to get recommendations from your wellness instructor, health education specialist, health care practitioner, or spiritual counselor. You also can talk to friends who have seen a therapist and find out whether they would recommend that person. And you can contact professional organizations or the Better Business Bureau to learn whether any consumer complaints are pending against a therapist. Most college campuses today have excellent counseling services, staffed by trained professionals who specialize in the problems commonly experienced by people your age. Spend some time learning where these services are on your campus. Talk with people in the student health center if you are unsuccessful in locating them, or discuss it with someone you know and trust.

Once you set up an appointment with a particular therapist, spend the first session interviewing him or her. Some counselors/therapists offer an initial consultation session at no cost to the patient. During your initial session, note whether the person really listens to what you say, asks thought-provoking questions, and seems to have a genuine interest in you. Notice how you feel, too. Are you comfortable talking with this person? Is this someone whom you feel you can really trust? If you are dissatisfied or uncomfortable, or simply don't feel right, find another therapist. It's pointless to invest time, money, and effort in a therapist whose interest or skill you questioned from the start. Remember, too, that the person your friend thought was great may not be suitable for you.

TABLE 9.4

Choices in Mental Health Counselors and Therapists

TYPE OF PROFESSIONAL	TRAINING	ADDITIONAL INFORMATION
Psychiatrist	M.D. degree Licensed physician	Can prescribe medication Accepts third-party payment May be affiliated with a clinic or hospital May charge $100+ per session, with a sliding scale sometimes available
Psychologist	Doctorate in counseling or clinical psychology	Must be licensed in most states Typically specializes in one or more areas Conducts individual or group sessions Accepts third-party payment Charges $50–100+ per session
Social worker	Master's degree in social work	Can counsel patients with emotional or social problems May be eligible for third-party payment Charges $35–75+ per session
Counselor	Two years graduate coursework or supervised practice May have degree in counseling, education, psychology, or related fields	Offers family, marital, drug, divorce, and other forms of counseling Charges widely varying fees

Sound Decision Making

NO LONGER INVISIBLE

"Why can't you be more like your older sister?" It seems to Lyn that she has been feeling the sting of those words since kindergarten. Her sister Samantha has always been a straight A student, athlete, and school leader; Lyn gets more Bs than As and thinks that she is as undistinguished as her sister is special. In high school, Lyn always had a small group of close friends, but when she gets to college she doesn't know a soul and is so shy she has a very hard time meeting people. Lyn feels mousy and invisible. After a few months of college, Lyn is so lonely she's ready to move back home with her parents even though she knows they would call her a failure for doing so.

One day when she goes to pick up her mail, Lyn sees a flyer for a support group for women with low self-esteem. She takes a copy of the address, and the night of the meeting she stands across the street and watches people go in, but she can't summon the nerve to join them. "What could I contribute?" she thinks. "They'd probably laugh me out of the room."

But the next week she goes back, and this time she does go in. Her stomach feels like it is twisted in knots, but as people begin to speak, she realizes that all the women in the room have feelings very similar to her own. And instead of laughing at Lyn, they ask friendly questions and seem interested in what she has to say. By the end of the evening Lyn feels more comfortable with the group, and she knows she is not the only one who feels invisible.

Over the next year, Lyn keeps attending the group and makes several close friends. They support each other as they make positive changes in their lives and help each other see their good qualities. Lyn discovers that she is an excellent listener and is the kind of person others go to in times of need. By her junior year, Lyn has come so far in overcoming her problems with self-esteem that she decides she wants to make a career out of helping others; her goal is to become a school counselor.

The best therapists attempt to get you to help yourself through a problem rather than allowing you to become dependent on them. If you find yourself coming back week after week without making any real progress, find another therapist. Just as with college instructors, there are effective and not-so-effective therapists. The interaction between the two of you is also important: The style of a therapist that is effective with someone else may not mesh with your individual needs.

Regardless of whether you choose to seek help from someone else or if you choose to try to help yourself through your problems, you have clearly reached a pivotal point headed toward a wellness perspective when you recognize that you need to take action or do something to get through a problem or improve your psychological health.

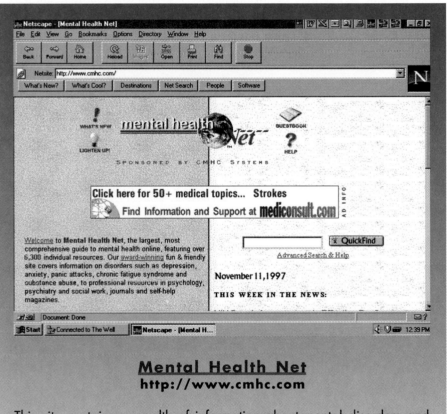

Mental Health Net
http://www.cmhc.com

This site contains a wealth of information about mental disorders and their treatments as well as resources for self-help. There are discussion and support forums on a number of topics such as depression and anxiety. The page lists weekly news updates of research and other information related to mental health, publishes its own electronic journal, *Perspectives,* and contains resources of interest to mental health professionals.

Critical thinking: Internet support groups are available for people suffering from dozens of mental health problems. What do you think are the pros and cons of participation in these forums? Can you think of any possible dangers?

Source: From Mental Health Net, 1998.

Lifestyle Choices: Plan for Action

Although each of us may fluctuate emotionally on a daily basis, we are remarkable, resilient beings, capable of calling on deep reserves of strength to get ourselves through even the toughest psychological adversity. Knowing how to call on our resources, how to cultivate our psychological strengths and minimize our weaknesses, and how to ask for help when necessary provide the basis for lifelong psychological wellness.

Begin by examining each of the following statements, describing your usual feelings and actions. By examining your responses, you may get a clearer picture of your own level of psychological wellness.

1.	I feel good about myself.	never	sometimes	usually	always
2.	I feel comfortable with others.	never	sometimes	usually	always
3.	I accept others for who they are.	never	sometimes	usually	always
4.	I am self-confident.	never	sometimes	usually	always
5.	I find meaning and purpose in my life.	never	sometimes	usually	always
6.	I make healthy choices.	never	sometimes	usually	always
7.	I am flexible and can adapt to situations.	never	sometimes	usually	always
8.	I am able to give love.	never	sometimes	usually	always
9.	I am able to receive love.	never	sometimes	usually	always
10.	I accept responsibility for my actions.	never	sometimes	usually	always
11.	I do not make excuses or rationalize personal mistakes/problems.	never	sometimes	usually	always
12.	I am able to meet the demands of life.	never	sometimes	usually	always
13.	I am concerned about the feelings of others.	never	sometimes	usually	always
14.	I have relationships that are satisfying and lasting.	never	sometimes	usually	always
15.	I respond in a positive way to life's problems.	never	sometimes	usually	always
16.	I plan ahead for future events.	never	sometimes	usually	always
17.	I establish realistic goals.	never	sometimes	usually	always
18.	I think before responding to my emotions.	never	sometimes	usually	always
19.	I experience emotions but am not overcome by them.	never	sometimes	usually	always

20. I recover in a reasonably short
period when exposed to stress
and strain.   never   sometimes   usually   always

Improving your psychological wellness can provide many personal challenges if you are really interested in *changing* the past behaviors and feelings
that have caused your problems. To begin this process, take a moment to
reflect on your answers to the previous statements. How would you charac-
terize your current psychological health? Do you think you have problems
in the way you view yourself? The way you view others? Your relationships? Your overall view of the world and of life? If you believe you have
a problem or if others have told you that you do, start with the area that
seems to be giving you the most difficulty. List the factors that you believe
influence you to think, feel, or behave negatively. Are they things from your
past? Your present? Which of these factors are changeable? Think about the
specific things that trigger your negative response. Can any of these things
be avoided? Changed?

Now that you have done some serious thinking about your psychological
health, consider which of the following action steps you might implement to
improve it.

1. *Practice "self-talk."* Focus on your strengths and giving yourself positive
   reinforcement or praise as many times per day as possible.

2. *Force yourself to get through one day without thinking one negative
   thought about yourself.* Block any negative comparisons with others,
   worries about others' perceptions, and so on. Don't worry about what
   the other person thinks. Practice your own positive affirmations.

3. *Don't allow yourself to be critical or negative about others.* Block negative thoughts and focus on the positive in other people. Practice giving
   praise to others and telling them how important they are to you, how
   good a job they have done, how nice they look, and so on.

4. *Don't dwell on any "woe is me" feelings.* Spend some time helping
   others who could really use it—for example, at a local hospital, home-
   less shelter, or humane society.

5. *Ask for help from your friends and family if necessary.* If you don't have
   someone to go to or if you can't afford a mental health professional, go
   to the city/county mental health service or to your minister, priest, rabbi,
   or spiritual counselor.

6. *Take at least one hour per day for yourself and enjoy life.* Block out
   thoughts of work, financial troubles, or other personal problems, and
   focus on the outdoors, a good book, music, or whatever else you really
   enjoy.

7. *Make time for friends and/or family.* Remember that the best way to
   have friends is to be a good friend. Listen to others and express a sincere interest in their well-being to attain the kind of social support network you'll need in both good and bad times.

8. *Plan for crisis.* Avoid problems by heading them off at the pass. Manage your time as if it really matters what you do with every moment of your day. Try to anticipate deviations or disruptions and have a contingency plan ready.

9. *Keep fit.* Avoid physical breakdowns by paying attention to your overall diet, exercise and stress levels, and other physical health parameters. Keep in mind that the best way to a sound mind is through a sound body, and vice versa (even though the presence of one does not necessarily guarantee the other).

10. *Keep in mind that no one is perfect.* Try to live life in a positive, productive way the majority of the time. Make it an ongoing goal to recognize and accept potential setbacks and to forge ahead through the bad times to get to the good times.

Start slowly and try to achieve one change per week and stick to that change. Once you think you're doing better in one area, move on to the next, and so on. Make a contract with yourself by putting your intentions in writing and signing it.

WEEK 1
This week I will make the following change:

_____

_____

_____

WEEK 2
This week I will make the following change:

_____

_____

_____

WEEK 3
This week I will make the following change:

_____

_____

_____

WEEK 4
This week I will make the following change:

_____

_____

_____

_____   _____

(signature)   *(date)*

Summary

Psychological wellness is difficult to define because it encompasses so many personality, biological, social, and environmental factors. What distinguishes you from everyone else is the result of a lifetime of experiences. Because so many intricate pieces must fall into place to determine your level of psychological wellness, it is difficult to prescribe a recipe for achieving wellness in this area.

Key concepts that you have learned in this chapter include these:

- Your level of psychological/emotional resilience, or ability to recover from upsets, is an important element of wellness.

- People who have a seemingly endless ability to respond positively to life's challenges are said to be psychologically well.

- Our ability to act rationally is referred to as our "mental health."

- Emotional health refers to the "feeling" aspect of our response to life.

- Social health, or our ability to relate to others, is another important dimension of psychological health.

- Internal influences on psychological well-being include the brain, hormones, heredity, and physical health.

- External influences on psychological well-being include maternal health, nurturing by parents, friendships, and socioeconomic conditions.

- Dysfunctional families may play a significant role in predisposing individuals to negative psychological well-being.

- Self-esteem, self-efficacy, locus of control, and self-concept are all important aspects of psychological wellness.

- Depression, suicide, and various anxiety disorders are among the more common psychological disorders faced by college students.

- Achieving psychological wellness takes time, effort, and the support of significant others in our lives.

- A variety of mental health professionals are available to help us overcome psychological problems.

References

Ackerman, R. *Perfect Daughters: Adult Daughters of Alcoholics.* Deerfield Beach, FL: Health Communications, 1989.

Alder, J. Road rage—You and other drivers. *Newsweek,* June 2, 1997: 70–71.

American Psychiatric Association. *Diagnostic and Statistical Manual of Mental Disorders,* 4th ed. Washington, DC: American Psychiatric Association, 1994.

Anderson, R., K. Kochenek and S. Murphy. Report of Final Mortality Statistics, 1995. *Monthly Vital Statistics Report, 45*(11), 1997.

Bandura, A. *Self-efficacy: The exercise of control.* New York: Freeman, 1997.

Bandura, A. Self-efficacy: Toward a unifying theory of behavioral change. *Psychological Review,* 84: 191–215, 1977.

Baranowski, T., and P. Nader. Family health behavior. In D. C. Turk and R. D. Kerns, eds., *Health, Illness, and Families: A Life-Span Perspective.* New York: Wiley, 1985, 51–80.

Bowers, B. Getting aggressive about road rage. *Best Review Property—Casualty Insurance Edition.* November 1997, 43–47.

Buechler, S., and C. Izard. On the emergence, functions, and regulation of some emotion expressions in infancy. In R. Plutchik and H. Kellerman, eds., *The Emotions: Emotions in Early Development,* Vol. 2. New York: Academic Press, 1983, 293–313.

Burgess, R., and P. Draper. The explanation of family violence: The role of biological, behavioral, and cultural selection. In L. Ohlin and M. Tonry, eds., *Family Violence.* Chicago: University of Chicago Press, 1989, 59–116.

Center for Science in the Public Interest. *Food and Mood.* Nutrition Action Health letter, 5–7 September 1992.

Ferguson, A. Road rage. *Time,* January 12, 1998: 64–9.

Fleming, J., and B. Courtney. The dimensionality of self-esteem. *Journal of Personality and Social Psychology,* 46: 404–421, 1984.

Hayes, E. *Why Good Parents Have Bad Kids.* New York: Doubleday, 1989.

Izard, C. E. On the autogeneses of emotions and emotion-cognition relationships in infancy. In M. Lewis and L. Rosenblum, eds., *The Emotions: Emotions in Early Development.* New York: Plenum, 1978, 389–413.

Kleinginna, P. R., and A. M. Kleinginna. A categorized list of motivation definitions with a suggestion for a consensual definition. *Motivation and Emotion,* 5: 263–291, 1981.

Mcdnick, S. A., et al. Biology and violence. In M. Wolfgang and N. Weiner, eds., *Criminal Violence.* Beverly Hills, CA: Sage, 1982, 21–80.

Mitchell, R., R. Cronkite, and R. Moos. Stress, coping and depression. *Journal of Abnormal Psychology,* 92: 433–448, 1983.

Rice, P. *Stress and Health,* 2nd ed. Pacific Grove, CA: Brooks/Cole, 1992, 97.

Robson, P. Improving self-esteem. *Harvard Mental Health Letter,* June 1990.

Rosenberg, M., and M. Fenley. *Violence in America: A Public Health Approach.* New York: Oxford University Press, 1991, 24–25.

Rosenham, D., and M. Seligman. *Abnormal Psychology,* 2nd ed. New York: Norton, 1989.

Rowe, J., and R. Kahn. *Successful aging.* New York: Pantheon Books, 1998.

Seligman, M. *Helplessness: On Depression, Development and Death.* San Francisco: Freeman, 1975.

Seligman, M. *Learned Optimism.* New York: Norton, 1991.

Werner, E. Resilient offspring of alcoholics: A longitudinal study from birth to age 18. *Journal of Studies on Alcohol,* 47: 34–40, 1986.

Woititz, J. *A Study of Self-Esteem in Children of Alcoholics.* Doctoral dissertation, Rutgers University, 1976, 53–55.

Laboratory 9.1

Assessing Psychological Well-Being

One of the first steps in achieving psychological well-being is to develop your own psychological wellness profile. Respond to each of the following statements to help identify your strength, potential problem areas, and areas for improvement. Circle the response that best describes you.

	Never	Sometimes	Usually	Always
1. I look forward to getting out of bed in the morning.	1	2	3	4
2. I get an adequate amount of sleep every day.	1	2	3	4
3. I manage stressful events in an appropriate way.	1	2	3	4
4. When I am feeling down, I have someone that I can talk to.	1	2	3	4
5. I am comfortable talking to other people that I don't know very well.	1	2	3	4
6. I have enough money to get by on.	1	2	3	4
7. I feel good about myself.	1	2	3	4
8. I trust most people when I meet them.	1	2	3	4
9. I am confident that I can get myself through a troubling time.	1	2	3	4
10. When things go wrong, it's usually my fault.	1	2	3	4
11. When I get angry, I yell at people close to me.	1	2	3	4
12. I tend to blame others for things that go wrong in my life.	1	2	3	4
13. I think life is not worth all its hassles.	1	2	3	4
14. I worry about things that never happen.	1	2	3	4
15. I am dissatisfied with my weight.	1	2	3	4
16. I wish I were better looking.	1	2	3	4
17. I feel that others get ahead by unfair means.	1	2	3	4
18. I think people are basically bad.	1	2	3	4
19. When things go wrong, someone else is to blame.	1	2	3	4
20. I am smarter and can take care of myself better than others.	1	2	3	4

Evaluation

Items 1–10:   An "always" response indicates a high level of psychological wellness. How many 4s did you circle? _____

Items 11–20: An "always" response indicates a low level of psychological wellness. How many 4s did you circle? _____

Did you have more high-level marks than low-level marks, or vice versa? Consider those areas that represent low-level psychological wellness. What can you do to improve in these areas?

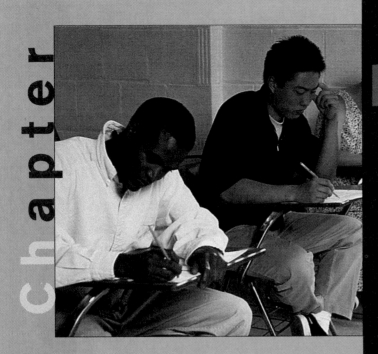

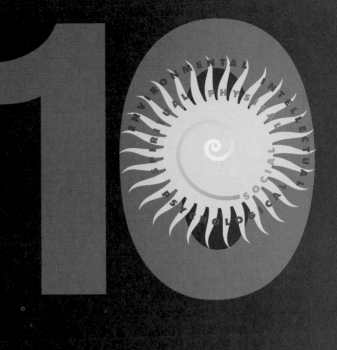

10

ENVIRONMENTAL · PHYSICAL · INTELLECTUAL · SOCIAL · PSYCHOLOGICAL

Stress and Well-Being: Facing Life's Challenges

One Student's View

I have found that stress can be a very common thing in a college lifestyle. Stressors come in small packages as well as big events. From an annoying habit of a roommate to the dreaded finals week, all stressors affect you and must be dealt with. This stress response can be positive as well as negative. A common response to stressors is to abuse drugs and alcohol. Although effective in the short run, they often cause more stress later. My most effective stress relief is to go for a long jog, put my mind at ease, and flow my stress response through a positive outlet.

—Josh Morrison

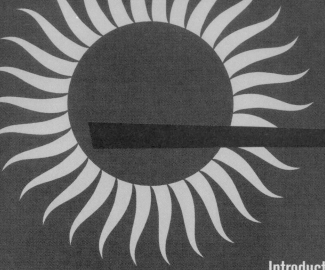

Introduction

How many times in the past week have you heard people saying that they're "stressed out," that they're exercising to reduce stress, or that their cold or headache was the result of too much stress? Every day we complain of being stressed by our families, roommates, jobs, relationships (or the lack of them!), finances, grades, and a host of other trials and tribulations. In fact, responses to a recent questionnaire that we distributed to students who use this text indicated that stress is the priority wellness issue for many of them. It's something we can't run from, hide from, or just ignore, and no matter how much we'd like to get rid of it, it is actually an essential part of human life. In this chapter, we examine what stress is, how it can affect your health and well-being, and, most important, what you can do to reduce your risks for the negative influences of stress.

Objectives

After reading this chapter, you should be able to

- **Distinguish between stress as a positive force and as a negative force in your life and in the lives of others**

- **Discuss the basic physiological changes caused by the stress response**

- **Understand the negative effects of chronic stress on body systems and overall health**

- **Explain the general adaptation syndrome and the impact of its three distinct phases on the body**

- **Describe eustress and its impact on health and well-being**

- **Identify the factors that increase individual susceptibility to stressors**

- **Discuss potential actions to control individual responses to stressors**

- **Identify and understand the role of selected stress buffers in reducing risk for stress and/or controlling potential harmful effects of chronic stress**

What Is Stress?

Normally, our bodies are in a state of internal physiological and psychological balance, or **homeostasis.** Even though there may be slight fluctuations in our dynamic range of human physiological responses, for the most part, our bodies just chug along doing what they need to do to keep us functioning and alert. Anything that disrupts the normal physiological and psychological balance of the body is a **stressor.** A stressor can be something external (someone actually chasing us down the street) or internal (the expectation that a threat lurks just around the corner). The **stress response** is a set of reactions or adaptations induced in the body by a stressor. Thus, **stress** refers to the disruption in normal physiological and psychological balance that is triggered by something in a person's environment or through something in his or her psychological reaction to an event or set of circumstances (stressors). In some instances, you may be perfectly aware that you are being subjected to a stressor; in others, it may be much more of a subconscious reaction. Regardless of the level of awareness, the important thing is that something in your immediate environment is signaling your body that it should be on the alert.

Although we often think that these stressors are negative and cause us harm, it is important to remember that some forms of stress, known as **eustress,** are usually the result of something positive going on in your life. For example, say that someone you are really attracted to walks up to you after class and asks you to go out for coffee or soda later in the afternoon. You begin to sweat, you blush, your heart starts to race. Sound familiar? It is actually the same type of physiological response you had when you heard a strange noise in the middle of the night. The difference is that one is caused by something you think of as positive or exciting and the other by something you perceive as a threat. First dates, graduation, weddings, births, the thrill of winning a championship game in athletics, and a host of other positive events are examples of eustress. In contrast, taking your SATs to get into college, getting into a shouting match with someone who gave you a "door ding" on your new car, the pressures of competition in athletics and classes, and a host of other negative stressors are often referred to as **distress.** Whether caused by positive or negative stressors, the stress response is crucial for surviving life's little ups and downs, crises, challenges, and excitements. So, what happens to us when we are really stressed by something? Can you be "scared to death?" Can you "stroke out" from too much pressure? Why is prolonged stress potentially harmful to the body? Although the human stress response is extremely complex, we try to provide you with basic information in the following sections that will help you understand your own stress response and the actions that you can take to reduce stress-related risks (Figure 10.1).

Reactions to Stress: A Mirror to Your Past

The idea of a balance between the body and its environment is a key to current perceptions about wellness, but it's hardly a novel idea. Over 2,000 years ago, Hippocrates described health as a harmonious balance with the world and disease as a challenge to that balance. And in the early 20th century, Walter Cannon, a noted physiologist who coined the term *homeostasis,* became convinced of its importance to the body.

homeostasis state of internal physiological and psychological balance

stressor anything that disrupts the normal physiological and psychological balance of the body

stress response set of reactions or adaptations induced in the body by a stressor

stress phenomenon of assorted stressors provoking a physiological and psychological response beyond homeostasis

eustress positive stressors prompting a stress response

distress negative stressors that prompt a stress response

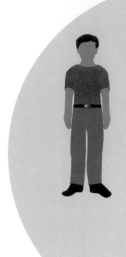

Stressed Students:
- Can't think clearly
- Have problems remembering facts
- Can't see the big picture
- Can't focus, tend to be easily distracted
- Tend to be grouchy/irritable/unpredictable
- May be disorganized or overly compulsive
- May be moody/have highs and lows
- May have difficulty sleeping
- May have problems with compulsive behaviors that may become addictions
- May not reach their potential in any area
- May be more prone toward health problems such as: depression, irritable bowel syndrome, acid stomach, chronic fatigue, aches and pains from arthritis, more headaches, sleep problems, allergy flare ups, skin problems, weight problems, increased risks for chronic diseases; more problems with infectious diseases such as the cold or flu

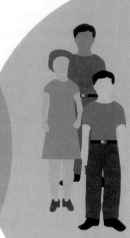

Stressed Friends:
- May be unpredictable/volatile
- May have problems with responsibility
- May have emotional problems
- May be "less available" for personal interactions
- May have any of the problems listed under Stressed Students
- May engage in destructive behavior patterns
- May be prone to violence/saying or doing things they normally wouldn't
- May be forgetful
- May have lots of problems with relationships/family
- May not be very tolerant of you

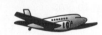

Stressed Communities:
- May be more prone to violence/higher rates of accidents/injuries
- May show signs of neglect/irresponsibility
- May lack support for poor, people in need, minorities
- May be prone to disruption/corruption
- May be breeding grounds for ill health

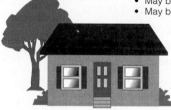

Figure 10.1

Each of us is affected by stress every day, in ways we may not even recognize. This "stress effect" may have far-reaching consequences.

general adaptation syndrome
series of physiological stages that the body progresses through as it adapts to a stressful situation

It was also Cannon who first described the body's reaction to stress. He and Hans Selye, another pioneering stress researcher, both recognized the "nonspecific" nature of the stress response. That is, regardless of the stressor, the body's reaction is the same: It stands ready for "fight or flight," as Cannon described it. This *fight-or-flight theory* was later referred to as the **general adaptation syndrome (GAS),** a series of physiological phases/stages that the body goes through when exposed to a stressor. In these stages, the body prepares either to fight or to flee in the face of adversity. In the first stage, known as the *alarm phase,* the heart begins to pound, the muscles tense, the mouth becomes dry, and a whole range of other physiological reactions occurs in body systems. The *resistance phase* of the GAS is noteworthy in that specific organs are targeted for dealing with various elements of the stressor. These target organs attempt to resist, and in some cases, chronic resistance and arousal trigger a malfunction or illness response.

Eventually, the body is unable to sustain it's resistive mechanisms and it enters the final *exhaustion phase* of the stress response. Normally, when energy reserves are depleted and exhaustion sets in, rest is necessary for recovery. Without adequate rest and proper nutrients to aid in recovery, the body reserves may become depleted and organ or system failures may result. Although researchers are now discovering some subtle differences in response to certain stressors, for all practical purposes Cannon's observation remains valid.

Whether the stressor is the physical predator that frequently threatened our ancestors or the fear that arises when our boss says, "I've got bad news," the body's neural and hormonal systems respond in the same way and go through the same types of GAS phases.

Ironically, researchers such as Hans Selye initially thought that the nonspecific stress response in his laboratory rats was a positive response: Emergencies arose and the body adapted. The "fittest" were able to adapt very effectively initially. In time, however, he discovered that stressed rats were also getting sick, particularly those rats that never seemed to get adequate relief from stressors. The body's "adaptation" was not an unqualified success after all. Thus, researchers began to ask questions about the negative as well as the positive consequences of the stress response (Sapolsky; Girdano et al.). For example, when are these adaptations helpful, and when do they fail and bring about disease? Why are psychological stressors stressful, and why do individuals differ in the quality of their stress response and their vulnerability to stress-related disease? All these concerns have implications for our lives today.

How the Stress Response Works

Although we seldom face dangers as menacing as someone chasing us down the street, we do face a continual barrage of threats to our ego, our relationships, our economic security, and our safety. In subtle, unconscious ways, the body responds by setting off an internal alarm that begins to mobilize body reserves to prepare for fighting or fleeing from battle. Regardless of whether the threat is real (a burglar jiggling your door handle in the night) or perceived (the suspicion that your boss is planning to fire you), the body responds in a predictable physiological pattern. In most cases, internal defense mechanisms and other body systems ward off the offending threat (we realize it's just the wind, not a burglar), and the body returns to normal fairly quickly after an initial dip in energy reserves. However, if the stressor is particularly strong or perceived as particularly menacing, or if our initial response is prolonged, the body will respond by activating certain systems. Consider the following example:

It's a dark and stormy night. As you walk across campus, you suddenly have the eerie sensation that someone is following you. You quicken your pace but sense that the person behind has speeded up, too. You begin to sweat, your breathing quickens, and your eyes dart here and there looking for other people or a place to run. You consider your options—to scream, to stop and confront the person, to run, or to stop and let the person pass—all within a few short seconds. Now, consider what is happening inside your body (see Figure 10.2). Initially, the *autonomic nervous system* (the division of the nervous system that responds involuntarily) sends a message to the *cerebral cortex*, the part of the brain that assesses the situation and tries to interpret a situation—in this case, a possible threat from the stranger. This interpretation derives from your past experiences, your knowledge of recent

Figure 10.2

The general adaptation syndrome: alarm phase

Source: Adapted from Donatelle and Davis, 1998.

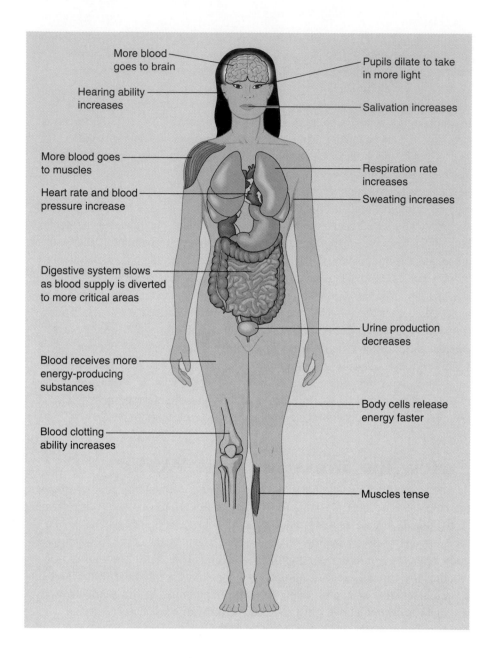

More blood goes to brain

Hearing ability increases

More blood goes to muscles

Heart rate and blood pressure increase

Digestive system slows as blood supply is diverted to more critical areas

Blood receives more energy-producing substances

Blood clotting ability increases

Pupils dilate to take in more light

Salivation increases

Respiration rate increases

Sweating increases

Urine production decreases

Body cells release energy faster

Muscles tense

incidents in the area, and your resulting expectations (Pearlin and Skaff). This is why some of you might really be stressed by an event that barely is noticed by your friends. *Perceptions* are an important part of your overall stress response. Fortunately, the message is also assessed by a highly complex region of the brain known as the *limbic system*. Impulses are sent from the brain to the body via a complex network of nerve fibers, known as the *reticular activating system* (RAS), which serves as yet another message filter and sorter of arousal messages. The RAS can reverberate with past messages long after the initial messages have passed. Unfortunately, in the case of chronic stress, chronic stimulation of the RAS may trigger a physiological stress response that continues to affect you long after the event that caused the response. Eventually, it is believed that this inability of the body to return to normal may be a contributor to persistent high blood pressure and other problems. As the cerebral cortex and the limbic system exchange messages, emotions of fear and anxiety may escalate or decline based on your perception of the threat. The limbic system will override the initial response

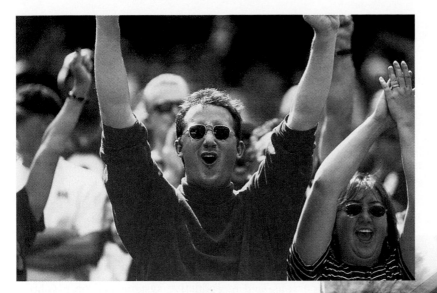

Both positive feelings (the euphoria associated with your team's victory) and negative (frustration while driving) result from the hypothalamus releasing stress hormones into the bloodstream.

and direct the body to return to normal, or it will prod the body to even greater response by calling the *hypothalamus* into play. The hypothalamus, in turn, stimulates the pituitary gland, and through their interaction, a complex assortment of stress hormones enters the bloodstream.

The hormone known as *ACTH* signals other glands to secrete specialized hormones in conjunction with the hypothalamus. Specifically, the hypothalamus stimulates the secretion of catecholamines, or hormones known as *epinephrine* (often called adrenaline) and *norepinephrine* (often called noradrenalin) from the adrenal glands at the top of the kidneys. Among the other, more significant adrenal hormones that are secreted are *cortisol* and *aldosterone,* which affect metabolic activity by increasing the availability of energy (in the form of glucose, fatty acids, and amino acids). Your body is undergoing the following changes:

- Increase in heart rate, blood pressure, and respiration

- Increase in blood volume, caused by a decrease in urine production and an increase in sodium retention

- Increase in metabolic activity and oxygen consumption, and the release of endorphins (natural opiates), which dull pain receptors

- Increase in the strength of muscular contractions, dilation of coronary arteries, dilation of pupils, constriction of the abdominal arteries, and movement of blood from nonessential to more essential areas

In other words, your fight-or-flight system is mobilized. Every sense in your body is aroused, and you are ready to take action. Any attacker would most likely be meeting you at your strongest, from a purely physiological point of view.

In times of crisis, then, your body responds to help you out. Just as the stress response prepares potential victims to save themselves from an attacker, it can also arouse conditioned athletes to perform at their peak during the crucial final seconds of a championship game. So what's the problem?

The Effects of Chronic Stress on Your Health

As we've seen, the stress response is an emergency system. Energy is mobilized and redirected from storage and from noncrucial functions (such as digestion, tissue repair, and reproduction) to those functions needed for fight or flight. Some of the body's functions are put on hold, and some are sent into hyper mode. This is fine in a true emergency, but when the stress response is activated too often or over too long a time (or for no physiological reason), the effects are not so beneficial.

Chronic stress can cause major problems with your physical and psychological health. Scientists are just beginning to unlock the complex web of stress-related physical and emotional interactions that actually cause or exacerbate conditions such as hypertension and diseases such as arteriosclerosis. They are also beginning to understand the effects of stress on the immune, digestive, cardiovascular, nervous, and reproductive systems and on psychological well-being (Elmharib; Leonard and Song; see Table 10.1).

Stress and the Body: Upsetting the Perfect Machine?

Scientists believe that the stress response disrupts the human body in several important ways, some of which have already been discussed. One exciting new area being explored relates to the effect of stress on the body's resistance to disease, particularly the ability of the immune system to fight infectious diseases. **Psychoneuroimmunology (PNI),** a new branch of scientific inquiry that has evolved in the past decade, is attempting to determine the intricate relationships among the mind, emotions, stress, and immune system. Preliminary investigations into this interrelationship provide striking evidence of a significant link between emotional duress and **immunocompetence,** the body's ability to ward off infectious agents and defend itself against illness successfully. In particular, this research has looked at the depletion of *t-cells* and *b-cells,* white blood cells that serve as major players in the body's resistance to selected diseases or to the proliferation of cancer cells (Rice; Baker; Dantzer and Kelly; Leonard and Song; Elmharib). Other studies have shown that susceptibility appeared to increase in cases in which the stressor was particularly intense, lasted for a longer-than-average time, and occurred with greater-than-expected frequency (Kiecolt-Glaser et al.; McNaughton et al.; Cohen and Williamson). For example, some researchers have theorized that women in particular may be more susceptible to some cancers immediately after experiencing major losses in their lives, the death of loved ones, stressors from multiple causes, and similar situations. In addition, some research, though controversial, has shown that positive emotions, social support, and other stress-relieving situations have served to bolster immune response and increase survival rates for cancer sufferers. Although much of this research is still in its infancy, the obvious implications for health—and wellness—are particularly exciting.

In addition to being implicated in immune functioning, stress appears to play a role in one's susceptibility to *hypertension,* an elevation in blood pressure higher then accepted levels (see Chapter 13). When the sympathetic nervous system is activated, as in a stress response, cardiac output is

psychoneuroimmunology new branch of scientific inquiry that is attempting to determine the intricate relationships between the mind and the immune system

immunocompetence body's ability to ward off infectious agents and defend itself against illness successfully

TABLE 10.1

Health Effects of Excessive Stress

Nervous System Effects
Hormonal imbalances leading to depression and emotional volatility
Muscular twitching and spasms
Increased agitation and mental arousal
Insomnia

Cardiovascular Effects/Hypertension
Increased fluid retention
Increased heart rate and intensified stroke volume
Increased blood volume
Increased blood pressure
Decreased urination
Increased cortisol levels and fatty acids in blood
Increased hormone secretion
Increased risk of atherosclerosis
Constricted blood vessels

Kidney Effects
Inhibited blood flow (vasoconstriction) and kidney function

Skin Effects
Dryness, itching, hives, acne

Gastrointestinal Effects
Slower blood flow and digestive activity in GI tract
Retention of food in stomach
Possible cancer development
Indigestion and nausea
Increased gastric juices, bad breath, indigestion
Diarrhea or constipation
Ulcer development
Increased likelihood of irritable bowel syndrome and colitis

Hyperglycemic States
Delay of or interference with insulin availability
Diabetes

Immunological Effects
Increased glucose, fatty acids, and amino acids in bloodstream
Increased risk of infection and cancer
Depletion of protein reserves for formation of white blood cells
Arthritislike conditions

Other Effects
Tension and migraine headaches
Increased drug use
Dysfunctional relationships
Reduced productivity

increased, with a resultant blood pressure increase. As epinephrine, norepinephrine, and renin from the kidneys combine to cause vasoconstriction and increased heart rate, blood pressure begins to rise. Chronic stress arousal may, in fact, lead to chronic hypertension.

Chronic stress has also been linked to the development of arteriosclerosis. Rosenman and Friedman were among the first researchers to link the development of atherosclerotic plaque—yellowish patches of cholesterol and other lipids that build up inside the arteries—with elevated stress levels. By studying cholesterol levels in accountants prior to and after the high-stress tax season, these researchers theorized that the stress of the job directly influenced cholesterol formation and subsequent plaque deposits (www.usatoday.com). However, much of this research remains controversial today, as researchers have explored other risk factors as possible contributors.

Gastrointestinal difficulties such as diarrhea, constipation, heartburn, gas, nausea, indigestion, irritable bowel syndrome, and ulcers may be due, in part, to excessive smooth muscle contraction during the stress response as well as to fluid imbalances brought about by the body's attempt to stabilize itself and/or by excess secretions of certain stress-related hormones. When the body is stressed, no internal system is left unscathed.

In addition, misuse of aspirin for stress-induced headaches and overconsumption of alcohol may cause additional gastrointestinal tract irritations. Indigestion and heartburn are common signs of too much stress in your life.

Scientists know a great deal about the many effects of stress on both the male and female reproductive systems. For example, stress-induced secretion

Perspectives

Is Reducing Mental Stress More Beneficial than Exercise in Preventing Heart Disease?

To ward off heart disease, the number one killer in America, we all know the routine: lose weight, cut the fat, get rid of the cigarettes, and exercise, exercise, exercise. Right? According to researchers at Duke University in North Carolina, learning to relax, reducing sadness, controlling hostility and anger, and feeling better about yourself in general may be even more important to that old risk-reduction formula. In fact, new research indicates that managing emotional and psychological stress can profoundly reduce the risk of coronary artery disease—which affects a staggering 13.5 million Americans each year and costs nearly $120 billion in treatment and lost productivity.

After a 5-year study of 107 patients with heart disease, the Duke researchers found that patients who learned to manage stress reduced their risk of having another heart attack or heart problems by 74% when compared to those patients whose treatment included only medications. Reducing mental stress also proved more beneficial than exercise. Researchers first gave the heart patients a battery of personality, physical, and mental stress tests. They filled out surveys, walked on treadmills, solved math problems in their heads, and wore heart monitors at home for 48 hours. Then the 107 heart patients were randomly divided into 3 groups. Forty received standard care only, meaning aspirin, medications to control heart arrhythmias or blood pressure, and so on. Thirty four were assigned to an exercise group in which they received their usual medications and worked out vigorously 35 minutes, 3 times per week. Thirty-three others came to an hour-and-a-half group therapy and stress management meeting once a week as well as taking their medications.

Over four months, the stress group learned about irritable and impatient Type A behaviors. Through biofeedback, sophisticated monitoring equipment that measures when muscles tense or relax, they began to recognize how their bodies seized up when they got angry or stressed. They learned to redirect the defeatist thoughts that often plague heart attack survivors and to focus on positive events. Researchers evaluated subjects over a 5-year period. In the group that had only standard care, 30% had additional heart troubles. In the exercise group, 21% had another heart attack or required surgery. But in the stress management group, only 9% had further problems!

Although these results represent only one study, from a select group of predominantly white male subjects, they raise interesting, important issues surrounding the importance of stress management programs in the risk-reduction/health-promotion programs of the future.

Source: From Schulte, 1997.

of hormones in women appears to result in a chain of events that reduces the likelihood of progesterone and estrogen secretion and formation of a viable egg (Sapolsky). Menstrual cycle irregularities also are common among highly stressed women. In men, stress-induced hormone secretion can result in decreased sperm production, among other effects (Fisher).

Stress and Psychological Well-Being

In our own lives, we can easily see the most basic relationship between stress and psychological factors. A physical stressor can become less stressful—and our stress response lessened—if we become psychologically conditioned to it. It is also obvious that stressors can be purely psychological; our minds can engender a stress response in the absence of any physical stressor. The effects of stress on our psychological health are numerous and fascinating (though in many ways they are more difficult to study than the physical health effects).

Behavior is one indicator of psychological well-being that often seems affected by chronic stress. Individuals experiencing chronic stress may become depressed, for example, and take mind-altering drugs or drink alcohol to drown out their problems. They may have trouble concentrating and thus do poorly in school or at work. What's more, they may find it extremely difficult to get along with others. The popular image of someone under stress as short-tempered, impatient, and preoccupied with personal needs and worries may be a true picture of how some individuals are affected by chronic stress. Others may find that, although their social health and spiritual well-being may suffer a bit, their productivity may actually increase in the presence of these stressors.

To a large degree, what happens to you when you are chronically stressed will depend on your background, your overall wellness, and your ingrained behavioral patterns. You may not be able to prevent all the negative health effects that stress may cause, but you can play a significant role in reducing your risks and improving your overall wellness profile. What makes one person become bedridden from a cold or the flu and another able to work and maintain normal daily activity even while ill? What makes one person physically assault someone or damage someone's property when stressed and another person decide to turn away from the conflict and go for a walk in the park? Although the response each of us makes is likely to be unique, many factors contribute to our overall stress response. Understanding these contributing factors may help us to make reasonable choices that can reduce our vulnerability to the effects of chronic stress.

What Are Your Risks for Too Much Stress?

The stress in our lives—stressors and our reactions to them—are influenced by a myriad of biological, sociocultural, environmental, and individual factors (see Table 10.2). College students, away from home for the first time or trying to manage the multiple roles of family, job, and college, may find that stress levels are explosive. Some of these factors may be impossible to control; others are within our reach. Many of them are influenced by things about you and your past that you seldom ever think about.

TABLE 10.2

Social Readjustment Rating Scale

RANK	LIFE EVENT	VALUE
1	Death of spouse	100
2	Divorce	73
3	Marital separation	65
4	Jail term	63
5	Death of close family member	63
6	Personal injury or illness	53
7	Marriage	50
8	Fired at work	47
9	Marital reconciliation	45
10	Retirement	45
11	Change in health of family member	44
12	Pregnancy	40
13	Sex difficulties	39
14	Gain of new family member	39
15	Business readjustment	39
16	Change in financial state	38
17	Death of close friend	37
18	Change to different line of work	36
19	Change in the number of arguments with spouse	35
20	Mortgage over $10,000	31
21	Foreclosure of mortgage or loan	30
22	Change in responsibilities at work	29
23	Son or daughter leaving home	29
24	Trouble with in-laws	29
25	Outstanding personal achievement	28
26	Spouse begins or stops work	26
27	Begin or end school	26
28	Change in living conditions	25
29	Revision of personal habits	24
30	Trouble with boss	23
31	Change in work hours or conditions	20
32	Change in residence	20
33	Change in schools	20
34	Change in recreation	19
35	Change in church activities	19
36	Change in social activities	18
37	Mortgage or loan less than $10,000	17
38	Change in sleeping habits	16
39	Change in number of family get-togethers	15
40	Change in eating habits	15
41	Vacation	13
42	Christmas	12
43	Minor violations of the law	11

Source: From Holmes and Rahe, 1967.

Culture

The cultural environment in which you are raised may have a major impact on your pattern of response to stress as you strive to live up to the cultural expectations of others. For example, Japan, which historically has featured a strong work ethic, long work weeks, a high regard for family honor and tradition, and few recreational outlets, also has high rates of drug abuse, tobacco use, suicide, and other stress-related problems. Similar patterns are evident in many subcultures in the United States. Although cultural influences are often ignored when considering our individual and collective responses to stressors, we must acknowledge that such influences may play a significant role in our stress-related behavior. Family values, attitudes, customs, religious beliefs, rituals, and behavioral patterns are all culturally influenced. By assessing those factors, you can obtain a better understanding of what you might need to change to reduce the impact of stressors in your life.

Environment

Although cultural factors may have a significant role in our individual stress responses, the physical environment also plays a major role. For example, people who live in unsanitary, unsafe, or inhospitable conditions typically suffer from many more stressors than those who do not (Kessler; Morris). Excessive noise, overcrowding, pollution, inaccessible health care facilities, and general environmental problems can exacerbate stress levels in even the most resilient individuals. Clearly, the same stressful event or situation may affect each of us differently in level and intensity. For example, the thought of sleeping on the streets would be a source of extreme stress for many people. However, those individuals who are faced with these conditions every day might wonder how people who are better off could consider their more privileged lives to be stressful in any way. Long lines, noisy study areas, difficulty finding parking, trouble getting an appointment with your instructor, and other stressors of college students may not seem serious to the person struggling for survival on the streets; however, for many people, such stressors may be enough to push them over the edge.

Social Factors

How many times in the past few days have you become upset over what another person said or did to you or, even worse, what you thought they might be saying? How often have you worried about how you "measured up" in a class, or on an athletic team, or with your friends or family members? How many times have you been concerned with how your body or hair or clothes looked? The way we interact with others and they with us, our communication methods (or the lack of them), our level of social acceptance, the expectations we place on others and they on us, our daily activity patterns, and a host of other interpersonal and intrapersonal social factors cause varying levels of stress in our lives. Being pressured to do things we don't want to do, such as going to a party hosted by someone we don't particularly like, and not being able to do things we do want to do because of internal and external pressures can be the source of significant turmoil.

In addition, certain social conditions influence your overall level of stress. Discrimination, unemployment or the possibility of unemployment, isolation from others, job-related stresses, lack of control, problems with your roommates, unsafe neighborhoods, and many other social forces may influence the nature and extent of stress that you experience. Adding any one of these social pressures to an existing high level of stress can significantly influence your stress load (Pearlin and Skaff).

Figure 10.3

Common stressors affecting your health

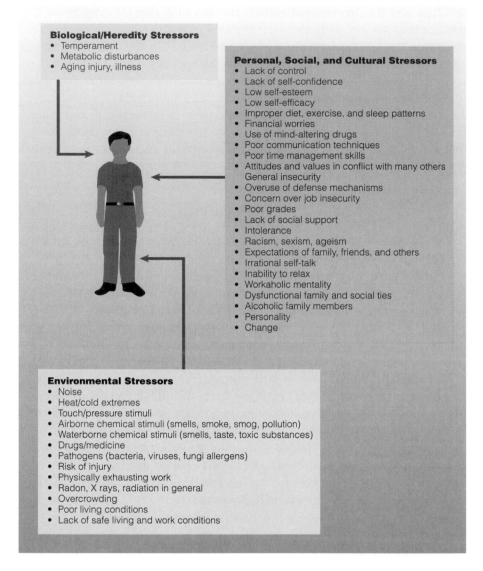

Biological/Heredity Stressors
- Temperament
- Metabolic disturbances
- Aging injury, illness

Personal, Social, and Cultural Stressors
- Lack of control
- Lack of self-confidence
- Low self-esteem
- Low self-efficacy
- Improper diet, exercise, and sleep patterns
- Financial worries
- Use of mind-altering drugs
- Poor communication techniques
- Poor time management skills
- Attitudes and values in conflict with many others General insecurity
- Overuse of defense mechanisms
- Concern over job insecurity
- Poor grades
- Lack of social support
- Intolerance
- Racism, sexism, ageism
- Expectations of family, friends, and others
- Irrational self-talk
- Inability to relax
- Workaholic mentality
- Dysfunctional family and social ties
- Alcoholic family members
- Personality
- Change

Environmental Stressors
- Noise
- Heat/cold extremes
- Touch/pressure stimuli
- Airborne chemical stimuli (smells, smoke, smog, pollution)
- Waterborne chemical stimuli (smells, taste, toxic substances)
- Drugs/medicine
- Pathogens (bacteria, viruses, fungi allergens)
- Risk of injury
- Physically exhausting work
- Radon, X rays, radiation in general
- Overcrowding
- Poor living conditions
- Lack of safe living and work conditions

Difficult homework assignments might be one cause of stress in a college student's environment.

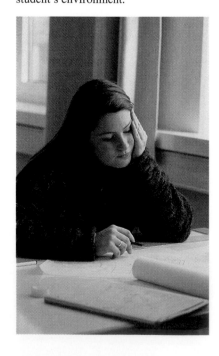

Stress Emotions: Frustration and Anger

Emotional wellness is the ability to feel and express the full range of human emotions, and to control them, not be controlled by them (Seaward). Ironically, from our earliest years, we are exhorted by society to not show our true feelings. Men are told that "big boys don't cry." We are told to "chill out" and not get "all worked up," and so on. By the time many of us reach adulthood, we have learned to conceal our outward displays of emotion the majority of the time. "Losing it" is not only not acceptable, it is often considered cause for social ostracism, so we are forced to brood inwardly about things that bother us rather than letting our emotions show. Many behavioral scientists believe that internalizing strong emotions can be a source of many stress-related problems, including depression, gastrointestinal upset, and hypertension (Hale, Greenberg, and Ramsey; Fisher; Felsten). On any given day, most of us get annoyed or angry about something. Recent studies of anger in the United States indicate that the average person experiences approximately 15 anger situations per day. Most of these episodes were based on violations of expectations, such as long lines at the checkout stand, rudeness by others, aggressive driving, or other daily problems (Seaward).

Have you ever gotten so angry by being cut off or delayed in traffic that you just wanted to bash your car into the car ahead of you? You are probably not alone if you have. Recent statistics quoted in the popular press estimate that as many as one-third of all highway fatalities today may be attributed to a phenomenon known as *road rage,* a stress-induced emotion that is generated when people are frightened or frustrated by the mass crush of traffic they must maneuver their way through on any given day of the week. Frustrations occur when we are blocked or held back from something we want to do or someplace we want to go. Emotionally, we respond to frustration with feelings of anger and aggression and with the nervous and hormonal responses that accompany them. Thus, frustration causes the stress response to zoom into action. Whereas normally reasonable people would not think of using their cars as weapons, the combination of problems at home, stresses at work, use of substances such as alcohol, and a tension-laden roadway can cause explosive results. This is just one example of frustration that provokes an angry reaction. Think about those long lines you stand in to register for classes or to buy textbooks, the difficulties you have in finding articles or books at the library, your shortage of money for buying the things you need, the long "busy" signals you experience when you are trying to get onto the Internet—and on and on. All these somewhat minor life frustrations can accumulate to produce major stress effects.

In its most basic form, anger is a survival emotion common to all animals. Darwin referred to this as **rage reflex.** He believed that this aggressive reaction was essential to the survival of all species. Whereas animals act instinctively to defend and protect themselves, their territory, or their young, humans have engineered the ability to combine conscious thought with the rage reflex to produce a hybrid of anger unparalleled in the animal kingdom. In that sense, human anger is a unique phenomenon in that we are the only species that can process anger into delayed revenge and behave aggressively for seemingly inexplicable reasons (Seaward). The concept of "getting even" takes on new dimensions for angry, stressed humans. Redford Williams, a well-known health behavioralist, indicates from his research on Type A behavior and health, that at least 20% of the American population has levels of hostile anger that can produce serious health problems and another 20% are teetering on the edge of illness due to the stress of unresolved anger (Williams & Stiegler; Williams & Williams; Felsten).

You can do some things to help you cope with anger-causing social stressors, but some factors may be beyond your control. Recognizing the things you can change in life and accepting those over which you have little control may be one of the biggest stress reducers of all. Also, remember that emotions such as anger are not always bad symptoms of stress. Instead, anger, when properly controlled, can be a signal to others that you have certain values and beliefs that you are willing to stand up for and defend adamantly. Anger has also been shown to be *cathartic* or relief-inducing if properly managed—when its use allows one to gain control of a situation, to avoid intense provocation by others, or to develop greater insight into the cause of the problem. For suggestions on ways you can better manage and control your own anger, see Table 10.3.

Changes in Personal Relationships

Although often given little attention in stress management classes, change in personal relationships is a significant source of stress for most of us. Family

rage reflex survival emotion common to many animal species

TABLE 10.3

Getting a Grip on Anger

Based on the works of Carol Tavris, Harold Weisinger, and Brian Seaward as well as this text's authors' perspectives on anger management, the following suggestions may help you manage some of your own anger experiences:

1. *Know your own anger style.* Take stock of your own anger situations. When something really gets to you, do you tend to hold your anger in? Do you have a short fuse and explode quickly? Do you get over your anger quickly, or does it stay with you for a long period of time? Note the things, if any, that really cause you to boil. Are there things today that make you more angry than they used to? Less angry than they used to? How did your parents and siblings show their anger? What kind of an anger style would you say your family has?

2. *Monitor your anger patterns over a period of days or weeks.* Keep a journal in which you note what makes you mad, what really brings it on, time of day, and so on. Do any patterns emerge?

3. *Assess your own anger philosophy.* What degree of anger display do you find acceptable in others? What kinds of anger displays are not acceptable? Why are some types of anger acceptable and others not? How long is it acceptable to stay mad?

4. *Learn to "chill out" before reacting.* Rather than jumping right into the fray with a sharp retort, threatening gesture, or nasty look, count to 20, force your mind to block out thoughts about the situation, take a quick walk to get a soda or cup of coffee, or do some other activity to divert your attention. Taking a time out helps defuse your anger and let you think more clearly. Instead of zipping off a nasty e-mail message or letter, write whatever you want to say and *save it* for 2 days. If you still want to send the message after thinking about it, reread the note to decide whether you might be able to change some wording to reduce possible repercussions. Think about other ways of resolving your situation rather than using an attack.

5. *Learn to express your feelings constructively.* Holding your tongue or reigning in your emotions is often a challenge, but in the long haul doing so is usually best. However, don't just suppress your true feelings. People who are most vulnerable to the negative aspects of stress-related illness are those who are constantly "stewing" about something but never resolve it directly. In other words, don't ignore, avoid, or repress your feelings. Anger has been compared to acid. It will eat away at you unless it is neutralized, and it is best neutralized by creative (constructive) expression. For example, instead of shouting at someone or saying, "This is really stupid and unfair. I can't believe you are doing this!" the more constructive approach would be to say, "Hey, I have some difficulties with this concept/issue. Have you thought about doing such and such in this way, so that such and such doesn't happen?"

6. *Plan ahead.* Some situations can be foreseen as potential anger provokers. Identify what these situations are and then find ways to minimize your exposure to them. If you know that standing in line at the post office really irritates you, try to find out what times of day are less busy and go to the post office then.

7. *Develop a support system.* Take time to develop trusting friendships with a couple of people who are nonjudgmental, who have values similar to yours, and whose opinions you value. Confide in them and share your honest thoughts. At the same time, you need to be willing to listen to them when they have difficulties. Rather than seeking allies or trying to get them to agree with you all the time, ask for their objective thoughts about a situation.

TABLE 10.3 Continued
Getting a Grip on Anger

Be prepared to accept their responses even when they don't match yours. Having someone you can talk to about anything without fearing judgment or criticism is an important aspect of social support—and we know that a good social support system is necessary to overall health and wellness.

8. *Learn to solve problems.* Always try to have a Plan B. If you have decided to take an action and it clearly isn't getting you anywhere, think of other options in advance and the limitations and strengths of various options. Learn to accept your decisions when you have tried several things and nothing seems to work. When all else fails, getting revenge is *not* a viable alternative. Revenge may make you feel better temporarily, but it does little to solve the underlying problem.

9. *Protect your health.* Keeping yourself in good health, getting adequate amounts of rest and exercise, and keeping your spirits up will do much to help you look on the brighter side more often than not. Give yourself time alone; take time to enjoy life; set aside time for work and for play. When you treat yourself well, you will probably be less bothered by or resentful about the minor offenses of others.

10. *Turn complaints into requests.* Pessimists tend to complain, whine, and moan. Anyone can complain. Complaining is a sign of victimization. When frustrated with a roommate or family member, rework the problem into a request for change with the person involved. Take a more optimistic outlook on your own perceptions. Don't be so demanding of people about their behavior and acknowledge that not all people are perfect. If there is something you don't like, ask the person involved if he or she could do things a bit differently to help you out. Also, acknowledge that in many cases when we place blame on others, we are partly to blame ourselves.

11. *Limit the amount of time you will waste with anger.* Learn to resolve issues that have caused you pain, frustration, or stress. Remember that when you let someone make you angry, you are giving that person the power to ruin your day. Now *that* should make you angry! Acknowledge that you are often angry because of your own values, fears, frustrations, or actions. If you are angry because your roommate always leaves dirty dishes in the sink, acknowledge that your family (probably your mom) would not have tolerated such a behavior and thus, you are bothered by it. Your roommate may never have had the luxury of someone who set such rules. You'll have to come up with a system that is acceptable for both of you and take responsibility for yourself. Try to focus on the few things that are really important and nonnegotiable in your roommate interactions. Let go of the little things.

12. *Learn to forgive.* Don't hold grudges for long periods of time about things that really are not that important. Acknowledge human weaknesses; let go of anger that arises out of jealousy, fear, poor self-concept, pressures to be liked, and other human frailties. As we all try to control our lives, our friendships, our successes, and our failures, there are times when we will probably make mistakes. Imagine what it would be like if your mother or father held a grudge against you for all the things you did in high school or all the things you said or did while growing up. Although we assume unconditional love from family members, we often treat them worse than we'd ever treat strangers on the street. We need to be resilient in our thinking and encourage others to try again to get things right. Assume that people can really do the right thing if challenged, and help challenge them to be better people by not holding them accountable for every misstep and action. Assume that people learn from their mistakes and try to learn from your own.

changes, such as divorces, separations, deaths, and other losses, can be major stressors for children and young adults. Changes in job, financial insecurities, and other problems that come about through moving, changes in family structure, and changes in the community can be sources of stress. Remember what it was like to leave the security and comfort of hometown and high school friends and arrive at a strange, large campus for the first time? Remember the initial shock of not having parents to give you money, cook your meals, check on your social life, and so on? All these changes in family relationships and structure and your interactions with friends can have particularly devastating stress effects. Often, these types of changes are considered *passages* and part of normal life transitions. However, without social support and social networks to rely on, without the love and security of the past, many college students have difficulty coping and drop out of college during the first year (Hale, Greenberg, and Ramsey; Fisher). At many universities today, increased attention is given to easing these separation pains for students through counseling services and campus-sponsored events to get students involved and linked with others.

The relationship changes just discussed can lead to significant stress; however, the stresses caused by "significant other" changes (break-ups, divorces, infidelity, death, physical and mental abuse, divorce, births, and so on) can wreak havoc on young adult lives. When these relationship changes or problems are superimposed on students who are pressured to go to classes and appear interested, concentrate on exams, complete part-time work, compete on athletic teams, and participate in student events, the overall load can lead even the most psychologically and physically healthy individuals to have problems. Stress overload can lead to depression, substance abuse, lots of colds and minor illnesses, and severe problems with productivity. The most progressive campuses have strong student support services that recognize the huge potential for problems and are ready to respond in times of crisis.

Individual Influences

Who you are as a person—physically, emotionally, intellectually—will have a significant impact on your overall stress levels. Your genetic makeup, health, life experiences, values, attitudes, beliefs, intelligence level, personality, and level of self-esteem, self-control, and self-efficacy all may influence how you are affected by stress.

The genetic makeup that you inherit may play a role in how you respond to potential stressors. Some theorists believe, for example, that the likelihood of our responding to a given situation in a particular manner may be subtly influenced by our inherited temperament.

Some experts suggest that temperament may determine our response pattern in one of three ways. First, activity patterns may vary tremendously from one person to the next: One person may be very active and assertive in interactions, and another will be extremely passive. Second, emotional responses in different people may vary greatly, Third, reactivity to stimuli may range from hypersensitivity, or being overly sensitive to all types of external stimulation, to hyposensitivity, or being much less likely to respond to stimuli than might be expected. Although temperament theory is somewhat controversial, some researchers believe that, like animals, humans may inherit a more passive or aggressive reactionary response (Loechlin et al.;

Johnson; Plomin et al.). In addition, other researchers suggest that genes may influence the stress response by the way they control the codes for the structure and function of organs and body systems. For example, hormonal levels may vary from one individual to another (Rice; Johnson; Plomin).

General biological functioning may also play a key role in stress responses, as may health status, age level, injury, illness, and other factors. If you are fit and healthy, your body systems may respond more effectively to real or perceived stressors, and chronic stress may not be as damaging.

Your life experiences, of course, also affect your response to stress (see Laboratory 10.1). Personal hardships and losses may cause you to develop unique defense mechanisms, to change your expectations and attitudes, and to make numerous other adjustments to life's ups and downs. Some people in these situations may become extremely depressed and even commit suicide.

MYTHS & CONTROVERSIES

Myth 1

Drinking and partying on the weekend is a good way to recover from a stressful week. Actually, drinking and drug use can cause more stress than they relieve. One or two drinks may make you feel more relaxed, but greater amounts of alcohol can make you do things you'll regret and may make you feel tense and irritable in the morning. Instead of relying on alcohol to help manage your stress, try talking with a friend, seeing a funny movie, or getting in a good workout.

Myth 2

Everyone should take stress vitamins regularly. The best advice we can give about taking any supplements is that usually they are not necessary. If you are eating a balanced diet from each of the food groups, getting adequate rest, exercising, maintaining adequate social interactions and social support, and paying attention to your spiritual side, stress vitamins are probably a waste of money. Your body will utilize only what it needs and excrete the water-soluble vitamins. Fat-soluble vitamins are probably already stored in adequate amounts in your body and you don't really need more. Only in times of extreme physical illness, extreme disruptions in your life, or situations when you find that eating is just not your priority are supplements of any kind really necessary.

Controversy 1

Stress is a product of our society, and certain racial and ethnic groups are just innately driven to be more stressed and hence, more violent. True, crime, delinquency, homicide, family violence, and gang-related acts of violence have often been linked to low socioeconomic status. However, rather than having anything to do with race or ethnicity, these problems have more to do with a disproportionate distribution of wealth and system support than they do with any specific racial group involvement. People who belong to the lower socioeconomic class and who live in persistent poverty not only are exposed to more stressors on a daily basis but may also be more vulnerable to stress. The poorer and less educated you are, the more likely you are to be exposed to hardships and the less likely you are to have the means to seek help or fight back. These people are at a disproportionately higher risk of stress due to poor housing, poor sanitation, crime-ridden streets, increased job insecurity, lack of access to health care, cutbacks in public health assistance programs and social services, and many related difficulties. Moreover, other studies link low income and lack of education with ineffective coping styles. Whether due to a strong belief in an external locus of control (see Chapter 9), to low self-esteem, to learned helplessness, or to other factors, many people in these groups find it impossible to cope with life's stressors. Whether poor coping skills promote increased difficulties or lead to the increased inability to cope remains unresolved.

Interestingly, suicide rates among young women of African-American descent are among the lowest of any racial/ethnic group. How, you might ask, could this be, particularly when persons in this group appear to have the highest risk from a purely socioeconomic standpoint? In part, their protective factor may be the net product of close family ties. When young African-American women get into trouble with early pregnancy or other crises, their families, particularly grandparents and other extended family members, are often quick to offer support, to help raise the child, and so on. Thus, this family system may actually help reduce risk from otherwise stress-laden lives.

MANAGING ◆ STRESS

Do

▲ Cultivate and appreciate simplicity in your life.

▲ Focus on the positive and pleasant aspects of situations; be an optimist.

▲ Find ways to keep in touch with friends and family, even when you are busy with school.

▲ Find time several times a week to exercise.

▲ Consider keeping a journal as a way to express yourself and get perspective on your problems.

▲ Get enough sleep and eat a balanced diet.

▲ Keep a list of priorities; get the important things done and don't sweat the small stuff.

▲ Respond actively to challenges and find a solution instead of giving up.

▲ Take time each day to savor a small ritual: fix a cup of tea, tend an herb garden, or play with a pet.

▲ Learn to say "no" to demands on your time if you are already booked up.

▲ Learn to recognize situations you can't change so you don't waste energy trying to change them.

▲ Find a stress-management technique (relaxation, exercise, meditation, etc.) you can practice regularly.

Don't

▼ Procrastinate; tackling that dreaded task will make you feel better in the long run.

▼ Rely on alcohol or drugs to relieve stress.

▼ Drink too many caffeinated beverages, which can cause irritability and fatigue.

▼ Get into the habit of rushing; it rarely saves time and can really boost your stress level.

▼ Ignore signs of stress overload such as chronic fatigue, headaches, indigestion, and sleep problems.

Others may forge ahead, looking for additional life experiences. Individuals raised in abusive families or in homes where an alcoholic family member routinely caused disruption, fear, and other psychological disturbances, for example, may find that they suffer from numerous negative stress reactions. They may be overly anxious about relationships, become agitated when someone raises his or her voice, or experience any number of unusual response patterns. Others may not show any of these adverse effects. Taking the inventory in Laboratory 10.1 developed by Holmes and Rahe, noted stress researchers, will help you assess your current stress load.

People who lack internal control or who have low self-efficacy, low self-esteem, or other identity problems (see Chapter 9) may find that their stressors are very difficult to deal with. Or they may lack the energy and motivation to try to overcome stressful situations.

As a result of genetic inheritance combined with personal history, family influences, and the like, one person may develop a more resilient personality type and demonstrate skills necessary to overcome stress whereas another may become mired in the same stressful event. In the 1960s and 1970s, stress researchers lumped people with certain personality characteristics into personality types (Rosenman and Friedman). The **Type A personality,** as typified by the overaggressive, driving, over-anxious, high-stress, easily angered individual, was thought to have an elevated risk for hypertension and heart disease (see also Chapter 13). By contrast, the **Type B personality,** as typified by the laid-back, nonaggressive, low-stress, low-anxiety individual, was thought to have a decreased risk for hypertension and heart disease. In the last decade, health researchers have discussed the **Type C personality,** the person who seems to thrive and reach peak performance under pressure. Type E personalities were yet another group to be singled out in the late 1980s and early 1990s. **Type E women** were women caught between the needs of family and career, women who were particularly vulnerable to excess stress. Although we could go through the entire alphabet characterizing yet another personality type susceptible to stress, most researchers give such typologies scant credibility today. We know that stress is a highly complex phenomenon and that putting people into little boxes with labels is likely to be inaccurate and not very helpful.

Today, most research supports the notion that people do not typically fall into such neat personality packages. Most of us can range from a raging Type A on the freeway, for example, to a nonaggressive, peaceful Type B elsewhere. In addition, many researchers today believe that Type A behavior per se is not what appears to elevate one's risk for heart disease but rather a common element of behavior seen in many **Type Ks** known as a "toxic core." Early researchers suggested that people who have a toxic core are hostile, angry, and basically cynical about life and other people (Williams and Stiegler). People who have more of the classic Type A profile actually are most likely to survive once they actually have a heart attack because of their "fighting" nature. Also, a person who is "psychologically hardy" is thought to be able to thrive on excessive stress and suffer few negative consequences (Kobasa, Solomon, and Temoshok). People who reflect this hardy personality in their daily activities may also be prone toward more sensation seeking and the taking of more calculated risks. Known as **Type R** personalities, these individuals appear to be more likely to confront their problems directly and work at resolving stressful situations before they become out of control.

As with many health-related theories, research on personality types is controversial. Many believe that labeling someone as having a particular type of personality is at best a superficial approach to explaining the complex

Type A personality typified by the overaggressive, driving, over-anxious, high-stress, easily angered individual thought to have an elevated risk for hypertension and heart disease

Type B personality typified by the laid-back, nonaggressive, low-stress, low-anxiety individual thought to have a decreased risk for hypertension and heart disease

Type C personality characterized by a person who thrives on stress

Type E woman woman driven by multiple demands from home, family, and career, often highly vulnerable to stress

Type K personality characterized by cynical hostility toward life in general; often related to a toxic core

Type R personality persons who reflect a hardy personality through sensation seeking and taking calculated risks. They are also more likely to confront problems.

ways that we respond to the nuances of life. After all, as you read this you may recognize that under different circumstances, you may be any one or a combination of several of these types.

Managing the Stress in Your Life

Once you recognize some of the sources of the stress in your life, you are partially on the way toward finding an effective way to manage it. Recognize which stressors are within your control and which are not. Worrying about the things you'll never be able to change is a needless waste of energy! Although that sounds good, we all worry far more than we should, even those of us who are supposed to know better!

Once you know what your stressors are, you can begin to take action toward reducing, modifying, eliminating, or changing them or learning to cope with them. Options include examining your self-talk, learning how to relax, and using stress buffers.

Examining Your Self-Talk

Robert Eliot, a well-known cardiologist specializing in stress physiology, gives the following advice for people considering how best to respond to the stressful aspects of daily life: " Don't sweat the small stuff—and remember, it's *all* small stuff." By keeping things in perspective and not allowing your mind to wreak havoc with your body, you can to some extent bring the negative effects of stress under control. Learning to think rationally about your situation and calm yourself down through consciously changing your self-talk (see Chapter 9) in a given situation is very important (see Laboratory 10.2). Through self-talk, we tell ourselves (consciously or unconsciously) what a particular event or action means. This internal conversation may influence our emotions, mental images, physical states, and behavior. Many of us have an irrational internal dialogue in which we subconsciously tell ourselves that we "should" or "must" behave in a particular way or achieve a particular level of excellence. These irrational conversations can cause us to impose unrealistic expectations on ourselves. For example, if you tell yourself that you "should" score an A on a given exam but aren't particularly knowledgeable on the subject or aren't really committed to putting in the extra time to study, this "should" statement may cause you undue levels of stress. And if your parents or others are imposing "should" statements on you—you "should" be an A student—your stressors may become overwhelming.

On any given day, you may spend a considerable amount of time talking yourself into worrying about things that never happen. Much of this worry stems from irrational thinking that causes you to exaggerate or distort the messages you receive from others. If you believe that others are untrustworthy and self-motivated, or that you are unable to handle a particular situation, these beliefs often become stressors for you, even if they are unfounded. According to Albert Ellis, a psychologist specializing in rational emotive therapy, our misperceptions and mistaken beliefs about the intentions, words, and actions of others and the things that we believe we "should" be doing all cause us unnecessary emotional trauma. A belief is irrational or unreasonable if it has the following characteristics: (1) It is *distorted* rather than *factual,* (2) it is *extreme* rather than *moderate,* and (3) it is *harmful* rather than *helpful* (see Laboratory 10.3).

A far healthier approach is to look around, try to see the true nature of a situation, and use factual self-talk to help yourself get through it. People who practice a more rational line of thinking work on adopting a positive outlook, which, admittedly, takes a good deal of self-discipline. They consciously force themselves to reframe their perception of what they thought happened. It's also important in a difficult situation to acknowledge rather than deny the emotional pain. We all know people who suffer silently because they believe they must not appear to be weak in a given situation. However, internalizing pain in this fashion is counterproductive because it merely increases stress levels.

In sum, keeping the major and minor crises in your life in perspective, acknowledging your pain or distress, and trying to balance your negative conversations with yourself about the "meaning" of these events with the positive events in your life may help you achieve a balanced stress reaction.

Learning to Relax

American culture traditionally places a high value on the notion of a hard day's work. However, many of us have a tough time moving from the "work and productivity" mode to the "relax and enjoy" mode. In recent years, researchers have become increasingly aware of the importance of relaxation to our overall health, particularly as a means of reducing the harmful effects of stress. The "relaxation response" is a natural and innate protective mechanism against *overstress;* it allows us to turn off harmful bodily effects and to counter the effects of the fight-or-flight response. This response to overstress brings bodily changes that decrease the heart rate, lower the metabolic rate, decrease the rate of breathing, relax muscles, slow down brain waves, and quiet the actions of key hormonal glands. Thus, by giving the body time to restore itself and to recuperate from the stresses of life, the relaxation response brings the body back into a healthier balance.

This relaxation response is a natural process that is invoked by your body every time you are stressed. Whereas the sympathetic nervous system acts to initiate the heightened awareness of the stress response, the *parasympathetic* or antagonistic branch of the autonomic nervous system acts to bring the chain of events back under control by quieting the hormonal stimulus triggered by the endocrine system.

Fortunately, the relaxation response is largely under your conscious control. You can initiate a relaxation response by practicing deep breathing, muscle relaxation, mental relaxation, and deep relaxation techniques. **Deep breathing techniques** consist of conscious steps taken to control the amount of air that is inhaled and exhaled. **Muscle relaxation techniques** typically consist of brief, on-the-spot tension reducers that involve contracting and relaxing various muscle groups. **Mental relaxation techniques** involve conscious procedures to change one's self-talk or to practice "blocking," "thought-stopping," or other, similar process-type methods.

Meditation, a common form of deep relaxation, is becoming more popular in the U. S. today.

deep breathing techniques
conscious steps taken to control the amount of air that is inhaled and exhaled

muscle relaxation techniques
brief on-the-spot tension reducers that involve contracting and relaxing various muscle groups

mental relaxation techniques
conscious procedures to change one's self-talk or to practice "blocking," "thought-stopping," or other, similar process-type methods

Deep relaxation techniques include any of several techniques designed to use various methods of tension control. Common forms of deep relaxation techniques include the following:

- *Meditation* typically consists of sitting or quietly reclining with your eyes closed for 10 to 20 minutes on average once or twice per day and mentally focusing on some object or event to quiet your body responses.

- *Biofeedback* teaches you to listen to and become aware of physiological activity in your body (heart rate, body temperature, blood pressure, and so on) through external monitoring devices or conscious recognition of body signals. After you gain awareness, you learn to bring these physiological responses under conscious control and thereby are able to lower blood pressure, body temperature, heart rate, and so on.

- *Autogenic relaxation* requires you consciously to imagine the warmth and feeling of your circulating blood and the warmth and weight of various body parts to achieve a highly relaxed state. For example, you would begin autogenic relaxation by saying "My right hand is becoming heavy and warm as the thick red blood pulses through it. I feel the heat in my fingers. My hand is becoming heavier . . . heavier . . . and the warmth is increasing in my fingers and hand" and so forth. This technique can be used progressively, starting with the tip of a body part, moving up the part, and gradually involving all the body. Imagination and concentration lead you actually to experience sensations of heat, heaviness, and eventual relaxation.

- *Visualization* is similar to autogenics in that you concentrate and induce a highly relaxed state by imagining a place of peace, quiet, and tranquility and putting yourself in that space. When stressed, a person practicing visualization might imagine sitting in the midst of a quiet forest with heavy snow drifting down peacefully.

- *Progressive muscle relaxation* requires you consciously to relax, one at a time, muscle groups in the hand, forearm, upper arm, shoulder, neck, trunk, and so on.

- *Hypnosis* is a process in which you are induced into a state of semisleep through the use of a "hypnotic suggestion" or device that aids in initiating the sleep-induced state. Although hypnosis has been widely used as a stress management technique, it has achieved mixed results and should be used only by persons trained in hypnotic techniques. (See Laboratory 10.4 for more on relaxation exercises.)

Using Stress Buffers: Inoculating Against Negative Stressors

Simply stated, a person who is in good health has a much better chance of resisting the harmful effects of stress than a person who is unwell. Stress buffers such as proper nutrition, adequate sleep, time management, and a fit, well-functioning body are all key elements of this stress resistance formula in that they tend to bolster your resources to fight the disease. Sometimes this bolstering of internal forces is referred to as *stress inoculation*, which operates in much the same way as a vaccination might aid you in resisting infectious diseases.

deep relaxation techniques
any of several techniques designed to utilize various methods of tension control, including meditation, biofeedback, autogenic relaxation, visualization, progressive muscle relaxation, and hypnosis

Sound Decision Making

STRUGGLING WITH PERFECTIONISM

Michael was an excellent student in high school, but he is having a hard time adapting to college. In addition to his studies, he is working 25 hours per week to make ends meet. Because he is always busy studying or working, he hasn't had much time to make friends at his new school. Lately, Michael has been feeling tired and irritable most of the time, and he is starting to think that maybe he just isn't college material after all. One day Michael goes to take a chemistry exam he's studied hard for. Even though he knows the material, he freezes up and the words seem to swim in front of his eyes. Michael fails the test, and tells his brother Jamal he's seriously thinking about dropping out of school.

Jamal has some personal experience dealing with stressful situations and recognizes that Michael needs to learn some ways to manage his stress. He suggests that the two of them work together on a stress-reduction plan. They agree on three goals for Michael: to reduce his negative self-talk and perfectionism regarding grades, to exercise several times a week, and to make more friends to socialize with.

Over the next 2 months, Michael becomes better at identifying instances of negative self-talk and substituting them with a review of all the positive things he's accomplished. He realizes that a few Bs aren't the end of the world, and he eases up on himself academically. Michael also joins an intramural volleyball team; he enjoys the exercise and the camaraderie at the pizza parlor after the games.

By the end of the semester, Michael is again feeling like he has the skills and abilities to succeed in college. Juggling the demands of study, work, and other activities continues to be a challenge, but Michael no longer feels that everything will collapse if he makes any small mistake. Michael smiles when he gets his grades: three As, and a B in chemistry.

Nutrition. Eating the right types of food and maintaining the proper weight are two of the most important stress management techniques you can employ. Carrying extra weight contributes to decreased energy levels and low self-esteem and other psychological problems that may increase emotional susceptibility to stressors. Going on crash diets, skipping meals, undereating, and trying other techniques to control weight contribute to a general malaise that can make stressors even more difficult to deal with. In fact, these dietary techniques may actually be stressors themselves. (For more information on a healthy diet, see Chapter 7.)

Excessive amounts of refined sugars in your diet may lead to increases in blood sugar levels in the bloodstream, hypersecretion of insulin to bring sugar levels down, and resultant sugar-related mood swings. However, research on the actual impact of these blood sugar levels on behavior for people of various ages in different settings is controversial. For those who already have trouble utilizing or producing insulin to reduce these sugar overloads (diabetics or prediabetics) and for children who suffer from other metabolic disturbances, excessive stress may lead to still more problems with regulation of blood sugar level and thus to increases in overall stress effects.

Excess sugar in the diet also may result in an ultimate reduction in the availability of certain dietary vitamins and minerals that are important to proper neurological functioning. For example, depletion of certain B vitamins, such as thiamin, niacin, and B_{12} may increase nervous reactivity, irritability, and general stress vulnerability. However, research indicating that vitamin supplements taken in these situations might serve as a stress reducer is inconclusive.

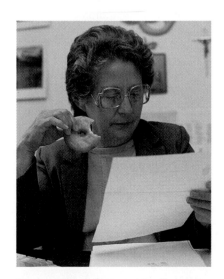

It's not only what you eat but how you eat that can influence your overall wellness.

STATS-AT-A-GLANCE
Exercise and Emotions

Exercise may be one of our best buffers against the undue effects of too much stress in our lives. Consider the following:

■ Of the nearly 700 respondents to a random survey of its readers by *Runner's World* magazine, 82% reported that running had enhanced their energy level, 73% said it had helped their life control, and 67% said it had increased their optimism (*Runner's World*).

■ Aerobic exercise was shown to improve cognitive functioning in formerly sedentary elderly patients. Specifically, after a 4-month exercise program, participants improved in mental flexibility, reaction, and memory-mental skills (*Runner's World*).

■ Among 15 moderately depressed men and women ages 26 to 53, depression scores were significantly lower after 10 weeks, 6 months, and 21 months in an exercise program (Sime).

■ Among undergraduate students, significant differences were noted between those who exercised three or more times per week aerobically and those who did not. Those who exercised more reported significantly better quality of life, fewer distress symptoms, less irritability, more internal control, less emotional tension and depression, more vitality and energy, higher self-esteem, more fun and playfulness, less loneliness, and more close friends (Schafer).

Other substances known as *sympathomimetic agents,* including caffeine-containing colas, coffee, chocolate, and teas as well as certain food colorings and preservatives stimulate increases in the metabolism and in levels of arousal. Although the actual result of ingesting these substances varies and some individuals appear to be tolerant of high doses, most people begin to demonstrate definable anxiety states at doses of about 720 mg of caffeine (the amount found in 5 to 6 cups of coffee or 12 to 15 colas). Clearly, many dietary variables affect your overall stress response.

Sleep. Although sometimes taken for granted, sleep is another of the major elements of your personal stress-buffering system. People who suffer from sleep deficits of one form of another are often extremely vulnerable to stressors of all types. Considerable evidence indicates that sleep deprivation results in increased vulnerability to emotional upset and increased susceptibility to disease.

Exercise. Exercise has long been regarded as a natural means of reducing or eliminating the negative effects of too much pent-up stress. More recently, a host of researchers have provided definitive evidence that exercise is related to decreases in hostility, tension, fatigue, depression, and emotional volatility, and to increases in self-esteem, energy levels, self-concept, locus of control, and a host of other stress-related factors (Johnsgard; Ungerleider et al.; Brown; Moses; Sime; Rice).

Psychological benefits of exercise for stress management include the following (Rice):

■ Release of pent-up emotions as exercisers' bodies move to return the stress response to normal or homeostasis

■ Creative problem solving during the exercise session and more constructive coping later as time spent exercising is used to focus thoughts and energy

■ Enhanced self-liking, self-acceptance, and self-esteem as exercisers begin to feel better about their appearance and accomplishments

■ Heightened internal control and self-confidence as exercisers find that they really can do what they set out to do

■ Feeling of well-being and calm "afterglow" from exercise

■ Mood stabilization as the parasympathetic nervous system regains control

■ "Time-away" benefit as the exercisers obtain a spiritual and emotional lift from the new environment

■ Decrease of negative thinking as an indirect result of improved self-esteem, increased self-confidence, and a positive emotional outlet

According to Rice, physiological benefits of exercise for stress management include the following:

■ Release of muscle tension

■ Burning off of stress-induced adrenaline, which leaves the bloodstream and is consumed in the muscles

■ Postexercise reduction of catecholamines

- Postexercise quieting of the sympathetic nervous system (the part that produces tension) as the parasympathetic system returns the body to homeostasis

- Production of beta-endorphins, the body's own morphine painkiller and source of pleasure

- Lower baseline tension level

- Faster recovery from acute stress as the body develops adaptive energy reserves

- Familiarity with and habituation to physiological arousal (see Stats-at-a-Glance)

Time Management. Do you remember those early years of your life when you could spend endless hours playing, watching television, or mindlessly watching your parents doing work? Do you ever wish to return to those carefree years when you didn't have to get a certain amount of work done on the weekend, be at work at a certain time, limit your time with friends because of all the work you have to do, or suffer certain consequences for not using your time effectively? Have you wondered why the days seem shorter and shorter as you get older, and why you seem to have less and less time to do what you want to do, and more and more time spent doing things that must be done? If so, you are not alone. So many people today seem to find that there just are not enough hours in the day to do everything they'd like to do. Fortunately, there are many methods for improving time management skills and organizing time so that you can both work and play (see Table 10.4).

TABLE 10.4

Fifteen Strategies for Time Management

1. Prioritize the things you need to do by developing a list of *must-dos*, *should-dos*, and *want-to-dos*, and allocate some time each day for each.

2. Break large tasks into small ones, with individual goals and deadlines for each.

3. Avoid distractions and possible diversions by finding a peaceful environment.

4. Learn to analyze why you think you should do something and to say no to things that are not really important to you.

5. Allow time to get where you are going, and take time to enjoy the environment on the way.

6. Delegate tasks to others whenever possible, and try to keep your own ego uninvolved.

7. Accept the fact that perfection is not always necessary and that others can do a good job, too.

8. Use your lunch hour for something enjoyable—meditating, taking a walk with a friend, reading, listening to music—that will slow you down and give you a chance to "get ready" for the rest of the day.

9. Find time and space to get away from other people each day and focus solely on yourself.

10. Practice effective listening by nodding to show interest and by not interrupting.

11. Avoid friends who delight in telling you how stressed or overworked they are, or change the subject when they start complaining about the pressures in their lives.

12. Leave time in your schedule for the unexpected, and if nothing unexpected happens, choose what you want to do next.

13. Plan ahead.

14. Don't procrastinate.

15. Never handle papers (bills, memos, requests, and so on) more than once. Read your correspondence, think about it, and take care of it.

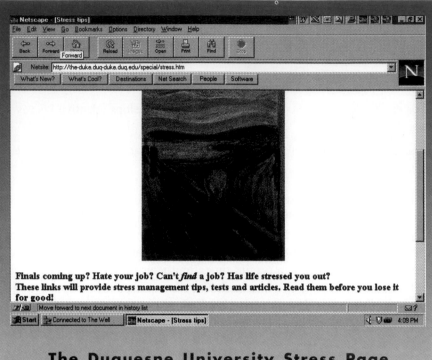

Finals coming up? Hate your job? Can't *find* a job? Has life stressed you out? These links will provide stress management tips, tests and articles. Read them before you lose it for good!

The Duquesne University Stress Page
http://the-duke.duq-duke.duq.edu/special/stress.htm

This page is especially devoted to the stress management needs of students. It provides a stress assessment, some quick stress-relief tips, special tips for students (don't take more than one five-credit course per term), and a focus on humor as a way to reduce stress.

Critical thinking: Lots of suggestions are given on this Web page and in this chapter on how to reduce stress. What works for you? What are your own top five ways to beat stress?

Source: From the Duquesne Duke and The Digital Duke Newspapers Website, 1998.

Lifestyle Choices: Plan for Action

Stress is an inevitable part of our world. You cannot run from it, hide from it, or ignore it out of existence. However, you can do many things to reduce the effects of stress in your life and/or channel potentially negative stress responses into positive challenges and opportunities for growth. Knowing how to plan for unavoidable stressors to reduce their impact and how to cope more effectively with stealth stressors that may catch you by surprise are important factors in enhancing your stress resistance.

Rate yourself on each of the following signs and symptoms of a stress-prone person. Such people often are overly critical of themselves and others and live life trying to keep up with their own perceptions of how things should and should not be.

1. I hate to admit when I am wrong.   never   sometimes   usually   always

2. I take life too seriously.   never   sometimes   usually   always

3. I feel overwhelmed with responsibilities.   never   sometimes   usually   always

4. I get impatient when things get out of order.   never   sometimes   usually   always

5. I easily find fault with others.   never   sometimes   usually   always

6. I easily find fault with myself.   never   sometimes   usually   always

7. I feel a tremendous need to be in control.   never   sometimes   usually   always

8. I worry about giving the wrong impression.   never   sometimes   usually   always

9. I have trouble making decisions.   never   sometimes   usually   always

10. I get upset by my lover/significant other's imperfections.   never   sometimes   usually   always

11. I believe that people should follow the rules.   never   sometimes   usually   always

12. I worry about things that might happen to embarrass me.   never   sometimes   usually   always

13. I worry about what others will think of me.   never   sometimes   usually   always

14. I believe that I should do better than my friends.   never   sometimes   usually   always

15. I find it difficult to control my anger when someone/something bothers me.   never   sometimes   usually   always

16. I drink more than I should when I am upset.   never   sometimes   usually   always

17. I find it difficult just to sit back and relax.   never   sometimes   usually   always

18. I become very disappointed when people let me down.	never	sometimes	usually	always
19. I find it difficult to sleep at night because of all of the things I need to get done.	never	sometimes	usually	always
20. I find that I'm always rushed and never seen to get things done on time.	never	sometimes	usually	always

By analyzing the items for which you circled "always" or "usually," you may discover underlying problems that you can work on to reduce stress in your life. Many of these involve changes in the way you view certain situations, in your behaviors to prevent or reduce the impact of a problem, and/or in the way you cope with a situation after it arises. After considering the areas that seem to cause difficulty for you, think about what you might do to change your thoughts, actions, or the environment (situation).

First, ask yourself how stressed you are on an average day. Are the things that are stressing you real events, or are they things that you think may be problematic? Are the majority of your stressors related to (1) your personal life (friends, lovers, colleagues, family members), (2) your environment/situation (finances, living situation, concerns over personal safety, and so on), (3) your psychological well-being (feelings about yourself and your appearance, confidence in your abilities, worry about what others may think of you, and so on), or (4) other factors in your life?

Next, ask yourself what three things are causing you the most stress/anxiety right now. Are these things that are actually happening, or are they things that you think might happen in the days ahead? What actions can you take to change the way you perceive or think about these stressors? What kinds of things are you telling yourself about them? What actions can you take to change the nature of the events that are actually causing you stress? (Would making a conscious effort to manage time more effectively, being more kind to others, being kinder to yourself, or taking any other actions help your situation?)

Now, make a list of all the things you think you must get done in the next week. Which of these will result in serious consequences if you don't get them done immediately? Move these items to the top of your list. Which of them do you think should be done but would not cause a crisis if not done immediately? Move these to the middle of the list. Which of them would be nice to get done but aren't really a big deal? Put these items on the bottom of your list. Who else could do these things? Learning to delegate to others is often a difficult task for the stress-prone perfectionist in all of us. Consider: Do they really need to be done at all? If you can't find someone willing to do them, and you can't do them yourself, either forget about them or admit that you can't do any more and go on with your life. Asking for help is often difficult, but it is a sign of maturity and reflects a realistic perspective on life.

Now that you have done some serious thinking about the stressors in your life, consider how many of the following stress-reducing steps you ought to implement.

1. *Do not allow yourself to be stressed by "little things" in your life.* Continually "sweating the small stuff" can waste your time and cause you to have little energy for the really important things in life. Stop harping at your friends and family about insignificant things. Don't allow yourself to dwell on minor mistakes and imperfections in others. If your self-talk about others is negative, block it out of your mind. Focus on the positive and let the little things be little things.

2. *Get rid of the "what if's" and "if only's" in your vocabulary.* Focus on the here and now. If you've messed up or made a mistake, forget it and focus on how much smarter and wiser you will be next time. Learn from your bad experiences and avoid similar problems in the future.

3. *Treat time as a precious resource.* If you find that a day has gone by and you haven't accomplished much or had much fun, make a list of where the hours went. By putting this down on paper, you will be able to see how much time you spent relaxing, how much time you spent talking to friends, how much time you can't account for, and how much time you may have spent doing things that were not on your must-do or nice-to-do list. Plan your next day, hour by hour. Stick to your task and avoid interruptions. When you have accomplished one task, give yourself a break and then move on to the next. If you feel too pressured, take time for a phone call to a friend, a walk, a favorite TV program, or whatever you enjoy, and then get back on your schedule. Allow time in whatever schedule you plan for you.

4. *Analyze your "self-talk."* If your conversations with yourself are mostly negative, consciously try to refocus on the good things about yourself, others, and life in general.

5. *Learn by example.* Pick out someone whom you admire and who seldom seems to be frazzled and/or distraught by life. Ask this person how he or she finds time to get everything done, how he or she maintains such a positive attitude about things in life, and so on. Try to assess what things you could improve on.

Like everything else in your life, your proneness to stress is probably a result of years of learned responses and adaptation. If your parents and family were uptight screamers and were always in a state of high anxiety, you may have learned many of your current behaviors from them. You may be stressed by your beliefs and habits rather than by real threats. If your current situation has included dramatic changes requiring that you be highly vigilant and cope with excessive numbers of stressors, you may need to call on hidden reserves and the support of others to get you through. Knowing when things are becoming overwhelming and then reaching out to others is a sign of positive stress management and control. Changing lifelong patterns of stress responses takes time, conscious effort, and planning. Work on each area that seems to be giving you problems. Once you seem to be managing one area more effectively, tackle another. Write down what you intend to do and try hard to stick to your plan.

WEEK 1

This week, I will concentrate on making the following change to reduce stress in my life:

_____

_____

WEEK 2

After reassessing my progress in week 1, I will make the following change:

_____

_____

WEEK 3

I will assess how I feel about the changes that I have made in weeks 1 and 2. I will continue trying to

_____

_____

_____   _____

(signature)   *(date)*

Summary

Exercise, nutrition, sleep patterns, time management, relaxation habits, self-talk, and a host of other factors can influence your overall susceptibility to the negative consequences of excessive stress and help you to achieve that harmonious balance that Hippocrates was talking about. Stress is an inevitable part of our everyday experiences as human beings. It can be viewed as a challenge, and methods can be found to manage or control its possible negative effects. The choice is yours.

Key concepts that you have learned in this chapter include these:

■ Normally, our bodies are in a state of balance or homeostasis; too many stressors cause this balance to be disturbed and negative health consequences can result.

■ Not all stressors are negatives; a certain amount of stress in your life may increase your performance and motivate you to try harder.

■ The prolonged effects of too much stress may affect several systems of the body, including the cardiovascular, immune, and digestive systems.

■ Specific responses to too much stress include decreased resistance to disease, increased susceptibility to hypertension, blood vessel occlusion, and ineffective digestive processes.

■ An individual's response to negative stressors is determined mainly by heredity, overall health, environmental supports, psychological health, emotional resiliency, and self-talk.

■ Risk factors for stress include, but are not limited to, culture, environment, social support and social interactions, individual characteristics from biology and social environment, personality, socioeconomic status, and access to health care.

■ Anger is an important stress response that must be controlled.

■ Learning to relax and practicing relaxation techniques are important factors in one's ability to cope with life's stresses.

■ It is possible to inoculate yourself against stress, thereby reducing your risk. Stress buffers including nutrition, sleep, exercise, social support, and time management are examples of buffers that will aid in reducing your risks.

References

Armstead, C., et al. Relationship of racial stressors to blood pressure response and anger expression in black college students. *Health Psychology,* 8: 541–556, 1989.

Baker, G. Invited review: Psychological factors and immunity. *Journal of Psychosomatic Research,* 31: 1–10, 1987.

Brown, R. Exercise as an adjunct to the treatment of mental disorders. In W. Morgan and S. Goldson, eds., *Exercise and Mental Health.* Washington, DC: Hemisphere, 1987, 131–137.

Cannon, W. The Wisdom of the Body, 2nd ed. New York, NY: W. W. Norton & Co., Inc. 1939.

Cohen, S., and G. Williamson. Stress and infectious disease in humans. *Psychological Bulletin,* 109: 5–24, 1991.

Dantzer, R., and K. Kelly. Stress and immunity: An integrated review of relationships between the brain and the immune system. *Life Sciences,* 44: 1995–2002, 1989.

Eliot, R. *Is It Worth Dying For?* Video produced and distributed by the American Heart Association, 1988.

Ellis, A. Reason and Emotion in Psychotherapy. New York, NY: Stuart Press, 1962.

Elmharib, N. A. Psychological stress, depression, and some aspects of human immunity: A meta-analysis of studies published between 1981 and 1991. *Desasat-Nafseyah,* 3: 335–372, 1993.

Felsten, G. Hostility, stress, and symptoms of depression. *Personality and Individual Differences,* 21: 461–467, 1996.

Fisher, S. *Stress in Academic Life: A Mental Assembly Line.* Buckingham, England: Open University Press, 1994, 106.

Girdano, D., G. Everly, and D. Dusek. *Controlling Stress and Tension.* Needham, MA: Allyn & Bacon, 1997.

Greenberg, W., and D. Shapiro. The effects of caffeine and stress on blood pressure in individuals with and without a family history of hypertension. *Psychophysiology,* 24: 151–156, 1987.

Hale, J., J. Greenberg, and S. Ramsey. Assessment of college student stress and stress management needs: A pilot study. In J. H. Humphrey, ed., *Human Stress: Current Selected Research,* Vol. 4. New York: AMS Press, 1990, 77–88.

Holmes, T. H. and R. Rahe. The Social Readjustment Rating Scale. *Journal of Psychosomatic Research.* 11: 213–218, 1967.

Johnsgard, K. *The Exercise Prescription for Depression and Anxiety.* New York: Plenum Press, 1989.

Johnson, D. Can psychology ever be the same again after the human genome is mapped? *Psychological Science,* 1: 331–332, 1990.

Kessler, R. Stress, social status, and psychological distress. *Journal of Health and Social Behavior,* 20: 259–272, 1979.

Kiecolt-Glaser, J., et al. Marital quality, marital disruption, and immune function. *Psychosomatic Medicine,* 49: 13–34, 1987.

Kobasa, S., S. Maddi, and S. Kahn. Hardiness and health: A prospective study. *Journal of Personal and Social Psychology,* 42: 68–177, 1982.

Leonard, B., and C. Song. Stress and the immune system in the etiology of anxiety and depression. *Pharmacology, Biochemistry and Behavior,* 54: 299–303, 1996.

Loechlin, J., L. Willerman, and J. Horn. Human behavioral genetics. *Annual Review of Psychology,* 39: 101–133, 1988.

McNaughton, M., et al. Stress, social support, coping, resources, and immune status in the elderly. *Journal of Nervous and Mental Disease,* 178: 460–462, 1990.

Morris, C. *Understanding Psychology.* Englewood Cliffs, NJ: Prentice-Hall, 1997.

Moses, J. Light exercise may yield more mental benefits. *Family Practice News,* 19: 51, 1989.

Pearlin, L., and M. Skaff. Stress and the life course: A paradigmatic alliance. *The Gerontologist,* 36: 239–247, 1996.

Plomin, R. The role of inheritance in behavior. *Science,* 248: 183–188, 1990.

Plomin, R., J. DeFries, and G. McClearn. *Behavioral Genetics: A Primer.* New York: Freeman, 1990.

Rice, P. *Stress and Health.* Pacific Grove, CA: Brooks/Cole, 1992.

Rosenman, R., and M. Friedman. *Type A Behavior and Your Heart,* New York: Fawcett, 1974.

Runner's World. Up with people, 1989.

Sapolsky, R. N. Neuroendocrinology of the stress-response. In J. B. Becker et al., eds., *Behavioral Endocrinology.* Cambridge and London: MIT Press, 1992.

Schafer, S. *Stress management for wellness,* 2nd ed. New York: Harcourt Brace Jovanovich, 1989, 265.

Selye, H. The stress concept today. In I. L. Kutash, L. B. Schlesinger, et al., eds. *Handbook on Stress and Anxiety.* San Francisco: Jossey-Bass, 1980, 127–133.

Selye, H. The Stress of Life. 1956. McGraw Hill New York.

Selye, H. *Stress Without Distress.* Philadelphia: Lippincott, 1974.

Seaward, B. *Managing Stress.* Sudbury, MA: Jones and Bartlett, 1997.

Sime, W. Exercise in the prevention and treatment of depression. In W. Morgan and S. Goldson, eds., *Exercise and Mental Health.* Washington, DC: Hemisphere, 1987, 137–141.

Stoney, C., M. Davis, and K. Mathews. Sex differences in physiological responses to stress in coronary heart disease: A causal link? *Psychophysiology,* 24: 127–131, 1987.

Tavris, C. *Anger—The Misunderstood Emotion.* New York, NY: Simon & Schuster, 1982.

Ungerleider, S., K. Porter, and J. Foster. Mental advantages for masters. *Running Times,* 156, 18–20, 1989.

Weisinger, H. Weisinger's Anger Work-Out Book. New York, NY: William Morrow, 1985.

Williams, R., and L. Stiegler. Hostility tied to heart trouble. Paper presented at annual scientific meeting of the American Heart Association, Dallas, 1990.

Williams, R. and Williams, V. *Anger Kills.* New York, NY: Harper Perennials, 1994.

www. usatoday.com 125 (2623), April 1997, 7. Stress and Personality Affect Cholesterol: Society for the Advancement of Education. ISSN: 0161-7389.

Laboratory 10.1
Student Stress Scale

The Student Stress Scale is an adaptation of Holmes and Rahe's Life Events Scale, modified to apply to college-age adults. It can provide a rough indication of stress levels and possible health consequences for teaching purposes.

In the Student Stress Scale, each event, such as beginning or ending school, is given a score that represents the amount of readjustment a person has to make as a result of the change. In some studies, people with serious illnesses have been found to have high scores on similar scales.

To determine your stress score, add up the number of points corresponding to the events you have experienced in the past 12 months.

1.	Death of a close family member	_____	100
2.	Death of a close friend	_____	73
3.	Divorce of parents	_____	65
4.	Jail term	_____	63
5.	Major personal injury or illness	_____	63
6.	Marriage	_____	58
7.	Getting fired from a job	_____	50
8.	Failing an important course	_____	47
9.	Change in the health of a family member	_____	45
10.	Pregnancy	_____	45
11.	Sex problems	_____	44
12.	Serious argument with a close friend	_____	40
13.	Change in financial status	_____	39
14.	Change of academic major	_____	39
15.	Trouble with parents	_____	39
16.	New girlfriend or boyfriend	_____	37
17.	Increase in workload at school	_____	37
18.	Outstanding personal achievement	_____	36
19.	First quarter/semester in college	_____	36
20.	Change in living conditions	_____	31
21.	Serious argument with an instructor	_____	30
22.	Getting lower grades than expected	_____	29
23.	Change in sleeping habits	_____	29
24.	Change in social activities	_____	29
25.	Change in eating habits	_____	28
26.	Chronic car trouble	_____	26
27.	Change in number of family get-togethers	_____	26
28.	Too many missed classes	_____	25
29.	Changing colleges	_____	24
30.	Dropping more than one class	_____	23
31.	Minor traffic violations	_____	20

Total Stress Score   _____

Evaluation

>300   You're at high risk for developing a health problem.

150–300   You have a 50-50 chance of experiencing a serious health change within 2 years.

<150   You have a 1-in-3 chance of a serious health change.

Source: From Holmes and Rahe, 1967.

Laboratory 10.2

Learning to "Hear" Your Own Negative Self-Talk

1. Think of a compliment that someone has tried to give you in the past few days (for example, "You really look nice" or "You did a super job"). How did the compliment make you feel? What did you say to the other person? What did you say to yourself?

2. When was the last time someone outwardly criticized you? What was your external reply? Your internal reply?

3. Think about a task or project that you wanted to do. What did you tell yourself about your ability to do it? What, if anything, were you worried about?

4. What beliefs about yourself have you shared with very close friends? Were these beliefs positive or negative?

5. How do you feel when you hear others talk about how good they are at something or how smart or good-looking they are? Are you comfortable praising and/or saying positive things about yourself around other people? Why or why not? What worries you about self-praise? What do you think would be an acceptable form of self-praise? Under what circumstances would you be likely to tell others how well you've done at something?

Sometimes, positive self-talk is very difficult to do. We worry about seeming to brag about ourselves. We worry that if we are too positive, we'll look like fools if we don't perform as well as we've said we would. Learning to be positive about ourselves and to others often takes practice. It also may mean that we have to "undo" a lifetime of negative self-directed conversations. By affirming our positive attributes and repeating them to ourselves, we can make them a part of our makeup. Rather than having to proclaim them to the world, we enable them to become apparent in more subtle ways: through a new self-confidence and a more positive and in-control attitude. Practice making the following statements whenever negative, self-deprecating thoughts enter your mind. In time, you may find that they are actually quite believable.

- I thrive on challenge.

- This is an opportunity for me, not a threat.

- Yes, this has been painful, but I have learned a lot from it.

- I may be slow, but I come through when I need to.

- I am a special and unique person.

- I like who I am and I'm getting better all the time.

- I can do it if I just concentrate.

- I am confident and deserve a chance.

- I have high ideals and believe that . . .

- I thrive under pressure and do my best work when challenged.

- I have more talent and skills than even I have yet discovered.

- I like who I am and feel good about myself.

- I like who I am, how I think, and what I feel.

- I love life and want to enjoy every moment.

- I am intelligent and I have a great sense of humor.

At first, you may feel a little silly saying good things about yourself. Instead of trying to find evidence for why these comments are stupid, try to find examples of things about you that prove them to be true. Don't let negative thoughts about you invade your mind, and stop worrying about what you may not be. Focus on your best qualities, and others will begin to see them, too.

Laboratory 10.3

Combating Common Irrational Beliefs

On any given day, each of us subjects ourselves to undue amounts of stress by our self-talk about the meaning of the event we are experiencing. The following list of 20 irrational beliefs summarizes some of the major statements that we commonly make to ourselves. For each statement, circle the appropriate option.

1. Other people and outside events upset me.

   strongly disagree   disagree   undecided   agree   strongly agree

2. I am thin-skinned by nature—I was born that way.

   strongly disagree   disagree   undecided   agree   strongly agree

3. I cannot control my thoughts and feelings.

   strongly disagree   disagree   undecided   agree   strongly agree

4. I cannot change. I am too old, too set in my ways, beyond hope.

   strongly disagree   disagree   undecided   agree   strongly agree

5. It is imperative that I be accepted by others, especially by those who are important to me.

   strongly disagree   disagree   undecided   agree   strongly agree

6. Most people are bad and cannot be trusted.

   strongly disagree   disagree   undecided   agree   strongly agree

7. If things do not go my way, it will be catastrophic.

   strongly disagree   disagree   undecided   agree   strongly agree

8. The only way to reduce my stress is to shape up the people around me who do such dumb things.

   strongly disagree   disagree   undecided   agree   strongly agree

9. It is easier to avoid responsibilities and difficulties than to face them.

   strongly disagree   disagree   undecided   agree   strongly agree

10. My early childhood experiences determine my emotions and behavior, and there is little I can do about it.

    strongly disagree   disagree   undecided   agree   strongly agree

11. I deserve to be upset and depressed over my shortcomings.

    strongly disagree   disagree   undecided   agree   strongly agree

12. I am fully justified in being aggravated over others' shortcomings, deficiencies, and blunders.

    strongly disagree   disagree   undecided   agree   strongly agree

13. I should be thoroughly competent in all respects.

    strongly disagree   disagree   undecided   agree   strongly agree

14. Justice should always triumph, and I am fully justified in feeling angry when it does not.

    strongly disagree   disagree   undecided   agree   strongly agree

15. I should do perfectly in nearly anything I attempt.

    strongly disagree   disagree   undecided   agree   strongly agree

16. There usually is one solution to a problem, and it is intolerable when this solution is not found or followed.

    strongly disagree   disagree   undecided   agree   strongly agree

17. I have a clear idea how other people should be and what they should do most of the time.

    strongly disagree   disagree   undecided   agree   strongly agree

18. Others should treat me kindly and considerately at all times.

    strongly disagree   disagree   undecided   agree   strongly agree

19. I have a right to expect a relatively pain-free and trouble-free life.

    strongly disagree   disagree   undecided   agree   strongly agree

20. When people around me are upset, it is usually because of something I have said or done.

    strongly disagree   disagree   undecided   agree   strongly agree

Do any of the above sound familiar? For many of us, these irrational beliefs become so embedded in our thinking patterns that we spend many of our waking hours in turmoil over one thing or another.

For each statement to which you responded "strongly agree," consider what might be the underlying fallacy. Is it distorted rather than factual? Is the view extreme rather than moderate? Is the result harmful rather than helpful? How could you change this self-talk into a statement that is more positive and wellness oriented?

Laboratory 10.4

Learning to Relax

AUTOGENIC RELAXATION TECHNIQUES

1. Recline or sit in a comfortable position in a quiet place and close your eyes.

2. Begin with the 6-second quieting response (see the second part of the laboratory).

3. Repeat each of the following stages three to six times in a 30- to 60-second period. Go slowly and try not to move on to the next stage until you "feel" the relaxed sensation. Repeat each statement as many times as necessary, in any order you'd like. (Note: Although we have indicated only one to two repetitions for each statement, you may find that it is most effective to repeat each statement several times, speaking slowly and concentrating on each statement and its effect on the body.)

Stage 1

My right arm is feeling heavy.

My right arm is feeling heavy.

My left arm is feeling heavy.

  "   "   "   "   "

Both arms are feeling heavy.

My right leg is feeling heavy.

  "   "   "   "   "   "

My left leg is feeling heavy.

  "   "   "   "   "   "

Both legs are feeling heavy.

Stage 2

My right arm is feeling warm.

(Continue the sequence outlined in Stage 1.)

Stage 3

My heartbeat is regular, slow, and calm.

My heartbeat is regular, slow, and calm.

(Repeat as necessary.)

Stage 4

My breathing is slow, calm, and relaxed. I feel the air slowly enter my nose, and the air that I am exhaling is warm and moist.

(Repeat as necessary.)

THE 6-SECOND QUIETING RESPONSE

This relaxation technique is very easy to perform, shouldn't make you feel uneasy, and typically has noteworthy results. Use it as a quick tension reliever whenever you feel the symptoms of stress or feel a bit "wired."

1. Inhale a long, deep, slow breath through your nose. (Feel the flare of your diaphragm and/or the expansion of your abdominal area.)

2. Hold the breath for 2 to 3 seconds.

3. Exhale slowly and completely. (You may open your mouth wide if you are in an appropriate location.)

4. As you exhale and air is being forced out of your lungs, let your jaw and shoulders drop. Feel the muscles of your arms and shoulders begin to relax.

5. Repeat.

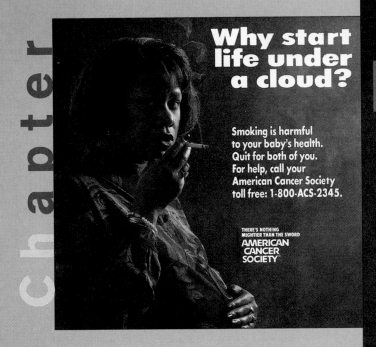

Why start life under a cloud?

Smoking is harmful to your baby's health. Quit for both of you. For help, call your American Cancer Society toll free: 1-800-ACS-2345.

THERE'S NOTHING MIGHTIER THAN THE SWORD
AMERICAN CANCER SOCIETY

chapter

11

Addictive Behavior: Substance Use and Abuse

One Student's View

I joined a 12-step program seven years ago, thoroughly beaten down from drug addiction. Through Narcotics Anonymous meetings, actively working through the steps, and living by the spiritual principles of honesty, open-mindedness, and willingness, I have a life again. I'm currently pursuing a BA degree, and I'm excited about my future.

—Jeanne Miffit

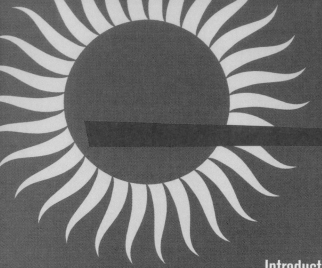

Introduction

We all practice literally hundreds of behaviors on a daily basis and use many different products and substances to sustain and enhance our lives. For most of us, the variety and access we have to these resources is part of the American dream, but for some, these wants and needs can become problematic. In our quest for happiness, our desires and habits may become abusive and addictive. Fortunately, most behaviors we practice and substances we use do not lead to abuse and addiction. No one sets out to be an addict, but if the combination of personal factors and characteristics of the substance or behavior are right, the end product may be abuse or addiction.

Use of a substance or practice of a behavior is predicated by a variety of factors including curiosity, modeling of adult behavior, peer pressure, availability, and favorable attitudes toward use. People who use a substance or try out a behavior and find that experience pleasurable often repeat the experience. This is not an unusual process; it is how we learn to enjoy and come to know a variety of experiences in life. We exercise, practice good eating habits, practice stress management skills, use seat belts, enjoy a cup of coffee, and discuss life's challenges with friends. Abuse, on the other hand implies that use of the substance or practice of the behavior is persistent despite adverse consequences. Abuse may be related to genetic factors, chemicals located in the brain, lack of social skills, poor self-concept, lack of connectedness to family and community, academic failure, and rebellion.

When a person with a predisposition to abuse connects with a substance or

Objectives

After reading this chapter, you should be able to

- **Describe the use and abuse of the most commonly used drugs on college campuses**

- **Summarize the alcohol use patterns of college students**

- **Explain the physiological and behavioral effects of alcohol, tobacco, caffeine, marijuana, cocaine, and methamphetamine**

- **Discuss the risks associated with using smokeless tobacco and cigars**

- **Discuss how alcohol use adversely affects the health of a fetus**

- **Define and explain the concept of addiction**

- **Name and discuss five criteria for addiction**

- **Describe the disease, biological, and psychosocial models of addiction**

- **Discuss the difference between substance and process addictions**

- **Explain the impact of addiction on families**

- **Describe the role of intervention, treatment, and relapse in the successful management of addiction**

behavior that is physically and/or psychologically addicting, the end result is often addiction. In this chapter, you will learn about substance abuse and the process of addiction. You will learn to recognize abusive and addictive patterns of use in yourself and others. Resources and strategies for overcoming abusive and addictive behaviors are included to help you work toward your wellness goals. Ultimately, a high level of wellness depends on your ability to know yourself, recognize your limitations, make choices, and set limits.

When a Habit Is More Than a Habit: Defining Addiction

Practically any behavior or mood-altering substance taken to an extreme can become addictive. Wellness behaviors that are practiced in moderation can help prevent these addictive tendencies. Those of us who run for 30 minutes four or five times per week and watch the amount of fat and sugar in our diets are practicing healthful behaviors. But when does a habit become more than a habit? When do we cross the threshold and pass from healthy habits to addictive behaviors or actions?

One way to look at the difference between habits and addictive behaviors is to examine *wants* versus *needs*. For example, a normal person may want occasionally to have a drink or buy a lottery ticket. By contrast, an alcoholic needs that drink to feel normal, and the compulsive gambler needs to buy that lottery ticket to feel good. Regardless of the type of addiction, people who become addicted cross the line between choosing and needing to use a substance or engage in a behavior. In the case of chemical addictions, addicts often use as the result of physical responses to chemicals and/or psychological reactions to physical cravings. People may have many reasons for using chemicals or engaging in addictive behaviors, but they do not do so with the goal of becoming dependent. Most people stumble into their addictions blindly. Alcohol, cocaine, gambling, food, excessive spending, sex, exercise, work—all are potential addictions in our society. But what is an addiction? Investigators in the early 1970s who compared substance abuse (addiction to a drug) with other types of habitual behaviors concluded that there are commonalities. Thus, an **addiction** is a pattern of reliance on a substance or behavior to produce mood change regardless of consequences.

The Addictive Process

Addiction is a process that evolves over time. It begins when an individual repeatedly seeks relief through a substance or event from unpleasant feelings or situations. Yoder states that "the process of addiction begins with shame and low self-esteem—we believe that we are not good enough." The addictive process is based on the fallacy that something outside of us can make us whole. This destructive view gives the addict a false sense of security and feeling of power that comes from the habit.

addiction pattern of reliance on a substance or behavior to produce mood change regardless of consequences

STATS-AT-A-GLANCE
Addiction and Substance Abuse

■ Teenagers and young adult drivers (ages 16–29) who were arrested for driving while intoxicated (DWI), were four times more likely to die in future crashes involving alcohol than were those who had not been arrested for DWI (U.S. Department of Health and Human Services, 1996).

■ Nearly half of all college students binge drink. (Binge drinking is defined as five or more drinks at a time for men, four or more drinks for women.) On a national scale, this is about three million students (Wechsler et al., 1994).

■ The number of college women who drink to get drunk has more than tripled in the past 10 years, rising from 10% to 35% (Wechsler et al., 1996).

■ Recent campus statistics show that alcohol is involved in about two-thirds of all violent behavior, almost half of all physical injuries, about one-third of all emotional difficulties among students, 40% of all academic problems, and 28% of all drop outs (Eigen; Anderson).

■ In 1994, the rate of illicit drug use was highest among persons 18 to 21 and 16 and 17 years old (National Household Survey on Drug Abuse, 1994).

■ Smoking prevalence rates among Vietnamese men are nearly 73%, the highest in the world, largely because of intensive marketing efforts by tobacco companies in that country (JAMA, 1997).

■ Excessive alcohol consumption causes more than 100,000 deaths annually in the United States (*Scientific American*, 1996).

The addictive process generally progresses through five stages: (1) no involvement, (2) experimental involvement, (3) regular involvement, (4) regular involvement with harmful consequences, and (5) compulsive involvement (see Figure 11.1). Keep in mind, however, that it is not simply the number of times a person uses a substance or performs a behavior that reflects a problem. What happens to that person when he or she is using is also an important marker. For example, your roommate may drink only once a month, but if he gets into fights and can't control his behavior during those monthly episodes, then his drinking is a problem.

As the addictive process continues, the person's whole life is affected: Relationships, schoolwork, job performance, and health all deteriorate. The addict may initially begin to pull away from family and friends and start skipping classes (Table 11.1 lists some common characteristics of addictions). Soon the process affects the addict's ability to sleep, causing confusion and fatigue. Over time, the intensity of the craving or the desire to repeat the behavior becomes all-consuming. Early recognition and treatment of the problem is essential. The longer an addiction remains untreated, the more difficult the recovery process will be.

Substance Use and Abuse

It is safe to say that in the late 1990s drug use remains a significant problem for both college students and the general population. Alcohol is the most important problem drug for most college students, but other drugs pose risks for certain students. Typically, students understand the dramatic effects that illicit drug use has had on many people's lives from loss of employment to deterioration of personal relationships. Realizing this, college students have generally moved away from using the most dangerous illegal drugs. The two categories of illicit drugs that have shown an increase in the past several years on campuses have been hallucinogens and marijuana. Our focus here is on alcohol, nicotine, caffeine, and some of the most common illicit drugs used by college students.

Alcohol

An estimated 70% of Americans consume alcoholic beverages regularly whereas consumption patterns are unevenly distributed throughout the drinking population. Ten percent of drinkers are heavy drinkers and account for half of all the alcohol consumed. The remaining 90% of the drinking population are infrequent, light, or moderate drinkers. According to the U.S. Department of Health and Human Services, 100,000 people die from alcohol-related causes each year. Furthermore, alcohol accounts for 44% of all deaths from motor vehicle crashes, one-third of all drownings, and about half of all deaths caused by fire. Alcohol is linked to half of all homicides, a third of all suicides, and two-thirds of all assaults. In addition, social workers report that alcohol is a factor in nearly 50% of domestic violence cases.

College Students and Alcohol Use. A recent report on college student drinking found that 85% of college students drink alcoholic beverages. Alcohol abuse by college students usually follows a pattern of binge

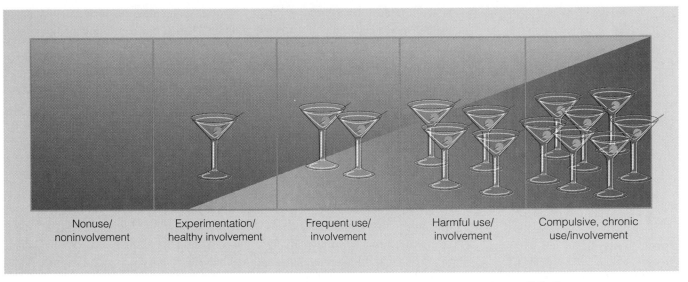

| Nonuse/
noninvolvement | Experimentation/
healthy involvement | Frequent use/
involvement | Harmful use/
involvement | Compulsive, chronic
use/involvement |

Figure 11.1

Addictions are often described in terms of five progressive stages. According to these stages, the amount of use and the frequency of involvement in the addictive behavior determine the extent of the addiction.

drinking. Binge drinking refers to the consumption for men of five drinks in a row and for women of four or more drinks in a row. It was found that 44% of U.S. students engaged in binge drinking behavior. Other significant findings of this report include the following:

- Drinking patterns established in high school often persist in college. Compared to other students, college students who were binge drinkers in high school were almost three times more likely to be binge drinkers in college.

- Being white, involved in athletics, or a resident of a fraternity or sorority made it more likely that a student would be a binge drinker.

TABLE 11.1
Characteristics of Addictions

- Erratic mood swings
- Euphoric responses to an activity
- Obsessive thoughts about or constant craving for a substance or activity
- Concerns expressed by friends or family member about particular behaviors
- Physiological and/or psychological withdrawal symptoms when unable to have the drug or be involved in the activity
- Denial and dishonesty to conceal involvement or support the activity
- Alienation from old friends
- Sharp drop in grades or job performance
- Loss of motivation and ambition
- Loss of control
- Rebellious or irritable behavior
- Changes in eating or sleeping habits
- Sudden withdrawal or emotional distance

■ Compared to non-binge-drinkers, a higher percentage of binge drinkers had experienced alcohol-related problems since the beginning of the school year. (See Table 11.2).

Non-binge-drinking students are also affected by the drinking of their classmates. These are called "secondhand binge" effects. It is now clear that not only the binge drinker experiences consequences of binge drinking: non-binge students are also highly affected. On a high-binge-drinking campus (where 50% or more of students are binge drinkers), the overwhelming majority of students (87%) who live on campus experienced one or more problems as a result of others' binge drinking. Non-binge-drinking students were twice as likely as those at low-binging schools to be insulted or humiliated; to be pushed, hit, or assaulted; and to experience unwanted sexual advances from drinking students. Students at high-binging campuses were two-and-one-half times as likely to sustain property damage, to end up taking care of a drunken student, and to have their study or sleep time interrupted by classmates' drinking.

Use, Moderate Use, and Abuse. Two-thirds of all American adults are classified as drinkers. These individuals enjoy an occasional alcoholic beverage equaling no more than one or two drinks per week (one drink is defined as ½ oz of rum, rye, scotch, brandy, gin, etc.; 12-oz bottle of

TABLE 11.2
What Bingers Do to Themselves

The information in the chart below illustrates the strong relationship between binge drinking and a variety of alcohol-related health, social, and academic problems. Frequent bingers are defined as those who binged three or more times in the past two weeks.

	NON-BINGE DRINKERS	BINGERS	FREQUENT BINGERS
Had a hangover	30%	75%	90%
Did something they regretted later	14%	37%	63%
Missed a class	8%	30%	61%
Forgot where they were or what they did	8%	26%	54%
Got behind in school work	6%	21%	46%
Argued with friends	8%	22%	42%
Engaged in unplanned sexual activity	8%	20%	41%
Had unprotected sex	4%	10%	22%
Got hurt or injured	2%	9%	23%
Damaged property	2%	8%	22%
Got into trouble with campus/local police	1%	4%	11%
Required treatment for alcohol overdose	<1%	<1%	1%

Source: From Harvard School of Public Health, 1995.

normal strength beer; 3 oz of fortified wine; or 5 oz of table wine). Others are defined as moderate drinkers, meaning they drink no more than two drinks each day for most men and one drink each day for women. These cut-off levels are based on the amount of alcohol that can be consumed without causing problems, either for the drinker or society. The alcohol abuser is the individual who drinks more than three drinks per day. This group also includes binge drinkers. Alcohol abusers view alcohol as something other than a beverage to be consumed at meals or used in a celebratory fashion. Alcohol abusers often use alcohol as a means of altering emotions, to help them sleep, or to cope with life's stresses. Does this mean that only individuals who are alcohol abusers have problems with alcohol? The answer is no. Individuals who use alcohol even at the infrequent or moderate-use levels and experience negative consequences of their alcohol use as result are considered problem drinkers.

Blood Alcohol Concentration. A drinker's blood alcohol concentration level depends on weight and body fat, the water content in the body tissues, the concentration of alcohol in the beverage consumed, the rate of consumption, presence of food in the stomach, and the volume of alcohol consumed. Heavier people have larger body surfaces through which to diffuse alcohol; therefore, they have lower concentrations of alcohol in their body than do thin people after drinking the same amount. Because alcohol does not diffuse as rapidly into body fat as into water, alcohol concentration is higher in a person with more body fat. Because a woman is likely to have more body fat and less water in her body tissues than a man of the same weight, she will be more intoxicated than a man after drinking the same amount of alcohol.

Body fat is not the only contributor to the difference in alcohol metabolism between men and women. Women appear to have half as much alcohol dehydrogenase as men. Alcohol dehydrogenase is the enzyme that breaks down alcohol in the stomach before it has a chance to get to the bloodstream and the brain. With less alcohol dehydrogenase action, women absorb about 30% more alcohol into the bloodstream then men, despite an identical number of drinks and equal body weight. Another factor contributing to the difference in alcohol metabolism between men and women is the menstrual cycle. Alcohol is absorbed more quickly during the premenstrual phase of a woman's cycle.

Knowing your alcohol concentration level is not only worthwhile from a wellness standpoint; it has legal implications as well. State drunk driving laws set a maximum blood alcohol concentration above which it is illegal to operate a motor vehicle. See Table 11.3 comparing blood alcohol levels by weight, sex, and number of drinks. This table provides an estimation of blood alcohol levels; many other factors may cause variation in these rates. You should always err on the side of caution when estimating blood alcohol levels.

Fetal Alcohol Syndrome. Fetal alcohol syndrome (FAS) is a condition acquired by the fetus as a result of the mother's drinking alcohol during her pregnancy. Alcohol passes through the placenta within minutes of consumption in a concentration equal to that in the mother's bloodstream. Because of the underdeveloped nature of the fetal liver, this alcohol is oxidized much more slowly than the alcohol in the mother. During this time of slow detoxification the fetus is certain to be exposed to the toxic effects of alcohol.

TABLE 11.3

Calculation of Estimated Blood Alcohol Concentration (BAC)

Body Weight: Calculations are for people with a *normal* body weight for their height, free of drugs or other affecting medication, and neither unusually thin nor obese.

Drink-Equivalents: 1 drink equals:
1½ ounces of rum, rye, scotch, brandy, gin, vodka, etc.
1 12-ounce bottle of normal-strength beer
3 ounces of fortified wine
5 ounces of table wine

Using the chart: Find the appropriate figure using the proper chart (male or female), body weight, and number of drinks consumed.

Then subtract the time factor (see Time Factor Table below) from the figure on the chart to obtain the approximate BAC. For example, for a 150-lb. man who has had 4 drinks in two hours, take the figure .116 (from the chart for males) and subtract .030 (from the Time Factor Table) to obtain a BAC of .086%.

Time Factor Table
Hours since first drink

	1	2	3	4	5	6
Subtract from BAC	.015	.030	.045	.060	.075	.090

MALES

NUMBER OF DRINKS

IDEAL BODY WEIGHT (LBS)	1	2	3	4	5	6	7	8	9	10
100	.043	.087	.130	.174	.217	.261	.304	.348	.391	.435
125	.034	.069	.103	.139	.173	.209	.242	.278	.312	.346
150	.029	.058	.087	.116	.145	.174	.203	.232	.261	.290
175	.025	.050	.075	.100	.125	.150	.175	.200	.225	.250
200	.022	.043	.065	.087	.108	.130	.152	.174	.195	.217
225	.019	.039	.058	.078	.097	.117	.136	.156	.175	.195
250	.017	.035	.052	.070	.087	.105	.122	.139	.156	.173

FEMALES

NUMBER OF DRINKS

IDEAL BODY WEIGHT (LBS)	1	2	3	4	5	6	7	8	9	10
100	.050	.101	.152	.203	.253	.304	.355	.406	.456	.507
125	.040	.080	.120	.162	.202	.244	.282	.324	.364	.404
150	.034	.068	.101	.135	.169	.203	.237	.271	.304	.338
175	.029	.058	.087	.117	.146	.175	.204	.233	.262	.292
200	.026	.050	.076	.101	.126	.152	.177	.203	.227	.253
225	.022	.045	.068	.091	.113	.136	.159	.182	.204	.227
250	.020	.041	.061	.082	.101	.122	.142	.162	.182	.202

Source: From Evans and O'Brien, 1991.

The amount of disability to the child can range from severe physical deformity (e.g., small head, widely spaced eyes), heart problems, clumsiness, low birth weight, behavioral problems, and stunted growth to mental retardation. Alcohol is the number one cause of mental retardation in the Western world.

Is there a safe limit to the number of drinks a pregnant woman can drink? As with many drugs, the effects of alcohol on the fetus are dose related. There is no precise blood alcohol threshold level above which damage occurs and below which there is no damage. Instead, the frequency and severity of defects progressively increase as the amount of drinking increases. Therefore, the safest plan for pregnant women is to avoid drinking alcohol altogether.

Alcoholism. Alcoholism is characterized by a compulsion to drink. Tolerance, dependence, and withdrawal symptoms must be present to qualify a drinker as an alcoholic. One of the early warning signs of alcohol abuse is frequent drinking, although this is often overlooked because it is considered socially acceptable. The traditional boasts of being able to "hold one's liquor" or to "drink anyone under the table" are now recognized as statements of possible addiction. Another warning sign of alcohol abuse is blackouts. A **blackout** is a chemically induced state of amnesia in which a person may appear to be normal to the casual observer but is unable to recall the events during a particular drinking episode. Any blackout episode should be taken very seriously.

Dependence on alcohol increases until it consumes the person's life. In response to problems at work, poor grades, and failed relationships, the alcohol abuser often sinks into depression. A drinking spiral develops as the alcoholic person uses alcohol to medicate feelings of depression or low self-esteem. This pattern of behavior continues until the person destroys himself or herself or seeks help.

The alcoholic individual who decides to quit drinking will experience withdrawal symptoms, which can include hyperexcitability, confusion, sleep disorders, and convulsions. In extreme cases, he or she may suffer from **delirium tremens (DTs),** a severe syndrome characterized by confusion, delusions, agitated behavior, and hallucinations brought on by withdrawal from alcohol. For the long-term alcohol abuser, medical supervision is usually necessary. **Detoxification,** the process of halting dependence on alcohol (or other drugs), is commonly carried out in a medical facility where the patient can be monitored to prevent fatal withdrawal reactions. Withdrawal takes 7 to 21 days, after which the alcohol abusers begin treatment for the psychological aspects of addiction.

A variety of treatments are available, including intensive hospital-based programs and family, individual, and group therapy. On some college campuses, student health centers have opened their own treatment programs. One of the most widely recognized treatment programs, Alcoholics Anonymous (AA), has over a million members worldwide. Since 1935, AA has provided support for individuals who decide to quit "cold turkey" as well as those undergoing other forms of treatment. In addition, support groups are available for family members of alcoholic people. Al-Teen serves youths under age 20; Al-Anon helps adult relatives and friends of alcoholics to understand the disease and discover ways to contribute to the recovery process.

Tobacco and Nicotine

According to the American Cancer Society, approximately 62 million people are addicted to nicotine. The U.S. Surgeon General has described cigarette smoking as the "chief preventable cause of death in our society" (U.S.

blackout chemically induced state of amnesia

DTs set of withdrawal symptoms characterized by agitation, confusion, and nervous activity

detoxification process of halting alcohol dependence in a facility where possible adverse effects are monitored

Sound Decision Making

AN ATHLETE FOR SOBRIETY

Shane learned to party hard in high school, and he looked forward to the new freedoms of college. Once on campus he rushed a fraternity known for its drinking and wild parties. For a couple of years, Shane seemed to have it all: he maintained reasonable grades, played for the varsity soccer team, had a great girlfriend, and drank more than his share of the house keg every weekend. Then, over the course of a month, things seemed to unravel. First, his girlfriend broke up with him; then he got suspended from the soccer team for hosting a party where minors were served alcohol; then he flunked a final exam in a class critical to his major because he was hung over the morning of the test. Confused about this turn of events, Shane had a long heart-to-heart conversation with Coach King about what was going on in his life. They came to see that many of the bad things in Shane's life could be traced to his drinking.

Shane did some soul searching to decide what was really important to him. He realized that athletics and graduating from college were most important in the short-term, and that he wanted some day to own his own business and to have a family. He decided he needed to clean up his act if he was going to meet any of these goals. Coach King helped him make a list of the things that would help him stop drinking: he needed to move out of the frat house, become better friends with some people who weren't into drinking, and consider joining a campus group called Athletes for Sobriety.

Moving out of the fraternity was incredibly difficult for Shane; he felt as if he were betraying his friends. But he promised to stay active in some aspects of fraternity life, and found off-campus housing with two other guys from the soccer team who also wanted a peaceful living environment. He felt awkward the first time he went to a meeting of Athletes for Sobriety, but he soon found that he had a lot in common with the men and women in the group, and they helped each other find ways to stay sober in a campus environment that didn't always seem to encourage sobriety.

Looking back on his college experience during his senior year, Shane could see how much he'd grown up. He was still active in his fraternity, but in a new capacity as director of community service projects. And he served as a peer counselor to freshman athletes on how to deal responsibly with alcohol and drugs. Shane feels lucky that he stopped drinking when he did, and he feels confident that he will meet his goals for the future.

Department of Health and Human Services, 1990a). To put things in perspective, more people die from smoking-related diseases than from alcohol, cocaine, heroin, suicide, homicide, car crashes, and AIDS combined (American Heart Association). Over 400,000 Americans die annually as a result of smoking. Despite all the efforts to curb nicotine addiction, thousands of young people start smoking each year.

Nicotine is a powerful, addicting drug. The 1987 Surgeon General's report, "Nicotine Addiction," announced that cigarettes are as addictive as heroin, cocaine, or alcohol. An example of the addictive power of nicotine is illustrated by people who find themselves addicted after having smoked as few as three packs of cigarettes. Tolerance to nicotine develops quickly. When smokers are deprived of nicotine they experience withdrawal symptoms that include nervousness, irritability, depression, headaches, and lack of concentration.

Why people begin smoking given all the known adverse health effects is a question frequently asked. The answer is not simple. Many smokers find that smoking relaxes them. Others find that smoking increases their concentration and helps make them more productive. Smoking can also be used as a means of weight control, but someone who has learned to rely on nicotine as an appetite suppressant will have an especially difficult time quitting.

For some smokers, Yoder claims the physiological withdrawal from nicotine is easier than the loss of their smoking rituals. Typical rituals include a cigarette with the morning cup of coffee, after each meal, with a beer, or in the car. Consider this: A pack-a-day smoker lights 20 cigarettes per day, 140 cigarettes per week, and 7,200 cigarettes per year. Because smokers often reach for a cigarette without consciously deciding to do so, smoking rituals compound their difficulty in trying to quit.

Cigarette smoking is not the only form of tobacco that poses a health risk to its users. Smokeless tobacco, also know as snuff and chew, is becoming increasingly popular with young males. Once the tobacco is placed in the mouth, nicotine and other compounds are absorbed through the mucous membranes and into the bloodstream. In a matter of minutes, blood levels of nicotine are comparable to those seen in cigarette smokers. Chewing and the use of snuff cause problems ranging from bad breath to cardiovascular disease and cancer. The presence of leukoplakia, thick and rough precancerous white spots, can appear on the gums, tongue, or inner cheek of chewers. Many health experts believe that smokeless tobacco use has serious life-threatening consequences. If current patterns of smokeless tobacco use continue, there is potential for an oral cancer epidemic.

One of the newest trends is smoking cigars. Cigar magazines and shops are catering to a new form of smoking chic. In part as a result of the glamorization of cigars, consumption of large cigars has risen 44% from 1993 to 1996 ("Cigar Smoking Among Teenagers"). Like cigarettes, cigar smoking can cause cancers of the oral cavity, larynx, esophagus, and lungs and chronic obstructive pulmonary disease.

In recent years, millions of people have quit smoking. Of those who did, 90% have quit "cold turkey." The majority of smokers want to quit; approximately one-third of smokers attempt to do so each year. Unfortunately, 90% or more of these attempts fail. Although the majority quit all at once, others use self-help programs or nicotine gum or patches as a means of easing withdrawal. Long-term success rates are generally highest with clinic-based programs, which provide professional supervision and support. The major barriers to success include high stress levels, social norms that make smoking acceptable, and presence of family members and peers who smoke.

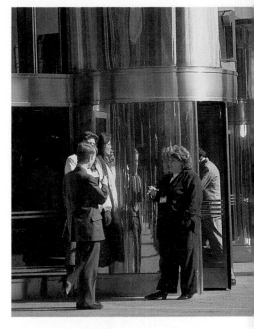

In a scene that is becoming more common, smokers indulge their nicotine addiction outdoors.

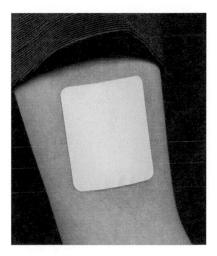

Nicotine patches such as this one can help smokers gradually decrease their cravings while avoiding severe withdrawal symptoms.

Caffeine

Caffeine is probably the most common drug used by adults and children in our society. A tasteless drug found in chocolate, some soft drinks, coffee, tea, and some aspirin and over-the-counter medications, caffeine is a powerful stimulant. In healthy, rested people, a dose of 100 milligrams (about 1 cup of coffee) increases alertness, banishes drowsiness, quickens reaction time, increases heart and respiratory rates, and stimulates urinary output.

Moderate use of caffeine is generally harmless, but overconsumption can produce a toxic reaction known as *caffeinism*. A 300-mg dose for many people produces sleep disruption, nervousness, headaches, heart palpitations, and gastric disturbances. Some women indicate that caffeine increases incidence of premenstrual syndrome and fibrocystic breast disease.

Caffeine is a habit-forming drug, and those who try to stop "cold turkey" often experience withdrawal symptoms. Headaches, lethargy, and irritability are common symptoms that typically diminish over a period of several weeks.

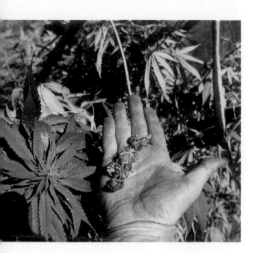

The marijuana hemp plant (cannabis sativa) contains the psychoactive compound THC.

Marijuana

There is no question that marijuana is the most commonly used illicit drug in the United States. Of the estimated 13 million Americans (12 years and older) who use illicit drugs, 10 million use marijuana. It is also the most commonly used illicit drug on college campuses. Recent statistics indicate that between 1992 and 1994, the rate of marijuana use among youths 12 to 17 years of age has nearly doubled. Use of marijuana by young people rose 105% from 1992 to 1994 and 37% between 1994 and 1995. At the Phoenix House Foundation 10 years ago, 13% of adolescents sought treatment for marijuana; today that figure has risen to 40%.

The main psychoactive drug in marijuana is THC (delta-9 tetrahydro-cannabinol). Marijuana is derived either from the cannabis sativa or cannabis indica (hemp) plants. The THC levels in marijuana are the key to determining how powerful a high the marijuana will produce. The THC levels of the 1960s are considerably different from today's levels. THC levels have risen from such lows as 1% to 5% to levels reaching 8% or higher.

The immediate short-term effects associated with the use of marijuana are diminished inhibitions and impaired perception of time and distance. At low doses, marijuana users typically experience euphoria and heightening of subjective sensory experiences. With moderate doses the effects become more pronounced and the user can experience impaired memory function, disturbed thought patterns, and lapses of attention. People who use high doses of marijuana have a feeling of depersonalization, an experience in which the mind seems to be separated from the body. Many people experience other sensations such as marked sensory distortion and changes in body perceptions (arms and legs feel extremely light). Physiologically, marijuana causes an increase in heart rate, up to 50% faster than normal in some cases. Certain blood vessels in the eye dilate, giving the smoker bloodshot eyes.

What are the long-term effects of marijuana? It is a very good question—but not simple to answer. Marijuana is a very complicated drug. Instead of being one compound like alcohol or cocaine, it is made up of more than 400 components, making it much more complex to understand. It will take many more years of research to determine the precise psychological and physiological effects of marijuana. One of the biggest long-term threats to users' health is the risk of irritation to the lungs and respiratory tract. Other potential long-term effects include gum disease; increased risk of cancer of the tongue, jaw, mouth, and lung; and impairment of the immune system.

Addiction to marijuana does not meet all the classic definitions of addiction. Although regular marijuana users certainly develop a tolerance, it has not been well established whether there is withdrawal associated with discontinued use. Marijuana can become a priority in the user's life, interfering with other activities, family, and friends.

Cocaine

Cocaine is the second most common used illicit drug in the United States. A central nervous system stimulant, cocaine is perhaps one of the most potent drugs. It is derived from leaves of the coca shrub, which is harvested in Central and South America. Cocaine is usually snorted, but it can be injected or smoked. The effects last from 5 to 30 minutes, then the user starts to crash. Users of cocaine experience a quick sense of euphoria. Cocaine can reach the brain in less than 3 minutes when snorted, in 30 seconds when inhaled, and in less than a second when injected. This sense of euphoria subsides quickly, causing the user to seek more cocaine. Users of cocaine develop tolerance quickly and need purer and purer forms of the drug to get the same effect.

Freebasing and the use of crack cocaine are the most common techniques used for maximizing the psychoactive effects of cocaine. Freebasing requires the conversion of cocaine by separating the drug from the parent compound by mixing it with water and ammonium hydroxide. The cocaine base is then separated from the water using a fast-drying solvent such as ether, leaving a pure cocaine freebase. The freebase then is smoked through a water pipe over a high temperature torch. This practice involves inherent danger. The ether used in this process is extremely volatile and may explode. Freebase cocaine reaches the brain in seconds and is considerably more dangerous than snorted cocaine. The high is more intense and reached more quickly. When the high disappears, it leaves the user craving more of the drug. Addiction to freebasing develops quickly and many people who freebase become severely addicted and experience health problems and financial difficulties.

The use of crack cocaine has evolved from the technique used to freebase. Crack is made by combining cocaine hydrochloride with common baking soda. This mixture makes a paste that when dried produces small, crystal-like rocks. These rocks are ready to smoke by placing them in cigarettes, joints, or pipes. Because crack is such a pure form of cocaine, it produces a rapid and intense euphoria. This high is always followed by an intense crash and subsequent searching for another high. Addiction to crack takes less time to develop than an addiction to snorting cocaine. Some users report addiction to crack after using just a couple of times.

The physical effects of cocaine, smoking crack, and freebase include dramatic increase in heart rate and blood pressure, loss of appetite that can lead to dramatic weight loss, convulsions, muscle twitching, irregular heart beat, even eventual death due to an overdose. Other effects of cocaine include temporary relief of depression, decreased fatigue, talkativeness, increased alterness, and heightened self-confidence. Again, however, as the dose increases, users become irritable and apprehensive, and their behavior may turn paranoid or violent. The intense high for the body can be overwhelming for the body's systems, causing convulsions, respiratory arrest, cardiac arrest, and death. Injecting cocaine can lead to increase risk of HIV, hepatitis B, and other infections due to the sharing of needles. There is overwhelming scientific evidence that users can quickly develop a strong psychological dependence. There is also considerable evidence that cocaine use produces a physiological dependence.

Amphetamines are a group of synthetic chemicals that are also central nervous system stimulants. Some of the more common names for this group of drugs are "crank" and "ice." "Ice" is a smokable, high potency form of methamphetamine. "Crank" is another form of methamphetamine that can be smoked, snorted, injected, and eaten. Both of these increasingly popular forms of methamphetamine are relatively inexpensive compared to crack. Their highs can last from 8 hours to several weeks. Some of the effects of "crank" and "ice" include an increased sense of euphoria, excessive energy, insomnia, violent behavior, and in some cases psychosis and permanent brain damage. Injecting also increases the risk of HIV infection and other blood-borne diseases from contaminated needles.

amphetamines group of synthetic chemicals known for their stimulant effects on the body

Other Drugs

Several other illicit drugs that are worth mentioning include heroin and LSD. The United States is currently experiencing a resurgence of heroin use. Purer and less expensive than the heroin of the 1980s, the heroin available today is now pure enough to snort or smoke. Heroin is a highly addictive narcotic that depresses the central nervous system. Many health problems related to heroin use are caused by uncertain dosage levels, use of unsterile equipment, or the use of heroin in combination with other drugs such as alcohol and cocaine. Typical problems include skin abscesses, inflammation of veins, overdose, heart valve infection, malnutrition, and hepatitis B.

Signs and symptoms of heroin use include euphoria, drowsiness, respiratory depression, and nausea. Withdrawal from heroin takes approximately one week. Withdrawal symptoms include runny nose, muscle cramps, insomnia, and loss of appetite. Elevation in blood pressure, respiration rate, and temperature occur as withdrawal progresses.

LSD is one of the most commonly known psychedelic drugs. LSD, frequently referred to as acid, is sold on the street in many forms, including tablets, pellets sometimes called microdots, gelatin chips known as windowpanes, and thin squares of absorbent paper soaked in liquid LSD called blotter acid. Like heroin, LSD use has also experienced resurgence of popularity. The comeback of LSD can be attributed to several factors. First, the potency is weaker, making reactions more manageable. Second, the packaging is attractive to young people; sometimes blotter paper features cartoon characters, stars, moons, and dragons. Last, it is affordable; a hit costs about $3 to $5 in most areas of the country.

The effects of LSD are dependent on the dose; the user's personality, mood, and expectations; and the surroundings in which the drug is used. The effects of the drug are usually felt within 30 to 90 minutes. The physical effects include dilated pupils, increased body temperature, increased heart rate and blood pressure, sweating, loss of appetite, sleeplessness, dry mouth, and tremors. Euphoria is a common psychological state produced by the drug, but dysphoria (a sense of evil and foreboding) may also be experienced. The drug also shortens attention span, causing the mind to wander. Thoughts may be interposed and juxtaposed as well. The user may be able to experience several thoughts simultaneously.

There is no evidence that LSD creates a physical dependence, but it may well create a psychological dependence. Many LSD users become depressed for one or two days following a trip and turn to the drug to relieve their depression. The result is a cycle of LSD use to relieve post-LSD depression, which often leads to psychological addiction.

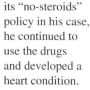

Ex-steroid user Steve Coursin, who played football for both the Pittsburgh Steelers and the Tampa Bay Buccaneers, sued the NFL. He claimed that because the NFL did not enforce its "no-steroids" policy in his case, he continued to use the drugs and developed a heart condition.

Anabolic Steroids

The use of anabolic steroids by weight lifters in the Eastern bloc dates back to the 1950s, and the practice has been spreading ever since. Anabolic steroids are compounds that are closely related chemically to the male sex hormone testosterone. They are used primarily to promote muscle size and strength. These **ergogenic aids** are used primarily by young males and females to increase their strength and power, reduce the amount of recovery time needed between workouts, improve their speed, and increase their weight. These attributes are thought to enhance their athletic performance and/or improve their physical appeal. Anabolic steroids are commonly administered to the body via injection into the belly muscles or orally with a pill.

Most steroids used illegally are obtained through the black market from underground sources. The quality and purity of such drugs are questionable at best. It is estimated that 17% to 20% of college athletes use steroids. An estimated one million noncompetitive body builders are thought to use steroids.

Steroid users subject themselves to more than 70 side effects ranging in severity from liver cancer to acne and encompassing psychological as well as physical reactions. The parts of the body that are most seriously affected by steroids are the liver and the cardiovascular and reproductive systems. In males, steroids can cause breast growth, testicular atrophy, prostate enlargement, sterility, and impotence. In females, irreversible masculine traits (deepening of the voice, male pattern baldness, and increased facial and body hair) can develop along with menstrual irregularities, breast reduction, and an enlarged clitoris. Psychological effects in both sexes include aggressive, combative behavior known as "roid rage" and depression. Some side effects may not show up for years, such as heart attacks and strokes, and some might not even be recognized as side effects, such as failure to achieve full height potential because of arrested bone development during adolescence.

In addition to the physical dangers, steroid use can lead to a vicious cycle of dependence. Users commonly take drugs in cycles that last from 4 to 18 weeks followed by a lengthy break. It is during this period when the user experiences shrinking, a phenomenon so abhorrent to those obsessed with size that they panic and begin using the drugs again in even larger doses. Many users "stack" their drugs, taking as many as three to five pills and injectables at once; some report taking as many as 14 drugs simultaneously. When steroid users stop, they often experience deep depression. This depression often occurs when users have a break in their cycle. It is compounded by the absence of the feeling of euphoria and invincibility that occurs with use.

In 1990, Congress passed the Anabolic Steroids Control Act to combat the growing problem of anabolic steroid use. It is illegal to possess or distribute anabolic steroids for nonmedical purposes under the federal law. Steroids are considered a Schedule III drug under the Controlled Substances Act. Penalties for use include up to five years in prison and a $250,000 fine for the first offense and 10 years in prison and $500,000 fine for subsequent offenses.

Process Addictions

Process addictions are any series of activities or interactions on which a person becomes dependent. Common process addictions include exercise, gambling, spending and borrowing, and sex.

Exercise

Most people would agree that some form of regular exercise contributes to wellness. However, some individuals have difficulty realizing when their exercise habits have gotten out of control (see Laboratory 11.1). Simply put, exercise addiction is too much of a good thing. A by-product of the 1970s jogging boom, exercise addiction reflects our stressful, fast-paced lifestyle. In

ergogenic aids substance that enhances athletic performance

addition, Americans are obsessed with thinness and body image, and exercise becomes another means for trying to achieve that "perfect" look.

What causes this compulsion to exercise beyond what is suggested for health benefits? There are two schools of thought on exercise compulsion. Thoren and Floras suggest that it results from the release of endorphins, which produce a "natural high" not just during the activity but several hours afterward. McMurray argues that no relationship exists between endorphins and "runner's high" and that "runner's high" results from an increase in adrenaline or the release of built-up stress. In short, running does such a good job of relieving stress that some people cannot do without it.

Regardless of which theory is correct, exercise addiction appears to be another means of achieving a desired emotional state through extreme behavioral patterns. People who exercise compulsively often place their running ahead of their families and jobs. Yates and colleagues found similarities between the personalities of anorexics (see Chapter 8) and addicted runners. As with anorexics, persons addicted to running tended to be self-effacing, hardworking high achievers from affluent families who were uncomfortable with anger and unable to express emotion. These runners felt they must keep proving themselves.

Often exercise addicts continue to exercise while experiencing unhealthy weight loss as well as excruciatingly painful injuries. They can develop chronic muscle soreness and fatigue, early degenerative arthritis, anemia, and a depressed immune system response. Eventually, kidney damage and muscle breakdown can occur unless they take time off from their exercise routine. Fortunately, only a small percentage of runners reach self-destructive extremes. For some addicted exercisers, the realization that they no longer have control over their exercise patterns is enough to make them switch to another activity or to exercise in moderation. Others consult qualified sports psychologists who are trained to help people who overindulge in endurance sports.

Gambling

Gambling is not only legal in many states, it is encouraged as a way to solve economic shortfalls. From riverboats and cruise ships to gas stations and grocery stores, you're urged to roll the dice, buy a ticket, or pull a tab. Gambling has changed dramatically since the 1970s and 1980s. Then the average age of compulsive gamblers was 30 to 55; today it is 17 to 70. America's gambling habit has grown from about $80 billion a year in 1986 to $300 billion in 1991.

The intense concentration, the excitement, and the feeling of being taken in beyond one's control give gambling its addictive allure. By current estimates, between 3% and 11% of the population experience problems with gambling. Compulsive gambling is sometimes called a hidden illness because it produces no smell on the gambler's breath, no stumbling, and no slurring of speech. A profile of the typical gambling addict shows a white male age 17 to 34 who is married, has a high school

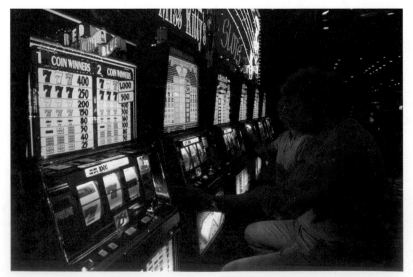

The popularity of gambling in the United States has grown in the last few decades.

diploma, and earns $20,000 to $50,000 annually. Compulsive gamblers are thought to be bright, aggressive, hardworking, successful people who love to take risks. Predisposing factors for compulsive gambling may include childhood trauma, abuse, and unresolved grief issues.

On average, it can take 8 years to progress from a recreational gambler to a compulsive gambler. In 1980, the American Psychiatric Association accepted pathological (compulsive) gambling as a "disorder of impulse control." This illness is a diagnosable, treatable disorder. It is a progressive disorder that is characterized by three phases: (1) the winning phase, (2) the losing phase, and (3) the desperation phase.

There are many inpatient and outpatient treatment programs for gambling addicts. Many gamblers find support groups beneficial and succeed in recovery using the 12-step program provided by Gamblers' Anonymous (GA). Gambling addicts have a high recovery rate, with 80% engaging in treatment successfully overcoming their habit.

Spending and Borrowing

We live in a society that urges us to use installment financing and credit cards to satisfy the "I want it now" syndrome. In short, we are encouraged to spend now and worry later. Advertisers constantly promote unneeded but attractive products that we are told we cannot live without. For those who cannot control or resist buying or borrowing, this type of pressure can prove destructive.

Compulsive spenders or shoppers go on wild shopping sprees, a behavior over which they have no control. These sprees produce a feeling of euphoria, relieve pain, and provide a way of escaping from feelings of worthlessness, helplessness, powerlessness, and anxiety. Often compulsive spenders use material possessions to meet their emotional needs. Compulsive debtors repeatedly borrow money from friends, family, or the bank.

A common factor found in both these addictions is low self-esteem, which often develops as the result of being brought up in a family in which the parents were themselves addicted to gambling, spending, or substances. The compulsive spender and debtor begin the addictive cycle by seeking instant gratification or relief from anxiety. This leads to a craving for buying things until, finally, the addict loses control over spending. Each indulgence leads to greater anxiety and guilt, which in turn is relieved by going on another spending spree.

Treatment for compulsive shoppers and debtors is available through Debtors Anonymous, which uses a 12-step approach to help members confront their problem and develop ways to keep track of and plan their spending. The key to recovery is learning new ways to handle money. Treatment may also include both personal and financial counseling, in which spenders and debtors learn healthier ways to build self-esteem and become financially responsible.

Sex

Healthy sex is fulfilling; it is an expression of love and a means of renewing emotional intimacy. Like most other compulsive behaviors, sexual addiction is a self-destructive twist on a normal life-enhancing activity. For sex addicts, sex is not a pleasurable pastime or an expression of love but a driving compulsion.

A definition of sexual addiction depends less on the behavior itself and more on the person performing the behavior. For example, the occasional "peeping Tom" or "flasher" is not necessarily a sex addict, even though each of these individuals is involved in a deviant and illegal activity. The difference, experts at the Do It Now Foundation say, lies in the ability of the person to control sexual feelings and postpone sexual actions—something sex addicts cannot do. They go on "binges" every few months or spend the day sizing up people and places for sexual opportunities. Eventually, the pursuit of sex becomes their prime objective, more important than work, family, friends, health, and safety.

Sex addiction may have a biological basis. Researchers at the Do It Now Foundation have identified a specific chemical in the brain, phenylethylamine, that is responsible for the thrill and euphoria that accompanies falling in love. Sex addicts may not be addicted to sex so much as to the physical and psychological arousal triggered by repeated doses of phenylethylamine.

According to the Do It Now Foundation, another theory of sex addiction takes a psychosocial approach, tying it to a cycle of abuse. Many sex addicts have experienced some form of abuse or neglect as a child, suffer from consequent low self-esteem, and feel they are to blame for what has happened to them. They attempt to meet their self-esteem needs through a wide range of sexual behaviors. According to this theory, four distinct steps may signal problems in controlling sexual behavior:

1. *Preoccupation.* The person constantly searches for new sexual prospects or situations.

2. *Ritualization.* The person repeats an activity or situation to keep the arousal level high.

3. *Compulsion.* The individual continues to engage in sexual activity despite harmful consequences and a sincere desire to stop.

4. *Despair.* The person experiences guilt or shame over the inability to stop, or remorse for pain inflicted on others.

Stopping sexual addiction begins with the recognition that one is out of control. Groups such as Sex Addicts Anonymous, Sexaholics Anonymous, and Sex Abusers Anonymous can offer support. Rebuilding relationships with others is often accomplished through family and individual counseling. Also, sex addicts must learn how to manage stress, because stress can trigger periods of compulsive sexual activity.

Addictive Characteristics

Aspects of drug addiction that can also be applied to nondrug addictions include tolerance, withdrawal, dependence, and craving. **Tolerance** refers to the decreasing effect of a drug with repeated administrations so that ever larger doses are needed to elicit the desired result. **Withdrawal** refers to a physical disturbance or cluster of symptoms that occur when an addict cuts down on or stops using a drug. Experiencing withdrawal when a drug is stopped indicates that physical **dependence**—preoccupation with or craving for a drug—has developed, so that the addict actually requires it to function normally. Finally, **craving** refers to the strong desire to continue taking a drug. Whereas withdrawal reflects the development of physical dependence, craving indicates psychological dependence. Psychological dependence occurs when the drug (or other habitual activity) produces a feeling of satisfaction and the desire to continue the pattern of behavior to produce pleasure and avoid discomfort.

In recent years, the recognition that people can become addicted not only to substances but also to mood-altering events has broadened the concept of addiction. While **process addictions**—addictions to a process or activity—do not always produce the classic symptoms associated with tolerance, withdrawal, and craving, they do manifest in predictable ways. Process addicts find that they must increase the frequency and intensity of an activity to get the desired effect. Many process addicts also experience withdrawal when they are not able to participate in an exhilarating event.

Criteria for Addictions

All addictions share certain behavioral criteria: compulsion, loss of control, continued involvement, denial, cessation or control of abuse, and the tendency to relapse.

- *Compulsion* refers to the irresistible impulse to act, regardless of how irrational the motive. For an exercise addict this would mean an overwhelming need to work out every day. For a jogging addict who missed a day of running, this might mean feelings of depression and the urge to do twice as much the next day to make up for the missed workout.

- *Loss of control* reflects the inability to resist the desire to repeat the behavior. Perhaps the biggest illusion people have about addictions is that they are in control and can stop whenever they choose.

- *Continued involvement* involves maintaining a behavior or activity in spite of adverse consequences. For example, alcohol abusers drink even if their relationships fail, they are forced to drop out of school, or they are fired from a job. Sex addicts risk their health and even their lives by placing themselves in situations that increase their risk for sexually transmitted diseases.

- *Denial* is the hallmark of addiction whereby the addict is unable to perceive or unwilling to admit that a problem exists. Because addicts do not want to be in touch with their thoughts and feelings, they mask anything unpleasant by taking a drug or engaging in other self-destructive activities.

- *Cessation, or control of abuse,* occurs when the addict decides to enter a treatment program, seeking counseling, or quit on his or her own. The point at which addicts seek help varies from individual to individual.

- The *tendency to relapse* commonly occurs following a period of abstinence. It is not unusual for people to go through treatment or therapy several times before they finally break an addiction. Those who learn to confront their emotions and develop healthful coping mechanisms are more likely to be successful in their treatment program.

tolerance refers to the decreasing effects of a drug with repeated administrations, so that ever larger doses are needed to elicit the desired result

withdrawal physical disturbance or cluster of symptoms that occur when an addict cuts down on or stops using a drug

dependence preoccupation with or craving for a drug

craving strong desire to continue taking a drug

process addictions addictions to a process or activity

Models of Addiction

Everyone is *potentially* an addict. What, then, determines why some people become addicted and others do not? Most experts agree that addictions are the result of the interaction between personality, environment, culture, and biology. Of the many theories that have been developed to explain the origin of addiction, three models stand out: (1) the disease, (2) the biological, and (3) the psychosocial

Disease Model

Formerly, being an addict was regarded as a social failing. Addicts' behaviors were viewed as immoral, and their lack of control was thought to reflect a weak will. By contrast, the disease model of addiction, first expressed in the 1950s, views addiction as a chronic illness. This model is based on Jellinek's claim that alcoholism is a progressive and potentially fatal disorder.

The disease model has been the subject of debate centering around the question of whether an addiction truly constitutes a disease. The most compelling argument against this model is the fact that individual alcoholics fail to display consistent patterns of addiction, and thus no single cause has ever been established for alcoholism. Opponents also argue that the model absolves those addicted of responsibility for their actions. In any case, the disease model has fostered greater acceptance and compassion in the treatment of addicts while encouraging recovery.

Biological Model

The biological model views addiction as resulting from a biochemical, metabolic, or genetic disorder. Addiction is a consequence of genetic deficiencies in brain hormones and/or neurotransmitters that cause addicts to react differently from nonaddicts to the same drug or experience. For example, according to Greeson, food addicts may select simply carbohydrates that boost their level of serotonin (a neurotransmitter). For them, serotonin functions as a mood-altering substance. Other research reported by the U.S. Department of Health and Human Services has shown that children of alcoholic parents are four times more likely than children of nonalcoholic parents to become alcoholics themselves, even if raised by nonalcoholic adoptive parents. Presumably, this is because they metabolize alcohol differently or have biochemical imbalances that are genetically predetermined.

Psychosocial Model

Many factors in the environment can contribute to addictive tendencies: life stresses, family and peer relationships, social and cultural mores, and media messages, to name a few. By examining the influence of each of these factors in our own lives, we can better understand the forces that motivate our behavior and affect our overall wellness.

Life Stresses. We all face stressful life events that challenge our coping skills and psychological resilience. Divorce, marriage, death of a loved one, physical or sexual assault, sudden illness, or loss of a job are just a few examples of stressful life events that can trigger addictive behavior. We cannot escape stress altogether, but we can develop coping skills and establish a strong social support system that discourages addictive behavior.

Family Relationships. Those persons (including partners and friends) who love, care, and support us as we mature serve as our "family." Through such family members we initially develop social attachments, the enduring emotional ties that bind us to our most intimate companions. Most of us have at least one family member with whom we developed a strong social bond that taught us the value of a caring human relationship. Some of us, however, may have developed our strongest social attachments to objects (expensive cars and clothes), events (horse races), or behaviors (beer drinking) that ultimately became addictions. When stress becomes overwhelming, we seek comfort from the behaviors that have come to meet our emotional needs.

Peer Relationships. The impact of peers is greatest during our adolescent and young adult years, when we are struggling to identify a sense of self and at the same time fit into our chosen peer group. The wants and needs of the self and that of the peer group are often in conflict. For instance, you may believe that getting drunk is not the best way to deal with ending a relationship, but faced with the stress of such an event, you may relinquish your decision-making powers to others. They may persuade you to use healthful coping methods, or they may encourage negative coping behaviors, which can develop into addictions.

Social and Cultural Mores. Mores are the accepted customs of a social group that are ingrained in a way of life. Within the context of our social or cultural group, certain behaviors are either reinforced or discouraged. For example, in cultures in which alcohol use is associated with special occasions or ceremonies, and intoxication is viewed as socially unacceptable, rates of alcoholism typically are low. Likewise, in areas of the world where the ideal female body type is not thin, women do not compulsively diet and worry about their weight. When striving for wellness, we must recognize that social and cultural influences can be positive in some regards and negative in others.

Media Messages. Media messages can have a great impact on our perception of what behaviors are socially acceptable. In addition, media images portray and define success, popularity, and "in-group" behavior in many subtle ways. When we do not or cannot fit the media's image of

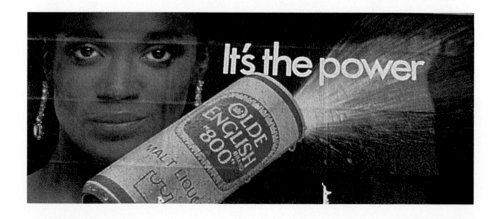

Media messages linking products such as alcohol to power, sexuality, and financial success can encourage addictive behaviors.

happiness and success, we may try to cope in negative ways. Indeed, some of our coping mechanisms, which can lead to addictive behavior such as smoking, drinking, or overeating, are actually encouraged through media messages. The message the media sends to the consumer is that unhealthy choices are acceptable; for those with a tendency toward addiction, such messages serve to sanction their abuse.

Relationships and Addiction

Yoder estimates that 15% of Americans are chemically addicted—10% to alcohol and 5% to either legal or illegal drugs. If each addict affects three family members, then 60% of the population is either addicted or directly affected by someone else's addiction.

Dysfunctional Families

The effect of addiction on the family has been described by Bradshaw, who says the family is "where we see ourselves for the first time. In families we learn about emotional intimacy. We learn what feelings are and how to express them. Our parents model what feelings are acceptable and family authorized and what feelings are prohibited." **Dysfunctional families** are families that are emotionally unhealthy. In dysfunctional families children learn a set of unspoken rules from an early age: Don't talk, don't trust, and don't feel. These rules keep the family from having to deal with real issues. The degree to which families are healthy or unhealthy depends on a number of factors (see Table 11.4).

Dealing with the far-reaching effects of addiction can strain the entire family. When one member of the family is an addict, other family members unconsciously adapt by adjusting their own behavior. To minimize their feelings about the addict, or out of love for the addict, family members can take on various dysfunctional roles that actually help perpetuate the addiction. For example, children in dysfunctional families can take on at least one of the following roles:

- *Family hero:* tries to divert attention away from the problem by being too good to be true

- *Scapegoat:* draws attention away from the family's primary problem through delinquency or misbehavior

- *Lost child:* becomes passive and quietly withdraws from upsetting situations

- *Mascot:* disrupts tense situations by using comic relief

In the past decade, we have come to recognize the unique problems of adult children of alcoholics (ACOAs). Having grown up with an addicted parent who was not able to provide adequate nurturance, ACOAs often must cope with problems such as the inability to develop social attachments, the need to be in control of all emotions and situations, low self-esteem, and depression.

Not all individuals who have grown up in dysfunctional families have lifelong problems. Why are some children more resilient than others? Steve

---

dysfunctional families families that are emotionally unhealthy

TABLE 11.4

Factors Contributing to Different Family Types[a]

IDEAL	DYSFUNCTIONAL
Members trust and value one another.	Members distrust one another.
Members are close.	Members are isolated.
Physical health is encouraged/ supported.	Physical health is neglected.
Individuality and interdependence are encouraged.	Personalities/boundaries between members are confused.
Child development and adaptation is appropriate.	Child development is impaired and maladaptive.
Communication is comfortable and clear.	Communication is vague and contradictory.
Problems are negotiated/resolved.	Problems are blamed/unresolved.
Values are consistent and clear.	Values are vague and inconsistent.
Members treat one another with dignity and respect.	Members verbally, physically, and sexually abuse one another.
Privacy is respected.	Privacy is denied/invaded.
Basic honesty prevails.	Secrecy, denial, and lies prevail.
The family is relaxed at most times.	The family constantly has a high stress level.
Members are sensitive to and supportive of individual feelings.	Members are insensitive to and inhibiting of individual feelings.
The family interacts well with the community.	The family avoids interaction with the community.
The general mood is warm, affectionate, optimistic, confident, and casual.	The general mood is hopeless, lonely, fearful, confused, and tense.
Parents/guardians are positive and mutually supportive as a couple and share responsibility for guidance and discipline.	Parents are in conflict (which may be hidden but is felt by all).
Each parent is an individual and has a separate relationship with each child.	Parents are distracted by unresolved issues in their own family of origin.
Parents work as an "executive team": Kids are kids and parents are parents.	Parents depend on the kids and often use them to fight each other.

[a]Characteristics are all relative. What is unhealthy in one family may be more healthy in another, depending on ethnic, cultural, or other important factors.

Source: From Sacred Heart General Hospital, 1988.

MYTHS & CONTROVERSIES

Controversy | **Is the concept of codependency useful in treating addiction?** Codependency has turned into an industry. Best-sellers and treatment groups abound. The Hazelden Foundation runs rehabilitation centers and publishes books, manuals, and pamphlets for recovering addicts and codependents. Melody Beattie's *Codependent No More* has sold more than 1.5 million copies. Mainline publishers are now producing books with essentially the same message.

The codependency movement offers help to people in distress, but is it the best kind of help? In the 1950s, the wives of heavy drinking men were singled out by researchers as being active collaborators in their husbands' addictions or actually the cause of it. Women who were married to heavy drinkers, according to the theory, had personality disorders: They were "Suffering Susans," "Controlling Catherines," "Wavering Winifreds," and "Punitive Pollys" who chose alcoholics to satisfy their own neurotic needs. (Never mind that the wives of nondrinkers might have these same "neuroses.") Such women, it was claimed, actually deteriorated when their husbands stopped drinking. They were "enablers"—that is, they secretly wanted their husbands to drink. They tried to "take over" if their husbands entered a hospital. In short, their misery was their own fault. But as scientific investigation later showed, the wives of alcoholics had personalities of all types. They were no more likely to be dysfunctional than other wives. And they actually felt better if their husbands quit drinking.

Nevertheless, as one feminist scholar, Betty Tallen, has written, "codendency accurately describes what many of us experience in our lives"—namely, what many women experience as wives, lovers, or children of alcoholics. But, as she also points out, the literature of codependency holds that you cannot control the behavior of the addicted person—indeed, that you cannot even criticize this behavior. Thus, according to adherents of this theory, families of alcoholics cannot even hold them responsible for the abuse. Somehow the victim must get well by dint of pure self-analysis, meditation, and prayer without reference to the social, economic, legal, and psychological forces that create dysfunctional families in the first place.

The truth is that very little is known about the psychological dynamics of families of alcoholics or other addicts. The literature of codependency is based on assertions, generalizations, and anecdotes. Of course, self-treatment for addicts or their families has been a largely positive development, and some people have no doubt been helped by thinking of themselves as codependents. Yet, as a recent article in the *Journal of Studies on Alcohol* reports, such labeling can be beneficial—or destructive. To start without the slightest shred of scientific evidence and casually label large groups as diseased may be helpful to a few, but it is potentially harmful and exploitive as well.

Source: Excerpted and adapted with permission from the University of California at Berkeley Wellness Letter © Health Letter Associates, 1990. To order a subscription, please call 800-829-9170.

Wolin, a family therapist, suggests that these children are able to reframe their parents' drinking and its consequences as a challenge. These children survive in three ways: (1) marrying into nonalcoholic families, (2) distancing themselves from their parents, or (3) creating their own family rituals to replace the disastrous childhood attempts at holidays, family dinners, and vacations. They enter adulthood armed with emotional strengths and valuable career-oriented skills.

Codependency

A **codependent** has been described as a person whose self-worth is based on another person (or place or thing), and who becomes obsessed with or addicted to controlling that person (or place or thing). Codependents are unable to separate their own feelings from their partners'.

Codependency is often learned growing up in a family in which one or more members are addicts. The hallmark of codependency is **enabling:** any action, or lack of action, that allows someone else to continue addictive behavior. The habit of enabling prevents the addict's recovery because that person never has to experience the consequences of his or her behavior. It

codependent person whose self-worth is based on another person and who becomes obsessed with or addicted to controlling that person

enabling any action, or lack of action, that allows someone to continue addictive behavior

intervention planned process of confrontation with the intent to break down the denial of the addict

can take both active forms (making excuses, throwing away drugs) and passive forms (saying/doing nothing). For example, suppose your roommate phones your professor and says that you cannot take your exam because you are sick with the flu, when in reality you are extremely hung over. In this case, your roommate is enabling your drinking behavior by protecting you from its negative consequences.

Recovery from codependency begins with people accepting responsibility for their own behavior, regardless of whether the addict's behavior changes. Codependents have to learn that they did not cause the addiction, cannot control it, and cannot cure it. They also must learn to set limits and stick with them—for example, no longer riding in a car when a partner is drunk or on drugs and sticking with that decision regardless of what the partner says or threatens. In 1985, Codependents Anonymous was founded to provide support for those people experiencing problems maintaining healthy relationships. Counselors can also help by offering group, individual, or family therapy. (See the Myths and Controversies box.)

Strategies to Overcome an Addiction

The most difficult step for addicts to take is acknowledging they have a problem. Addicts typically use denial as a defensive mechanism to separate themselves from the painful reality of their actions. Addicts in denial are unable to see the truth and recognize the devastation their behavior is having on their life. The turning point is when addicts realize that they need and want help.

Intervention is a planned process of confrontation with the intent to break down the denial of the addict. Interventions are conducted by significant people in the life of the addict. The idea is to chip away at the addict's defenses until the person sees the problem. However, this must be done in a caring way, without attempting to punish the addict; otherwise, it can be dangerous or useless, or even making things worse. (See the Do's and Don'ts box.)

Treatment

Treatment strategies vary from addiction to addiction. Some addictions are more complicated to treat than others, especially long-standing ones. Both inpatient and outpatient treatment options are available for those with alcohol and substance addictions, and are becoming more common for people with food and sex addictions as well. Inpatient treatment programs appear to be most beneficial for addicts with multiple addictions, little social support, or a history of relapse. Combining individual counseling, group and family therapy, and education, and providing an aftercare program that involves some type of self-help support group appears to offer the addict the best chance for recovery.

Thousands of individuals currently follow programs base on AA's 12-step recovery program. These programs provide peer support and give recovering individuals a sense of purpose to continue with their life. Participants in these programs identify themselves by first name only and spend the meeting time

HELPING ◆ A ◆ LOVED ◆ ONE WITH ◆ AN ◆ ADDICTION

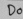

Do

▲ Provide information relevant to the addiction.

▲ Be supportive; the greatest gift you can give is a listening ear with no strings attached.

▲ Suggest that the addict get help, but be prepared for denial, resistance, and stubborn, sullen hostility.

▲ Try to convince the addict that recovery has more advantages than the disorder.

▲ Realize recovery is the addict's responsibility, not yours.

▲ Be kind to yourself; you are a good person doing the best you can.

Don't

▼ Nag, plead, beg, threaten, or manipulate; you will get stuck in a power struggle, and you will lose.

▼ Criticize or shame the addict, because he or she will withdraw.

▼ Pry or give advice unless asked.

▼ Overestimate what you can accomplish; you can provide support and encouragement, but you can't make people change when they don't want to.

sharing information about how their addiction has affected their lives. Program members are urged to place their faith and control of their lives in the hands of a "higher being" and to take life one day at a time.

The 12-step approach is now used for many addictions besides alcohol. Approximately 200 different types of programs are estimated to use AA's philosophical approach. These include Gamblers Anonymous, Sexaholics Anonymous, Debtors Anonymous, Workaholics Anonymous, Overeaters Anonymous, Narcotics Anonymous, Smokers Anonymous, and Cocaine Anonymous.

Not every 12-step meeting is the same. Because the person in recovery must feel comfortable with the group, he or she might have to try several groups before finding the right one. Many college campuses have 12-step programs that meet on a regular basis. The best way to find these groups is to contact the counseling center. Other 12-step groups typically advertise their meeting locations in local newspapers. In addition, many other types of support groups can be found through hospitals, clinics, and social service agencies. Check your local phone book and newspaper for meeting times and locations.

While there is no consensus on the "perfect" treatment, any form of treatment should have the same basic goals:

- To promote healthy physical and emotional functioning in everyday life

- To develop self-support, stress management, problem-solving, decision-making, and coping skills

- To maintain an adequate level of motivation and a desire to continue with the new behavior

- To build self-esteem

- To learn to deal positively with failure

- To provide support that reinforces new behavior

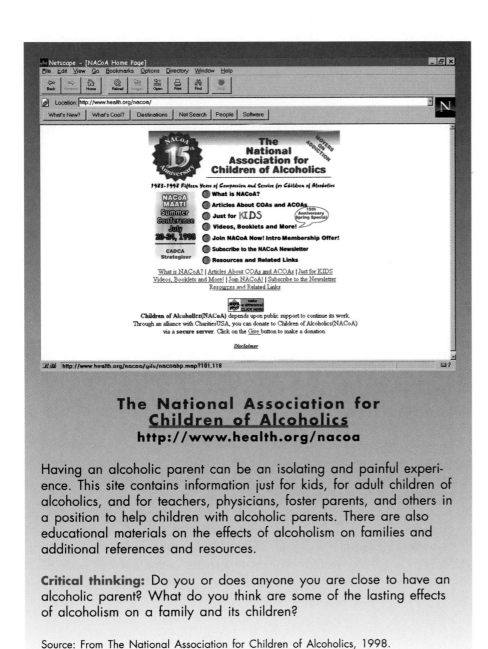

The National Association for Children of Alcoholics
http://www.health.org/nacoa

Having an alcoholic parent can be an isolating and painful experience. This site contains information just for kids, for adult children of alcoholics, and for teachers, physicians, foster parents, and others in a position to help children with alcoholic parents. There are also educational materials on the effects of alcoholism on families and additional references and resources.

Critical thinking: Do you or does anyone you are close to have an alcoholic parent? What do you think are some of the lasting effects of alcoholism on a family and its children?

Source: From The National Association for Children of Alcoholics, 1998.

TABLE 11.5

A Six-Step Plan for Preventing Relapses

1. *Stop, look, and listen.* You must stop the rush of events or behavior and pay attention to your situation. If possible, retreat to a quiet place to contemplate what you are doing.

2. *Keep calm.* It doesn't pay to become guilty or to chastise yourself; these reactions only prompt more addictive behavior. Nor will panic help you get back on track.

3. *Renew your commitment.* Instead of giving up on your plan to stay non-addicted, now is the time to reassert your desire and your commitment to be free of the addiction. Remind yourself of your success up to this point.

4. *Make an immediate plan.* You had a plan for licking your addiction from which you temporarily departed. Start right now to map out how you will proceed from here.

5. *Ask or look for help.* Look for support from whomever you count on. Now is the time to turn to friends and helpers. In doing so, you will let them know that you are serious and that you don't want to let them down.

6. *Review the relapse situation.* After your slip, instead of punishing yourself, analyze the elements in the situation that created your slip. There is much to learn from this to avoid it in the future.

Source: From Marlatt and Gordon, 1985.

Relapse

Addicts are prone to high relapse rates. For example, people who have successfully quit smoking have probably tried to quit at least four times before achieving that success. Marlatt and Gordon report that roughly 60% of alcoholics relapse within 3 months of treatment, as do about 75% of cocaine addicts. In short, it is extremely difficult to break a pattern of behavior that has come to dominate a person's life.

The person seeking optimal wellness must not only confront the addiction but also guard against the tendency to relapse. There are four major reasons for relapse: (1) failure to recognize and control personality traits (such as compulsiveness, perfectionism, and passive aggressive tendencies), (2) a limited view of recovery and the belief that all that is needed is weekly attendance at an AA or other support group meeting, (3) the tendency to substitute one addiction for another, and (4) the inability to avoid environmental factors that have fostered addictive behaviors in the past.

Relapse is best prevented when treatment programs target the weakness of an addicted individual and work to develop relevant coping strategies (see Table 11.5). Recovery work must include a strong commitment to self-discovery, improved self-esteem, and personal growth. Without this commitment to these important aspects of wellness, long-term recovery is unlikely.

Lifestyle Choices: Plan for Action

What role, if any, does substance use play in your life? Remember that a person does not have to be an addict to be an abuser of substances. An analysis of whether you or someone you know is abusing a substance is just as important as trying to ascertain whether someone has an addictive relationship with a substance. The following questions are designed to point out symptoms of abuse.

- Have you ever though you couldn't have a good time or fit in without using substances like alcohol, tobacco, or drugs?

- Do you avoid friends or family members when you are trying to use a substance?

- Have you noticed frequent mood swings ranging from withdrawal to angry flare-ups?

- Has your school or job performance been affected by your substance use?

- Has anyone ever told you that you should cut down on your substance use?

- Have you ever tried to stop or control your substance use?

- Do you ever tell yourself you can stop using substances whenever you want to?

- Do you continue to use substances despite negative consequences?

- Do you continue to use alcohol, tobacco, or drugs even though you are aware of the dangers they may pose to your health?

- Have you ever felt physical or psychological discomfort when trying to quit using substances?

If you answered yes to any of these questions, you may need help for substance abuse. If you do not have a problem with alcohol, tobacco, or drugs, review the process addictions covered in this chapter and consider whether any of them pose a problem for you.

Summary

Addiction is a difficult concept to define because there are so many different types of addiction and theories of causation. The complex interrelationships among your physiological makeup and family, social, and environmental influences all play a part in determining your susceptibility to developing an addiction. Learning to recognize your own limitations, make responsible choices, and set limits can help you manage your level of psychological wellness.

Key concepts that you have learned in this chapter include these:

- Approximately 85% of college students drink alcohol and 44% of students binge drink.

- Two-thirds of all Americans are classified as drinkers.

- Many factors affect the rate of absorption of alcohol into the bloodstream.

- Alcohol is the number one cause of mental retardation in the Western world.

- Alcoholism involves extensive problems with alcohol, usually involving tolerance, dependence, and withdrawal.

- Smoking is the largest preventable cause of ill health and death in the United States.

- The majority of smokers who quit, quit "cold turkey."

- Caffeine is probably the drug most commonly used in our society.

- Caffeinism is a toxic reaction to the overconsumption of caffeine.

- Marijuana is the illicit drug most commonly used in the United States.

- Marijuana in low doses usually causes euphoria and a relaxed attitude; very high doses may produce feelings of depersonalization and sensory distortion.

- Cocaine is a central nervous system stimulant. It produces an intense sense of euphoria. It can be sniffed, snorted, or injected.

- Amphetamines are a group of synthetic chemicals also called central nervous system stimulants.

- "Crank" and "ice" are both forms of methamphetamine, an inexpensive alternative to crack cocaine.

- Heroin is a highly addictive narcotic that depresses the central nervous system.

- LSD is one of the most commonly known psychedelic drugs. Its effects on the user include an altered sense of time, disorders of vision, and changes in mood.

- Everyone has the potential for becoming an addict.

- Aspects of drug addiction that can also be applied to process addictions include tolerance, withdrawal, dependence, and craving.

- All addictions share certain behavioral criteria: compulsion, loss of control, continued involvement, denial, cessation or control of abuse, and the tendency to relapse.

- Theories that have been developed to explain the origin of addiction include the disease model, the biological model, and the psychosocial model.

- Environmental factors that can contribute to addictive tendencies include life stresses, family and peer relationships, social and cultural mores, and media messages.

- The most common addictive substances are alcohol, drugs, nicotine, and caffeine.

- Common process addictions include exercise, gambling, spending and borrowing, and sex.

- Families that are emotionally unhealthy are called dysfunctional.

References

American Cancer Society. Facts on Lung Cancer, 1996, 5.

American Heart Association, American Cancer Association, and American Lung Association. *Smoke-Free Class of 2000 Facts.* Dallas: American Heart Association, 1995.

Anderson, D. *Breaking the Tradition on College Campuses: Reducing Drug and Alcohol Misuse.* Fairfax, VA: George Mason University, 1994.

Bradshaw, J. *The Family.* Deerfield Beach, FL: Health Communications, 1987, 6.

Cigar smoking among teenagers—United States, Massachusetts, and New York, 1996. *Morbidity and Mortality Weekly,* 46(20), 1997.

Eigen, L. D. Alcohol practices, policies, and potentials of American colleges and universities. *Office of Substance Abuse and Prevention White Paper,* 1991.

Liska, K. *Drugs and the Human body, with Implications for Society,* 3rd ed. New York: Macmillan, 1990, 306–307.

Marlatt, G. A. Cognitive assessment and intervention procedures for relapse prevention. In G. A. Marlatt and J. R. Gordon, eds., *Relapse Prevention.* New York: Guilford Press, 1985, Table 4.2.

Marlatt, G. A. and J. R. Gordon. *Relapse Prevention.* New York: Guilford Press, 1985.

McMurray, R. G. Rethinking the high in the runner's high. *Psychology Today,* 18(5): 8, May 1984.

National Clearinghouse for Alcohol and Drug Information. *The Fact Is . . .* Rockville, MD: National Clearinghouse, n.d.

Prochaska, J. O., and C. C. DiClemente. Toward a comprehensive model of change. In W. R. Miller and H. Heather, eds., *Treating Addictive Behaviors.* New York: Plenum Press, 1986, 25.

Roots of addiction. *Newsweek,* 20 February 1989.

Schrof, J. Pumped up. *U.S. News & World Report,* 1 June 1992, 56–58.

Sommers, I. Pathological gambling: Estimating prevalence and group characteristics. *International Journal of Addictions,* 23: 477–490, 1988.

Thoren, P., and J. S. Floras. Endorphins and exercise: Physiological mechanisms and clinical implications. *Medicine and Science in Sports and Exercise,* 22(4): 417–428, 1990.

U.S. Department of Health and Human Services, Public Health Service. *Healthy People 2000,* National Health Promotion and Disease Prevention Objectives. Washington, DC: U.S. Government Printing Office, 1990a.

U.S. Department of Health and Human Services. *Seventh Special Report to Congress on Alcohol and Health.* Washington, DC: U.S. Government Printing Office, 1990b, 22–24, 44.

U.S. Department of Health and Human Services: NIAAA Alcohol Alert, No. 13 (PH 297). Washington, DC; U.S. Government Printing Office, July 1991.

U.S. Department of Health and Human Services. *Injury Control Update,* 1(1): 13, 1996.

Wechsler, H., G. W. Dowdall, A. Davenport, and W. DeJong. Binge drinking on campus: Results of a national study. *Bulletin Series,* Center for Alcohol and Other Drug Prevention, 1996.

Wechsler, H., G. W. Dowdall, A. Davenport, and W. DeJong. Health and behavioral consequences of binge drinking in college. *Journal of the American Medical Association,* 272 (21): 1672–1677, 1994.

Welles, C. American's gambling fever: Everybody wants a piece of the action—but is it good for us? *Business Week,* 112, 24 April 1989.

Wolin, S. J., and S. Wolin. *The Resilient Self.* New York: Dillard, 1993, 97.

Yates, A., K. Leehey, and C. M. Shisslak. Running an analogue of anorexia? *New England Journal of Medicine,* 308: 253, 1983.

Yoder, B. *The Recovery Resource Book.* New York: Simon & Schuster, 1990, 2,3, 32, 59, 128.

Laboratory 11.1

Assessing Your Level of Alcohol Use

Having the facts is only part of making careful decisions about alcohol use. Analyze your attitudes and behavior by answering the following self-assessment questions.

1. Are you unable to stop drinking after a certain number of drinks?

2. Do you need a drink to get motivated?

3. Do you often forget what happened while you were "partying" (have blackouts)?

4. Do you drink or "party" alone?

5. Have others annoyed you by criticizing your alcohol use?

6. Have you been involved in fights with your friends or family while you were drunk or high?

7. Have you done or said anything while drinking that you later regretted?

8. Have you destroyed or damaged property while drinking?

9. Do you drive while high or drunk?

10. Have you been physically hurt while drinking?

11. Have you been in trouble with the school authorities or the campus police because of your drinking?

12. Have you dropped or chosen friends based on their drinking habits?

13. Do you think you are a normal drinker despite friends' comments that you drink too much?

14. Have you ever missed classes because you were too hungover to get up on time?

15. Have you ever done poorly on an exam or assignment because of drinking?

16. Do you think about drinking or getting high a lot?

17. Do you feel guilty or self-conscious about your drinking?

If you answered "yes" to three or more of these questions, or if your answer to any of the questions concerns you, you may be using alcohol in ways that are harmful. Do not waste your time blaming yourself for past binges or any other alcohol-related behavior. If you think you have or might be developing problems in which drinking plays a part, act now. You can get help.

Source: From American College Health Association, 1988.

Laboratory 11.2
Rating Your Level of Exercise Addiction

On a scale of 1 to 10, with 10 being the strongest and 1 the weakest, give an objective weight to each of the following statements as they apply to you and your endurance fitness. Then total your numbers and check the ratings at the end of the test.

_____ 1. Aerobic fitness is important to me. I'm positive I'll be engaged in one or more endurance sports for the rest of my life.

_____ 2. I cannot go a day without an endurance workout.

_____ 3. If it becomes downright impossible to get my workout in today, I can always double up tomorrow.

_____ 4. Until I get my workout in, I am impossible to be around.

_____ 5. A little pain proves there's progress being made.

_____ 6. If 5 hours of exercise per week is good, 10 hours is twice as good.

_____ 7. Warm-up and cool-down are important, but it's what comes in the middle of a workout that counts.

_____ 8. As far as endurance training goes, more is always better.

_____ 9. One of my favorite topics of discussion is my workouts.

_____ 10. Regularity at any cost is the key to all fitness.

_____ 11. If I can't run for an hour it is not worth going at all.

_____ 12. I feel most comfortable with myself when I'm running.

_____ 13. You're not a real runner until you've done a marathon.

_____ 14. Rest is for the weary, not for the strong.

_____ 15. Triathlons are important because they allow you to do more training with impunity.

_____ 16. To be the best you can possibly be is what's most important in life.

_____ 17. A person who has nothing to prove has already made a point.

_____ 18. If you don't even try, you have already lost.

_____ 19. Relaxation is OK after you have completed your workout.

_____ 20. It is best never to miss a workout.

_____ TOTAL

Evaluation

20–40   Very few people involved in aerobic activities are likely to score in this category.

41–80   A person who pursues aerobic fitness according to the minimum recommended requirements and who maintains fitness strictly for the health benefits is likely to fall into this category.

81–120   This range is neutral. It includes people who occasionally increase their training to take part in a particular event or increase their training when the weather improves.

121–160   Most aerobic athletes fall into this category. They are involved in fitness for more than health benefits and they regularly pursue competitive goals.

161–200   At this level one's commitment to aerobic activities and sports tends to cross over into obsessive and compulsive behavior. Aerobic training becomes more important than anything else in life. It is the focal point of each day.

Source: From Benyo, 1990.

Laboratory 11.3

Assessing Your Gambling Behavior

The following are some questions you should ask yourself if you feel you may have a problem with gambling. These are the Twenty Questions of Gamblers Anonymous.

1. Do you lose time from work or school due to gambling?
2. Does gambling make your home life unhappy?
3. Does gambling affect your reputation?
4. Do you ever feel remorse after gambling?
5. Do you ever gamble to get money with which to pay debts or otherwise solve financial difficulties?
6. Does gambling cause a decrease in your ambition or efficiency?
7. After losing, do you have a strong urge to return and win more?
8. After a win, do you have a strong urge to return and win more?
9. Do you often gamble until your last dollar is gone?
10. Do you ever borrow to finance your gambling?
11. Do you ever sell anything to finance gambling?
12. Are you reluctant to use "gambling money" for normal expenditures?
13. Does gambling make you careless about the welfare of your family?
14. Do you ever gamble longer than you planned?
15. Do you ever gamble to escape worry or trouble?
16. Do you ever commit, or consider committing, an illegal act to finance your gambling?
17. Does gambling cause you to have difficulties sleeping?
18. Do arguments, disappointments, or frustrations create within you an urge to gamble?
19. Do you have an urge to celebrate good fortune by a few hours of gambling?
20. Do you ever consider self-destruction as a result of your gambling?

If you answer "yes" to at least seven (7) of the twenty questions you could have a compulsive gambling problem.

Source: From Gamblers Anonymous, Inc.

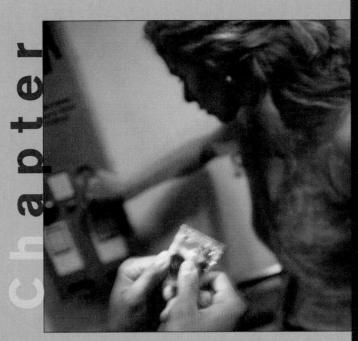

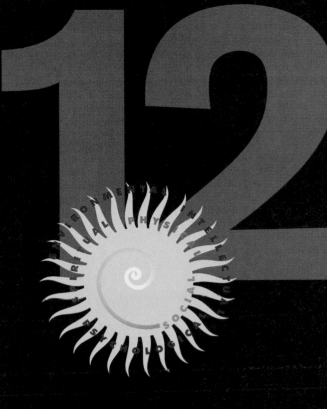

chapter

12

AIDS and STDs

One Student's View

Today it is more important than ever before to be careful in sexual relationships. Before you're even with your significant other, you have to set boundaries for yourself as far as what type of behavior you are willing to participate in. If you choose to be open to the possibility of sex of any kind, it is up to you to provide yourself with protection. You can't rely upon the other person to show up with a condom, so protect yourself.

—Catherine Arnold

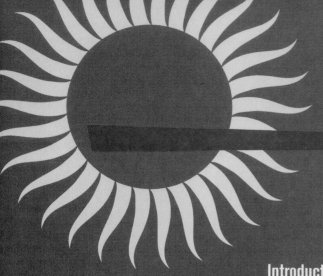

Introduction

Sexually active individuals today face risks to their health and well-being that previous generations seldom had to consider. Our parents may have worried about getting pregnant or contracting a venereal disease if they had sex. If they did pick up such a disease, however, they were confident they could be treated and, barring complications, cured. Now, with the rapid spread of human immunodeficiency virus (HIV) and acquired immune deficiency syndrome (AIDS) and the epidemic incidence of other sexually transmitted diseases (STDs), things have changed. As we enter a new century, every sexually active person must be aware of the possibility of contracting a serious illness—one that could lead to sterility, chronic pain and disfigurement, and even death.

In this chapter you will find answers to some basic questions about STDs. You may be wondering, for example, how a single adult might form a healthy, relatively risk-free intimate relationship. Which STDs should you be most concerned about? Can you protect yourself on a date without carrying a flashlight, rubber gloves, and a magnifying glass to detect suspicious sores, bumps, and/or discharges? Do you need to have a box of condoms, spermicides, and antibacterial creams and lotions in case you decide to go beyond a simple goodnight kiss? Is there such a thing as "safe" sex, even in the most committed relationship? Is all the recent concern about AIDS and other STDs justifiable, or is it just media hype?

In this chapter you will learn about the symptoms, diagnosis, and treatment for the most common STDs, including those that are caused by bacteria and those that are caused by viruses. You will also learn ways in which you can significantly

Objectives

After reading this chapter, you should be able to

■ **Define what is meant by sexually transmitted diseases (STDs) and explain why these diseases have reached epidemic proportions in the United States**

■ **Identify the main high-risk behaviors that increase your risk of acquiring an STD**

■ **Describe the basic functions of your immune system and other ways that your body defends itself against infection**

■ **Name the most common types of pathogens and identify which of these can cause STDs**

■ **Identify the four most common types of bacterially caused STDs and the three most common types of virally caused STDs, and describe the symptoms, diagnosis, and treatment for each**

■ **Explain the distinction between HIV and AIDS and describe how HIV is transmitted, what stages it progresses through, and how it is diagnosed and treated**

■ **Explain how you can use preventive strategies to decrease your chance of acquiring HIV or another type of STD**

reduce your risk of becoming infected. As you translate this knowledge into responsible action, you can greatly reduce your risks of contracting (or spreading) STDs, despite their prevalence in our society. If you want more information about any of these diseases, you can consult the resources listed at the end of the chapter.

The Epidemic of Sexually Transmitted Diseases (STDs)

More Americans are infected by STDs than ever before. Reports by the Centers for Disease Control and Prevention indicate that today one out of every six American adults has an STD. The economic burden of the STD epidemic is illustrated in Table 12.1. The statistics for young people are especially alarming: As many as 86% of all STDs occur among 15- to 29-year-olds.

Although most STDs can be cured if treated early in the infection cycle, these diseases should always be taken seriously. Without proper medical attention, some STDs can lead to severe and permanent damage such as blindness, cancer, heart disease, chronic pain, and even death (Eng and Butler). STDs are the main cause of preventable sterility in this country and also can cause serious complications during pregnancy, such as miscarriage, uterine infection, and premature delivery. Some of these diseases can also be transferred from a pregnant woman to her fetus during pregnancy, causing numerous problems for the newborn.

STDs and Overall Wellness

Sexually transmitted diseases (STDs), sometimes called *venereal diseases,* are infections contracted through sexual contact with an infected person. You may have gathered from media reports that AIDS and a few of the better-known STDs, such as herpes and syphilis, are the only ones you need to be concerned about, but over 25 different diseases are known to be spread through sexual contact. In fact, STDs are among the most common contagious diseases in the United States. The Centers for Disease Control and Prevention estimate that approximately 50% of Americans will contract at least one STD by the time they reach their thirties.

A number of factors explain the rapid spread of STDs (Crooks and Baur). Since the "sexual revolution" of the 1960s, sexual activity has increased among young people, the group most frequently affected by STDs. Casual attitudes toward sexuality as well as a tendency to have a greater

TABLE 12.1

Annual Direct and Indirect Costs of Major STDs in the United States

Selected Major STDs	$10 billion
STDs and HIV infections	$17 billion

Source: Institute of Medicine, 1996.

sexually transmitted diseases (STDs) infections contracted through sexual contact with an infected person

number of sex partners have provided more opportunities for the spread of disease. Furthermore, because STDs are not always accompanied by obvious symptoms, many people pass the disease on without ever knowing that they themselves have been infected. Changing trends in contraceptive use may also be a factor. Birth control pills, now used more often than condoms or vaginal spermicides, do not provide even the limited protection against STDs offered by these more traditional methods.

If you consider the factors that make STDs a growing health problem, you can easily see how these diseases affect all the components of wellness. Whereas the diseases themselves affect your physical health, your patterns of social interaction influence your likelihood of contracting an STD. From a psychological standpoint, if you are feeling emotionally balanced and secure, you will be less likely to engage in high-risk behavior without weighing all the consequences. Becoming educated about STDs (which might be considered an aspect of your intellectual wellness) can make a significant difference in your overall wellness levels. If you take the time to become informed about the risks of STDs, you will be in a better position to make appropriate choices to reduce your risks. And passing this information along to others who are less informed can contribute to a healthier environment for all of us.

Risk Factors for STDs

STDs are spread primarily through intimate sexual contact with an infected person. Vaginal intercourse, oral-genital contact, and anal intercourse are the most common ways of spreading these diseases. In rare instances, STDs may

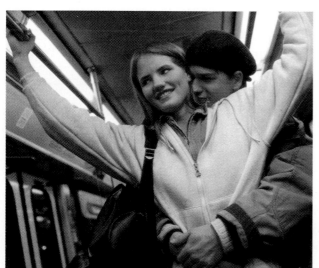

Intimate sexual contact with an infected person greatly increases your risk for being infected with an STD.

be spread through deep kissing and through contact with body sores. Some STDs also can be transmitted from mother to fetus, as mentioned previously, or through blood transfusions.

It is possible to have more than one STD at a time. In fact, being infected with one STD can significantly increase your risk for HIV infection. Each of the over 25 different types of STDs is caused by a specific **pathogen,** or disease-causing agent, has a different pattern of symptoms and prognosis, and requires a different type of treatment. Therefore, receiving treatment for one type of STD does not necessarily mean that a second infection will also be cured. Typically, bodily fluids, including semen, vaginal secretions, and blood, are the routes of pathogen transmission.

These pathogens do not discriminate. STDs can affect people from all socioeconomic levels, ages, ethnic and racial groups, and geographic regions. Whether you are a male or a female, or heterosexual, bisexual, or homosexual, you are at increased risk for an STD if you engage in high-risk behaviors such as the following:

■ *Having sexual intercourse with multiple partners or with persons who have had sex with multiple partners.* The more partners you have, the less likely you are to know fully about their sexual histories. Furthermore, if each of them has had many partners, your risk increases proportionately.

■ *Having unprotected sex.* Research has shown that blood and semen, and vaginal, cervical, and anal secretions are highly infectious for most STDs, particularly HIV. Saliva, clear fluids from sores and wounds, and other body secretions have been implicated in HIV transmission but typically are considered to be high-risk fluids only for less serious STDs. Although no form of protection against STDs is foolproof, using condoms and pathogen-killing spermicides make sex safer for those involved (see Table 12.2).

- *Taking drugs intravenously.* Some STDs also can be transmitted through the sharing of infected needles. Drug use in which there is an exchange of body fluids from shared needles has been demonstrated to be a high-risk behavior for HIV as well as some forms of hepatitis.

- *Using alcohol or other drugs to excess.* Excessive alcohol or drug consumption can reduce users' inhibitions, which in turn can lead to an increased likelihood of negative sexual outcomes, including STDs.

Although these high-risk behaviors may predispose you toward a variety of STDs, other factors also play an important role in determining individual risk. Perhaps the greatest factor that influences susceptibility to disease is the overall health of your immune system. In general, the healthier you are, the better your body systems are able to defend against invaders. Use Laboratory 12.1 to assess your risk for STDs and HIV.

The Body's Defense System

Every minute of every day, there are millions of pathogens resting on the surfaces of the skin and the body openings, waiting for an easy mode of entry. The vast majority of them die, are killed by environmental conditions, or are destroyed by specific disease-fighting agents in the body. Numerous physical, chemical, and immunological defenses protect us against these invaders.

Physical and Chemical Defenses. Perhaps the single most important early defense system is the skin itself. Layered to provide an intricate web of barriers, our skin allows few pathogens to enter. Only if there are cracks or breaks in the skin can pathogens gain easy access to the body.

The linings of the body provide another method of protection. Mucous membranes found in the respiratory tract and other linings of the body trap and engulf invading organisms through the action of specific enzymes. Cilia—hairlike projections found in the lungs and respiratory tract—move in a waving action to sweep unwanted invaders from their space. Tears, ear wax,

TABLE 12.2	
Choose Your Own Thoughts	
EXCUSE	**REALITY**
Safer sex reduces sexual pleasure.	We'll feel more relaxed, have more peace of mind, and thus enjoy sex more.
Condoms are not a guarantee against HIV/STDs, so why bother?	Condoms are the best protection available for anal/vaginal sex.
My partner may think I don't trust him/her.	This shows I care for myself as well as my partner.
Putting on a condom interrupts sex.	Putting on a condom can be an erotic process.

pathogens
disease-causing agents

The spread of sexually transmitted diseases like AIDS has led to billboard campaigns to advertise the importance of safe sex.

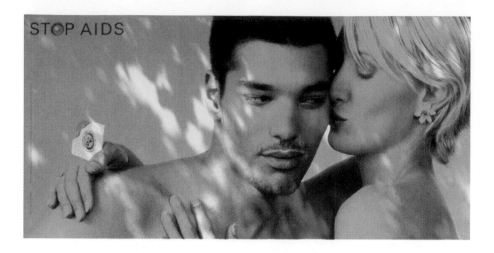

STOP AIDS

and nasal and other secretions found at body entrances contain enzymes, organic substances designed to destroy or neutralize invading pathogens.

The Immune System. If a pathogen is able to survive the initial lines of defense, it faces an even more complex and specialized network of defenses. The **immune system** is the body's natural defense mechanism against a variety of invading substances, such as bacteria, viruses, fungi, and protozoa. Unless the body can protect itself against these pathogens, they can multiply, often very rapidly, and cause disease.

A key property of the immune system is its ability to distinguish foreign substances from the body's own, healthy molecules. Any molecule capable of triggering an immune response is called an **antigen** (short for "antibody generating"). Antigens can be found on viruses, bacteria, fungi, or parasites as well as on the surface of cells within the body that have ingested pathogens or on cells from another individual.

When the body is invaded, it responds by forming substances called **antibodies,** highly specialized proteins that are matched to the specific antigen, much like a key to a lock. Once an antigen breaches the initial body defenses, the body begins a process of antigen analysis. In this process of **humoral immunity,** the body considers the size and shape of the invader, verifies that the antigen is not part of the "self," and begins to produce a specific antibody to destroy or weaken the antigen. This process takes place primarily in the bodily fluids and represents an indirect (that is, through the action of antibodies) defense mechanism.

Cell-mediated immunity, on the other hand, involves the launching of a more direct attack against invading pathogens at the cellular level. It is characterized by the formation of **lymphocytes,** white blood cells that can attack and destroy foreign substances.

Two types of lymphocytes in particular play a role in the immune response. *B-lymphocytes (B-cells)* are primarily involved in humoral immunity, whereas *T-lymphocytes (T-cells)* are involved in cell-mediated immunity. Different types of T-cells help your immune system in a variety of ways.

Some T-cells, known as *helper T-cells,* direct the activities of the immune system and help other cells to mount an immune response. These cells are essential for activating B-cells and other T-cells as well as *macrophages* (white blood cells). Another type of T-cell, called a *killer T-cell,* directly attacks infected or malignant cells and helps the body get rid of these unwanted cells.

immune system body's natural defense mechanisms against a variety of invading substances, such as bacteria, viruses, fungi, and protozoa

antigen any molecule capable of triggering an immune response

antibodies highly specialized proteins formed by the body that are matched to specific antigens

humoral immunity process whereby the body considers the size and shape of an invader, verifies that the antigen is not part of the "self," and begins to produce a specific antibody to destroy or weaken the antigen

cell-mediated immunity launching of a more direct attack against invading pathogens right at the cellular level

lymphocytes white blood cells that can attack and destroy foreign substances

After an initial attack by a pathogen, some T- and B-cells remain as *memory T- and B-cells,* enabling the body to quickly recognize and respond to subsequent attacks by the same organism. For this reason, once you have survived some types of infectious disease, you become *immune*—meaning that you will probably not develop that disease again.

Immunizations have been developed for many infectious diseases as a way to create immunity for people without their ever having to experience the illness. Although many infectious diseases can be prevented through immunizations, vaccinations are unfortunately not available for most STDs. Even more important, your body does not provide lasting immunity to these diseases. This means that you can catch them over and over again, each time you are exposed.

The Invaders. If you are in good health, observe proper sanitation habits, practice sensible dietary and exercise regimens, get enough rest, control undue stress, and avoid toxic substances that may weaken your defenses, your likelihood of getting an infectious disease is greatly reduced. However, if your immune system is weakened, or if you are exposed to powerful pathogens, your chances of becoming ill are greatly increased. The most common forms of pathogens affecting people of all ages today are these:

- *Bacteria.* Single-celled organisms that are not visible to the naked eye, bacteria can cause any number of serious diseases. Fortunately, bacterial diseases are among the most readily treatable, using a wide array of drugs called antibiotics. Bacterially caused STDs discussed in this chapter include gonorrhea, syphilis, chlamydia, and chancroid (see Figure 12.la).

- *Viruses.* Parasitic organisms approximately one five-hundredth the size of bacteria, viruses cause infections that are difficult to treat due to an extremely limited pharmaceutical arsenal. Treatment for many viruses is *palliative,* meaning that physicians are able to treat only the symptoms rather than actually destroying the virus. Virally caused STDs discussed in this chapter include herpes, hepatitis B, genital warts, and HIV (see Figure 12.lb).

- *Fungi.* Hundreds of species of fungi inhabit our environment—from those that are multicellular, such as molds, to those that are unicellular, such as yeasts. Most fungi serve useful purposes in the environment, but many cause infections on entering the human body. The skin, mucous membranes, and respiratory tract are particularly susceptible to these pathogens. Vaginal yeast infections are caused by fungi: They may be transmitted sexually, although generally they are not (see Figure 12.1c).

- *Protozoa.* Microscopic, single-celled organisms, protozoa are generally associated with tropical diseases, such as malaria and African sleeping sickness. Trichomoniasis is caused by a protozoan type of parasite called Trichomonas vaginalis. Trichomoniasis is the most common parasitic STD in the United States (see Figure 12.ld).

Regardless of the type of pathogen that attacks the human body, several conditions conducive to infection must be present for disease to occur. First, the pathogen must be virulent enough to overcome the host's defenses and proliferate (multiply). Second, the host's immune system must be compromised in some manner so that the defenses are not strong enough to ward off infection. Finally, the environment itself must be such that the organism

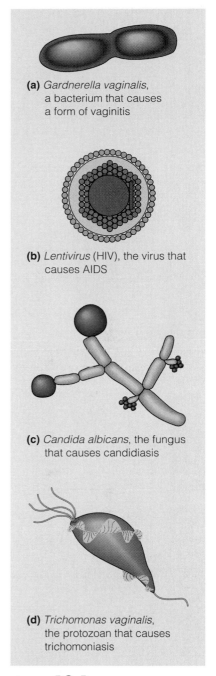

(a) *Gardnerella vaginalis,* a bacterium that causes a form of vaginitis

(b) *Lentivirus* (HIV), the virus that causes AIDS

(c) *Candida albicans,* the fungus that causes candidiasis

(d) *Trichomonas vaginalis,* the protozoan that causes trichomoniasis

Figure 12.1

The four most common forms of pathogens affecting people are **(a)** bacteria, **(b)** viruses, **(c)** fungi, and **(d)** protozoa.

is able to proliferate. For example, the pathogens that cause STDs thrive in warm, dark, moist body surfaces, such as those found in the membranes of the reproductive organs.

In the following sections, we examine the patterns of infection characteristic of the most common STDs. However, there are some general warning signs that may indicate the presence of infection. Some of these signs are particular to women, some to men; others are common to both sexes (see Table 12.3). If you or your partner notices any of the signs or symptoms listed in Table 12.3, seek medical attention. The steps to follow are outlined in Table 12.4. As always, be vigilant in protecting yourself and your partner from transmitting any possible infection. Remember, too, that not all STDs have observable signs or symptoms such as those listed in Table 12.3.

Bacterially Caused STDs

Although many bacterially caused STDs are treatable, the passage of time has produced some extremely virulent strains of "super bugs" that have become resistant to modern medicine. Some mimic minor ailments common among adults and therefore often go untreated for long periods. Others have mutated to the point that even the most powerful pharmaceutical weapons are unable to bring them under control.

Gonorrhea

Although the overall incidence of gonorrhea, popularly known as "the clap," has declined in the past two decades, it is still among the most prevalent STDs in the United States today. Although 326,000 new cases of gonorrhea were reported in 1996, this disease is believed to be seriously underreported by family physicians. According to the Centers for Disease Control and Prevention, a more accurate estimate would be one million new cases annually.

Underreporting of gonorrhea cases may be in part because most women and some men are *asymptomatic* (have no visible or noticeable symptoms) during the early stages of infection. In fact, about four women in five are asymptomatic and therefore less likely to seek treatment than men (Nevid). Even without symptoms, however, gonorrhea is transmissible to other sexual partners. For people who are sexually active, other risk factors for gonorrhea include low socioeconomic status, urban residence, ethnic minority status, early onset of sexual activity, and previous history of an STD.

The *Neisseria gonorrhea,* a bacterial pathogen, primarily infects the linings of the urethra, genital tract, pharynx, and rectum. **Gonorrhea** may be spread to other body areas, such as the eyes, anus, or rectum, by the hands or through exchanges of bodily fluids. If untreated for a long time, this disease may also spread to the prostate, testicles, bladder, and kidneys in men, and to the ovaries and fallopian tubes in women, leading to sterility. In some cases, it may also be spread to newborn babies, in whom it can be particularly damaging to the eyes. In rare cases, gonorrhea can enter the bloodstream and spread throughout the body, invading the heart, liver, and brain.

Symptoms. The *incubation period* (time between the initial infection and the development of symptoms) for gonococcal infection in men is usu-

gonorrhea bacterial STD that commonly affects the linings of the urethra, genital tract, pharynx, and rectum

TABLE 12.3

Signs or Symptoms of STDs

MEN AND WOMEN

■ Sores, bumps, or blisters near the sex organs, rectum, or mouth

■ Burning or pain during urination

■ Swelling or redness in the throat

■ Fever, chills, and aches

■ Swelling in the area around the sexual organs

WOMEN ONLY

■ Unusual discharge or smell from the vagina

■ Pain in the pelvic (lower belly) area or deep inside the vagina during sex

■ Burning or itching around the vagina

■ Bleeding from the vagina other than during regular menstrual periods

MEN ONLY

■ A drip or discharge from the penis

TABLE 12.4

Personal Action: What to Do if You Have Contracted an STD

■ Consult with your physician or health professional as early as possible.

■ Take all medication as directed.

■ Educate yourself about the infection.

■ Notify sexual partners who may have infected you or whom you may have infected.

■ Abstain from sexual contact during an active infection.

■ Seek support for emotional problems.

■ Pay attention to your general health.

ally 1 to 5 days, but may be up to 2 weeks. About 60% of those infected experience *dysuria* (painful or difficult urination) and a profuse, pus-laden discharge from the penis. Some men have little discharge, however, and others may have no discharge at all. If untreated, these symptoms will disappear after a few weeks; this is no guarantee, however, that the disease has been defeated by the immune system. Only in rare cases does the immune system eradicate gonorrhea without medical treatment.

For females, the incubation period is longer, usually 6 to 10 days. Early symptoms include inflammation of the cervix, which can produce a green or yellow discharge. The majority of women either have no symptoms of the disease or overlook their symptoms. Many women do not show symptoms until the following menstrual period, when they may experience chronic pain or other symptoms due to acute inflammation of the pelvis (see the section on pelvic inflammatory disease).

Diagnosis. For gonorrhea to be diagnosed, a sample of the discharge is examined in a laboratory. Cultures also may be taken from other potentially infected sites for more conclusive evaluation. For example, it is important to examine cultures from the throats and anuses of people who have engaged in oral-genital sex or anal intercourse because infections at these sites are often asymptomatic. Persons who are sexually active with multiple partners can request that they be examined for gonorrhea during routine physical examinations, even if symptoms are not present.

Treatment. Historically, penicillin was the treatment of choice for persons infected with gonococcal bacteria. Over time, however, penicillin-resistant strains of the gonococcal bacteria have made this treatment less effective. Today, treatment may involve such drugs as tetracycline (for those who are allergic to penicillin or who also have another bacterially caused STD) or, more commonly, spectinomycin, cefixime, or ceftriaxone. Since 1989, a single intramuscular injection of ceftriaxone has been considered the treatment of choice for eradicating gonorrhea.

Regardless of the drug regimen prescribed, afflicted individuals must follow recommended procedures carefully to ensure that the bacteria have been completely destroyed. Most antibiotic regimens are prescribed in *therapeutic doses,* meaning that only the minimal amount of a drug needed to obtain the desired results is given. Failure to comply with this minimal regimen often means that the bacteria will continue to spread as well as infect others. Because disappearance of the symptoms of gonorrhea does not necessarily mean that all bacteria have been eradicated, it is important to get a negative culture 3 to 7 days after completing the cycle of antibiotics.

Syphilis

Syphilis has been described in one form or another throughout history; people from biblical and ancient Roman times, the royal families of the Old World, and historical figures in the United States have all reportedly been afflicted with the disease. After peaking in the United States after World War II, syphilis rates began to rise again in the 1970s. This increase was short-lived, and rates began to decline again after 1982, largely as a consequence of changing lifestyles and the adoption of less risky sexual practices among bisexuals and homosexuals due to widespread concern over the AIDS epidemic. However, syphilis rates have risen substantially among heterosexuals since 1986. The increased rate in this population, especially in urban areas, is ostensibly due to the rise in illicit drug use, particularly crack cocaine, and the frequent exchange of sexual services for drugs. The increasing rate of syphilis among adults has been followed by an alarming increase in congenital syphilis in many urban areas.

Symptoms. Syphilis is caused by a corkscrew-shaped spirochete (bacterium) known as the *Treponema pallidum,* which thrives in dark, moist areas. It is transmitted through contact with bacteria-laden mucus from these areas. Fortunately, the organism is fairly fragile and dies quickly on exposure to air and temperature extremes. As a result, transmission from toilet seats and other, similar types of contact is virtually impossible.

syphilis bacterial STD characterized by four stages: primary, secondary, late, and tertiary

The incubation period for the disease is 10 days to 3 months, with an average of 3 weeks. Generally, untreated syphilis consists of four stages: primary, secondary, latent, and tertiary.

Primary syphilis begins at the site where the bacteria entered the body. There the organism multiplies and a tissue reaction called a *chancre* develops. About the size of a dime, the chancre is painless and oozing with bacteria. Typically, this chancre appears 3 to 4 weeks after infection, although it may not appear at all. Chancres can occur at any site where bacteria break through the body's defenses; the penis and vagina are common sites, and the throat, mouth, breast, and anus are less common ones. The chancre usually heals without treatment 1 to 5 weeks after it first appears. Even though the person may have no symptoms, the disease can be transmitted to others.

Secondary syphilis occurs 1 to 12 months after the chancre disappears. Symptoms include a rash; white patches on the skin and the mucous membranes of the mouth, throat, or genitals; hair loss; lymph node enlargement; fever; and headache. Because many of these symptoms are similar to those caused by other ailments, they are often overlooked. Even without treatment, these symptoms usually resolve themselves. Nevertheless, a person in this stage is highly infectious.

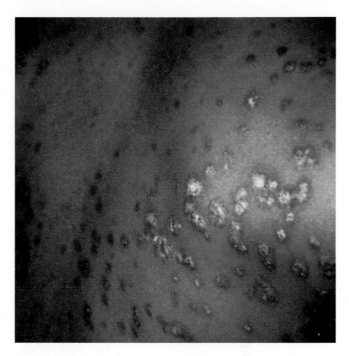

The characteristic body rash of secondary syphilis.

Latent syphilis occurs as the secondary stage symptoms disappear. The latent stage can last for many years, during which time the syphilis pathogens may or may not continue to multiply. During this stage the spirochetes begin to complete their destruction on an internal level. Occasionally, when the immune system is stressed as a result of other ailments, symptoms can recur. However, these usually are ignored as minor ailments.

Although the individual is no longer contagious after a year at this stage, fetal transmission can occur at any time. Death, blindness, deafness, and disfigurement are possible fetal consequences, particularly if the fetus is infected during the first trimester. Occasionally, the baby born to an infected mother shows no signs of the disease at birth but develops a rash, runny nose, or other problems weeks after birth.

Tertiary or late syphilis occurs 3 to 40 years after syphilis pathogens first enter the body. The health consequences can be very serious, including heart and central nervous system damage, blindness, deafness, paralysis, premature senility, severe mental disturbance, and death.

Diagnosis. Because the Treponema organism cannot be cultured, a sample of the chancre is viewed with a dark-field microscope during the primary stages. Similar procedures can be used for diagnosis during the secondary stage; in addition, blood samples can be checked to detect bacteria that have entered the bloodstream. As the disease progresses to the late stages, dark-field microscopic examination becomes difficult and a cerebrospinal fluid exam may be necessary.

Treatment. Treatment for all stages of syphilis is penicillin G. If the individual has had the disease for less than a year, a single dose may be sufficient. If the disease has been present for more than a year, the treatment is weekly injections of penicillin for 3 weeks. Those who are allergic to penicillin can take doxycycline, tetracycline, or erythromycin, usually for 2 weeks. The earlier a person obtains treatment, the greater is the likelihood of a complete cure. If the disease has damaged nervous tissue or other body organs, the residual effects may be lifelong. It is important to remember that not all antibiotic therapies work the first time. Undergoing a follow-up evaluation and abstaining from intimate relations for at least 1 month after treatment is an essential part of the treatment regimen.

Chlamydia

Chlamydia is the most frequently reported infectious disease in the United States and affects an estimated 4 million Americans each year (see Table 12.5). The rate of infection is highest among teenagers, especially girls. The organism is believed to infect over 10% of all college students and is at epidemic levels in many regions of the country. Accurate reports of the number of chlamydia cases are difficult to obtain because the disease is often asymptomatic and therefore infected persons do not seek treatment. As many as 80% of women infected and 50% of men do not show symptoms, according to the Centers for Disease Control and Prevention.

Chlamydia is caused by *Chlamydia trachomatis,* a microorganism that is classified as a bacterium but grows within cells much like a virus. **Chlamydia** is spread mainly through sexual contact but also can be transmitted by hand from the infected site. Like gonorrhea, chlamydia infection can be transmitted from mother to infant during passage through the infected birth canal, although this does not always occur.

Symptoms. In males, chlamydia is estimated to cause about half the cases of *epididymitis* (infection of the tube leading from the testicles) and *nongonococcal urethritis* (NGU; infection of the urethra) (Potts). Some men experience early symptoms of frequent, painful, and difficult urination as well as a watery, pus-like discharge from the penis. Symptoms of epididymitis include heaviness or swelling of the testicles and inflammation of the scrotum; symptoms of NGU include painful urination and discharge from the penis.

Among females, chlamydia is the leading cause of *pelvic inflammatory disease (PID)* and *cervicitis* (inflammation of the cervix). The Centers for Disease Control and Prevention estimates that chlamydia is the cause of approximately half of the 1 million cases of PID reported in the United States each year. When the infection remains in the lower reproductive tract, the disease tends to be asymptomatic, but some women experience a yellowish discharge, itching of the genitals, and painful urination. When the disease

chlamydia bacterial STD spread mainly through sexual contact but also by hand from the infected site

TABLE 12.5	
Chlamydia Cases	
Actual Reported Chlamydia Cases in 1996	498,884
Estimated Chlamydia Cases in 1996	3 to 5 million
Source: Centers for Disease Control and Prevention	

reaches the upper reproductive tract, causing PID, symptoms may include disrupted periods, abdominal pain or discomfort, fever, nausea, and headache.

It is important to note that people with chlamydia who show no symptoms may unknowingly infect their sexual partners. If the disease goes undetected for long periods of time, serious consequences can result. For example, males can experience damage to the prostate gland, seminal vesicles, and Cowper's gland. Females can suffer damage to the cervix and fallopian tubes, ectopic pregnancies, premature need for a hysterectomy, and a host of other complications.

Diagnosis. Historically, chlamydia organisms have been difficult to culture because of their unique characteristic of viral-like reproduction and growth only within living host cells. However, inexpensive nonculture diagnostic methods have been developed and are available at most student health centers and other walk-in clinics. Many physicians recommend chlamydia testing for individuals with multiple sexual partners and for sexually active young adults who complain of vague symptoms or problems that might be STD related.

Treatment. Like gonorrhea and many of the other bacterially caused STDs, chlamydia is easy to treat if it is detected before significant damage has been done. A week of tetracycline or doxycycline for men and nonpregnant women and erythromycin for pregnant women and newborns typically cures the disease. Penicillin is not effective. Noncompliance with the prescribed treatment and failure to abstain from sexual intercourse until a clean bill of health is obtained, however, often results in a "Ping-Pong" infection chain between sexual partners.

Chancroid

Chancroid is an acute bacterial infection that is on the increase among young adults in the United States. Chancroid occurs most frequently in men (more than 90% of reported cases), particularly those who are not circumcised. As with most other STDs, many cases go unreported.

Symptoms. Anywhere from 3 to 14 days after infection, the primary sore typically appears. This sore is inflamed and painful, and it often spreads to form several painful, pus-filled, pimple-like sores on the genitals, particularly on the underside of the foreskin of the penis. These lesions eventually rupture and form painful, soft, crater-like ulcers that emit a foul-smelling discharge. Although women often do not have symptoms, when they do occur they often are internal (in the vagina and cervix) and go undetected. This infection can spread to regional lymph nodes in both sexes and cause profuse swelling and pain.

Diagnosis and Treatment. Because of the ulcerative sores, chancroid is often confused with other STDs such as herpes and syphilis. Diagnosis involves analyzing a culture taken from the ulcer or sore to confirm the presence of the chancroid bacteria. If a positive test is obtained, the infection is treated with a 1-week supply of oral erythromycin or a single intramuscular injection of cefriaxone. As with most STDs, sexual partners should be treated at the same time and both partners should abstain from sexual intercourse until they have tested negative for the disease.

chancroid acute bacterial STD that is on the rise among young adults in the United States

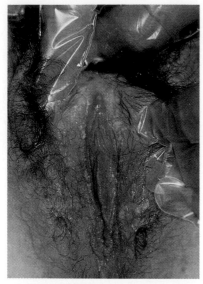

a

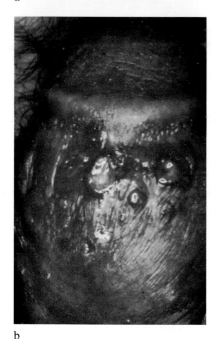

b

(a) genital herpes can raise blisters on the labia or (b) the penis.

herpes general term for a family of STDs characterized by blister-like sores or eruptions on the skin, ranging from mildly uncomfortable to extremely serious

Virally Caused STDs

Although bacterially caused STDs pose a significant threat to many Americans, the virally caused STDs are of increasing concern to public health professionals.

Herpes

Herpes is a general term for a family of diseases characterized by blister-like sores or eruptions on the skin. These infections may range from mildly uncomfortable to extremely serious and can affect persons of all ages, socioeconomic conditions, and races. The Centers for Disease Control and Prevention has identified several different strains of the Herpes simplex virus (HSV). The most common form, HSV-1, causes the cold sores and fever blisters on the lips to which over 90% of all Americans have been exposed and have antibodies for by the age of 5 years.

Genital herpes (herpes that affect the genitals) is one of the most common STDs in America today. In most cases it is caused by the herpes simplex virus type 2 (HSV-2). However, 20% to 50% of genital herpes cases are caused by HSV-1. Infections caused by either type of herpes virus are difficult to distinguish from each other without serologic (blood) testing. Practically speaking, the symptoms for these diseases are essentially the same, and both types can be spread to other locations on the body. For example, you can get an HSV-2 infection on the lip or an HSV-1 infection on the genitals by engaging in oral-genital sex or simply by touching a sore and then scratching or rubbing elsewhere. For this reason, it is important to avoid touching herpes sores and to wash your hands with soap and water if you do touch a sore.

In spite of years of extensive research, genital herpes continues to plague millions of Americans. The Centers for Disease Control and Prevention estimates that 4 out of 5 adults have orofacial herpes (HSV-1) and 1 in 6 has genital herpes. The legacy of herpes is particularly devastating for those who become infected because it is a lifelong illness: Once you get it, it typically never goes away.

Most people never develop serious complications as a result of herpes infection. Women with herpes are believed to be at an increased risk for developing cervical cancer, although there are other risk factors. Babies born to women with herpes may become blind or even die as a result of exposure to the virus.

Like many other STDs, herpes is spread by direct skin-to-skin contact. For example, if you have a cold sore and kiss someone, you can transfer the virus from your mouth to his or hers. Similarly, if you have active genital herpes and engage in vaginal or anal intercourse, you can infect your partner. In addition, if you have a cold sore and put your mouth on your partner's genitals (oral sex), you can give that person genital herpes.

Symptoms. Symptoms of herpes usually develop 2 to 20 days after contact with the virus, although it can take much longer. In some people, the initial attack from the herpes virus is so mild that it goes unnoticed. In others, the initial attack causes visible, blister-like sores that may itch, burn, or tingle. Flu-like symptoms are also common and may include swollen glands, headache, muscle aches, and fever. Herpes may also infect the urethra, causing painful urination for up to several weeks. The virus eventually retreats into the nervous system and lies dormant there.

Some people have frequent recurrences; others may go years without another outbreak. Usually, the sores recur in the same location as the virus travels back down the nerve to the skin surface. Many factors can trigger a recurrence, including the presence of other illnesses, surgery, stress, fatigue, skin irritations such as sunburn, diet, and hormonal changes such as those that occur in the menstrual cycle. In fact, some women have reported serious flare-ups of the disease every month with their menstrual cycle.

Can herpes be contracted when no sores are present? Generally, the most infectious period for herpes occurs when sores are present. However, herpes also can be spread during the *prodromal period* (before sores are present), when a person often experiences characteristic burning, tingling, and itching at the site of infection (Mertz et al.). At this time, the virus may be shedding, and even if the person is asymptomatic, he or she can transmit the virus to someone else. Likewise, during the later, dormant period, the virus can be transmitted.

Diagnosis and Treatment. Diagnosis of herpes is usually based on the presence of symptoms or on subsequent confirming tests conducted by a laboratory. Although herpes is incurable, oral Zovirax (acyclovir), when taken at the first signs of an outbreak, has been effective in reducing the frequency and duration of the symptoms. Continuously administered acyclovir also helps to suppress or reduce the duration of recurrent episodes of herpes in individuals who are prone to recurrences.

During an outbreak, the infected area must be kept as clean and dry as possible. Aspirin and ice packs also help relieve pain and itching temporarily. Preventive health behaviors, such as controlling stress, avoiding sunburn, getting enough rest, and generally practicing those health/wellness activities likely to bolster your body's defenses can help prevent recurrences.

Studies have shown that the herpes virus does not pass through latex condoms; thus, wearing a condom is an important preventive measure. However, even regular condom use does not guarantee safety. Much depends on the location of the sores and the potential drift of bodily fluids to other locations. For example, wearing a condom during intercourse will do little good if you engage in heavy petting and inadvertently transmit the virus to your eyes, mouth, or other body parts via your hands. In general, commonsense rules for sexual practices and preventive behaviors for other STDs also apply to herpes prevention (see the section "Protecting Yourself from STDs and HIV").

Hepatitis B

Hepatitis is a general term meaning inflammation of the liver that can result in liver cell damage or death. There are two main types of hepatitis: nonviral, such as alcohol-induced, and viral infection (hepatitis A, B, C, D, and E), which is the most frequent cause.

The hepatitis B virus (HBV) infects about 300,000 Americans per year, and approximately two-thirds of the cases are from sexual transmission through infected blood and other bodily fluids. Risk factors for hepatitis B infection include having more than one sex partner in the past 6 months, sharing needles, and being recently diagnosed with another STD.

hepatitis inflammation of the liver

Most people's immune systems are able to successfully eliminate the virus from the body after initial infection and thereafter have lifetime immunity. However, about 5% to 10% of the people who get infected with HBV become *chronic carriers,* which means they have a lifelong HBV infection and are infectious. In this state, hepatitis B can lead to chronic liver disease, cirrhosis, and liver cancer. It is estimated that there are one million chronic carriers in the United States.

Symptoms. Fifty percent of men and women have mild or no symptoms after initial infection with HBV. For those with symptoms, nausea, fever, malaise, joint pains, loss of strength, *pruritus* (severe itching), dark urine, and pale stools may be present a few weeks to 6 months after initial infection. A person is highly contagious 4 to 6 weeks before symptoms appear.

Treatment. Treatment consists of bed rest until the person is free of symptoms, usually 4 to 8 weeks. Zero intake of alcohol is advised during this time because alcohol is metabolized by the liver.

Although there is not a cure for chronic hepatitis B, there is a preventive vaccine that has been available since 1982. As very few of the 28 million Americans "at risk" were vaccinated during the years following vaccine availability, the Centers for Disease Control and Prevention recommended newborn immunization.

Sound Decision Making

LEARNING TO LIVE WITH AN STD

When Kendra started dating Paul at the beginning of their freshman year of college, everything seemed perfect. He was kind, handsome, and fun to be with, and they both shared a small-town background and values. They got to know each other slowly over a couple of months before the issue of sexual intimacy came up. Both of them had had sex with one other person before, in high school. Kendra saw no risk factors with Paul, so she didn't suggest they use condoms when they finally made love. Two weeks later, Kendra came down with what seemed like the flu, and she noticed some itchy blisters on her labia.

Panic stricken, Kendra went to the school health center where a diagnosis of genital herpes was made. The nurse-practitioner told her that there is no cure for herpes and that she could have outbreaks frequently, or possibly never again. She gave Kendra a prescription for Zovirax and told her to keep the affected area clean and dry. Kendra felt sad and angry at the same time; how could this happen to a nice girl like her?

The next day, she confronted Paul with the news of her herpes diagnosis. Paul admitted that he had contracted the disease from his previous girlfriend, but didn't tell Kendra because he was afraid she wouldn't want to go out with him. He thought that since he didn't seem to be having an outbreak of sores, he couldn't pass the virus on to Kendra. Kendra was furious with his deception and, despite Paul's pleading, ended their relationship.

Kendra had another outbreak of herpes sores right around final exam time. She managed to get her test dates changed, but learned firsthand that stress can trigger a recurrence of symptoms. After that, her outbreaks came less frequently—only about once a year. When Kendra started dating Jim during her junior year, she told him about her sexually transmitted disease well before they decided to have sex. Jim was initially put off by this information, but he really cared about Kendra. When they did become sexually involved they were careful to use condoms every time and even found ways to make condom use a fun part of their lovemaking.

Genital Warts

Genital warts, also known as *venereal warts* or *condylomas,* are growths caused by a group of viruses known as human papillomaviruses *(HPVs).* A person becomes infected when an HPV penetrates the skin or mucous membrane during the exchanges of bodily fluids that accompany sexual contact. Local friction during intercourse may be partially responsible for tiny abrasions that allow the virus to penetrate the skin's defensive barrier.

Over 20 million American women are estimated to have genital warts, and approximately 75% of their partners are also infected (Zazove, Caruthers, and Reed). Moreover, rates of HPV infection have been escalating rapidly, especially among young, sexually active men and women. For example, a survey of female undergraduate students found that 46% were infected with HPV (Bauer et al.).

HPV is transmitted during vaginal, anal, or oral-genital contact. The incubation period is usually 2 to 3 months but can be as brief as 3 weeks. The HPV that causes genital warts may be among the most virulent of all STDs, with over 60% of exposed sexual partners developing the disease after a 2- to 3-month incubation period. The infection can also be passed from mother to fetus during passage through an infected birth canal. Infected infants can develop acute HPV infections in their respiratory tracts that cause lifelong health problems.

Genital warts also can result in serious health problems for the person infected, including urinary obstruction, *dysplasia* (changes in cells that can lead to development of cancer), and cancers of the cervix, vagina, vulva, penis, and anus.

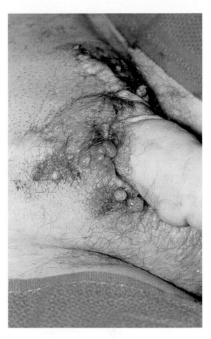

Genital warts on the penis.

Symptoms. Symptoms of genital warts vary considerably, with many people being asymptomatic. Warts range in size from small, itchy bumps on the genitals to large, cauliflower-like growths capable of obstructing urinary or reproductive activity. Typically, these warts are of two different types: flat warts and full-blown warts. Flat warts are whitish-gray, flat growths that do not protrude from the surface of the skin; full-blown warts are soft, pink to reddish-brown, discrete growths that occur singly or in clusters.

Diagnosis. In females, warts are often internal and may not be detected unless a skilled physician notes abnormalities during a routine Pap exam. Abnormal Pap smear results may prompt a diagnostic *colposcopy,* in which a vinegar-like solution is applied to the vaginal walls and cervix making any warts visible. The area is then viewed through a magnifying instrument known as a *colposcope.* A similar but newer instrument, known as a cerviscope, projects an image of the viewing area on a screen and is believed to be much more sensitive in detecting warts than a colposcope. The *DNA probe* is an even newer diagnostic technique that can analyze the genetic makeup of a wart.

A male can make a preliminary at-home diagnosis of genital warts by wrapping his penis in a vinegar-soaked cloth, waiting 5 minutes, and checking for white-bleached areas indicating flat-wart infections. A confirming diagnosis, however, must be made by a physician.

Treatment. If left alone, occasionally warts will eventually go away. However, while they are present, they not only are infectious but also may cause complications for the person infected.

genital warts growths caused by a group of viruses that penetrate the skin or mucous membrane during the exchanges of bodily fluids that accompany sexual contact

STATS-AT-A-GLANCE

Estimated New STD Cases Each Year in the United States:

- Chlamydia — 4,000,000
- Trichomoniasis — 3,000,000
- Gonorrhea — 1,100,000
- Genital Warts — 1,000,000
- Genital Herpes — 500,000
- Hepatitis B — 300,000
- Syphilis — 120,000
- HIV — 40,000

Source: Centers for Disease Control and Prevention

Treatment for genital warts involves removal of the wart. This can be accomplished by applications of *topical* (used on the skin, not ingested) agents such as podophyllin, trichloroacetic acid, and 5-fluorouracil cream. Podophyllin is quite toxic and should be used with extreme care, particularly if the person infected is pregnant. Surgical options include laser surgery, electrosurgery, surgical excision, and cryosurgery, in which the affected area is "frozen" and the warts fall off after a period of time.

Pelvic Inflammatory Disease

Although technically not an STD, pelvic inflammatory disease represents one of the most serious consequences of many STDs. **Pelvic inflammatory disease (PID)** is an acute inflammation of the lining of a woman's fallopian tubes or uterus. It can cause severe pain in the lower abdominal cavity, menstrual irregularities, fever, nausea, painful intercourse, recurring infection, ectopic pregnancy, and severe depression. Infertility results if scarring of the fallopian tubes is severe enough.

Approximately one out of every seven women of child-bearing age has PID, with about one million new cases reported annually (Handsfield and Hammerschlag). Gonorrhea and chlamydia are the two leading causes of PID, responsible for up to one-half of all PID cases. Genital herpes and other recurrent STDs can also create a chronically inflamed reproductive tract with all the aforementioned symptoms. Nonsexual invasions by other pathogens, such as yeast infections, and chronic irritations, such as those caused by an intrauterine device (IUD), are among the many other conditions that might predispose a woman to PID. Research suggests that cigarette smokers are twice as likely as nonsmokers to contract PID (Scholes et al.).

Diagnosis of PID is complicated by the failure of many women to notice symptoms before scarring has occurred. Treatment involves intensive antibiotic therapy and sometimes hospitalization.

HIV and AIDS

The 1980s left us with one of the deadliest legacies of modern times, **acquired immune deficiency syndrome (AIDS).** In the spring of 1981, a significant number of gay men in California and New York came down with a series of symptoms that indicated a steadily weakening immune response. Patients typically developed a vast number of debilitating infections that ultimately led to a painful death. It took researchers 3 years to isolate the virus that caused these strange symptoms: the **human immunodeficiency virus (HIV),** which is actually a *retrovirus,* meaning that it reverses the usual flow of genetic information during reproduction. Although progress has been made on developing treatments for the disease, which are extending longevity rates, AIDS remains a deadly epidemic.

pelvic inflammatory disease (PID) acute inflammation of the lining of a woman's fallopian tubes or uterus

acquired immune deficiency syndrome (AIDS) series of symptoms indicating a steadily weakening immune response and leading to a number of debilitating and ultimately fatal infections

human immunodeficiency virus (HIV) virus that causes AIDS

MYTHS & CONTROVERSIES

Myth 1 **Homosexuals and IV-drug users are the only people at risk for HIV infection.** It is true that the majority of reported cases of HIV infection are among homosexual or bisexual men or intravenous drug users. However, the rate of infection is currently increasing faster in women than in men; in 1996 there was a 15% *decrease* in deaths among men and a 3% *increase* in deaths among women. AIDS is also the sixth leading cause of death in children age 1 to 4 in the United States. The fact is that anyone who has unprotected vaginal, oral, or anal sex, or who shares needles, is at risk for HIV infection.

Myth 2 **HIV can be transmitted by casual contact with an infected person, by mosquitoes, or by donating blood.** In fact, the AIDS virus has never been transmitted by food and drink, insect bites, or sneezing, and it cannot penetrate intact human skin. There is no risk of infection in giving blood. HIV can be spread only by sexual intercourse or the exchange of blood with an infected person. There is no known risk of infection in daily life outside of these situations.

Myth 3 **The success of the new HIV-fighting drugs means the AIDS crisis is over.** The effects of protease inhibitor drugs are indeed dramatic, but they are not a cure and their long-term success has yet to be determined. Many researchers believe that they will extend the healthy lives of people infected with HIV, but their effects may diminish over time. And millions of HIV-positive people in the United States and especially around the world cannot afford these expensive drugs. HIV is still a serious threat to our health, and prevention techniques like safer sex should still be practiced.

Prevalence of HIV/AIDS

HIV has spread virtually unchecked since its discovery. At least 40,000 people will become HIV infected each year in the United States (Rosenberg). Through June 1997, a cumulative total of 612,078 persons with AIDS were reported to the Centers for Disease Control and Prevention. Estimates are that 239,000 of these persons are living with AIDS (had tested positive for HIV, had a defining opportunistic disease, and/or had a *CD4 lymphocyte*—that is, helper T-cell—count of 200 cells or less per cubic millimeter of blood).

To be more accurate, and to counteract the stigma often associated with the label "AIDS," many health professionals and the Centers for Disease Control and Prevention now use the term *HIV disease* to describe the series of symptoms a person demonstrates after infection. HIV disease has replaced the previous label of *ARC (AIDS-related complex),* commonly applied during the 1980s to individuals who tested positive for the virus but did not have AIDS.

In addition to those with AIDS, close to one million Americans are believed to be infected with HIV, many of them undiagnosed (see Figure 12.2). The World Health Organization (WHO) has estimated that 22.6 million people worldwide are HIV-infected (see Table 12.6). Assuming the present rate of spread, that number is expected to reach 30 to 40 million by the year 2000. Moreover, AIDS was the second leading cause of death among men age 25 to 44, and the eighth leading cause of overall deaths in the United States in 1996 (see Table 12.7). Over 90% of the newly infected adults will have acquired their infection through heterosexual intercourse.

Despite a massive educational campaign and media attention in the late 1980s, which seemed to slow the tide of the disease in some populations, AIDS remains a major health concern (Mann). The disease is spreading most rapidly among women, adolescents, and people of color (Farmer). Sociocultural taboos related to sexuality, social inequities, public apathy, an attitude of "it can't happen to me," and increased numbers of intravenous drug users who share needles and people who engage in sex in exchange for drugs are believed to contribute to this epidemic.

Figure 12.2
Reported Cases and Known Deaths from AIDS, United States, 1981–1996. The extreme rise in reported cases in 1993 is due to a change in the definition of AIDS, which broadened the list of conditions reportable as AIDS and included measures of immune-system function.

Source: National Center for Health Statistics. National Vital Statistics System.

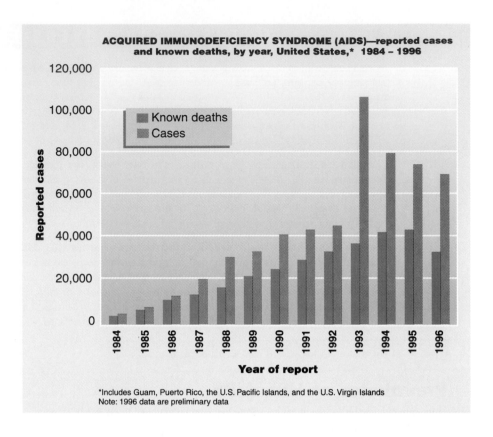

ACQUIRED IMMUNODEFICIENCY SYNDROME (AIDS)—reported cases and known deaths, by year, United States,* 1984 – 1996

*Includes Guam, Puerto Rico, the U.S. Pacific Islands, and the U.S. Virgin Islands
Note: 1996 data are preliminary data

TABLE 12.6

Estimated Number of Persons Living with HIV/AIDS at the End of 1996, by Region

■ North America	750,000
■ Western Europe	510,000
■ Eastern Europe & Central Asia	50,000
■ Caribbean	270,000
■ Latin America	1.3 million
■ Middle East	200,000
■ Sub-Saharan Africa	14 million
■ Southern & Southeastern Asia	5.2 million
■ Australia & New Zealand	13,000
Global Total:	**22.6 million**

Source: World Health Organization

HIV Transmission

Like many other STDs, the AIDS virus must enter the body by breaching one of its many defenses. Mucous membranes in the genital organs and anus appear to be the most likely entry points. However, once in the body, the virus spreads rapidly through all bodily fluids, including blood, semen, and

TABLE 12.7

HIV Infection as a Cause of Death in the United States

MALES		FEMALES		COMBINED
RANK OF HIV AS CAUSE OF DEATH				
All males	8th	All females	14th	8th overall cause of death in the United States
White	9th	White	not listed	Not among top 10 causes of death
Black	3rd	Black	6th	Not listed

AGE GROUP FOR MALES AND FEMALES (ALL RACES)

	RANK OF HIV AS CAUSE OF DEATH
1–4 years	7th
5–14 years	7th
15–24 years	6th (after accidents, homicides and legal intervention, suicide, cancer, and heart disease)
25–44 years	2nd (after accidents)
45–64 years	8th

Source: National Center for Health Statistics. *Preliminary Data: 1996 Mortality Statistics.*

vaginal secretions. These fluids are considered high-risk fluids for infection because they can be transmitted between partners. Other bodily fluids, such as tears, breast milk, and saliva, can also carry the virus, but transmission via these fluids is less likely. Nevertheless, these low-risk fluids should be considered in a personal prevention program. Deep kissing (French kissing) and other low-risk fluid exchanges with persons who have engaged in high-risk behaviors (shared needles, had sex with multiple partners) should be avoided. Anal intercourse also should be avoided because the virus can be transmitted through small abrasions in the rectal tissue.

Unprotected sexual intercourse or other exchanges of body fluids (such as needle sharing) with an HIV-positive person are the most likely means of infection, but the virus can be transmitted in other ways. For example, persons who received a blood transfusion prior to 1985, when the Red Cross mounted a massive blood-screening campaign, were at risk for contracting the disease. Mother-to-infant transmission is also possible either in the womb or during the baby's passage through the birth canal. Although breast-feeding has been implicated as a possible means of spreading the virus after birth, recent evidence indicates that it is not the breast milk but rather bleeding nipples caused by overzealous nursing by infants that may be the route of transmission.

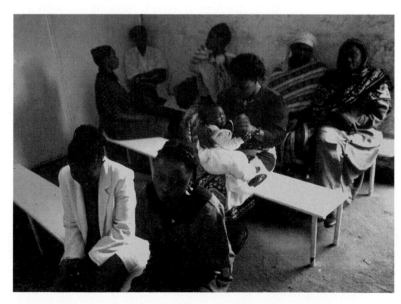

In Majengo, a suburb of Nairobi, 95% of prostitutes are thought to be HIV-positive. These prostitutes wait in the clinic for their checkups.

Perspectives

AIDS and Public Policy

If you were trying to come up with an issue that (1) struck fear in the hearts of people; (2) caused people to focus on the most intimate of sexual acts; (3) involved illegal drug abuse in some cases; (4) played on people's innermost beliefs about morality, sexual behaviors, sexual orientation, and divine punishment for "sins of the flesh"; (5) caused parents to react violently to protect their children from what they perceived as incorrect education; and (6) involved the medical, legal, research, and education systems and the general public in a struggle over policy and procedure, what would you discuss? Probably AIDS. The following are just some of the controversial issues related to this highly charged topic.

■ At what age, if any, should schools bear the responsibility for AIDS education? Should condoms be given to schoolchildren? Should they be freely available to minors in restrooms?

■ As death rates from AIDS decline, should the money spent on AIDS research decline also? Or should the money be used for research into other diseases that kill more people than AIDS? Should the money be used instead to fund programs to prevent transmission of HIV in the first place?

■ Who or what is responsible for the AIDS epidemic? Gays? Haitians? People of African descent? Plants? Animals? Viral warfare gone awry? Do we really know? Does it matter?

■ Should people with AIDS be required to wear identifying bracelets or be tattooed?

■ Should health care workers be required to tell patients they are HIV-positive?

■ Should patients be required to tell health care providers that they are HIV-positive on treatment?

■ Should HIV-positive people be quarantined? Fired from their jobs? Lose their health insurance?

■ Should health insurance companies be able to drop AIDS patients from their policies? How about people with cancer? Recurrent STDs?

■ Should spouses, partners, doctors, public health workers, or employers be notified of an individual's positive HIV test?

■ Should employers be allowed to screen employees for HIV prior to hiring?

■ Should HIV-positive foreigners be allowed into the United States?

■ What are the rights of persons with AIDS in terms of employment, housing, marriage licenses, mandatory notification of partners, and health care?

■ Who should pay for HIV-infected individuals' health care costs?

■ Should people be allowed to sue the person who infected them with HIV?

■ Should AIDS patients be given experimental drugs that have not yet received FDA approval if they are near death?

■ Should HIV-infected fetuses be aborted?

What do your responses tell you about your own biases? Do you think you would feel differently if you knew the person involved? If the person was a consenting adult? Rape victim? Homosexual? Heterosexual? Hemophiliac? Prostitute? Young child? Your brother or sister?

Stages of HIV Infection

Like most viruses, HIV lives only within the cell it invades and dies almost immediately on exposure to air, water, or other surfaces. Once it has entered a host cell, the virus begins to change the genetic structure of that cell by commandeering the cellular activities so they can be used for its own replication purposes. Although the body responds by developing antibodies to protect itself from HIV—a process known as *seroconversion*—it is typically unable to mount an adequate defense. The shortest known time between exposure to the virus and seroconversion is 27 days.

After seroconversion, the virus multiplies rapidly, invading the bloodstream and cerebrospinal fluid, destroying CD4 lymphocytes, and weakening the body's ability to fight off other *opportunistic infections.* Opportunistic infections are caused by pathogens that usually find it difficult to flourish in someone with a healthy immune system. However, when infected with HIV, the body's immune system is progressively weakened to the point that these organisms can gain a foothold. In fact, most people with HIV do not actually die from AIDS; they succumb to any number of invading pathogens. For example, the person might develop a life-threatening strain of pneumonia that would otherwise cause few problems. Other common opportunistic infections include herpes, Kaposi's sarcoma (a rare form of cancer), tuberculosis, and a variety of fungal and bacterial infections.

Once someone has become HIV-infected, that person is "HIV-positive" and is fully capable of transmitting the virus to others. In fact, an individual is highly infectious in the first 60 days after initial infection, even though he or she may not show HIV antibodies on a test. Although many people equate an HIV-positive diagnosis with AIDS, the two are not synonymous. Not everyone who has been infected with HIV has developed AIDS. In some cases asymptomatic HIV-positive individuals have outlived several sexual partners whom they infected with the virus. Nevertheless, the vast majority do develop symptoms sooner or later.

Symptoms of HIV disease may appear as soon as 1 month after seroconversion, or they may not occur for many years. If symptoms are severe enough, the person can be diagnosed with AIDS at any time. Although the length of time for progression to AIDS varies considerably, the median time period is 10 years for adults who do not get treatment. Without treatment, babies infected with HIV may live less than 2 years, and in small children the disease typically progresses 3 to 4 years later. As new treatments are becoming available, many patients with HIV disease are living longer without developing AIDS, and many are living longer after a diagnosis of AIDS.

Symptoms

As stated previously, a person may go for months or years after seroconversion without showing symptoms. The initial symptoms of HIV disease vary considerably, depending on the state of an individual's immune system and the particular opportunistic infections at work. Some typical symptoms include unexplained weight loss, fever, night sweats, loss of appetite, chronic fatigue, swollen lymph nodes, diarrhea, headaches, and chronic cough. Many of these symptoms are also associated with other, less serious ailments and therefore do not necessarily indicate the presence of HIV.

Diagnosis

The most commonly used test to detect HIV antibodies is a blood test known as the ELISA, which is considered 99% accurate. A seronegative result means that HIV is not present; a seropositive result indicates the presence of HIV. Because of the serious implications of a false negative result (that is, measuring negative when the result should be positive), the ELISA is designed to be highly sensitive to the presence of HIV. Generally, the test is administered three times to make a clear diagnosis. Because it can produce false positive results (that is, measuring positive when such is not the case), confirming tests are conducted using the Western Blot technique. Tests for HIV that involve the analysis of saliva and urine samples are also available.

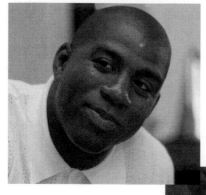

(a) Magic Johnson, for whom triple-drug therapy has worked well.

(b) The protease inhibitor Crixivan is one element of this man's expensive drug regimen.

Treatment

The development of new antiretroviral drugs provides increasing options for "drug cocktail" combination therapy against disease progression in persons living with AIDS and has prolonged symptom-free living in HIV-positive individuals. The number of deaths from AIDS in the United States dropped for the first time in 1996. The decline in death rates reflects new and better drug treatments, improvements in the clinical management of HIV-infected people, and a slowing of HIV infections that began in the late 1980s among white homosexual men. This progression holds the promise that HIV/AIDS can become a manageable condition and that people with HIV will live longer than in earlier years.

Treatment guidelines for HIV/AIDS are constantly evolving. There are currently two categories of anti-retroviral drugs: reverse transcriptase inhibitors, such as Retrovir (AZT) and Hivid (ddC), and protease inhibitors such as Crixivan (Indinavir). The latest clinical data suggest that the best treatment is a three-drug combination: two reverse transcriptase inhibitors and a protease inhibitor. Because there is no standard protocol, and because the course of HIV disease varies greatly, the National Institutes of Health and Public Health Service recommend that HIV/AIDS treatment should be individualized with each patient and each physician. In addition, there are many more drugs forthcoming in other categories that attack HIV at different points in its reproductive cycle; these will need to be considered.

In spite of the positive aspects of the recent breakthroughs in HIV treatment, HIV/AIDS remains a serious, life-threatening disease. There are people who have intolerable side effects to all available therapies or who become resistant to the anti-HIV drugs or fail to respond. The failure rate of the current treatment regimens is about 10% to 20% for patients (Cohen). HIV-infected individuals face other issues as well: difficult treatment decisions, drug interactions, demanding treatment schedules, lack of data about efficacy, and the cost of and access to drugs. A typical drug regimen that includes a protease inhibitor is extremely expensive, costing $12,000 to $16,000 a year (Waldholz). Treatments for specific HIV-related illnesses and prophylactic drugs for opportunistic diseases add even more to the total cost. The World Health Organization estimates that worldwide, 90% of people do not have access to HIV antiretroviral drugs.

Because the new hope offered by the recent breakthroughs in treatment is out of reach for most people in the world due to its enormous cost, a preventive vaccine seems to offer most prospects for access. In 1997, President Clinton declared the development of a preventive HIV vaccine "a new national goal." Although some vaccines are being tested in animal studies or small human safety studies, there are many obstacles: the complex nature of HIV; its fast mutating and replicating abilities; its resistance to drugs; and legal, financial, and ethical questions of safety and testing in humans (Bangham and Phillips).

The best hope for stemming the tide of HIV disease lies with individuals. Although most people have heard the guidelines for preventing infection countless times, many ignore commonsense recommendations. The increasing numbers of cases in heterosexuals provides strong evidence of this fact. Table 12.8 provides a summary of all the STDs, their symptoms, and treatment.

Protecting Yourself from STDs and HIV

For many of you, trying to find the safest and most satisfying way to relate to another person without putting yourself at risk emotionally or physically may be difficult. This is particularly true if you have trouble differentiating between what it means to have an "intimate relationship" and what it means to have an "intimate sexual relationship." Intimate relationships typically have three characteristics: (1) behavioral interdependence, or the mutual impact that partners have on each other as their lives become closely intertwined; (2) need fulfillment, or the need to have someone who can share feelings and concerns and who can be relied on to give help or reassurance;

TABLE 12.8

Common STDs

DISEASE	PATHOGEN	INCUBATION PERIOD	SYMPTOMS	EFFECTS	TREATMENT
Genital herpes (HSV-2)	Virus	2–12 days	Itching; small fluid-filled blisters; pain and fever	Infant death and disability	Acyclovir to relieve symptoms and frequency of attacks
Genital warts	Papilloma virus	1–20 months	Warts on genitals or other body parts	Cervical cancer; sterility	Physician removal
Chlamydia	Bacterium	5–7 days or more	Urinary burning; vaginal or urethral discharge; or asymptomatic	Sterility; pelvic inflammatory disease (PID); preterm delivery; tubal pregnancy	Antibiotics
Candida	Yeast	Variable	Itching; white discharge (also known as thrush)	Transmissible to fetus during birth	Prescription drugs
Gonorrhea	Bacterium	2–8 days or more	Urinary burning; vaginal or urethral discharge	Sterility; PID	Antibiotics
Syphilis	Bacterium	10–90 days	Distinct stages ranging from chancre to death	Diffuse, from skin rash to heart and nervous system damage to sterility	Antibiotics
Trichomoniasis	Protozoan	4–20 days	Irritation, itching; frothy, odorous discharge	Sterility; PID	Prescription drugs
HIV/AIDS	Virus	Variable	Immune system breakdown	Increased susceptibility to infectious diseases/death	Palliative
Hepatitis B	Virus	45–160 days	Fever; nausea; jaundice	Liver damage	Palliative; vaccine to prevent

AVOIDING ◆ STDs

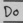 Do

▲ Use a condom *every time* you have vaginal, oral, or anal sex.

▲ Learn to use condoms properly to obtain maximum protection.

▲ Limit your number of sexual partners.

▲ Get to know potential sexual partners and talk honestly about your sexual histories.

▲ Avoid sexual contact with people who have HIV or an STD, or who have engaged in risky behavior in the past.

▲ Get checked periodically for STDs if you are sexually active.

▲ Know the symptoms of STDs and get prompt treatment for any STD you contract.

▲ Make sure any needles used for tattoos, piercing, acupuncture, or anything else are sterile.

▲ Educate yourself and others about the risks of STDs and HIV on your campus.

Don't

▼ Have unprotected sex of any kind.

▼ Assume that because someone looks nice and clean that he or she can't have an STD.

▼ Assume that risks of STDs don't apply to you; if you are sexually active they *do* apply.

▼ Let the expectations of your friends or sexual partners cause you to ignore your own feelings about your sexuality.

▼ Drink or use drugs in sexual situations; they may make you more likely to engage in high-risk behaviors.

▼ Share needles, syringes, or anything that could have blood on it.

▼ Spread prejudice or hysteria about people with HIV infection.

and (3) emotional attachment, or feelings of love and affection for another person. By contrast, intimate *sexual relationships* focus on genital contact and may have some, all, or none of the above characteristics, depending on individual circumstances. Moving too quickly from an intimate relationship to an intimate sexual relationship can create emotional stress as well as increase your risk of acquiring an STD.

General Guidelines

If you do choose to have an intimate sexual relationship, the following guidelines developed by the Centers for Disease Control and Prevention can significantly reduce your risk, and your partner's, of becoming infected with HIV. Although these preventive measures apply specifically to HIV disease, they also are effective for the majority of STDs.

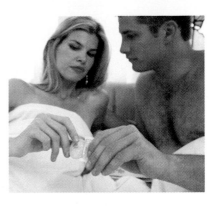

Communicating with your partner about condom use or other protective measures should be done prior to an intimate sexual encounter.

1. *Know your partner.* Although celibacy is the best way to protect yourself, it is not a viable alternative for most adults. The next best means of protection is through maintenance of a monogamous sexual relationship. If you and your partner have been faithful to each other for at least 5 years, neither of you is at risk, whether you are involved in a heterosexual or homosexual relationship. Unless you are *absolutely* certain that neither of you has been exposed to HIV during past relationships, you must use protective behavior. Although your partner may attempt to verify his or her safety by showing you negative HIV antibody test results, keep in mind that there is a "window" period after infection. During this time, although the test may be negative, the person may be beginning to seroconvert. Sex during that time can result in infection.

2. *Communicate with your partner.* Do not be afraid to ask questions or to obtain information. If your partner refuses to discuss these issues with you or to use condoms or other protective measures, it may be time to ask some serious questions about the level of concern or caring in your relationship.

3. *Get a blood test.* If you have been involved in any of the high-risk activities discussed previously, and if you are considering a sexual relationship with another person, you should have a blood test to learn whether you have been infected. If you test positive, you should tell your sexual partner.

4. *Protect yourself and your partner against infection.* If your partner has tested positive for HIV, or you suspect that he or she has been exposed by previous heterosexual or homosexual behavior or has used intravenous drugs with shared needles, a condom and spermicide containing nonoxynol-9 (which kills HIV and other infectious agents) should always be used during sexual intercourse (vaginal or anal). You also should use a condom and a spermicide if you have had sex with more than one partner or with a person who has had multiple partners.

5. *Avoid high-risk sexual behavior.* If you or your partner is at high risk, avoid oral contact with the penis, vagina, or rectum. Also avoid all sexual activities that could cause cuts or tears in the linings of the rectum, vagina, or penis.

6. *Learn to say no to sex and drugs.* This is especially important during the teen years and when you are not certain about the risks your partner may be

exposing you to. Table 12.9 shows some barriers to being able to "just say no" in certain communities, such as the poor, drug users, and adolescents.

7. *Avoid sex with prostitutes.* Infected male and female prostitutes are frequently also intravenous drug abusers; therefore, they may infect clients by sexual intercourse.

Condoms

After abstinence, no other method has been as widely promoted as the use of condoms in protecting against HIV infection or infection with a number of STDs. Are condoms as effective as claimed by many? Probably not. It is important to remember that condoms were initially developed as a method of birth control. Although they make sex "safer" than no protection at all, there is no such thing as totally "safe" sex. Even under ideal conditions in which an individual used the condom correctly and the condom itself remained intact, pregnancies have been reported. Human error in use and problems with the condom itself could also leave a person susceptible to HIV or other STD infections.

Factors associated with lack of condom effectiveness include the following: (1) failure to put the condom on in time, (2) failure to use the condom on an "every time" basis, (3) failure to unroll the condom properly, (4) having the condom come off during intercourse, and (5) breakdown of the condom.

The following recommendations may substantially lower your risk of possible infections while using a condom:

1. Decide ahead of time that you will not have sexual relations without using a condom. Insist on it and make sure that at least one of you has one with you.

2. Never reuse a condom.

3. Purchase latex condoms rather than natural membrane or other types of condoms. Latex condoms have been shown to provide superior protection in laboratory tests.

TABLE 12.9

Disproportionate Effect of STDs on Poor and Minority Communities

Some psychosocial, cultural, and economic realities that are barriers to STD prevention:

- Poverty

- Homelessness

- Addiction to drugs and alcohol

- Mental illness

- Prostitution

- Limited access to health care

- Cuts in Medicaid and social programs

4. Store condoms in a cool, dry place, out of direct sunlight—and out of your wallet.

5. Don't use old condoms. If a condom appears brittle or sticky, or if the package is battered from being stored in the bottom of a purse or glove compartment, don't chance it—purchase a new one.

6. Put on the condom before there is any contact between genital organs.

7. Put the condom on properly. Hold the tip of the condom and unroll it onto the erect penis leaving space at the tip to collect semen. If you have questions about how to do this properly, ask health professionals at your student health center or clinic.

8. Apply a water-based lubricant with a spermicide to provide additional protection in case of possible condom failure or displacement of the condom during intercourse. Do not use massage oils, petroleum jelly, oil-based lubricants, cooking oils, or other non-water-based products on the condom because they may weaken the latex.

9. If the condom breaks, tears, or comes off, replace it immediately, wash the genitals if possible, and apply a spermicide directly to the areas of contact. These extra precautions may provide an extra measure of protection.

10. After ejaculation, withdraw the penis while still erect. Be sure to hold the base of the condom so that it doesn't slip off during withdrawal.

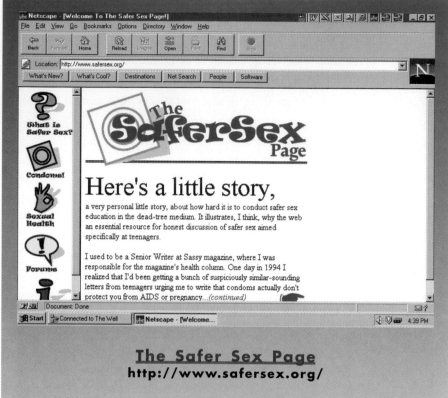

The Safer Sex Page
http://www.safersex.org/

Do you have questions about safer sex practices but aren't sure who to ask? The Safer Sex Page contains information on condom use and other safer sex techniques, women's health issues, HIV and other sexually transmitted diseases, and contraception. There is also a forum to discuss issues related to safer sex and resources for counselors and others who educate on safer sex issues.

Critical thinking: Do you think education is enough to convince you and your peers to practice safer sex? What kinds of information would be most helpful to people you know? If you think education isn't enough, what else would help?

Source: From Filkins, 1998.

Lifestyle Choices: Plan for Action

Of the top ten most frequently reported infectious diseases in 1996 in the United States, five were STDs. Overall, STD prevalence is highest in young adults. One danger to your health and well-being is becoming complacent and accepting the risk of contracting a sexually transmitted infection. However, acknowledging that safer sex practices reduce the number of all STDs and the incidence of HIV, and acting on that knowledge with healthy sexual behavior, will significantly reduce your risks of disease and contribute to your overall wellness.

Summary

In this chapter you have learned about the various STDs and how they can threaten your well-being. Because many of the more than 25 known STDs, including HIV, are spreading rapidly, now more than ever individuals must act cautiously and responsibly in their sexual behavior.

Key concepts that you have learned in this chapter include these:

- STDs, also called venereal diseases, are infections one can get from sexual contact with an infected person.

- Factors that put an individual at high risk for STDs include having sexual intercourse with multiple partners or with persons who have had sex with multiple partners, having unprotected sex, injecting drugs and sharing needles, and using alcohol or other drugs to excess.

- The immune system is the body's main natural defense mechanism against a variety of invading substances, but the skin, mucous membranes, and various enzymes also provide physical and chemical defenses against infections.

- Bacteria, fungi, viruses, and protozoa are the main types of pathogens that can cause STDs.

- Bacterially caused STDs include gonorrhea, syphilis, chlamydia, and chancroid; virally caused STDs include herpes, hepatitis B, genital warts, and HIV disease.

- Pelvic inflammatory disease (PID), an acute inflammation of the lining of a woman's fallopian tubes or uterus, can cause severe pain, menstrual irregularities, and infertility.

- The term *HIV disease* describes the series of symptoms a person demonstrates after infection with the AIDS virus.

- Unprotected anal or vaginal intercourse with an HIV-infected person is the most common means of infection, but HIV also can be transmitted by sharing needles with an HIV-infected drug user, through a blood transfusion (prior to 1985), and from mother-to-fetus contact.

- Protective measures against HIV disease or other STDs include getting to know your partner beforehand, communicating about your concerns, using a condom and spermicide if you or your partner have had other relationships in the past 5 years or have injected drugs, and getting a blood test to determine whether you are infected.

References

Alters, S., and W. Schiff. Essential Concepts for Healthy Living. Pacific Grove, CA: Brooks/Cole, 1998.

Bangham, C., and R. E. Phillips. What is required of an HIV vaccine? *Lancet,* 350 (9091): 1617, 1997.

Bauer, H., et al. Genital human papillomavirus infection in female university students as determined by a PCR-based method. *Journal of the American Medical Association,* 265: 472–477, 1991.

Centers for Disease Control and Prevention. Pelvic inflammatory disease: Guidelines for prevention and management. *Morbidity and Mortality Weekly Report,* 40: 1–26, 1992.

Centers for Disease Control and Prevention. Summary of Notifiable Diseases, United States. *Morbidity and Mortality Weekly Report,* 45(53), 1997.

Cohen, C. Guidance offered in drug combination choices. *AIDS Alert,* 12(12): 135, 1997.

Crooks, R. and K. Baur. *Our Sexuality,* 7th ed. Pacific Grove, CA: Brooks/Cole, 1998.

Eng, T. R., and W. T. Butler, eds. *The Hidden Epidemic: Confronting Sexually Transmitted Diseases.* Washington, DC: National Academy Press, 1996.

Farmer, P. Social inequalities and emerging infectious diseases. *Emerging Infectious Diseases,* 2(4): 259–269, 1996.

Handsfield, H., and M. Hammerschlag. Chlamydia: The challenge is diagnosis. *Patient Care,* 15 February 1992, 69–84.

Kessler, W. J., and W. Cates. The epidemiology and prevention of sexually transmitted diseases. *Urologic Clinics of North America,* February 1992.

Mann, J. M. *AIDS in the World II.* New York: Oxford University Press, 1996.

Mertz, G., et al. Risk factors for the sexual transmission of genital herpes. *Annals of Internal Medicine,* 116: 197–202, 1992.

National Center for Health Statistics. *Preliminary Data: 1996 Mortality Statistics Report.* Hyattsville, MD: U.S. Department of Health and Human Services, 1997.

Nevid, J. S. *Choices: Sex in the Age of STDs,* 2nd ed. Boston: Allyn & Bacon, 1998.

Potts, J. Chlamydial infection: Screening and management update. *Postgraduate Medicine,* 19: 120–126, 1992.

Rosenberg, P. S. Scope of the AIDS epidemic in the United States. *Science,* 270(5240): 1372, 1995.

Royce, R. A., A. Sena, W. Cates, and M. S. Cohen. Sexual transmission of HIV. *The New England Journal of Medicine,* 336(15): 1072–1077, 1997.

Scholes, D., et al. Smoking and pelvic inflammatory disease. *American Journal of Public Health,* 10, 1992.

Schulte, J. M., et al. Chancroid in the United States, 1981–1990: Evidence of underreporting of cases. *MMWR CDC Surveillance Summaries,* 29 May 1992.

Waldholz, M. Precious pills: New AIDS treatment raises tough question of who will get it. *Wall Street Journal,* 3 July 1996, p. 1.

World Health Organization. *Emerging and Other Communicable Diseases.* Geneva: Division of Emerging and Other Communicable Diseases Surveillance and Control, 1997.

Zazove, P., B. Caruthers, and B. Reed. Genital human papillomavirus infection. *American Family Physician,* 43: 1279–1291, 1991.

Laboratory 12.1

Assessing Your Risk for an STD and/or HIV Disease

Like many other areas of health, there are things that you currently are doing that may put you at an increased risk for disease. Rate yourself on each of the following items. Which behaviors listed below may increase your risk?

1. I am sexually abstinent or maintain a monogamous relationship.

   not applicable   never   sometimes   usually   always

2. I am comfortable discussing intimate topics with my friends.

   not applicable   never   sometimes   usually   always

3. I am comfortable talking about my sexual past with potential partners and asking them about their sexual past.

   not applicable   never   sometimes   usually   always

4. I avoid sexual relationships with people I do not know very well.

   not applicable   never   sometimes   usually   always

5. I avoid sexual intercourse with persons I am not in a monogamous relationship with.

   not applicable   never   sometimes   usually   always

6. If a new relationship was becoming sexual, I would discuss the topic of STDs with that person before engaging in sexual intercourse.

   not applicable   never   sometimes   usually   always

7. I refuse to have sex with a partner who does not think that wearing a condom is important.

   not applicable   never   sometimes   usually   always

8. I avoid sexual relationships with people who have had many sexual partners.

   not applicable   never   sometimes   usually   always

9. I feel comfortable discussing my sexual relationships with a close friend.

   not applicable   never   sometimes   usually   always

10. I take time to find out about STDs and check for possible symptoms.

    not applicable   never   sometimes   usually   always

11. If I found out that I had an STD, I would immediately notify my partner.

    not applicable   never   sometimes   usually   always

12. If I found out that I had an STD, I would go to a doctor or STD clinic immediately.

    not applicable   never   sometimes   usually   always

13. If I had symptoms that seemed potentially STD-related, I would go to the student health center on campus.

    not applicable   never   sometimes   usually   always

14. If someone I loved had an STD, I would refuse to be intimate with that person until he or she was treated.

    not applicable   never   sometimes   usually   always

15. I avoid having sex with persons who inject themselves with needles.

    not applicable   never   sometimes   usually   always

Evaluation

To how many of these statements did you answer "always" or "usually"? To which ones (if any) did you answer "never" or "sometimes"? For these latter statements, what actions could you take to change your behavior?

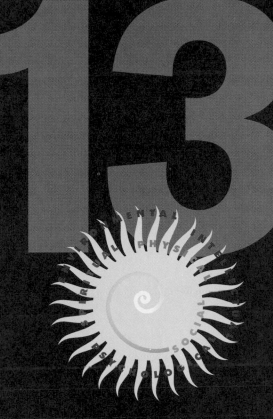

13

Chronic Diseases

The Student's View

My great-grandmother, grandmother, and mother all have diabetes. My great-grandmother and grandmother are insulin-dependent. I could not imagine having to stick myself or have someone else stick me with a needle every day of my life. So, I decided that since I am severely at risk because I am Afro-American, it runs in my family, and I am overweight, I need to do something. I started by first taking this course to get some info on health and nutrition. Then I started working with my doctor on exercise and a diet to put me at lower risk. I have been sticking with it and am feeling better physically and mentally.

—Aretha Pearson

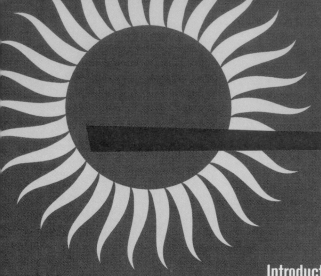

Introduction

Since the early 1900s, our society has made tremendous strides in conquering childhood diseases. People are living longer and life expectancy has nearly doubled over the last century. Now that we have significantly improved the quantity of life, quality of life has become a focus in today's prevention-oriented society. For example, national objectives spelled out in *Healthy People 2000* (U.S. Department of Health and Human Services) emphasize disease prevention and health promotion through modification of lifestyle. Although society has not achieved the national objectives of *Healthy People 2000*, increased awareness and improved behaviors among the U.S. population are promising. Further, new research is identifying strategies for exercise and other healthy choices that are more user-friendly, thus easier for individuals to adopt. These strategies are outlined in the more recent *Healthy People 2010* (U.S. Department of Health and Human Services) recommendations.

Research has consistently shown that lifestyle choices have a significant influence on the prevalence of many common chronic diseases. A **chronic disease** is any disease that develops over time as the body's ability to resist potential pathogens and environmental threats begins to diminish. As it ages, the human body tends to lose some of the resilience characteristic of youth and becomes progressively more susceptible to illness. In some cases, younger people never develop a strong ability to resist disease and find themselves facing a chronic ailment early in life. Many of the factors that contribute to chronic diseases are physical in nature. For example, high blood pressure predisposes a person to heart disease, and lack of calcium to osteoporosis. However, a variety of psychological, social, and environmental factors also come into play. For example, the psychological need to overeat can be a contributing factor in diabetes, stress can contribute to heart disease or cancer, and chemicals in the environment can cause cancer.

Objectives

After reading this chapter, you should be able to

- Define cardiovascular disease, cancer, diabetes, and osteoporosis

- Describe the prevalence of cardiovascular diseases, cancer, diabetes, and osteoporosis

- Identify risk factors for cardiovascular disease, cancer, diabetes, and osteoporosis

- Discuss ways to reduce your risk for cardiovascular disease, cancer, diabetes, and osteoporosis

- Describe the different treatments for cardiovascular disease, cancer, diabetes, and osteoporosis

In this chapter, you will learn about the major chronic diseases affecting people today: cardiovascular (heart) diseases, cancer, diabetes, and osteoporosis. You will become familiar with factors affecting your risk for developing these diseases. In addition, you will learn how to reduce your risk by making appropriate lifestyle choices.

Cardiovascular Diseases

The good news about cardiovascular diseases is that the number of people dying from them has been declining over the past 30 years. For most of the 20th century, the number of deaths due to cardiovascular disease increased each year. This trend has reversed as a result of improvements in the diagnosis and treatment of the diseases and increases in the number of people exercising and eating more healthful diets. The bad news about cardiovascular diseases is that they are still the leading cause of death in the United States. The American Heart Association reports that more people die from heart disease than from the next seven leading causes of death combined. (See the Stats-at-a-Glance.)

Heart disease takes many forms, including coronary artery disease (CAD), hypertension (high blood pressure), and stroke. High blood pressure is the most prevalent form of heart disease—50 million Americans have it, compared with 14 million who have CAD and 4 million who have suffered a stroke. However, CAD is responsible for the most deaths—approximately 500,000 each year, compared with 158,000 from stroke and 40,000 from high blood pressure. For this reason, much of our discussion of cardiovascular diseases will focus on CAD and the underlying disease process that causes it: atherosclerosis.

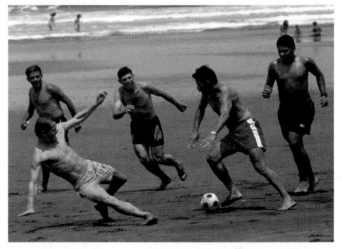

Lifestyle choices play a big role in chronic disease.

Defining the Diseases

Coronary artery disease (CAD) is a condition in which the arteries that carry blood to the heart have been damaged by atherosclerosis, resulting in a reduction of blood flow to the heart muscle. **Atherosclerosis** is the progressive narrowing and hardening of the arteries due to the formation of **plaque,** which is the accumulation of fat, connective tissue, and other substances in the inner lining of the arterial walls. Plaque can collect until it occupies more than 75% of the diameter of an artery or, in extreme cases, completely blocks the flow of blood through an artery (see Figure 13.1). A brief review of the physiology of the heart will demonstrate why CAD can be so deadly.

The function of the heart is to pump blood, first to the lungs to pick up oxygen and release carbon dioxide, and then throughout the rest of the body. Some of the blood is circulated back to the heart, through the coronary arteries, to provide the **myocardium**—the muscular wall of the heart or, collectively, the muscle fibers of the heart—with needed oxygen and nutrients (see Figure 13.2). Because the heart is constantly pumping, the myocardial fibers extract and use most of the oxygen carried in the blood that passes through the coronary arteries. These fibers require even more oxygen when the heart

chronic disease any disease that develops over time

coronary artery disease (CAD) condition in which the arteries that serve the heart have been damaged by atherosclerosis

atherosclerosis progressive narrowing and hardening of the arteries due to the formation of plaque

plaque accumulation of fat, connective tissue, and other substances in the inner lining of the arterial walls

myocardium muscular wall of the heart; collectively, the muscle fibers of the heart

STATS-AT-A-GLANCE:
Cardiovascular Diseases

■ Since 1900, cardiovascular disease has been the #1 killer in the United States every year but one (1918).

■ Cardiovascular diseases claimed 960,592 lives in 1995 (41.5% of all deaths), which is more than the number of deaths caused by cancer, accidents, pneumonia, influenza, homicides, and HIV (AIDS) combined.

■ Each day, more than 2,600 Americans die from cardiovascular diseases, an average of one death every 33 seconds.

■ An estimated 1,100,000 Americans will have a heart attack this year, and about one-third of them will die.

■ If all forms of cardiovascular disease were eliminated, life expectancy would increase by almost 10 years. If all forms of cancer were eliminated, the gain would be 3 years.

■ Of the approximately 50 million Americans who have high blood pressure, one-half are not on therapy and another 27% are on inadequate therapy.

■ The cost of cardiovascular disease in 1998—including the cost of physician and nursing services, hospital and nursing home services, medications, and lost productivity resulting from disability—will be $274.2 billion.

■ Heart attack is the primary killer of American women.

Source: American Heart Association

works harder—for example, during exercise or periods of stress. To deliver more oxygen to the myocardial fibers, the coronary arteries must widen to increase the volume of blood reaching the myocardium. Because the supply of blood through the coronary arteries is critical to the functioning of the heart, which, in turn, is critical to the functioning of the body, anything that compromises myocardial blood supply jeopardizes your well-being. For people with CAD, the amount of blood that can pass through the coronary arteries may not be enough to nourish the myocardial fibers.

The condition in which cells in the heart receive an insufficient supply of blood is called **ischemia.** Deprived of oxygen, ischemic myocardial fibers cannot contract effectively, and this reduces the pumping ability of the heart; if the ischemia persists, the affected fibers die. **Myocardial infarction (MI),** or "heart attack," refers to the death of a region of the myocardium due to an insufficient supply of blood. A heart attack can be fatal when the compromised heart fails to pump enough blood to supply the brain and other vital organs with the oxygen and nutrients they require. If the infarcted area of the heart is not large, the victim can survive because the remaining healthy myocardium can still pump adequate amounts of blood.

Myocardial ischemia can also cause *ventricular fibrillation,* in which the fibers of the heart contract in an uncontrolled, uncoordinated, and ineffective manner. This, too, can be fatal because a fibrillating heart is unable to keep blood flowing throughout the body. A person can survive ventricular fibrillation with the help of cardiopulmonary resuscitation (CPR) while awaiting emergency care. The normal contraction rhythm of the heart can often be reestablished with a *defibrillator,* which sends a jolt of electricity across the heart to make all the fibers contract at once.

Myocardial ischemia can occur without resulting in a heart attack. These episodes of ischemia cause chest pain known as **angina pectoris** and are often brought on by emotional stress or physical exertion. Rest usually relieves the symptoms of angina. When a person experiences a bout of angina, he or she can take nitroglycerine tablets to expand the blood vessels and reduce the work of the heart, thus reducing the myocardial oxygen demand.

Some heart attacks are caused by the formation of a blood clot *(thrombus).* If the thrombus is attached to plaque on the artery wall, it can grow until it blocks the vessel, or it can dislodge from the plaque and block the vessel at a narrower point downstream. Emergency treatment of heart attacks caused by blood clots includes the administration of clot-dissolving drugs such as streptokinase or tissue plasminogen activator (TPA). A common household medication, aspirin, has been found to inhibit the formation of blood clots. A large study of middle-aged male physicians found that those

Figure 13.1

(1) In a healthy artery, blood flows unobstructed. **(2–4)** Atherosclerosis results in the progressive formation of plaque on artery walls and thus in restricted blood flow.

Source: From Brannon and Feist, 1997.

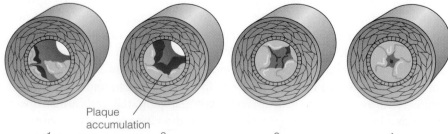

Plaque accumulation

1   2   3   4

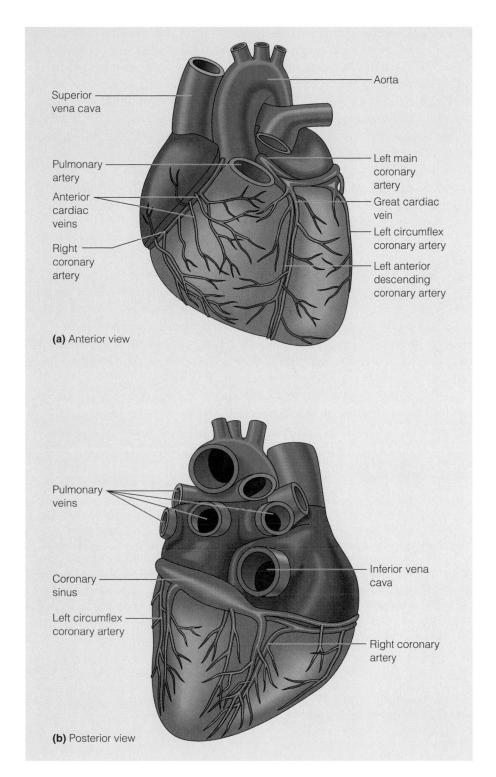

Superior
vena cava

Aorta

Pulmonary
artery

Left main
coronary
artery

Anterior
cardiac
veins

Great cardiac
vein

Left circumflex
coronary artery

Right
coronary
artery

Left anterior
descending
coronary artery

(a) Anterior view

Pulmonary
veins

Coronary
sinus

Inferior vena
cava

Left circumflex
coronary artery

Right coronary
artery

(b) Posterior view

Figure 13.2

The coronary circulation (the coronary arteries are in red, the coronary veins in blue). The coronary arteries transport blood, carrying oxygen and nutrients, to the myocardium.
Source: From Marieb, 1992.

taking one aspirin tablet every other day had 47% fewer heart attacks than those who did not take the aspirin (Physicians Health Study Research Group). Because aspirin can irritate the stomach, it is recommended that anyone considering taking it on a regular basis consult a physician first.

Most people associate CAD and heart attacks with the elderly. Although 70% of all heart attacks occur in those over age 65, the disease process actually begins long before that. For example, fatty streaks, the precursor of atherosclerotic plaque, have been found in the coronary arteries of children.

ischemia condition in which cells receive an insufficient supply of blood

myocardial infarction "heart attack"; the death of a region of the myocardium due to an insufficient supply of blood

angina pectoris chest pain caused by myocardial ischemia

In the early and middle stages of the disease, heart disease symptoms are not evident, as the arterial **lumen** (the open space in the interior of a blood vessel) is sufficient to allow adequate blood flow. This is the silent phase of CAD. However, as plaque build-up continues, the lumen grows progressively smaller. As shown in Figure 13.3, with 70% or more of the lumen blocked with plaque, ischemia, angina, infarction, and, ultimately, heart failure can occur. Studies tracking the appearance and progression of CAD risk factors in children demonstrate that atherosclerotic fatty streaks and plaque were more evident at this young age in those who had high blood cholesterol levels. These findings underscore the importance of adopting a healthy lifestyle now, including physical activity, not smoking, and a good diet, to slow or prevent the progression of the disease.

Risk Factors

The exact causes of atherosclerosis and CAD are not known, but researchers have identified several major risk factors that are definitely associated with the development of these diseases, including smoking, hypertension, high blood cholesterol, and physical inactivity. Having one of the major risk factors for CAD increases your chance of developing heart disease; having several risk factors present at once sharply increases your risk of a heart attack (see Figure 13.6). You will have an opportunity to evaluate your risk for heart disease by completing the RISKO assessment in Laboratory 13.1.

lumen open space in the interior of a blood vessel

MYTHS & CONTROVERSIES

Myth 1

The biggest threat to women's health is breast cancer. Actually, the leading cause of death among women is heart disease. Polls indicate that women tend to overestimate their risk of dying of breast cancer and to underestimate their risk of heart disease. In 1995, the mortality rate for CAD for women was three times higher than that for breast cancer; in every year since 1984, cardiovascular disease has claimed more women than men (see Figures 13.4 and 13.5, respectively). Women have a greater incidence of high cholesterol, physical inactivity, and overweight— each a CAD risk factor. With a better understanding of their risk for heart disease, women can more readily see the value in becoming more physically active and adopting a diet that is conducive to lowering blood cholesterol and maintaining optimal body weight. Breast cancer is the second most common cause of cancer death in women, after lung cancer. Smoking is a major risk factor for both lung cancer and heart disease.

Controversy 1

Are certain personality types more prone to cancer and heart disease? Current research suggests that people who have a chronically hostile and cynical attitude toward life are more likely to develop heart disease than people who are calmer. These people seem to have trouble shutting down the stress response when they encounter everyday irritations, and the result is higher blood pressure and more heart disease. A theory has been advanced that there is also a personality type that is prone to cancer, the so-called "Type-C personality." These people are said to express anger rarely, to put others' needs ahead of their own consistently, and to try to please everyone. However, this theory is very controversial and more research is needed to understand the relationship between personality traits and cancer.

Controversy 2

Is being religious good for your health? The answer seems to be "yes." In studies looking at the effects of religious commitment on health, 75% showed a positive effect, including lower rates among religious individuals of depression, hypertension, and heart disease. The critical factor seems to be the intensity of religious conviction; those with the strongest ties to a religious community are the healthiest. The reason for this effect is unclear, but researchers speculate that strongly religious people tend to have less social isolation than others and may also have a healthier lifestyle than the general population.

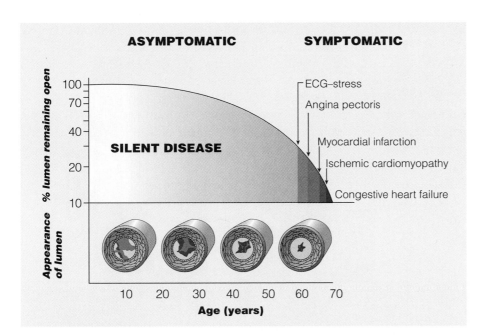

Figure 13.3

Atherosclerotic plaque build up progresses over many years without the appearance of symptoms. Serious symptoms can occur when 70% or more of the lumen is blocked.

Source: From Berenson et al., 1989.

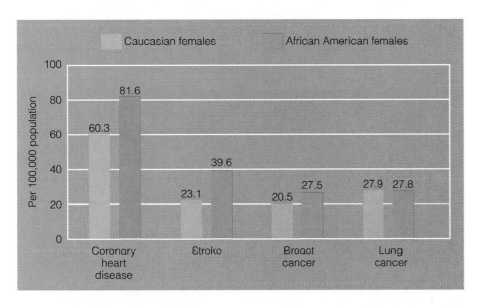

Figure 13.4

Age-adjusted death rates for coronary heart disease, stroke, breast cancer, and lung cancer for Caucasian and African-American females; United States, 1995.

Source: Reproduced with permission. *Heart and Stroke Facts: 1988 Statistical Supplement,* 1997. Copyright American Heart Association.

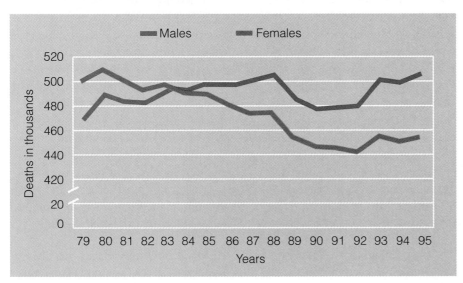

Figure 13.5

Cardiovascular disease mortality trends for males and females; United States, 1979–1995.

Source: Reproduced with permission. *Heart and Stroke Facts: 1988 Statistical Supplement,* 1997. Copyright American Heart Association.

Figure 13.6

There is a sharp increase in the overall risk for a heart attack when multiple risk factors are present.
Source: Framingham Heart Study Section 37. The Probability of Developing Certain Cardiovascular Diseases in Eight Years at Specified Values of Some Characteristics (Aug. 1987).

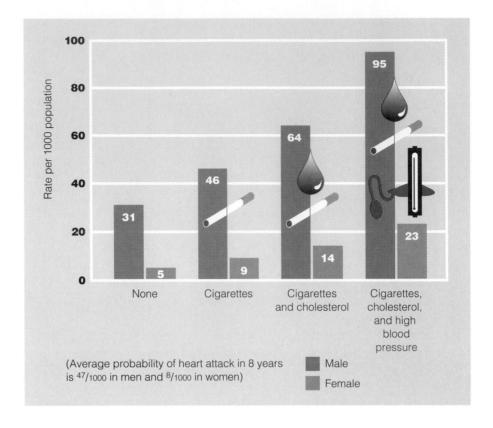

(Average probability of heart attack in 8 years is $^{47}/_{1000}$ in men and $^{8}/_{1000}$ in women)

Smoking. Smokers have more than twice the risk of having a heart attack as nonsmokers, and among all individuals who have a heart attack, smokers are more likely to die from it than are nonsmokers. Although the number of smokers has declined over the past 20 years, too many people still smoke—an estimated 23% of all adult females and 28% of adult males. Smoking contributes to CAD through at least two mechanisms: (1) facilitating the creation of plaque by injuring the lining of the artery walls, and (2) increasing the likelihood of blood clot formation.

Research indicates that a combination of smoking and oral contraceptives further increases the risk of CAD. The American Heart Association reports that female smokers who use birth control pills are much are more likely to have a heart attack or a stroke than women who neither smoke nor take oral contraceptives.

Being exposed to secondhand, environmental tobacco smoke at home or at work increases a person's risk of death from CAD by up to 30%. For this reason, many states and communities have prohibited smoking in the workplace and in public buildings. We are now less likely to encounter secondhand smoke in public settings, but passive smoking continues to occur at home. It is estimated that approximately 40% of American children are exposed to secondhand smoke at home in their first decade of life. When we give up smoking to improve our own health, we also improve the health of those around us.

Your chance of avoiding CAD increases as soon as you break the smoking habit. Even if you once smoked up to a pack of cigarettes per day, after 3 years of nonsmoking your risk of death from heart disease will be comparable to that of someone who never smoked, other factors being equal.

Hypertension. Hypertension (high blood pressure) places your heart and arteries under constant stress, thus predisposing you to CAD. This condition affects one American in four; it can lead to kidney damage or the rupture of small vessels in the eye, with resulting loss of peripheral vision. It can also enlarge and weaken the heart, reducing its pumping effectiveness. The injurious effects of hypertension on the arteries accelerate the athero-sclerotic process, making a person more susceptible to heart attack and to **stroke**—damage to the brain due to inadequate blood supply or a ruptured blood vessel (a "brain attack").

The underlying cause of high blood pressure is not understood for over 90% of those who have it, but the condition can be detected easily and most cases can be controlled. Do you know your blood pressure? Because 45% of those with high blood pressure are unaware of it, regular blood pressure checks are advised. As discussed in Chapter 3, the peak blood pressure reading, which occurs when the heart contracts and pumps blood into the arteries, is called *systolic pressure*. The lower blood pressure reading, which occurs when the heart rests between heart beats, is called *diastolic pressure*. Table 13.1 gives the values for normal and high blood pressure readings. If you have a reading that indicates mild hypertension, you should confirm this value with several more readings over the next few months. If your blood pressure reading is in the severe range, you should see your doctor immediately.

High Blood Cholesterol. The amount and type of cholesterol you have in your blood may place you at risk for developing CAD. Because cholesterol cannot be dissolved in blood, lipid-protein complexes, known as **lipoproteins,** transport cholesterol and trygliceride through the blood. Two lipoproteins account for most of the cholesterol in circulation in the blood: *low-density lipoprotein (LDL)* and *high-density lipoprotein (HDL)*.

LDL delivers cholesterol to the cells throughout the body and therefore is responsible for a buildup of cholesterol in the tissues and arteries. HDL picks up cholesterol from throughout the body and delivers it to the liver, where it is processed or excreted from the body. As a result of their different functions, these two lipoproteins have opposite effects on your overall risk for CAD. If you have a high level of LDL, you have an increased risk of CAD; if you have a high level of HDL, you have a reduced risk of CAD.

Evaluating your CAD risk based on cholesterol levels is done in two stages. The first step is to determine your total cholesterol level. The desired level for total cholesterol is less than 200 milligrams (mg) per decaliter (dL;

TABLE 13.1

Values for Normal and Hypertensive Blood Pressures

	SYSTOLIC PRESSURE (MM HG)	DIASTOLIC PRESSURE (MM HG)
Normal	< 140	< 85
High normal	—	85–89
Mild hypertension	140–159	90–104
Moderate hypertension	—	105–114
Severe hypertension	> 160	> 115

stroke "brain attack"; damage to the brain due to an inadequate blood supply or a ruptured blood vessel

lipoproteins lipid-protein complexes that transport cholesterol and triglycerides through the blood

100 milliliters) of blood. With a total cholesterol level below 200 mg/dL, your risk of CAD is considered to be low.

If your total cholesterol is greater than 200 mg/dL, however, the second step in the evaluation is to determine your LDL level. Table 13.2 gives the classifications for total cholesterol and LDL levels according to the National Cholesterol Education Program Adult Treatment Panel. This panel recommends that your LDL level be below 130 mg/dL. Evaluating your HDL level is done by determining what proportion of your total cholesterol is in the form of HDL. If the value for HDL is greater than 30% of the value for total cholesterol, then you have a desirable level of HDL.

Physical Inactivity. Studies have repeatedly demonstrated that physically active people have a lower incidence of CAD than those who are inactive. An ongoing study of Harvard alumni has found that those men who expend an additional 2,000 kilocalories per week beyond the energy used for sedentary living have a significantly lower incidence of death by CAD, cancer, and other diseases, and they have a 1- to 2-year greater life expectancy than their inactive counterparts (Paffenbarger et al.). A review of the research on CAD and physical inactivity found that a sedentary lifestyle places people at a risk for CAD that is comparable to the risk they would have if they had high blood pressure or high cholesterol levels, or if they smoked (Powell et al.). A person with any one of these risk factors has approximately twice the risk of heart attack than would be the case without the risk factor. For this reason, the American Heart Association has designated physical inactivity one of the major CAD risk factors.

Contributing Factors. The contributing risk factors for CAD do not show as strong or as well established an influence as the major risk factors. Some of the contributing risk factors cannot be changed: heredity (family history), age, and sex. Children whose parents develop CAD prior to age 55 are more likely to develop it themselves. African Americans have a higher rate of hypertension than Caucasians; although this does not appear to increase their incidence of heart attacks, it does contribute to a higher prevalence of strokes among this racial group.

Age and Sex. Figure 13.7 depicts the incidence of heart attacks in men and women as they age. For both sexes, heart attacks dramatically increase with age, but the increase occurs at a later age for women than it does for men. One factor that accounts for this difference is that women typically have high levels of HDL. The female sex hormone estrogen stimulates HDL

TABLE 13.2

Classification Based on Total Cholesterol and LDL Levels in the Blood

CHOLESTEROL (MG/DL)		LDL (MG/DL)
< 200	Desirable	< 130
200–239	Borderline high	130–159
> 240	High	> 160

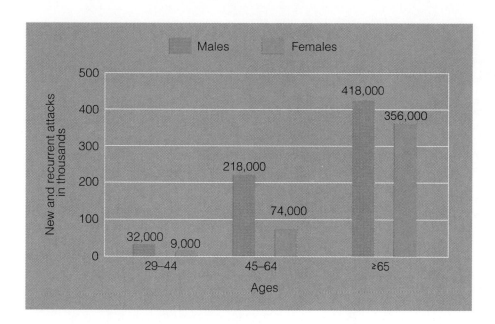

Figure 13.7

The estimated annual number of Americans, by age and sex, who experience a heart attack. The incidence of heart attacks is greater for men than for women, but the difference in incidence between the sexes is greatly reduced after age 65.

Source: Reproduced with permission. *Heart and Stroke Facts: 1988 Statistical Supplement,* 1997. Copyright American Heart Association.

formation, but this risk-lowering advantage is lost when estrogen production is reduced after menopause. Thus, postmenopausal women have almost three times as many heart attacks as premenopausal women. In addition, women over 65 years of age are more likely to die from their heart attacks as are men.

Diabetes. Diabetes mellitus is another unalterable risk factor because it cannot be cured once a person develops it. (The disease process of diabetes is discussed later in this chapter.) Diabetes accelerates the development of atherosclerosis by causing a disruption in the lining of the arterial walls and/or by causing abnormalities in lipoprotein levels. More than 80% of people with diabetes die of some form of CAD (American Heart Association).

Obesity. An excessive amount of body fat (as described in Chapter 8) is associated with hypertension, high cholesterol levels, diabetes, and CAD. Previously, the association between obesity and CAD was thought to be indirect, operating through the risk factors just discussed. However, the Framingham Heart Study, a long-term study that has generated much of what we know about CAD risk factors, established that obesity exerts an independent influence on the development of CAD. Reducing body fat can be very beneficial for health because it lowers not just CAD risk but also blood pressure, cholesterol levels, and the risk for diabetes.

Stress. As discussed in Chapter 10, stress is thought to be a predisposing factor for CAD, although the mechanism by which it exerts its effects is not understood. Stress is a fact of modern life, and people have quite individualized ways of experiencing and reacting to it. The relationship between stress and CAD is not simple and straightforward, however. For example, one study evaluating the association between job-related stress and heart disease noted that stress alone did not predict a person's risk for CAD. The lack of control people felt in their jobs was also associated with their risk for CAD. Thus, executives and supervisors who had positions of authority had fewer adverse health consequences from their stress than those lower in the power structure who had to follow the orders of their supervisors.

Influencing the Progression of CAD

Coronary artery disease has a very long silent phase, in which the plaque build-up in the coronary arteries has not advanced to the point that a person experiences the symptoms of heart disease. Evidence from the Bogolusa Heart Study and other projects that have evaluated the arteries of children and young adults who have died from accidents or homicides or were wartime casualties have demonstrated that the development of fatty streaks and plaque begins early in the life span. It is probably accurate to assume that the disease is already established in you, although you cannot know to what extent without performing sophisticated laboratory tests. Picturing your coronary arteries already collecting fat and cellular debris along their walls can be somewhat unsettling. However, you also know that plaque has to build to an advanced stage before it is likely to result in a coronary event. Therefore, a wise course would be to adopt a wellness lifestyle now that will minimize your CAD risk factors and slow the progression of the disease. Components of this lifestyle are outlined in the Prevention section of this chapter: don't smoke, exercise, eat wisely, and maintain your optimal body weight.

Treatment

The first steps to improving coronary health are to adopt a "heart-healthy" diet, reduce excess body fat, learn stress-reduction techniques, exercise regularly, and quit smoking. These lifestyle changes are recommended if you're at risk for CAD or if you have symptoms.

Perhaps the most effective step is to lose excess body weight. Reducing your daily intake of sodium to 1.5 to 2.5 grams per day is also recommended. Regular aerobic exercise can help to lower blood pressure, although there is some conflicting research regarding its effectiveness. Because exercise can assist you in losing weight and has many other health benefits, seeing whether it will also lower your blood pressure is worthwhile.

When CAD symptoms are more serious or fail to respond sufficiently to changes in diet and exercise, your doctor may prescribe medications to lower your blood pressure or cholesterol levels or to relieve symptoms of angina. Medications for hypertension include diuretics, beta-blockers, calcium channel blockers, and angiotensin converting enzyme (ACE) inhibitors. Cholesterol-lowering medications include lovestatin, niacin, and clofibrate.

If atherosclerosis has progressed to the point that one or more of the coronary arteries are severely narrowed or entirely blocked, surgery may be required. Blood flow to the myocardium can be restored by *coronary artery bypass graft (CABG) surgery,* in which blood vessels from other regions of the body are grafted to the coronary arteries to provide an alternate channel for blood flow. Another procedure to increase the flow of blood through a narrowed artery is *percutaneous transluminal coronary angioplasty (PTCA),* in which a tube is inserted into the artery and inflated to expand the vessel at the site of plaque buildup. In 1995, approximately 573,000 CABG surgeries and 419,000 PTCA procedures were performed, with each procedure costing an average of $44,820 and $20,370, respectively.

Prevention

You cannot totally prevent the atherosclerotic process, but you can slow its progress. Your best bet for avoiding CAD is to minimize your risk factors.

Because many of these risk factors are the result of lifestyle choices you make, making the right choices will have a profound effect on the health of your heart and on your overall wellness. The heart-healthy lifestyle choices include the following:

1. *Do not smoke.*

2. *Stay physically active.* This helps to lower your blood pressure, your blood cholesterol levels, and your body fat. It will increase your HDL levels, reduce your risk of developing diabetes, and strengthen your bones. Exercise is also an effective stress-reducing activity.

3. *Maintain your appropriate body weight.* This will reduce your blood pressure, cholesterol levels, and risk for diabetes.

4. *Eat a diet low in fat (particularly saturated fat), cholesterol, and sodium (salt)* (see Chapter 7). A low-fat diet helps lower cholesterol levels and helps you maintain an appropriate body weight. A low-salt diet helps to lower blood pressure.

5. *Regularly monitor your blood pressure and blood cholesterol levels.* You should have your blood pressure checked once or twice a year. If your total cholesterol and LDL levels are in the recommended ranges, you should have them rechecked within 5 years. If they are high, recheck them yearly to assess the effectiveness of the lifestyle changes you have made. Most university student health centers, community health clinics, and hospitals offer blood lipid screening for under $30.

Cancer

During the past 50 years, perhaps no other disease has instilled greater fear than cancer. Part of the reason for this concern may be that cancer kills more people annually than AIDS, accidents and homicide *combined* (American Cancer Society, Facts and Figures). Many of these deaths could be prevented. In spite of major advances in cancer diagnosis, treatment, and long-term survival for some cancers, the disease continues to strike people of all ages, races, and socioeconomic backgrounds. (See Stats-at-a-Glance.) Typically, cancer develops over time, making it more common among persons as they age, particularly those over 50. However, the young are major targets for some cancers, such as childhood leukemia and skin cancer. Although cancer is fairly rare among this age group, most people are surprised to discover that it is the chief cause of death by disease in children under the age of 15. Other cancers, such as ovarian, breast, and testicular cancer, are attacking an increasing number of young adults, especially those with a genetic tendency for the disease and whose lifestyle choices are not optimal.

As you can see from Figure 13.8, deaths from lung cancer have increased dramatically over the past 60 years, whereas mortality rates for uterine and stomach cancer have declined. More recently, there have been epidemic rises in the incidence of breast, prostate, and skin cancers among selected segments of the population. Although these figures may seem rather bleak, particularly for some cancers, note that nearly half (4 out of 10 overall) of those who are treated for cancer survive at least 5 years without a recurrence of symptoms. The American Cancer Society

STATS-AT-A-GLANCE
Cancer

- Cancer is the second leading cause of death in this country, exceeded only by heart disease.

- One in every four deaths in the United States is due to cancer—more than 1,500 deaths per day.

- In the United States, men have a 1 in 2 lifetime risk of developing cancer; for women, the risk is 1 in 3. (Lifetime risk refers to the probability that you will develop or die from cancer in your lifetime.)

- Scientific evidence suggests that up to one-third of the 560,000 cancer deaths in 1997 were related to nutrition. For example, a high intake of fat is related to many cancers, such as cancer of the colon and prostate.

- Lung cancer is the primary cancer killer for men and women, followed by prostate cancer for men and breast cancer for women.

- In the early 1900s, few cancer patients had any hope of long-term survival. In the 1930s about one in four was alive five years after treatment. Today, approximately 4 in 10 of those who will develop cancer will live 5 years or more.

- The National Cancer Institute estimates that overall costs for cancer were $104 billion in direct and indirect costs in 1997. Of course, these, estimates do not estimate the "human" value of the loss of loved ones.

Source: From American Cancer Society, 1997.

Figure 13.8
Cancer death rates by type, in the
United States over the last 60 years.
Source: From American Cancer Society,
1993.

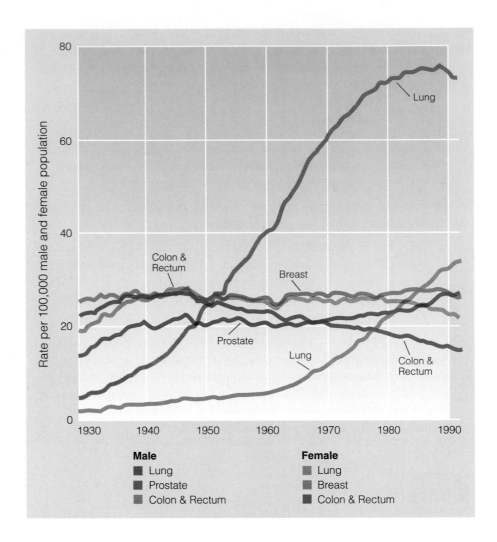

and the National Cancer Institute consider *5-year survival* as equivalent to
being cured. Although cancer is common in Americans of all racial and
ethnic groups, the rate of cancer occurrence (often called the incidence
rate) varies considerably from group to group. Among men, cancer rates
are highest among African Americans, followed by whites whose rates are
about 16% lower. Cancer incidence rates for American Indian men in New
Mexico are the lowest, and rates among Asian men are also low. Among
women, the differences in rates across racial and ethnic groups are less
pronounced than among men. Rates are highest among Alaska-Native
women, followed closely by white women (American Cancer Society,
Cancer Facts and Figures).

Defining the Disease

The term **cancer** refers to over 100 different types of cancer-like diseases
characterized by abnormal and uncontrollable cell growth. The result is
tumors, masses of abnormal tissue that grow rapidly and that can be either
benign (noncancerous) or *malignant* (cancerous). Although benign tumors, or
cysts, can become so large that they interfere with circulation or other functions, they are not life threatening. By contrast, malignant neoplasms (new
growth) can invade surrounding structures, infiltrating blood vessels, organs,
nerves, or the lymphatic system.

cancer group of over 100 different
types of diseases characterized by
abnormal and uncontrollable cell
growth

tumor mass of abnormal tissue that
grows rapidly and that can be either
benign or malignant

metastasis process by which
cancerous cells from a malignant
tumor travel from the primary site to
distant ports of the body to form new
tumors

Sound Decision Making

CONFRONTING AND CONTROLLING YOUR RISK FACTORS

Joseph had always been close to his father, so he was devastated when the older man had a heart attack at age 54. Joseph's father eventually recovered with lots of support from his family, but he continued to have chest pain. In talking with his father about the event, Joseph learned that three of his four grandparents and two uncles also had had heart attacks or severe chest pain. Joseph did some reading at his school library about heart disease and realized that he himself had many risk factors: he had a strong family history of early heart disease, he was male, he was overweight and ate a high-fat diet, and he was African-American. In fact, most of these risk factors applied to Joseph's brothers and sisters as well.

When the family gathered for Thanksgiving a few weeks later, Joseph made a proposal to the group. He suggested that the family legacy of early heart disease should stop with his generation, and that he and his brothers and sisters should start a campaign to educate themselves about their own risk of heart disease and to make lifestyle changes that would greatly reduce their risk of the disease. His siblings were skeptical at first, but Joseph's parents were enthusiastic and convinced them to give it a try. Joseph's plan was simple in some ways. The two siblings who smoked should stop; all should eat a lower fat diet, get some exercise every day, watch their weight, and get their blood pressure and cholesterol checked. The brothers and sisters would form an informal support group and call on each other for encouragement.

Joseph had some difficulties at first in changing his eating habits. He had never thought much about what he ate, and it seemed that now he had to scrutinize everything that went into his mouth. But he found that trading tips and recipes with others in his family helped, and they began having weekly healthy dinner gatherings together. They also spent some weekend afternoons going for walks. The group support and the clear goal of avoiding cardiovascular disease in the future kept Joseph's motivation high.

Six months later, Joseph had lost 30 pounds and was close to his ideal weight. His siblings had all lost weight too, and one of them had successfully quit smoking. An unexpected benefit to the family was how close they felt to each other; they had met their goals together for their common good. As the family gathered to celebrate Joseph's father's birthday the next year, they felt they all had a lot to be thankful for, and the fat-free cake wasn't half bad.

Malignant cancer cells destroy healthy cells by disrupting the normal nucleic structure of cellular RNA and DNA (the genetic programming of the cell). Cells from a malignant tumor can travel from the primary site to distant parts of the body to form new tumors in a process known as **metastasis.** If a cancer metastasizes quickly or if it is not diagnosed until it has already spread, the chances of effective treatment are drastically reduced. Thus, early detection, particularly for virulent (invasive) forms of cancer such as *melanoma* (skin cancer) and ovarian and testicular cancers, is critical to possible treatment or cure. The poor, or those without adequate insurance that allows for early screening, are disadvantaged when it comes to early access and often have poorer prognoses because of tumor spread and level of invasiveness.

Cancerous tumors are generally classified according to the type of tissue in which they originate. There are four major types of cancer:

1. Carcinomas

2. Sarcomas

3. Lymphomas

4. Leukemias

Carcinomas, the most common group of cancers, develop in the outer layers of body tissue (*epithelial* tissue such as the linings of the skin, stomach, intestines, breasts, lungs, or uterus) and metastasize primarily through the lymphatic system. The lymphatic system is a one-way network of drainage vessels that absorbs excess fluid that has escaped from the blood and returns it to the bloodstream.

Sarcomas, the second-largest group of cancers, develop primarily in fibrous and connective tissues, such as those found in bones and joints, and metastasize through the blood. **Lymphomas** develop and spread via the lymphatic system and can seriously impair the body's ability to form and effectively utilize white blood cells as part of the body's immune system. The fourth type of cancer, leukemia, is different from the three preceding types; rather than forming a solid mass, **leukemia** affects the blood-forming cells of the body; it is referred to as a nonsolid tumor and is characterized by an abnormally high number of white blood cells. Cancers are also commonly known by the body part they affect (for example, breast, brain, colon) (see Figure 13.9).

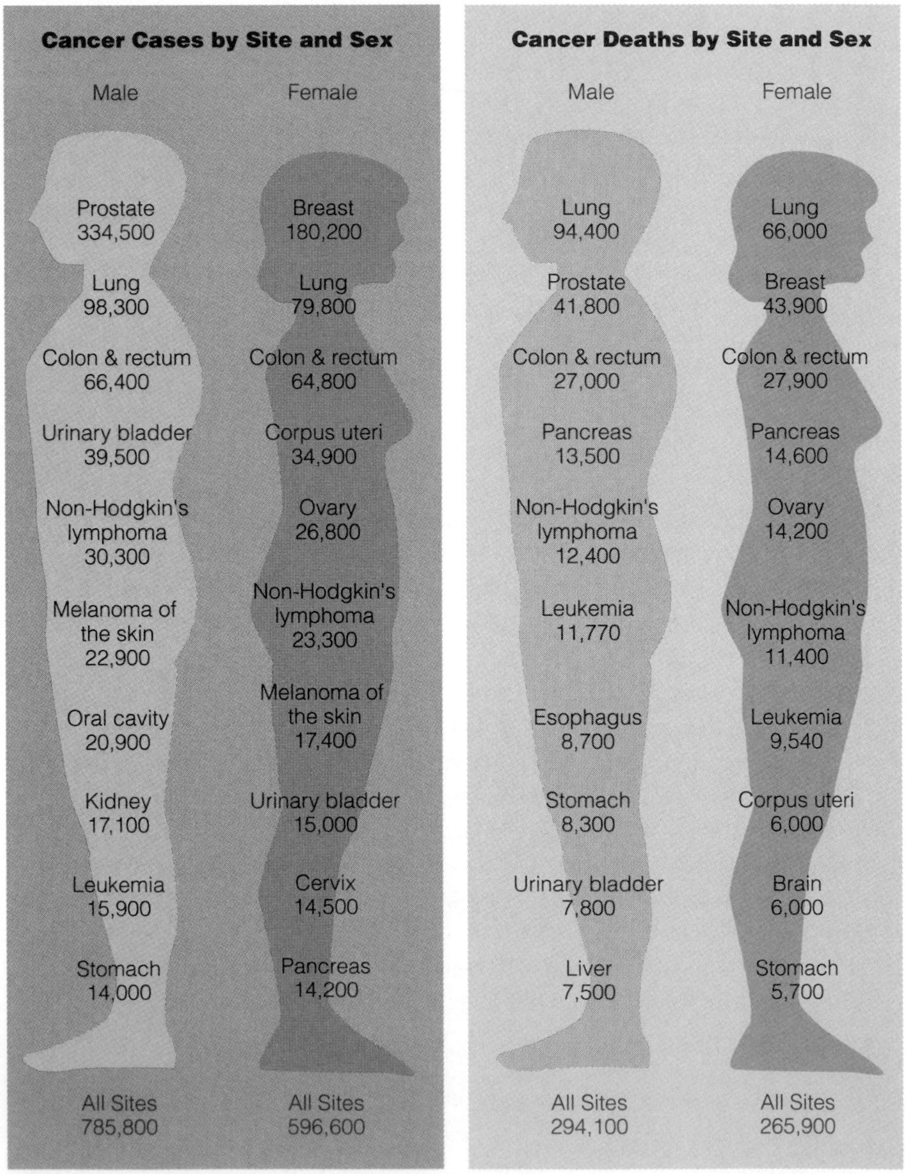

Figure **13.9**

Leading Sites of New Cancer Cases and Deaths—1997 Estimates*
*Excluding basal and squamous cell skin cancer and in situ carcinomas except bladder.
Source: From American Cancer Society, 1997.

Cancer Cases by Site and Sex

Male	Female
Prostate 334,500	Breast 180,200
Lung 98,300	Lung 79,800
Colon & rectum 66,400	Colon & rectum 64,800
Urinary bladder 39,500	Corpus uteri 34,900
Non-Hodgkin's lymphoma 30,300	Ovary 26,800
Melanoma of the skin 22,900	Non-Hodgkin's lymphoma 23,300
Oral cavity 20,900	Melanoma of the skin 17,400
Kidney 17,100	Urinary bladder 15,000
Leukemia 15,900	Cervix 14,500
Stomach 14,000	Pancreas 14,200
All Sites 785,800	All Sites 596,600

Cancer Deaths by Site and Sex

Male	Female
Lung 94,400	Lung 66,000
Prostate 41,800	Breast 43,900
Colon & rectum 27,000	Colon & rectum 27,900
Pancreas 13,500	Pancreas 14,600
Non-Hodgkin's lymphoma 12,400	Ovary 14,200
Leukemia 11,770	Non-Hodgkin's lymphoma 11,400
Esophagus 8,700	Leukemia 9,540
Stomach 8,300	Corpus uteri 6,000
Urinary bladder 7,800	Brain 6,000
Liver 7,500	Stomach 5,700
All Sites 294,100	All Sites 265,900

*Excluding basal and squamous cell skin cancer and in situ carcinomas except bladder.
American Cancer Society Surveillance Research, 1997.

carcinomas cancer type that develops in outer layers of body tissue and metastasizes primarily via the lymphatic system

sarcomas cancer type that develops in fibrous and connective tissues, such as bones and joints, and metastasizes through the blood

lymphomas cancer type that develops and spreads via the lymphatic system

leukemia cancer type that affects the blood-forming cells of the body

Risk Factors

Oncologists—doctors who specialize in cancer research and treatment— believe that many cancers have no single cause. In all likelihood, cancer is a *multifactorial* disease, influenced by a variety of factors. The following are some of the currently proposed theories of cancer risk.

Environmental Exposure. Numerous factors in the environment can increase your risk for cancer. **Carcinogens,** or cancer-causing agents, include a vast array of substances, such as asbestos, tobacco, alcohol, radiation, auto emissions, gases, petroleum products, chemicals used as food preservatives or additives, dyes, and ultraviolet light (for example, sunlight) (World Cancer Research Fund; Potter). If you work in an environment where carcinogens are present, you are at increased risk of exposure. It is the job of industrial hygienists, safety officers, health promotion and health education specialists, consumer groups, and environmental protection agencies to keep potentially lethal substances out of the air you breathe, the water and food you drink and eat, and the substances you touch. Knowing what these carcinogenic agents are and trying to avoid them as much as possible can protect you against risks that government, public health, and consumer groups are unable to control. Recent bans on indoor tobacco smoke in restaurants, bars, and public places in California and Oregon are designed to reduce the risk of direct and indirect (passive) exposure to the potentially harmful effects of tobacco carcinogens.

Genetics. The question of whether people can inherit a gene that makes them more susceptible to cancer has been the subject of much research. Scientists have identified a variety of **oncogenes**—genes that appear to cause cancer growth. However, because oncogenes are also present in normal cells, other factors must be present if cancer is to develop. Cancers that have been linked most closely to genetic causes include breast, colon, brain, and kidney cancer. In each of these types of cancer, if a primary relative (mother, father, or sibling) develops cancer, other family members may run an increased risk.

Viruses. Researchers have also investigated the relationship between certain viruses and cancer. For example, the herpes 11 virus has been strongly associated with the development of cervical cancer, and the hepatitis B virus has been linked with liver cancer. The virus that causes AIDS (HIV) has been linked to the subsequent development of a cancer known as Kaposi's sarcoma, which systematically damages the blood vessels.

Chronic Irritation. Substantial evidence suggests that certain precancerous chronic irritations increase cancer risks. For example, chewing tobacco can irritate linings of the mouth, leading to the development of whitish-colored patches known as leukoplakia. Irritants caused by daily shaving or cutting facial moles, bra straps that abrade underlying tissue or moles, and many similar occurrences may precipitate the development of cancer.

Lifestyle Factors. Although you may have little influence over environmental, viral, or genetic risks for cancer, you can change many of the lifestyle factors, such as diet, smoking, or stress, that are believed to affect your risk.

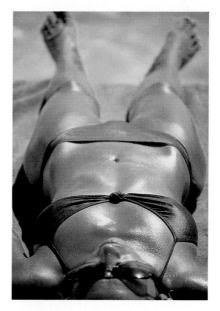

You can decrease your risk of some kinds of cancer by controlling environmental factors. Ultraviolet light—which has provided this person with a deep suntan—is a known carcinogen.

carcinogens cancer-causing agents
oncogenes genes that appear to cause cancer

Diet. As many as 35% of all cancer deaths can be attributed to dietary factors. Studies by the American Cancer Society, the National Cancer Institute, the National Academy of Sciences, and others have shown a strong association among a high-fat diet, obesity, a sedentary lifestyle, and cancer development (Willet and Trichopoulos; Hunter and Willet; Kolonel; Kono and Hirohata; Steinmetz and Potter; Kearney et al.) High-fat diets are particularly implicated in breast, colon, and prostate cancer. Whether the diet itself or the tendency to obesity among those with high-fat diets causes cancer remains in question. However, the combined effects of these two risks appears to be a major factor in cancer development.

Whereas high-fat diets increase risk, certain foods, particularly those with high fiber content, appear to reduce risk. Foods containing large amounts of vitamins A and C, and cruciferous vegetables (those in the cabbage family) appear to be most beneficial. In particular, foods containing certain micronutrients such as the *antioxidant group,* have gained increasing attention as possible protectors of DNA; hence, their reported beneficial effects in protection against cancer. Much of this research continues to remain controversial because of difficulties in studying exact dosages and chemical structures as well as other problems in research methodology (Cancer and Nutrition). Some studies show positive effects; others show no effects at all.

Tobacco Use. Tobacco use, responsible for over 87% of all lung cancer deaths, is the second major lifestyle factor contributing to cancer risk (American Cancer Society, *Cancer Facts and Figures*). Smoking itself is believed to be the most preventable cause of death in our society today, conservatively estimated to be related to about 419,000 deaths in the United States each year (American Cancer Society, *Cancer Facts and Figures*). Although the number of cardiovascular deaths is declining, smoking-related cancer deaths continue to rise. Since 1987, more women have died each year from lung cancer than breast cancer, which for over 40 years was the major cause of cancer death in women (American Cancer Society, *Cancer Facts and Figures*). In addition to lung cancer, smoking increases a person's risk of cancers of the mouth, throat, esophagus, larynx, pancreas, bladder, and cervix. Nor do you have to be a smoker yourself to be at risk; exposure to passive smoke, also known as sidestream or secondhand smoke, from someone else's smoking can also increase your risk of lung cancer and heart disease. In fact, each year, over 3,000 nonsmoking adults die of lung cancer as a result of breathing the smoke of others' cigarettes (American Cancer Society, *Cancer Facts and Figures*). Add to that the number of nonsmokers who die of heart disease from others' smoke and the numbers of asthmatics and others who suffer from exposure to the smoke of others, and the arguments for policies against sidestream exposure become clear.

Although most people are familiar with the general concept that cigarette smoking is harmful, increasing numbers of young adults are turning to alternatives to cigarettes. Use of smokeless tobacco has increased dramatically, with significant concern being shown over the practice of "dipping snuff" or putting a moist tobacco powder between the cheek and gum. These practices are leading to major increases in oral cancers—cancer of the cheek, gum, and tongue, in particular.

In addition to smokeless tobacco, 1994 marked the first annual increase in *cigar consumption* in the United States. Tobacco bars, celebrity endorsements, a distorted image of sophistication, and the misconception that cigar smoke is healthier than cigarettes because it isn't inhaled all contribute to this increase. But consider the following:

- Most of the same carcinogens and cancer-producing chemicals found in cigarettes are found in cigars.

- Overall cancer deaths among men who smoke cigars are 34% higher than among nonsmokers.

- Studies have shown that all tobacco users are 5 to 10 times more likely to get cancer of the mouth or throat than their nonsmoking counterparts.

- Cigar smokers have 4 to 10 times the risk of nonsmokers of dying from laryngeal, oral, or esophageal cancers. (American Cancer Society, *Cancer Facts and Figures*)

In addition to the potentially harmful effects of tobacco, consuming large amounts of alcohol is believed to substantially increase a person's risk for oral, throat, and liver cancer.

Stress. Increasing attention is also being directed at the role of chronic stress in the development of cancer. Much of this research is inconclusive, but many studies suggest that stress can reduce the ability of the immune system to form infection-fighting white blood cells, thus interfering with overall immune system functioning.

Treatment

In general, treatments for cancer are less invasive and provide more choices for patients than ever before, particularly for those who live near a medical facility that specializes in cancer and who have access to this care through health insurance. For example, whereas radical mastectomy (surgical removal of the breast as well as surrounding tissue) used to be commonly performed, patients now tend to receive more moderate treatments involving a combination of limited surgery, chemotherapy, or other treatment regimens. Whereas a diagnosis of colon cancer typically meant removal of the entire colon and a lifetime of discomfort with external bags for removal of body wastes just a decade ago, patients now typically experience only partial removal of the intestine, with therapy to prevent recurrence. Supportive devices, bags, and other items have become so refined that most cancer patients have few of the difficulties experienced by previous generations. New blood tests, enzyme tests, and other diagnostic/imaging techniques have meant much earlier diagnosis for many and a faster return to health.

Although treatment techniques have improved dramatically, oncologists continue to rely on three primary methods: (1) *surgery,* to remove the tumor as well as surrounding tissue that might be affected; (2) *radiation therapy*, to destroy cancer cells; and (3) *chemotherapy,* or the administration of powerful chemicals, which also destroys cancer cells. A fourth type of therapy, *immunotherapy,* designed to strengthen the body's natural ability to fight the disease, is becoming more common.

None of the treatments for cancer is risk free. In fact, the more aggressive the treatment (due to the severity of the cancer), the higher is the risk and the worse the prognosis. Most treatments today include variations or combinations of the techniques. Going to your general practitioner might be fine for minor ailments; however, if you are diagnosed with cancer, it is in your best interest to seek treatment from an oncologist who works at a facility that routinely treats large numbers of patients with similar symptoms, with teaching hospitals in certain geographic locations having the best histories of success.

Prevention

For many of us, the term *prevention* has become a fairly common buzz word in the health and fitness world. We are encouraged to prevent heart disease by exercising, eating the right low-fat, high-fiber foods, and actively managing our stress levels. Unfortunately, prevention often implies something quick and easy that we can do to avoid a negative outcome, such as remaining alert while driving to prevent a head-on collision. The hard fact is that when we talk about preventing diseases such as cancer which have multiple causes, a quick fix of avoidance will not necessarily reduce your risk.

Prevention of cancer refers to the actions you take and the policies, programs, and services that are available to help you reduce the cumulative and additive threats from the disease at each age and stage of your life. Confusing? Think of it this way. Cancer is a slowly developing process in most cases, culminating in the disease after several decades of exposure to chemicals, lifestyle behaviors, genetic mutation, biological decline, and other events in your life. If you can act to reduce your risk or defer your own diagnosis for 10 to 20 years—for example, instead of getting cancer at 60, you develop it at 75 to 80—the impact of prevention is very significant. The lifestyle choices you make now can significantly reduce your risk of developing cancer and increase your years of health. Clearly, not all cancers are preventable. Some will happen for reasons that defy logic and the best methods of research that are available today. What is commonly believed is that many people have a certain number of precancerous or cancerous cells at any given time. It is quite possible that we cannot alter the course of many of these cells in spite of our best efforts. However, there are clear instances when the choices we make increase our risk and seem actually to help cancer cells in their invasion.

There are also instances when prevention is made more difficult because of the estimated 18% of Americans under age 65 and 14% of those over the age of 65 who lack access to health care. In these cases, lack of health education about risks, and the lack of early diagnostic screenings for breast, prostate, lung, and other cancers, can dramatically reduce your chances for a healthy lifespan.

Improving Lifestyle Behaviors. Often we are more attentive to our cars than to the way our bodies function. We systematically change the oil with only the best oil and filters, note every ding or scratch, investigate the reputation of our mechanic, and faithfully perform regular maintenance procedures. Yet when it comes to our bodies, we scarcely notice changes, wait until the last minute for medical assistance, ignore scheduled examinations, and choose our medical practitioners without investigating their credentials or philosophy. The following are some behaviors to incorporate in your lifestyle to reduce your risk of cancer:

1. *Remain vigilant.* If your family has a history of cancer, or if you live with a smoker or work in a hazardous environment, you need to pay particular attention to your body. Noticing subtle changes in the way things

"feel" is one way to increase your chances of obtaining an early diagnosis. If you know that your mother or sister has had breast cancer, it is especially important to listen to your body signals and have regular checkups. Although youth can be a protective factor, you should never ignore symptoms thinking "it could never happen to me" until it is much too late for effective treatment.

2. *Check your parts!* Regular self-examinations to check for changes in body parts that may be prone to cancer should be part of your routine. Breast self-examination, testicular self-examination, mole checks, lump checks, stool checks, and pain checks are important, yet often overlooked, procedures that can be easily performed by you or your intimate partner (see Figures 13.10 and 13.11). To help yourself recognize the possible presence of cancer, the American Cancer Society suggests that you remember the following warning signs (note that the first letters of each item taken together spell CAUTION):

    Change in bowel or bladder habits

    A sore that does not heal

    Unusual bleeding or discharge

    Thickening or lump in the breast or elsewhere

    Indigestion that persists or difficulty in swallowing

    Obvious change in a wart or mole

    Nagging cough or hoarseness

3. *Protect yourself from excessive exposure to ultraviolet light.* Use sunscreens with high SPFs (sun protection factors) and avoid exposure to ultraviolet light in tanning booths.

4. *Control your weight.* Obesity is a risk factor in the development of certain types of cancer. The longer you have been obese, the greater is your risk. Starting a weight-reduction program now may significantly reduce your risk.

5. *Eat a balanced, health-enhancing diet.* As already stated, what you put in your mouth in terms of fats and chemicals, as well as foods that protect you, may influence your risk.

6. *Avoid alcohol and tobacco.* Both of these substances are carcinogenic and show clear links to cancer promotion. In addition to breaking the habit yourself, avoiding bars and social situations where there is heavy tobacco smoke will reduce your risk.

7. *Exercise regularly.* Besides helping you avoid the risk of obesity, exercise stimulates immune functioning and may help your body defend itself against cancer and other threats.

8. *Manage excessive stress.* Although the jury is still out on this one, the general belief is that people who are subjected to high chronic levels of stress or who have serious emotional problems tend to have a higher rate of cancer development.

9. *Avoid excessive radiation and chemical exposure.* Most medical techniques that use radiation are safe, particularly when given according to recommended diagnostic guidelines. However, long-term or repeated

Look for Changes

At the Mirror

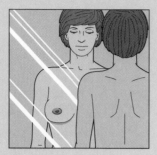 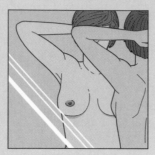 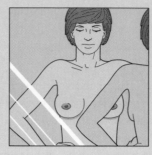 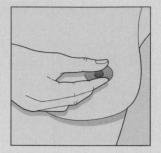

- First, relax, sitting or standing, whichever is comfortable.
- With your arms at your sides, look for changes in your breasts—lumps, thickenings, dimples, or skin changes.

- Next, raise your arms above or behind your head, again looking for the same changes.

- Now, with your hands on your hips, press down and tense your chest muscles. This will make any changes more prominent.

- Finally, squeeze each nipple gently for any discharge.

Feel for Changes

In the Shower   *Lying Down*

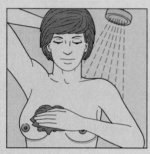 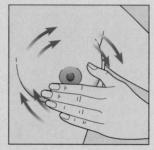 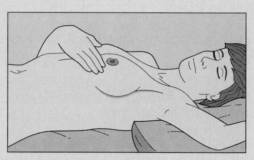

- Start by raising your right arm behind your head.
- With your left hand soaped and fingers held flat together, roll and press the breast firmly against the chest wall.

- Circle and feel a small portion of the breast at a time until the entire breast and underarm area have been checked.
- Now repeat, raising your left arm and checking your left breast with your right hand.

- Lie down on your back and get comfortable.
- Then place a pillow under your right shoulder.
- Now simply repeat the process you went through in the shower, examining your right breast with your left hand.
- Move the pillow under your left shoulder and examine your left breast with your right hand.

Signs of Breast Cancer

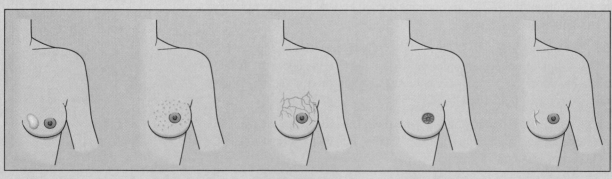

A lump—usually single, firm, and painless

Skin swelling—a portion of the skin on the breast taking on the appearance of an orange peel

Superficial veins—the skin surface veins on one breast becoming more prominent than the other

Inverted nipple—in a previously normal breast

Skin dimpling—a depression occurring in a localized area of the breast surface

Figure 13.10

The best time to examine your breasts is after your menstrual period. Source: From Customized Communications.

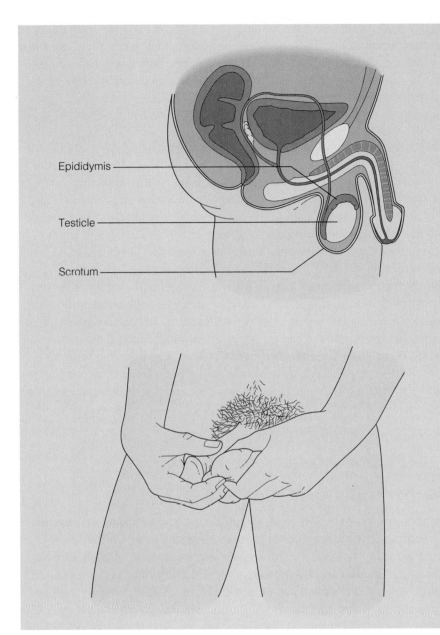

The testicular self-exam (TSE) should be performed after a hot bath or shower when the scrotal skin is relaxed, making it easier to find anything unusual. The procedure is simple and only takes a few minutes:

- Examine each testicle gently with both hands. The index and middle fingers should be placed underneath the testicle while the thumbs are placed on the top. Roll the testicle gently between the thumbs and fingers. One testicle may be larger than the other. This is normal.
- The epididymis is a cordlike structure on the top and back of the testicle that stores and transports the sperm. Do not confuse the epididymis with an abnormal lump.
- Feel for any abnormal lumps—about the size of a pea—on the front or the side of the testicle. These lumps are usually painless.
- If you find a lump, contact your doctor immediately. The lump may be due to an infection, and a doctor can determine the proper treatment. If the lump is not caused by infection, it is likely to be cancer. Remember that testicular cancer is highly curable, especially when detected and treated early. Note, too, that testicular cancer almost always occurs in only one testicle, and the other testicle is all that is needed for full sexual function.

Routine TSEs are important, but they cannot substitute for a doctor's examination. Your doctor should examine your testicles when you have a physical exam. You also can ask your doctor to check the way you do your TSE.

Epididymis

Testicle

Scrotum

Figure **13.11**

The best time to examine your testicles is after a hot bath or shower, when the scrotum is most relaxed.
Source: From Williams, 1993.

exposure to any form of radiation may increase your risk. Ask for a second opinion before undergoing a diagnostic test that exposes you to a high dose of radiation. Insist on the most modern equipment when such tests are necessary to ensure that you get the lowest dose possible. Make sure that X rays for dental checkups and other minor procedures are given by a licensed practitioner with equipment that has been checked on a regular basis.

Practicing Responsible Consumerism. Although much of what happens in the environment is beyond your control, you can exert an influence through your voting power, purchasing habits, and recreational choices. For example, you can have an impact on environmental decisions regarding clean air and water by paying attention to the voting records of your legislators. You can persuade companies to use fewer pesticides, chemicals, additives, preservatives, and other substances by buying environmentally safe products. You can influence the amount of fat in foods and the availability of more nutritionally sound choices by reading labels and purchasing only those foods that meet your standards. This type of responsible consumerism has led to the introduction of low-fat ice cream, unsaturated cooking oils, and other, healthier food choices in the marketplace. As little as 10 years ago, many of these products were virtually nonexistent; we had no choices.

Becoming an Advocate for Your Health. Today's health consumers and patients are more pro-active than ever before. They are beginning to question their medical care providers and to demand quality care in the confusion of managed care. Community education that teaches consumers about risks, about appropriate questioning of health care professionals, about advocacy for loved ones who may be vulnerable in a medical situation, and other activities only serve to increase the likelihood that should you develop cancer, you will have the best chance for survival. A person diagnosed with breast cancer can get on the Internet and connect to the best information available about cancer treatment options, facilities, and doctors known for their expertise in certain cancers. Taking the time to read widely, check your options, and question, question, question those who would be taking your life into their hands is your best opportunity to be your own advocate. Health care advocacy and wise consumerism are important parts in dealing with any chronic condition and are thus important components of overall health and wellness.

Diabetes

Chances are you either know someone or know of someone who has diabetes mellitus. It is the third leading cause of death in the United States and represents a major coronary health risk. Diabetics are highly susceptible to complications such as atherosclerosis, coronary artery disease, hypertension, infection, cataracts, blindness, and chronic kidney disease. Over 14 million Americans have diabetes. Of these, 1 million are insulin-dependent. According to the American Diabetes Association, an estimated 6 million individuals do not even know they are diabetic. (See the Stats-at-a-Glance.)

Defining the Disease

Diabetes mellitus is characterized by the abnormal metabolism of carbohydrates (i.e., sugars and starches) resulting in abnormally high blood sugar levels. **Type 1 diabetes** [formerly known as insulin-dependent diabetes mellitus (IDDM) and juvenile-onset diabetes] typically occurs in children and young adults who are slim but can occur at any age. **Type 2 diabetes** [formerly non-insulin-dependent diabetes mellitus (NIDDM) or adult-onset diabetes] is most common in obese individuals over age 40 but has recently been increasing among obese children. Of all diabetics, 90% have type 2 diabetes.

The typical physiologic response of a well person to a high-carbohydrate meal is the release of insulin as soon as blood glucose levels rise above normal. Glucose cannot readily enter muscle, liver, or adipose tissue cells where it can be utilized or stored. **Insulin**, a hormone produced in the pancreas, is required to "open the gates" of these cells (via receptors) to

Of the 14 million Americans who have diabetes, 1 million are insulin-dependent.

STATS-AT-A-GLANCE
Diabetes

■ Approximately 16 million Americans have diabetes but only half are diagnosed.

■ Of the 16 million, 15.3 million have type 2 diabetes and 700,000 have type 1.

■ Formerly considered "adult onset," type 2 diabetes is increasing in children, especially those who are obese.

■ Diabetes is the fourth leading cause of death by disease in the United States.

CHRONIC ◆ DISEASES

Do

▲ Quit smoking; this may be the most important single thing you can do to protect your health.

▲ Reduce or avoid high cholesterol and hypertension.

▲ Eat a healthy, low-fat diet.

▲ Stay active by finding a form of exercise you enjoy and can stick with for the long term.

▲ Maintain a healthy weight.

▲ Be sure to get enough calcium in your diet or take calcium supplements.

▲ Have regular cancer screenings, including breast self-exams and pap smears for women, and testicular self-exams for men.

▲ Limit your intake of alcohol to no more than two drinks per day.

▲ Keep your stress level under control.

▲ Stay out of the sun and use sunscreen regularly.

▲ Get your blood pressure and cholesterol level checked regularly.

▲ Know your hereditary risks for chronic diseases.

▲ Learn cardiopulmonary resuscitation (CPR) so you can help a person who has a heart attack.

▲ Protect yourself from possible environmental carcinogens and follow safety precautions when handling hazardous materials.

▲ See a physician if you see any warning signs of cancer.

Don't

▼ Think that you are too young to worry about heart disease or cancer; the habits you establish now may very well determine whether or not you are alive in 50 years.

▼ Think that genetics are destiny; your genes play a role in your chances of getting many diseases, but your lifestyle often plays an even bigger role.

▼ Rely on doctors to deal with chronic diseases; *you* are in charge of preventing diseases like cancer and heart disease.

▼ Neglect cancer screening tests or warning signs; see a doctor regularly.

diabetes mellitus disease characterized by the abnormal metabolism of carbohydrates (sugars and starches) resulting in abnormally high blood sugar levels

Type 1 diabetes [formerly termed insulin-dependent diabetes mellitus (IDDM) or juvenile-onset diabetes]; the form of diabetes caused by a lack of insulin production

Type 2 diabetes [formerly non-insulin-dependent diabetes mellitus (NIDDM) or adult onset diabetes]; the form of diabetes caused by a resistance to the glucose transport effect of insulin on cells

insulin hormone produced by the pancreas that facilitates the transport of glucose from the blood into muscle, liver, and adipose tissue cells

glucose, thereby reducing blood sugar levels and making glucose available for energy production (see Figure 13.12). Within 1 to 2 hours after the meal, blood glucose is back within normal range (80–110 mg/dl). Diabetics do not have the normal control over blood glucose. People with type 1 are unable to produce insulin. Those with type 2 can still produce insulin, but the cells of the body are resistant to its effect on glucose transport. As a result, a person with diabetes may need 4 to 5 hours for blood glucose to return to pre-meal levels.

The diagnosis of diabetes is fasting plasma glucose (FPG) levels. In acute, untreated stages, it is not uncommon for glucose levels to be over 600 mg/dl. However, there is new evidence that even slightly high FPG (>126 mg/dl) over a long period of time leads to serious complications. Hence, diabetes is now diagnosed at 126 mg/dl (American Diabetes Association). Recommendations are for FPG testing in all individuals at the age of 45 and, if normal (70–110 mg/dl), the testing is repeated at 3-year intervals. This new approach may help identify the millions of undiagnosed Americans. Further, the state between normal FPG (110 mg/dl) and diabetes (126 mg/dl) indicates impaired glucose metabolism and represents an important risk factor for future diabetes and cardiovascular disease.

Risk Factors

The main risk factors for diabetes are obesity, genetics, age, ethnicity, hypertension, and cholesterol/triglyceride levels. You can evaluate your risk for diabetes in Laboratory 13.2. Warning signs for the disease are shown in Table 13.3.

Genetics. The tendency to develop diabetes appears to be present at birth. Currently, a positive family history is the only known risk factor for type 1 diabetes. This type of diabetes is characterized by a reduction of insulin production by the pancreas. This pattern is thought to develop because an individual (1) is susceptible to a virus that destroys insulin-producing cells, (2) develops "killer" cells that attack these specialized cells, or (3) simply inherits faulty insulin-producing cells.

Obesity and Physical Activity. Although type 2 is also genetic, people run a greater risk of developing this disease if they are more than 20 pounds over normal weight and do not participate in regular aerobic exercise. Individuals whose weight is 50% greater than normal are five times more likely to develop diabetes than people of normal weight. In some obese

Figure 13.12

Insulin facilitates the transport of glucose across the cell membrane. Insulin binds to its receptor in the cell membrane and activates a carrier system (C) that transports glucose through the cell membrane to the interior cell.

Source: From Melvin H. Williams, Lifetime Fitness and Wellness, 3rd edition. Copyright © 1993 Wm. C. Brown Communications, Inc. Dubuque, IA. All rights reserved. Reprinted by permission of The McGraw-Hill Companies.

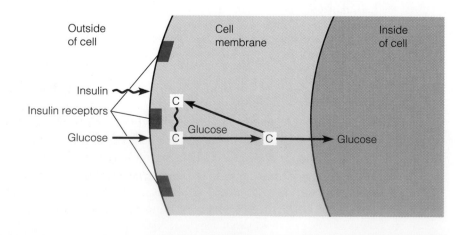

TABLE 13.3

The Warning Signs for Diabetes

INSULIN-DEPENDENT[a]	NON-INSULIN-DEPENDENT[b]
Frequent urination	Any of the insulin-dependent symptoms
Excessive thirst	Recurring or hard-to-heal skin, gum, or bladder infections
Extreme hunger	Drowsiness
Dramatic weight loss	Blurred vision
Irritability	Tingling or numbness in hands or feet
Weakness and fatigue	Itching
Nausea and vomiting	

[a]Usually occur suddenly
[b]Usually occur less suddenly
Note: If you experience any of these symptoms, discuss them with your physician.
Source: From American Diabetes Association, Inc., 1992

individuals, insulin is not produced when it is needed. Even if adequate insulin is present, glucose may still be unable to enter the target cells in these individuals.

Fasting Blood Glucose (FPG). Blood glucose of > 126 mg/dl is the cutoff point for diagnosing diabetes. The state between normal, 110 mg/dl, and diabetes is a risk factor for developing diabetes and cardiovascular disease.

Age. As noted previously, individuals over 40 years of age are more susceptible to type 2 diabetes, and although the disease develops over time its onset is typically observed in the older adult. Age combined with obesity further increases a person's risk of developing diabetes. This is most evident in recent reports that type 2 diabetes is becoming more prevalent in obese children.

Ethnicity. African Americans, Latinos, and Native Americans are especially prone to diabetes. The reason for this is not clear, but it is likely linked to lifestyle patterns of diet and physical activity.

Treatment

The goal of treatment for individuals with diabetes is to reduce blood glucose levels by increasing muscle, liver, and adipose cell uptake. For type 1, insulin, diet, and exercise are the triad of control (see Figure 13.13). Insulin is injected or delivered through a pump daily, diet is high in complex carbohydrates and low in simple sugar, and exercise consists of regular aerobic activity (at least three times per week) at an intensity level that can be maintained for at least 30 minutes per session. Weight control is not a part of the triad for type 1 diabetics because it is not the primary problem with this type of diabetes.

Type 2 diabetes can usually be controlled through a balanced program of diet, exercise, and weight control (see Figure 13.13). The diet should be similar to that for type 1 diabetes, keeping in mind the need to lose fat. Fat

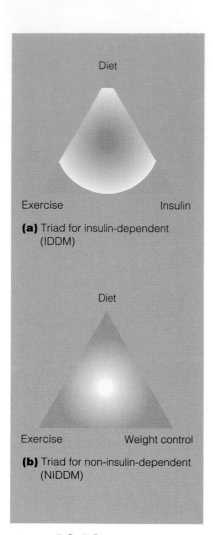

Diet

Exercise   Insulin

(a) Triad for insulin-dependent (IDDM)

Diet

Exercise   Weight control

(b) Triad for non-insulin-dependent (NIDDM)

Figure 13.13

A triad of control is the treatment prescription for both **(a)** insulin- and **(b)** non-insulin-dependent diabetes.

STATS-AT-A-GLANCE
Osteoporosis

- Approximately 25 million Americans have osteoporosis; 80% of these are elderly women.

- One out of every five men will suffer a fracture from osteoporosis.

- Hip fractures are responsible for 50% of nursing home admissions annually.

- Osteoporosis is responsible for over $14 billion of health care costs annually.

loss is associated with an increased sensitivity to insulin. The importance of aerobic exercise cannot be overemphasized for both types of diabetes. Through as yet unknown mechanisms, aerobic activity increases glucose uptake by muscle cells in the absence of insulin. Therefore, exercise itself acts like insulin does during the workout. The person with diabetes needs to recognize, however, that there is not a chronic "training effect" for insulin sensitivity. That is, blood glucose levels begin to creep up following the workout, indicating the need for consistency in an aerobic program.

People with diabetes must also take certain precautions when exercising. Because aerobic exercise can stimulate glucose intake much the way insulin does, it is possible for them to develop **hypoglycemia,** or low blood sugar, during activity. An individual with type 1 diabetes can maintain control of blood glucose during exercise by decreasing the dose of injected insulin and/or increasing the consumption of carbohydrates before and after exercise. This is particularly important for strenuous and prolonged activity. In addition, individuals with both type 1 and 2 diabetes need to carry a "sweet treat" in the event of hypoglycemia during exercise.

Prevention

As yet, type 1 diabetes cannot be prevented, but researchers are seeking answers to help individuals with this disease. However, you can reduce your risk for developing the most common form of diabetes, type 2, by making the following lifestyle choices:

1. *Maintain normal weight.* As discussed in Chapter 8, weight can be controlled through regular exercise and adherence to a diet low in sugar and fat.

2. *Engage in a regular program of aerobic fitness.* Aerobic fitness activities utilize blood glucose and enable cells to take up glucose even without insulin. Additionally, exercise, which increases your energy expenditure, is a key factor in helping you achieve and maintain your proper body weight (see Chapter 8).

3. *Have blood sugar tested beginning at age 45.* The most recent report from the American Diabetes Association recommends blood glucose testing beginning at age 45 and, if normal, repeated at 3-year intervals. This recommendation is based on evidence that the serious complications of diabetes begin far earlier than previously suspected.

4. *Recognize the warning signs for diabetes.* As with other chronic diseases, it is essential that you know the warning signs for diabetes (see Table 13.3). This is particularly important if you have a family history of diabetes. If you can catch the disease in its early stages, you can begin a treatment program and thus prevent or delay the progress of the disease.

Osteoporosis

The term *osteoporosis* conjures up the mental picture of an old woman with a humpback who has great difficulty moving about. However, such an image actually represents someone in the most advanced stages of the disease. Over half of American women 50 years and older can expect to suffer bone fractures due to osteoporosis. Of these fractures, one-third occur at the hip and often are serious enough to require hospitalization or nursing home care. In fact, 50% of nursing home admissions are due to hip fractures. The mortality associated with osteoporosis is from pneumonia and other bed rest infections that develop in hip fracture patients. Although it is considered a "woman's disease," osteoporosis also occurs in older men. In fact, of the men who reach 90 years, one in six has suffered a hip fracture.

Defining the Disease

Osteoporosis is characterized by low bone mineral content (BMC), which can lead to fractures of the vertebrae, hip, and wrist. **Bone mineral content** is the amount of calcium phosphate in bone tissue. Greater bone mineral is associated with stronger bones, which naturally are more resistant to fracture. Osteoporosis is considered a "silent" disease because fractures typically occur before any symptoms are noticed.

A definition of the types of bone that make up the skeleton is important to understand the disease. **Cortical bone,** or "compact" bone, comprises the long bones of the skeleton and contains minerals that are tightly packed together. **Trabecular** bone, or "spongy" bone, comprises a large proportion of the vertebrae and ends of long bones, and contains many trabeculae arranged in a network fashion resembling a sponge (see Figure 13.14). Trabecular bone is more susceptible to calcium loss than is compact bone for two reasons. First, it has more surface area exposed to the circulation, so the calcium within it is more available to meet the needs of the body. Second, it houses the body's red marrow. Because red marrow is very active metabolically, as it manufactures red blood cells at a very rapid rate, spongy bone is highly vulnerable to calcium losses.

Figure 13.14

As this cross-sectional view shows, in the lacy interior, called trabecular bone, minerals are crystallized around a protein matrix (network); the compact bone at the exterior of the shaft is cortical bone.

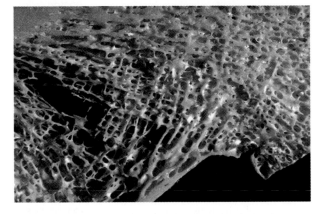

Risk Factors

When considering the risk factor profile of osteoporosis, remember that this disease results from a combination of risk factors. You can assess your risk for osteoporosis in Laboratory 13.3.

Genetics. There is evidence that people are more at risk for developing osteoporosis if they have a family history of the disease. Researchers in Australia have recently identified an "osteoporosis gene" that has been tagged as the main hereditary culprit in a person's developing the disease.

Frame Size. People who are thin or small framed are at greater risk for fractures in later life. They typically have less bone mineral density than those with larger builds.

Gender. Women are four times more likely to develop osteoporosis than men because of their generally smaller, lighter frame sizes and because they stop producing estrogen at menopause.

Race. White and Asian women suffer two to three times as many fractures as African-American and Hispanic women. This does not mean,

hypoglycemia low blood sugar levels

osteoporosis condition characterized by low bone mineral content which increases susceptibility to fractures of the vertebrae, hips, and wrists

bone mineral content amount of calcium phosphate in bone tissue

cortical bone "compact" bone that comprises the long bones of the skeleton and contains minerals that are packed tightly together

trabecular bone "spongy" bone that comprises a large proportion of the vertebrae and ends of long bones and contains many trabeculae arranged in a network fashion resembling a sponge

however, that African Americans and Hispanics are protected because they are also affected by the disease.

Aging. For both men and women, loss of trabecular bone begins at about age 30 and progresses at a rate of about 1% per year (see Figure 13.15). That means that by age 50, levels of bone mineral density could be about 20% lower than in young adulthood for both men and women. In menopausal women (about age 50), when estrogen levels fall dramatically, BMC loss accelerates to 2% to 5% per year for about 5 years, then slows down to the initial rate. This phenomenon accounts for the higher incidence of osteoporosis among women. Loss of compact bone does not begin until about age 50 and is more dramatic in women than in men.

Reduced Peak Bone Mass. Fracture risk is associated not only with BMC loss due to age but also with the maximum amount of bone mineral attained at maturity. This is called peak bone mineral content, or peak bone mass, and occurs at about 15 years of age. As illustrated in Figure 13.15, trabecular BMC in women is maintained for about 12 years following its peak. In cases of reduced calcium intake and amenorrhea (loss of menstrual periods) during adolescence, peak bone mass may never reach a high level.

Low Estrogen and Testosterone Levels. The hormones estrogen and testosterone have pronounced effects on bone. Boys and girls with low levels of these hormones have substantial deficits in BMC. The loss of blood levels of testosterone or estrogen during adult life leads to accelerated loss of BMC, an effect that is particularly marked when it occurs at an early age. Replacement of estrogen at menopause helps prevent further BMC loss and reduces the risk of osteoporotic fractures. Estrogen deficiency may have an overwhelming influence on bone mass even when adequate attention is given to other influences on bone health. For example, women athletes who experience amenorrhea lose BMC despite regular high-intensity exercise (Robinson et al.; Drinkwater et al.). Male endurance athletes can also experience lower testosterone levels as a result of training. Lowered testosterone can significantly reduce their BMC.

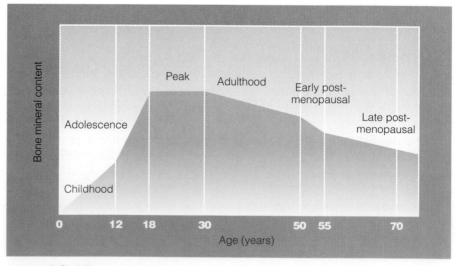

Figure 13.15

Bone mineral content changes in trabecular bone from childhood to old age in women.

Physical Inactivity. Although our understanding is incomplete concerning exactly how the skeleton is stimulated to increase its mineral content by exercise, we know that physical activity clearly has a positive effect on bone mass (Snow, Matkin, and Shaw). Conversely, when physical activity is diminished, BMC decreases. This is particularly striking during immobilization and bed rest, which are both accompanied by severe bone loss (Garland and colleagues; Krolner and Toft). The type of exercise that stimulates the formation of BMC at the clinically relevant sites of the hip and spine appears to be exercise that is weight bearing and is accompanied by high ground and muscle forces (jumping, stair climbing, step aerobics, racquet sports, weight lifting; Robinson et al.; Heinonen et al.; Snow-Harter et al.).

Inadequate Calcium Intake. Your skeleton can be considered a calcium bank because it stores 99.5% of the calcium in your body. During times of need, your system draws on this bank to support circulating calcium levels. The relationship between calcium intake and bone health is particularly strong during growth. For the skeleton to develop optimal peak BMC, it must have access to an adequate supply of calcium. With inadequate daily calcium intake, peak BMC will not reach the highest possible levels.

The recommended dietary calcium intake for adolescent boys and girls is 1,200 mg per day. This level is equivalent to four 8-ounce glasses of milk. Because 60% of final bone mass is deposited in the 2 to 3 years that define puberty, dietary inadequacy may reduce bone formation more at this time than any other. Statistics indicate that the calcium intake of American men corresponds to recommended levels at most ages but that median intake for American girls is substantially below recommended levels by age 11 and never recovers (Carroll and colleagues).

The National Institutes of Health (1994) have released updated recommendations for optimal calcium intake. For women, it is 1,200 mg/day to age 24, then, 1,000 mg/day thereafter until menopause. At this time, for women taking estrogen replacements, 1,000 mg/day is recommended; for women who are not taking estrogen replacements, the value is 1,500 mg/day. For men, the recommended amounts is 1,000 mg/day. Over the age of 65 years, for both men and women the recommended amount is 1,500 mg/day. Pregnant women and nursing mothers require 1,200 to 1,500 mg/day.

Smoking. People who smoke generally exhibit lower BMC than do nonsmokers. Women who smoke even less than one pack per day have been found to lose more bone than nonsmoking women (Krall and Dawson-Hughes). Although few studies have examined this factor, the consensus is that smoking does increase a person's risk for osteoporosis.

Alcohol Consumption. There is evidence that alcoholics have a significantly lower BMC than do nondrinkers (Chappard and colleagues). In particular, heavy alcohol intake (more than three drinks per day) is associated with low BMC.

Treatment

Because osteoporosis is most common in postmenopausal women, treatment is targeted at this population. Treatment typically includes hormone replacement therapy (estrogen/progestin combinations), increased calcium intake, and increased levels of weight-bearing exercise. Because estrogen therapy places a woman at higher risk for uterine cancer, anyone at risk for this type of cancer needs a different form of intervention. A new class of pharmaceuticals, called bisphosphonates, have been found to be extremely effective in improving bone strength; women who cannot take hormone replacement therapy are being treated with this drug. Keep in mind that none of these treatments reverses osteoporosis; rather, they all delay its progress. An osteoporotic fracture indicates that bone mineral levels are below a critical fracture threshold and other bones are more susceptible to fracture. It is not uncommon for a woman to have one vertebral fracture, then 6 months later suffer another. If treatment for low BMC can begin prior to the first fracture, further loss and fractures may possibly be prevented. With new technologies, women who are at highest risk for osteoporosis can be identified early enough to begin intervention strategies that can help prevent fractures. Dual energy X-ray absorptiometry is an excellent screening device that uses very low radiation to quantify the amount of mineral in bones.

Prevention

Prevention of BMC loss is the key to reducing a person's risk for osteoporosis. During young adulthood, the thought of a crippling bone disease may seem remote, but this is the best time to begin making lifestyle changes for prevention. By making lifestyle choices early on, you may be able to build BMC and slow age-related loss. Although your risk for osteoporosis is somewhat based on hereditary factors, preventive measures include the following:

1. *Increase physical activity levels.* Include weight-bearing and muscle-building exercises in your fitness program at least three times per week. Keep in mind that to build BMC, the exercise needs to overload (challenge) your system. In addition to increasing bone mass, exercise may help offset or reduce age-related BMC loss.

2. *Take dietary calcium.* Although taking added calcium in adulthood has not been shown to increase bone mass, it is important to ingest the RDA to provide your body with the necessary building blocks for bone. A high intake of phosphorus can reduce intestinal absorption of calcium. The ratio of calcium to phosphorus should be one to one, which is common in most dairy products. It is also important to reduce your intake of sodas, most of which have high levels of phosphorus and no calcium.

3. *Be wary of overexercising.* Overexertion, particularly in aerobic fitness activities, should be avoided because it can alter hormone levels.

4. *Keep alcohol consumption moderate.* Because high alcohol intake is detrimental to BMC, you should be moderate in your consumption of alcohol, particularly if you have any of the other risk factors for osteoporosis.

5. *Quit smoking.* The less you smoke, the more protection you offer your skeleton. Because drinking and smoking often go hand in hand, a reduction in one may trigger reduction or even cessation of the other.

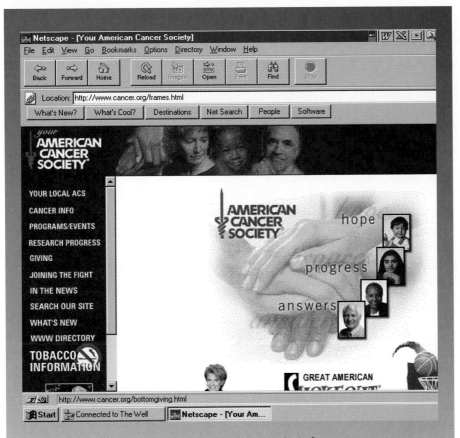

Netscape - [Your American Cancer Society]

File Edit View Go Bookmarks Options Directory Window Help

Back | Forward | Home | Reload | Images | Open | Print | Find | Stop

Location: http://www.cancer.org/frames.html

What's New? | What's Cool? | Destinations | Net Search | People | Software

your
AMERICAN CANCER SOCIETY

YOUR LOCAL ACS
CANCER INFO
PROGRAMS/EVENTS
RESEARCH PROGRESS
GIVING
JOINING THE FIGHT
IN THE NEWS
SEARCH OUR SITE
WHAT'S NEW
WWW DIRECTORY
TOBACCO INFORMATION

AMERICAN CANCER SOCIETY

hope
progress
answers

GREAT AMERICAN

http://www.cancer.org/bottomgiving.html

Start | Connected to The Well | Netscape - [Your Am...

American Cancer Society
http://www.cancer.org/frames.html

This site contains lots of information on all kinds of cancer and their prevention, diagnosis, and treatment. There is also news about research progress in treating cancer and ways for community members to get involved in the fight against cancer. The American Cancer Society sponsors the Great American Smokeout, and there is information on participating in this event.

Critical thinking: Recently there have been many lawsuits in the news against tobacco companies because smoking is responsible for the great majority of lung cancer. Should tobacco companies be held responsible for these lung cancer deaths? Or is each person solely responsible for his or her health behavior?

Source: From American Cancer Society, 1998.

Lifestyle Choices: Plan for Action

Lifestyle factors play a major role in the development of coronary artery disease (CAD), type 2 diabetes, and osteoporosis. Although the causes of cancer are not well understood, lifestyle factors such as diet, exposure to chemicals or ultraviolet light, and alcohol consumption or smoking have been linked with various forms of the disease. A wellness lifestyle not only improves your health and fitness in the present but also represents an important investment for your future well-being. Even though each of the chronic diseases discussed in this chapter is unique and distinct from the others, the following list shows that the lifestyle choices that reduce your risk of developing them are remarkably similar. The list is long and may seem daunting, but making just one healthy choice may markedly reduce your risk of developing one or more of the chronic diseases.

LIFESTYLE CHOICE	REDUCES RISK FOR
Keeping physically active	CAD, type 2 diabetes, cancer, osteoporosis
Maintaining proper body weight	CAD, type 2 diabetes, cancer, osteoporosis
Eating properly:	
Low-fat, low-cholesterol foods	CAD, cancer
Adequate fiber	CAD, cancer
Low-sodium foods	CAD
Adequate calcium and vitamin D	Osteoporosis
Not smoking	CAD, cancer, osteoporosis
Moderating alcohol intake	CAD, cancer, osteoporosis
Controlling life stresses	CAD, cancer
Avoiding exposure to ultraviolet light, chemicals, and radiation	Cancer
Monitoring blood glucose	Type 2 diabetes
Monitoring blood pressure, blood cholesterol	CAD
Breasts or testicles self-exam	Cancer

Summary

Although your susceptibility to four major chronic diseases—cardiovascular disease, cancer, diabetes, and osteoporosis—has a genetic link, it is also influenced by the lifestyle choices you make. Incorporating the lifestyle choices recommended in this chapter into your daily patterns will reduce your risk of developing these diseases and bring you that much closer to wellness.

Key concepts that you have learned in this chapter include these:

- In coronary artery disease, the arteries that serve the heart are damaged by atherosclerosis, a progressive narrowing of the artery due to the accumulation of plaque on the arterial walls.

- The major risk factors for cardiovascular disease include smoking, hypertension, high blood cholesterol, and physical inactivity; contributing risk factors include heredity, age, sex, diabetes, obesity, and stress.

- Improving coronary health means following a healthy diet, losing extra body fat, reducing stress, exercising regularly, and quitting smoking.

- Cancer is characterized by abnormal, uncontrolled cell growth in the form of either benign (noncancerous) or malignant (cancerous) tumors.

- The four major types of cancer are carcinomas, sarcomas, lymphomas, and leukemia.

- The major risk factors for cancer include environmental exposure, genetics, viruses, chronic irritation, and lifestyle factors such as diet, smoking, and stress.

- Your risk for developing cancer can be reduced by making lifestyle changes; listening to your body; performing self-exams; protecting against ultraviolet light; eating a healthy diet high in fiber; controlling your weight; exercising regularly; avoiding stress, alcohol, and tobacco; and being a responsible consumer.

- Diabetes mellitus is characterized by the abnormal metabolism of carbohydrates.

- Risk factors for diabetes include genetics, obesity, age, and ethnicity.

- Insulin, diet, and exercise are the triad of control for insulin-dependent diabetes; non-insulin-dependent diabetes can usually be controlled through a triad of diet, exercise, and weight control.

- Osteoporosis is characterized by low bone mineral content, which can lead to fractures, most commonly of the vertebrae, hips, and wrists.

- Risk factors for osteoporosis include a light skeleton, age, reduced peak bone mass, physical inactivity, insufficient calcium, low levels of estrogen or testosterone, smoking, and alcohol consumption.

- You can reduce your risk of osteoporosis by increasing your physical activity, taking calcium, quitting smoking, reducing alcohol consumption, and avoiding overexercising.

- Osteoporosis treatment involves hormone replacement therapy, increased calcium intake, and increased levels of weight-bearing exercise.

References

American Cancer Society. *American Cancer Society Dietary Guidelines Advisory Committee Guidelines on Diet, Nutrition and Cancer Prevention: Reducing the Risk of Cancer with Healthy Food Choices and Physical Activity.* Washington, DC: American Cancer Society, 1996.

American Cancer Society. *Cancer Facts and Figures.* Atlanta: American Cancer Society, 1997.

American Diabetes Association. Position statement: Nutritional recommendations and principles for individuals with diabetes mellitus: 1986. *Diabetes Care,* 10: 126–132, 1987.

American Diabetes Association, Scientific Committee Report, *Diabetes Care,* July 1997.

American Heart Association. *Heart and Stroke Facts.* Dallas: American Heart Association, 1996.

American Heart Association. *1998 Heart and Stroke Statistical Update.* Dallas: American Heart Association, 1997.

American Heart Association Medical/Scientific Statement. Cardiovascular diseases and stroke in African-Americans and other racial minorities in the United States. *Circulation,* 83: 1462–1480, 1991.

American Heart Association Medical/Scientific Statement. The cholesterol facts: A summary of the evidence relating dietary fats, serum cholesterol, and coronary heart disease. *Circulation,* 81: 1721–1733, 1990.

Berenson, G. S. et al. Risk factors in early life as predictors of adult heart disease: The Bogolusa Heart Study. *American Journal of the Medical Sciences,* 298: 141–151, 1989.

Berg, K. E. *Diabetic's Guide to Health and Fitness.* Champaign, IL: Life Enhancement, 1986.

Blumenthal, J. A., W. C. Siegel, and M. Appelbaum. Failure of exercise to reduce blood pressure in patients with mild hypertension. *Journal of the American Medical Association,* 266: 2098–2104, 1991.

Carroll, M. D., S. Abraham, and C. M. Dresser. Dietary intake source data, 1976–1980. DHHS pub. no. (PHS) 83–1681. Washington, DC: U.S. Government Printing Office, 1983.

Chappard, D., et al. Alcoholic cirrhosis and osteoporosis in men: A light and scanning electron microscopy study. *Journal of Studies in Alcohol,* 52(3): 269–274, 1991.

Chrischilles, E. A., et al. A model of lifetime osteoporosis impact. *Archives of Internal Medicine,* 151: 2026–2032, 1991.

Drinkwater, B. L., et al. Bone mineral content of amenorrheic and eumenorrheic athletes. *New England Journal of Medicine,* 311: 277–281, 1984.

Drinkwater, B., S. Grimston, D. Raab-Cullen, and C. Snow-Harter. ACSM position stand on osteoporosis and exercise. *Medicine and Science in Sports and Exercise,* 27(4): i–vii, 1995.

Fletcher, G. F., et al. Benefits and recommendations for physical activity programs for all Americans: A statement for health professionals by the Committee on Exercise and Cardiac Rehabilitation of the Council on Clinical Cardiology, American Heart Association. *Circulation,* 86: 340–344, 1992.

Franz, M. J. Exercise and the management of diabetes mellitus. *Journal of the American Diabetic Association,* 87: 872–882, 1987.

Fuster, V., et al. The pathogenesis of coronary artery disease and the acute coronary syndromes, part one. *New England Journal of Medicine,* 326: 242–250, 1992.

Fuster, V., et al. The pathogenesis of coronary artery disease and the acute coronary syndromes, part two. *New England Journal of Medicine,* 326: 310–318, 1992.

Garland, D. E., et al. Osteoporosis after spinal cord injury. *Journal of Orthopedic Research,* 10: 371–378, 1992.

Gilders, R. M., and G. A. Dudley. Endurance exercise training and treatment of hypertension: The controversy. *Sports Medicine,* 13: 71–77, 1992.

Guyton, A. C. *Textbook of Medical Physiology,* 9th ed. Philadelphia: Saunders, 1996.

Heinonen, A., P. Kannus, H. Slevanen, et al. Randomized, controlled trial of effect of high impact exercise on selected risk factors of osteoporosis fractures. *Lancet,* 348: 1343–1347, 1996.

Hunter, D. J., and W. C. Willett. Nutrition and breast cancer. *Cancer Causes and Control.* 7: 56–68, 1996.

Kearney, J., E. Giovanucci, E. B. Rimm, et al. Diet, alcohol and smoking and the occurrences of hyperplaslic polyps of the colon and rectum. *Cancer Causes and Control,* 6: 45–56, 1995.

King, D. S., et al. Effects of exercise and lack of exercise on insulin sensitivity and responsiveness. *Journal of Applied Physiology,* 64: 1942–1946, 1988.

Kleinman, J. C., et al. Mortality among diabetics in a national sample. *American Journal of Epidemiology,* 128: 389–401, 1988.

Kolonel, L. N. Nutrition and prostate cancer. *Cancer Causes and Control,* 7: 83–94, 1996.

Kono, S., and T. Hirohata. Nutrition and stomach cancer. *Cancer Causes and Control,* 7: 41–55, 1996.

Kovar, M. G., M. I. Harris, and W. C. Hadden. The scope of diabetes in the United States population. *American Handbook of Public Health,* 77: 1549–1550, 1987.

Krall, E. A., and B. Dawson-Hughes. Smoking and bone loss among postmenopausal women. *Journal of Bone Mineral Research,* 6: 331–338, 1991.

Krolner, B., and B. Toft. Vertebral bone loss: An unheeded side effect of therapeutic bed rest. *Clinical Science,* 64:537–540, 1983.

Marcus, R., et al. Menstrual function and bone mass in elite women distance runners: Endocrine metabolic features. *Annals of Internal Medicine,* 102: 158–163, 1985.

Martin, J. E., P. M. Dubbert, and W. C. Cushman. Controlled trial of aerobic exercise in hypertension. *Circulation,* 81: 1560–1567, 1990.

Morrison, N. A., et al. Prediction of bone density from vitamin D receptor alleles. *Nature,* 367: 284–287, 1994.

National Institutes of Health. Consensus Development Conference on Diet and Exercise in Non-Insulin-Dependent Diabetes Mellitus. *Diabetes Care,* 10: 639–644, 1987.

National Institutes of Health Consensus Report: Optimal Calcium Intake. NIH: Bethesda, MD, 1994.

Paffenbarger, R. S., et al. Physical activity, all-cause mortality, and longevity of college alumni. *New England Journal of Medicine,* 314: 605–613, 1986.

Physician's Health Study Research Group, Steering Committee. Preliminary report: Findings from the aspirin component of the ongoing Physicians' Health Study. *New England Journal of Medicine,* 318: 262–264, 1988.

Pollock, M. L., and J. H. Wilmore. *Exercise in Health and Disease.* Philadelphia: Saunders, 1990.

Potter, J. D. Nutrition and colorectal cancer. *Cancer Causes and Control,* 7(1): 127–146, 1996.

Powell, K. E., et al. Physical activity and the incidence of coronary heart disease. *Annual Review of Public Health,* 8: 253–287, 1987.

Riggs, B. L., and L. J. Melton. The prevention and treatment of osteoporosis. *New England Journal of Medicine,* 327(9): 620–627, 1992.

Robinson, T. L., and C. Snow-Harter, D. R. Taaffe, D. Gillis, J. Shaw, R. Marcus. Gymnasts exhibit higher bone mineral density than runners despite similar prevalence of oligo- and amenorrhea. *Journal of Bone Mineral Research,* 10: 26–34, 1995.

Siniske, S. J., et al. The physical and mechanical effects of suspension-induced osteopenia on mouse long bones. *Journal of Biomechanics,* 25: 489–499, 1992.

Snow, C. Osteoporosis and exercise in premenopausal women. *Bone,* 18: 51S–55S, pp.511–525 1996.

Snow, C. M., C. Matkin, and J. M. Shaw. Physical activity and risk for osteoporosis and associated fractures. In R. Marcus, J. Kelsey, and D. Feldman, *Osteoporosis.* Orlando: Academic Press, 1996.

Snow-Harter, C. Athletic amenorrhea and bone health. In *Medical and Orthopaedic Issues in Active and Athletic Women.* Philadelphia: Hanley and Belfus, 1994, 164–168.

Snow-Harter, C. Bone health and prevention of osteoporosis in active and athletic women. *Clinics in Sports Medicine,* 13(2): 389, 404, 1994.

Snow-Harter, C., et al. Muscle strength as a predictor of bone mineral density in young women. *Journal of Bone Mineral Research,* 5: 589–595, 1990.

Steinmetz, K. A., J. D. Potter. Vegetables, fruit and cancer prevention: A review. *Journal of American Dietetic Association.* 96: 1027–1037.

Ulrich, C. M., C. C. Georgiou, C. Snow-Harter, and D. Gillis. Bone mineral density and lifetime physical activity. *American Journal of Clinical Nutrition,* 63: 72–79, 1996.

U.S. Department of Health and Human Services. *Physical Activity and Health: A Report of the Surgeon General.*

Atlanta, GA: U.S. Department of Health and Human Services, Centers for Disease Control and Prevention, National Center for Chronic Disease Prevention and Health Promotion, 1996.

U.S. Department of Health and Human Services, Public Health Service. *Healthy People 2000*; National Health Promotion and Disease Prevention Objectives. DHHS Publication No. 91-50212. U.S. Government Printing Office, Washington, DC, 1990.

Vitug, A., S. H. Schneider, and N. B. Rudennan. Exercise and type I diabetes mellitus. *American Handbook of Public Health,* 16: 285–304, 1988.

Willett, W. C., and D. Trichopoulos. Summary of the evidence: Nutrition and cancer. *Cancer Causes and Control,* 7: 178–180.

World Cancer Research Fund. *Food, Nutrition, and the Prevention of Cancer: A Global Perspective.* American Institute for Cancer Research, 1997, 472–497.

RISKO — A Heart Health Appraisal by the American Heart Association

The RISKO Heart Health Appraisal is a quick way to evaluate your risk for coronary heart disease based upon your profile in three of the major risk factors (blood pressure, cigarette smoking, and blood cholesterol) and one of the contributing risk factors (body weight). Use the accompanying tables in each category to derive your score for that risk factor. Add these four scores together to compute your RISKO score, and use the guide to evaluate your risk based upon this score.

What Your Score Means

Note: If you're diabetic, you have a greater risk of heart disease. Add 7 points to your total score.

0–2	You have a low risk of heart disease for a person of your age and sex.
3–4	You have a low-to-moderate risk of heart disease for a person of your age and sex. That's good, but there's room for improvement.
5–7	You have a moderate-to-high risk of heart disease for a person of your age and sex. There's considerable room for improvement in some areas.
8–15	You have a high risk of developing heart disease for a person of your age and sex. There's lots of room for improvement in all areas.
16 & over	You have a very high risk of developing heart disease for a person of your age and sex. You should act now to reduce all your risk factors.

Some Words of Caution

■ RISKO is a way for adults who don't have signs of heart disease now to measure their risk. If you already have heart disease, it's very important to work with your doctor to reduce your risk.

■ RISKO is not a substitute for a thorough physical examination and assessment by your doctor. It's intended to help you learn more about the factors that influence the risk of heart disease, and thus to reduce your risk.

■ If you have a family history of heart disease, your risk of heart disease will be higher than your RISKO score shows. If you have a high RISKO score and a family history of heart disease, taking action now to reduce your risk is even more important.

■ If you're a woman under 45 years old or a man under 35 years old, your real risk of heart disease is probably lower than your RISKO score.

■ If you're overweight, have high blood pressure or high blood cholesterol, or smoke cigarettes, your long-term risk of heart disease is higher even if your risk of heart disease in the next several years is low. To reduce your risk, you should eliminate or control these risk factors.

How To Reduce Your Risk

Refer to the cardiovascular disease prevention section earlier in this chapter (pages 406–407).

MEN

1. Systolic Blood Pressure

If you **are not** taking anti-hypertensive medications and your blood pressure is . . .

124 or less	0 points
between 125 and 134	2 points
between 135 and 144	4 points
between 145 and 154	6 points
between 155 and 164	8 points
between 165 and 174	10 points
between 175 and 184	12 points
between 185 and 194	14 points
between 195 and 204	16 points
between 205 and 214	18 points
between 215 and 224	20 points

If you **are** taking anti-hypertensive medications and your blood pressure is . . .

120 or less	0 points
between 121 and 127	2 points
between 128 and 135	4 points
between 136 and 143	6 points
between 144 and 153	8 points
between 154 and 163	10 points
between 164 and 175	12 points
between 176 and 190	14 points
between 191 and 204	16 points
between 205 and 214	18 points
between 215 and 224	20 points

2. Blood Cholesterol

Locate the number of points for your total and HDL cholesterol in the table below.

		HDL							
		25	30	35	40	50	60	70	80
	140	4	2	0	0	0	0	0	0
	160	5	3	2	0	0	0	0	0
	180	6	4	3	1	0	0	0	0
	200	7	5	4	3	0	0	0	0
	220	7	6	5	4	1	0	0	0
TOTAL	240	8	7	5	4	2	0	0	0
	260	8	7	6	5	3	1	0	0
	280	9	8	7	6	4	2	0	0
	300	9	8	7	6	4	3	1	0
	340	9	9	8	7	6	4	2	1
	400	10	9	9	8	7	5	4	3

3. Cigarette Smoking

If you . . .

do not smoke	0 points
smoke less than a pack a day	2 points
smoke a pack a day	5 points
smoke two or more packs a day	9 points

4. Weight

Locate your weight category in the table below. If you are in . . .

weight category A	0 points
weight category B	1 points
weight category C	2 points

FT	IN	A	B	C
5	1	up to 162	163–250	251+
5	2	up to 167	168–257	258+
5	3	up to 172	173–264	265+
5	4	up to 176	177–272	273+
5	5	up to 181	182–279	280+
5	6	up to 185	186–286	287+
5	7	up to 190	191–293	294+
5	8	up to 195	196–300	301+
5	9	up to 199	200–307	308+
5	10	up to 204	205–315	316+
5	11	up to 209	210–322	323+
6	0	up to 213	214–329	330+
6	1	up to 218	219–336	337+
6	2	up to 223	224–343	344+
6	3	up to 227	228–350	351+
6	4	up to 232	233–368	359+
6	5	up to 238	239–365	366+
6	6	up to 241	242–372	373+

Total Score

WOMEN

1. Systolic Blood Pressure

If you **are not** taking anti-hypertensive medications and your blood pressure is . . .

125 or less	0 points
between 126 and 136	2 points
between 137 and 148	4 points
between 149 and 160	6 points
between 161 and 171	8 points
between 172 and 183	10 points
between 184 and 194	12 points
between 195 and 206	14 points
between 207 and 218	16 points

If you **are** taking anti-hypertensive medications and your blood pressure is . . .

117 or less	0 points
between 118 and 123	2 points
between 124 and 129	4 points
between 130 and 136	6 points
between 137 and 144	8 points
between 145 and 154	10 points
between 155 and 168	12 points
between 169 and 206	14 points
between 207 and 218	16 points

2. Blood Cholesterol

Locate the number of points for your total and HDL cholesterol in the table below.

		HDL							
		25	30	35	40	50	60	70	80
	140	2	1	0	0	0	0	0	0
	160	3	2	1	0	0	0	0	0
	180	4	3	2	1	0	0	0	0
	200	4	3	2	2	0	0	0	0
	220	5	4	3	2	1	0	0	0
TOTAL	240	5	4	3	3	1	0	0	0
	260	5	4	4	3	2	1	0	0
	280	5	5	4	4	2	1	0	0
	300	6	5	4	4	3	2	1	0
	340	6	5	5	4	3	2	1	0
	400	6	6	5	5	4	3	2	2

3. Cigarette Smoking

If you . . .

do not smoke	0 points
smoke less than a pack a day	2 points
smoke a pack a day	5 points
smoke two or more packs a day	9 points

4. Weight

Locate your weight category in the table below. If you are in . . .

weight category A	0 points
weight category B	1 points
weight category C	2 points
weight category D	3 points

FT	IN	A	B	C	D
4	8	up to 139	140–161	162–184	185+
4	9	up to 140	141–162	163–185	186+
4	10	up to 141	142–163	164–187	188+
4	11	up to 143	144–166	167–190	191+
5	0	up to 145	146–168	169–193	194+
5	1	up to 147	148–171	172–196	197+
5	2	up to 149	150–173	174–198	199+
5	3	up to 152	153–176	177–201	202+
5	4	up to 154	155–178	179–204	205+
5	5	up to 157	158–182	183–209	210+
5	6	up to 160	161–186	187–213	214+
5	7	up to 165	166–191	192–219	220+
5	8	up to 169	170–196	197–225	226+
5	9	up to 173	174–201	202–231	232+
5	10	up to 178	179–206	207–238	239+
5	11	up to 182	183–212	213–242	243+
6	0	up to 187	188–217	218–248	249+
6	1	up to 191	192–222	223–254	255+

Total Score

Source: From American Heart Association, 1994.

Laboratory 13.2

Assessing Your Risk for Diabetes

For each of the following statements, if you respond yes, enter the appropriate point total. If you respond no, enter 0.

1. I have been experiencing one or more of the following symptoms on a regular basis

excessive thirst	3	_____
frequent urination	3	_____
extreme fatigue	1	_____
unexplained weight loss	3	_____
blurry vision from time to time	2	_____

2. I am over 40 years old.　1 _____

3. I believe that I am more than 20% overweight.　2 _____

4. I am a woman who has had more than one baby weighing over 9 pounds at birth.　2 _____

5. I am of Native American descent.　1 _____

6. I am of Hispanic or African-American descent.　2 _____

7. I have a parent with diabetes.　1 _____

8. I have a brother or sister with diabetes.　1 _____

Evaluation

3–5　You are probably at low risk for diabetes. But don't just forget about it, especially if you're over 40, overweight, or of African-American, Hispanic, or Native American descent.

≥ 5　You may be at high risk for diabetes and may even already have diabetes. See your doctor promptly.

Source: Adapted from the American Diabetes Association National Service Center, 1660 Duke St., Alexandria, VA 22314.

Laboratory 13.3

Assessing Your Risk for Osteoporosis

For each of the following questions, check either yes or no.

1. *Do you have a family history of osteoporosis? (Have any of your female relatives broken a wrist or hip or had a dowager's hump?)*

   ❑ yes   ❑ no

2. *Did you go through menopause or have your ovaries removed by surgery before age 50?*

   ❑ yes   ❑ no

3. *Did your menstrual periods ever stop for more than a year for reasons other than pregnancy or nursing?*

   ❑ yes   ❑ no

4. *Did your ancestors come from England, Ireland, Scotland, Northern Europe, or Asia, or do you have a small, thin body frame?*

   ❑ yes   ❑ no

5. *Have you had surgery in which a part of your stomach or intestines was removed?*

   ❑ yes   ❑ no

6. *Are you taking or have you taken drugs like cortisone, steroids, or anticonvulsants over a prolonged period?*

   ❑ yes   ❑ no

7. *Do you have a thyroid or parathyroid disorder (hyperthyroidism or hyperparathyroidism)?*

   ❑ yes   ❑ no

8. *Are you allergic to milk products or are you lactose intolerant?*

   ❑ yes   ❑ no

9. *Do you smoke cigarettes?*

   ❑ yes   ❑ no

10. *Do you drink wine, beer, or other alcoholic beverages daily?*

    ❑ yes   ❑ no

11. *Do you do less than 1 hour of exercising such as aerobics, walking, or jogging per week?*

    ❑ yes   ❑ no

12. *Have you ever exercised so strenuously that you had irregular periods or no periods at all?*

    ❑ yes   ❑ no

13. *Have you ever had an eating disorder (bulimia or anorexia nervosa)?*

    ❑ yes   ❑ no

How Did You Do?

Did you have several yes answers? If so, you may have a very high chance of getting osteoporosis. It would be a good idea to talk with your doctor today so that you can work together to keep this disabling disease from happening to you.

Appendix A
Food Composition

FOOD DESCRIPTION	MEASURE	WT (G)	ENER (CAL)	PROT (G)	CARB (G)	DIETARY FIBER (G)	FAT (G)	FAT BREAKDOWN (G)			CHOL (MG)	CALC (MG)	IRON (MG)	SODI (MG)
								SAT	MONO	POLY				
BEVERAGES														
Alcoholic:														
Beer:														
Regular (12 fl oz)	1½ c	356	146	1	13	3	0	0	0	0	0	18	.11	18
Light (12 fl oz)	1½ c	354	99[1]	1	5	1	0	0	0	0	0	18	.14	11
Wine:														
Red	3½ fl oz	103	74	<1	2	0	0	0	0	0	0	8	.44	5
White medium	3½ fl oz	103	70	<1	1	0	0	0	0	0	0	9	.33	5
Carbonated:[2]														
Cola beverage (12 fl oz)	1½ c	370	152	0	38	0	<1	0	0	.1	0	11	.11	15
Diet cola w/aspartame (12 fl oz)	1½ c	355	4	<1	<1	0	0	0	0	0	0	14	.11	21[3]
Diet cola w/saccharin (12 fl oz)	1½ c	355	0	0	<1	0	0	0	0	0	0	14	.14	57
Lemon-lime (12 fl oz)	1½ c	368	147	0	38	0	0	0	0	0	0	7	.26	40
Pepper-type soda (12 fl oz)	1½ c	368	151	0	38	0	<1	.3	0	0	0	11	.15	37
Coffee, brewed	1 c	240	5[4]	<1	1	0	<1	0	0	0	0	5	.12	5
Coffee, prepared from instant	1 c	240	5[4]	<1	1	0	<1	0	0	0	0	7	.12	7
Fruit drinks, noncarbonated:[5]														
Fruit punch drink, canned	½ c	126	59	0	15	0	<1	0	0	0	0	10	.26	28
Gatorade	1 c	240	60	0	15	0	0	0	0	0	0	0	.12	96
Grape drink, canned	½ c	125	63	<1	16	<1	0	0	0	0	0	4	.13	1
Lemonade,														
frozen concentrate (6-oz can)	¾ c	219	396	1	103	1	<1	.1	t	.1	0	15	1.58	9
Tea:[2]														
Brewed, regular	1 c	240	2	0	1	0	<1	0	0	t	0	0	.05	7
Brewed, herbal	¾ c	178	2	0	<1	0	t	0	0	t	0	4	.14	2
DAIRY														
Butter: see Fats and Oils														
Cheese, natural:														
Cheddar	1 oz	28	114	7	<1	0	9	6	2.7	.3	30	204	.19	176
Cottage:														
Low sodium, low fat	1 c	225	162	28	6	0	2	1.4	.6	.1	9	137	.32	29
Creamed, large curd	1 c	225	232	28	6	0	10	6.4	2.9	.3	33	135	.32	911
Creamed, small curd	1 c	210	216	26	6	0	9	6	2.7	.3	31	126	.29	851
Cream	1 oz	28	99	2	1	0	10	6.2	2.8	.4	31	23	.34	84
Low fat	1 oz	28	65	3	2	0	5	3.1	1.4	.2	16	32	.48	84
Monterey Jack	1 oz	28	106	7	<1	0	9	5.4	2.5	.3	25	211	.2	152
Mozzarella, whole milk	1 oz	28	80	5	1	0	6	3.7	1.9	.2	22	146	.05	105
Mozzarella, part-skim milk,														
low moisture	1 oz	28	79	8	1	0	5	3.1	1.4	.1	15	207	.07	149
Parmesan, grated:														
Cup, not pressed down	1 c	100	456	42	4	0	30	19	8.7	.7	79	1375	.95	1861
Tablespoon	1 tbs	5	23	2	<1	0	2	1	.4	t	4	69	.05	93
Provolone	1 oz	28	100	7	1	0	8	4.8	2.1	.2	20	214	.15	247
Ricotta, whole milk	1 c	246	428	28	8	0	32	20.4	8.9	1	124	509	.93	206
Ricotta, part-skim milk	1 c	246	339	28	13	0	19	12.1	5.7	.6	76	669	1.08	308
Swiss	1 oz	28	106	8	1	0	8	5	2.1	.3	26	272	.05	74
low fat	1 oz	28	51	8	1	0	1	.9	.4	<.1	10	272	.05	74

[1]Calories can vary from 78 to 131 for 12 fl. oz.

[2]Mineral content varies depending on water source.

[3]Value for product sweetened with aspartame only; sodium is 32 mg if a blend of aspartame and sodium saccharin is used.

[4]Calorie values from USDA vary from 1 to 5 cal per cup.

[5]Usually less than 10% fruit juice.

(For purposes of calculations, use "0" for t, <1, <.1, <.01, etc.)

Food Composition

FOOD DESCRIPTION	MEASURE	WT (G)	ENER (CAL)	PROT (G)	CARB (G)	DIETARY FIBER (G)	FAT (G)	FAT BREAKDOWN (G)			CHOL (MG)	CALC (MG)	IRON (MG)	SODI (MG)
								SAT	MONO	POLY				
DAIRY — CONT.														
Cheese, cont.														
American	1 oz	28	106	6	<1	0	9	5.6	2.5	.3	27	174	.11	405
Swiss	1 oz	28	94	7	1	0	7	4.6	2	.2	24	219	.17	388
Velveeta cheese spread,														
low fat, low sodium	1 oz	28	51	7	1	0	2	1.3	0.6	.1	10	194	.12	2
Cream, sweet:	1 c	242	315	7	10	0	28	17.3	8	1	89	254	.17	98
Half & half (cream & milk):														
Tablespoon	1 tbs	15	19	<1	1	0	2	1.1	.5	.1	6	16	.01	6
Light, coffee or table	1 c	240	468	6	9	0	46	28.8	13.4	1.7	158	230	.1	95
Light whipping cream, liquid[1]	1 c	239	698	5	7	0	74	46.1	21.7	2.1	265	165	.07	82
Heavy whipping cream, liquid[1]	1 c	238	821	5	7	0	88	54.7	25.5	3.3	326	153	.07	89
Cream, sour, cultured:	1 c	230	492	7	10	0	48	29.9	13.9	1.8	102	267	.14	122
Tablespoon	1 tbs	14	30	<1	1	0	3	1.8	.8	.1	6	16	.01	7
Milk, fluid:														
Whole milk	1 c	244	150	8	11	0	8	5.1	2.3	.3	33	290	.12	120
2% low-fat milk	1 c	244	121	8	12	0	5	2.9	1.3	.2	18	298	.12	122
2% milk solids added[1]	1 c	245	124	9	12	0	5	2.9	1.4	.2	18	311	.12	128
1% low-fat milk	1 c	244	102	8	12	—	3	1.6	.8	.1	10	300	.12	123
1% milk solids added[1]	1 c	245	104	9	12	0	2	1.5	.7	.1	10	311	.12	128
Nonfat milk, vitamin A added	1 c	245	86	8	12	0	<1	.3	.1	t	4	301	.1	126
Buttermilk, nonfat	1 c	245	99	8	12	0	2	1.3	.6	.1	9	284	.12	257
Chocolate:														
Whole	1 c	250	208	8	26	3	9	5.2	2.5	.3	30	280	.6	149
2% fat	1 c	250	178	8	26	3	5	3.1	1.5	.2	17	285	.6	151
1% fat	1 c	250	157	8	26	3	3	1.5	.7	.1	7	288	.6	152
Milk shakes, chocolate (10 fl oz)	1¼ c	283	359	10	58	<1	10	6.5	3	.4	37	320	.88	275
Milk shakes, vanilla (10 fl oz)	1¼ c	283	314	10	51	<1	8	5.3	2.4	.3	31	345	.25	232
Milk desserts:														
Low-fat frozen dessert bars	1 ea	81	90	2	18	0	1	.2	.1	.4	1	82	.07	47
Ice cream, vanilla (about 10% fat):														
Cup	1 c	133	267	5	31	<1	15	9	4.2	.6	59	170	.12	106
Soft serve	1 c	173	372	7	38	<1	22	12.9	6	.8	157	227	.36	106
Ice cream, rich vanilla (16% fat):														
Cup	1 c	148	357	5	33	<1	24	14.8	6.9	.9	90	173	.07	83
Ben & Jerry's	½ c	106	230	4	21	0	17	10	—	—	95	150	.36	55
Ice milk, vanilla (about 4% fat):														
Cup	1 c	131	182	5	30	<1	6	3.5	1.6	.2	18	182	.13	111
Soft serve (about 3% fat)	1 c	175	221	9	38	<1	5	2.8	1.3	.2	21	275	.1	123
Sherbet (2% fat):														
Cup	1 c	193	266	2	59	0	4	2.2	1	.2	10	104	.27	89
Yogurt, frozen, low-fat[2]	½ c	87	138	3	21	0	5	3	1.4	.2	2	124	.26	76
Scoop	1 ea	79	78	4	16	0	<1	.1	t	0	1	137	.07	53
Yogurt, low-fat:														
Fruit added with														
low-calorie sweetener	1 c	241	122	11	19	1	<1	.2	.1	t	3	369	.61	139
Fruit added[3]	1 c	227	232	10	43	<1	2	1.6	.7	.1	10	345	.16	133
Plain	1 c	227	144	12	16	0	4	2.3	1	.1	14	415	.18	159
Yogurt, made with nonfat milk	1 c	227	127	13	17	0	<1	.3	.1	t	4	452	.2	174
Yogurt, made with whole milk	1 c	227	139	8	11	0	7	4.8	2	.2	29	275	.11	105

[1]Milk solids added, label claims less than 10 g protein per cup.
[2]Data is from 1992 USDA data on snacks and sweets.
[3]Carbohydrates and calories vary widely—consult label if more precise values are needed.
(For purposes of calculations, use "0" for t, <1, <.1, <.01, etc.)

Food Composition

FOOD DESCRIPTION	MEASURE	WT (G)	ENER (CAL)	PROT (G)	CARB (G)	DIETARY FIBER (G)	FAT (G)	FAT BREAKDOWN (G) SAT	MONO	POLY	CHOL (MG)	CALC (MG)	IRON (MG)	SODI (MG)
EGGS														
Raw, large:														
Whole, without shell	1 ea	50	74	6	1	0	5	1.5	1.9	.7	213	25	.72	63
White	1 ea	33	17	4	<1	0	0	0	0	0	0	2	.01	54
Yolk	1 ea	17	59	3	<1	0	5	1.6	1.9	.7	218	23	.59	7
Cooked:														
Fried in margarine	1 ea	46	92	6	1	0	7	1.9	2.8	1.3	211	25	.72	162
Hard-cooked, shell removed	1 ea	50	78	6	1	0	5	1.6	2	.7	212	25	.59	62
Scrambled with milk & margarine	1 ea	61	101	7	1	0	7	2.2	2.9	1.3	215	43	.73	171
FATS AND OILS														
Butter:														
Tablespoon	1 tbs	14	100	<1	<1	0	11	7.1	3.4	.4	31	3	.02	117[1]
Pat (about 1 tsp)[2]	1 ea	5	36	<1	<1	0	4	2.5	1.2	.2	11	1	.01	41[1]
Vegetable shortening:	1 c	205	1812	0	0	0	205	51.5	91.2	53.5	0	0	0	0
Tablespoon	1 tbs	13	115	0	0	0	13	3.3	5.8	3.4	0	0	0	0
Margarine:														
Imitation (about 40% fat), soft:	1 c	227	783	1	1	0	88	14.5	33	37	0	40	0	800[3]
Tablespoon	1 tbs	14	48	<1	<1	0	5	.9	2	2.3	0	2	0	49[3]
Regular, hard (about 80% fat):	½ c	113	812	1	1	0	91	14.8	42	29.6	0	34	0	1065[3]
Tablespoon	1 tbs	14	101	<1	<1	0	11	1.8	5	3.6	0	4	0	132[3]
Oils:														
Corn:														
Tablespoon	1 tbs	14	124	0	0	0	14	1.8	3.4	8.2	0	0	0	0
Olive:														
Tablespoon	1 tbs	14	124	0	0	0	14	1.9	10.3	1.2	0	<1	.05	<1
Safflower:														
Tablespoon	1 tbs	14	124	0	0	0	14	1.3	1.7	10.4	0	0	0	0
Sunflower:														
Tablespoon	1 tbs	14	124	0	0	0	14	1.5	2.9	9.2	0	0	0	0
Salad dressings/sandwich spreads:														
Blue cheese, regular	1 tbs	15	76	1	1	<1	8	1.5	1.9	4.4	3	12	.03	164
Low calorie	1 tbs	15	15	1	<1	<1	1	.2	.5	.4	<1	13	.08	180
French, regular	1 tbs	16	69	<1	3	<1	9	1.5	1.2	3.4	9	2	.06	219
Low calorie	1 tbs	16	21	<1	3	<1	1	.1	.2	.5	1	2	.06	126
Italian, regular	1 tbs	15	70	<1	1	<1	9	1	1.6	4.1	0	2	.03	118
Low calorie	1 tbs	15	16	<1	1	<1	1	.2	.3	.9	1	<1	.03	118
Ranch, regular	½ c	119	436	4	6	0	45	6.7	19.4	17	47	119	.31	522
Low calorie	2 tbs	28	60	0	2	0	5	1	—	—	10	20	0	240
Vinegar & oil	1 tbs	16	72	0	<1	0	8	1.5	2.4	3.9	0	0	0	<1
FRUITS AND FRUIT JUICES														
Apples:														
Fresh, raw, with peel:														
2¾" diam (about 3 per lb w/cores)	1 ea	138	81	<1	21	3	<1	.1	t	.1	0	10	.25	0
Apple juice, bottled or canned	1 c	248	116	<1	29	<1	<1	<1	t	<.1	0	17	.92	7
Applesauce, sweetened	1 c	255	193	<1	51	3	<1	.1	t	.1	0	10	.89	8
Apricots:														
Raw, w/o pits														
(about 12 per lb w/pits)	3 ea	106	51	1	12	2	<1	t	.2	.1	0	15	.57	1

[1]For salted butter, unsalted butter contains 12 mg sodium per stick or ½ c, 1.5 mg/tbs, or .5 mg/pat.
[2]Pat is 1: square, ⅓" thick; about 1 tsp; 90 per lb.
[3]For salted margarine.
(For purposes of calculations, use "0" for t, <1, <.1, <.01, etc.)

Food Composition

FOOD DESCRIPTION	MEASURE	WT (G)	ENER (CAL)	PROT (G)	CARB (G)	DIETARY FIBER (G)	FAT (G)	FAT BREAKDOWN (G)			CHOL (MG)	CALC (MG)	IRON (MG)	SODI (MG)
								SAT	MONO	POLY				
FRUITS AND FRUIT JUICES — CONT.														
Avocados, raw, edible part only:														
California (2 lb with refuse)	1 ea	173	306	4	12	6	30	4.5	19.4	3.5	0	19	2.04	21
Bananas, raw, without peel:														
Whole, 8¾″ long (175 g w/peel)	1 ea	114	104	1	27	2	1	.2	t	.1	0	7	.35	1
Blueberries:														
Fresh	1 c	145	81	1	20	4	1	t	.2	.3	0	9	.25	9
Frozen, sweetened	10 oz	284	230	1	62	6	<1	.1	.1	.2	0	17	1.11	3
Cherries:														
Sweet, red pitted, raw	10 ea	68	49	1	11	<1	1	.1	.2	.2	0	10	.26	0
Cranberry juice cocktail[1]	1 c	253	144	0[2]	36	<1	<1	.1	t	.1	0	8	.38	5
Cranberry juice, low calorie	¾ c	178	34	0	8	1	0	0	0	0	0	16	.07	5
Grapefruit:														
Raw 3¾″ diam (half w/rind = 241 g)														
Pink/red, half fruit, edible part	1 ea	123	37	1	9	2	<1	t	t	t	0	13	.15	0
White, half fruit, edible part	1 ea	118	39	1	10	2	<1	t	t	t	0	14	.07	0
Grapes, raw European (adherent skin):														
Thompson seedless	10 ea	50	35	<1	9	<1	<1	.1	t	.1	0	6	.13	1
Grape juice:														
Bottled or canned	1 c	253	154	1	38	2	<1	.1	t	.1	0	23	.61	8
Melons, raw, without rind and contents:														
Cantaloupe, 5″ diam (2⅓ lb whole with refuse), orange flesh	½ ea	267	93	2	22	2	1	.1	.1	.2	0	29	.56	24
Honeydew, 6½″ diam (5¼ lb whole with refuse), slice = 1/10 melon	1 pce	129	45	1	12	1	<1	t	t	t	0	8	.09	13
Oranges, raw:														
Whole w/o peel and seeds, 2⅝″ diam (180 g with peel and seeds)	1 ea	131	62	1	15	3	<1	t	t	t	0	52	.13	0
Orange juice:														
Fresh, all varieties	1 c	248	112	2	26	<1	<1	.1	.1	.1	0	27	.5	2
Canned, unsweetened	1 c	249	105	1	24	<1	<1	t	.1	.1	0	20	1.1	5
Peaches:														
Raw, whole, 2½″ diam, peeled, pitted (about 4 per lb whole)	1 ea	87	37	1	10	2	<1	t	t	t	0	4	.1	0
Pears:														
Fresh, with skin, cored:														
Bartlett, 2½″ diam (about 2½ per lb)	1 ea	166	98	1	25	4[3]	1	t	.1	.2	0	18	.41	0
Bosc, 2⅕″ diam (about 3 per lb)	1 ea	141	83	1	21	3[3]	1	t	.1	.1	0	16	.35	0
D'Anjou, 3″ diam (about 2 per lb)	1 ea	200	118	1	30	5[3]	1	t	.2	.2	0	22	.5	0
Pineapple:														
Fresh chunks, diced	1 c	155	76	1	19	2	1	t	.1	.2	0	11	.57	2
Plums:														
Fresh, medium, 2⅛″ diam	1 ea	66	36	1	9	1	<1	t	.3	.1	0	3	.07	0
Pomegranate, fresh	1 ea	154	105	1	27	5	<1	—	—	—	0	5	.46	5
Prunes, dried, pitted	10 ea	84	200	2	53	8[4]	<1	t	.3	.1	0	43	2.08	3
Prune juice, bottled or canned	1 c	256	182	2	45	3	1	t	.5	t	0	31	3	10

[1]Data here are from the newest USDA *Handbook 8–14* on beverages. These data are somewhat different from that presented in *Handbook 8–9* on fruits and fruit juices.

[2]The newest USDA *Handbook 8–14* data on beverages indicates "0" for protein.

[3]Dietary fiber data vary 2.4 to 3.4 g/100 g for fresh pears; 1.6 to 2.6 g/100 g for canned pears.

[4]Dietary fiber data can vary between 6 and 13 g for 10 prunes.

(For purposes of calculations, use "0" for t, <1, <.1, <.01, etc.)

Food Composition

FOOD DESCRIPTION	MEASURE	WT (G)	ENER (CAL)	PROT (G)	CARB (G)	DIETARY FIBER (G)	FAT (G)	FAT BREAKDOWN (G) SAT	MONO	POLY	CHOL (MG)	CALC (MG)	IRON (MG)	SODI (MG)
FRUITS AND FRUIT JUICES — CONT.														
Raisins, seedless:														
Cup, not pressed down	1 c	145	435	5	115	5	1	.2	t	.2	0	71	3.02	17
One packet, ½ oz	½ oz	14	42	<1	11	1	<1	t	t	t	0	7	.29	2
Raspberries:														
Fresh	1 c	123	60	1	14	5	1	t	.1	.4	0	27	.7	0
Strawberries:														
Fresh, whole, capped	1 c	149	45	1	10	2	1	t	.1	.3	0	21	.57	1
Frozen, sliced, sweetened:														
10-oz container	10 oz	284	272	2	74	5	<1	t	.1	.2	0	31	1.68	9
Tangerines, without peel and seeds:														
Fresh (2⅜" whole) 116 g w/refuse	1 ea	84	37	1	9	1	<1	t	t	t	0	12	.08	1
Watermelon, raw, without rind & seeds:														
Piece, 1" by 10" diam														
(2 lb w/refuse or 926 g)	1 pce	482	154	3	35	1	2	.6	.4	1.1	0	39	.82	10
BAKED GOODS: BREADS, CAKES, COOKIES, CRACKERS, PIES														
Bagels, plain, enriched, 3½" diam	1 ea	68	187	7	36	2	1	.1	.1	.5	0	50	2.43	363
Breads:														
Cracked wheat (¼ cracked-wheat														
& ¾ enr wheat flour):														
Slice (18 per loaf)	1 pce	25	65	2	12	2	1	.2	.5	.2	0	11	.7	135
Slice, toasted	1 pce	21	59	2	11	1	1	.2	.4	.2	0	10	.64	123
French/Vienna, enriched:														
Slice, 4¾ × 4 × ½"	1 pce	25	68	2	13	1	1	.2	.3	.2	0	19	.63	152
French, slice, 5 × 2½"	1 pce	35	96	3	18	1	1	.2	.4	.2	0	26	.89	213
Italian, enriched: 1-lb loaf	1 ea	454	1230	40	227	14	16	3.9	3.7	6.3	0	354	13.4	2648
Slice, 4½ × 3¼ × ¾"	1 pce	30	81	3	15	1	1	.3	.2	.4	0	23	.88	175
Mixed grain:														
Slice (18 per loaf)	1 pce	25	62	3	12	2	1	.2	.4	.2	0	23	.87	122
Oatmeal:														
Slice (18 per loaf)	1 pce	25	67	2	12	1	1	.2	.4	.4	0	16	.68	150
Pita pocket bread, enr, 6½" round	1 ea	60	165	5	33	1	1	.1	.1	.3	0	52	1.58	322
Pumpernickel:														
Slice, 5 × 4 × ⅜"	1 pce	32	80	3	15	2	1	.1	.3	.4	0	22	.92	215
Slice, toasted	1 pce	29	80	3	15	2	1	.1	.3	.4	0	22	.92	214
Raisin, enriched:														
Slice (18 per loaf)	1 pce	25	68	2	13	1	1	.3	.6	.2	0	17	.73	97
Rye, light:														
Slice, 4¾ × 3¾ × ⁷⁄₁₆"	1 pce	25	65	2	12	2	1	.2	.3	.2	0	18	.71	165
Slice, toasted	1 pce	22	62	2	12	2	1	.2	.3	.2	0	18	.68	160
Wheat (enr wheat & whole-wheat flour):														
Slice (18 per loaf)	1 pce	25	64	2	12	1	1	.2	.4	.2	0	26	.83	133
White:														
Slice (18 per loaf)	1 pce	25	67	2	12	1	1	.2	.4	.2	<1	27	.71	135
Slice, toasted	1 pce	22	64	2	12	1	1	.2	.4	.2	<1	26	.73	130
Whole-wheat:														
Slice (16 per loaf)	1 pce	28	69	3	13	2	1	.3	.5	.3	0	20	.94	147
Slice, toasted	1 pce	25	69	3	13	2	1	.3	.5	.3	0	20	.93	148
Cakes[1]:														
Angel food:														
Piece, ¹⁄₁₂ of cake	1 pce	53	137	3	31	1	<1	.1	t	.2	0	74	.28	397

[1]Excepting angel food cake, cakes were made from mixes containing vegetable shortening, and frostings were made with margarine. All mixes use enriched flour. (For purposes of calculations, use "0" for t, <1, <.1, <.01, etc.)

Food Composition

FOOD DESCRIPTION	MEASURE	WT (G)	ENER (CAL)	PROT (G)	CARB (G)	DIETARY FIBER (G)	FAT (G)	FAT BREAKDOWN (G) SAT	MONO	POLY	CHOL (MG)	CALC (MG)	IRON (MG)	SODI (MG)
BAKED GOODS: BREADS, CAKES, COOKIES, CRACKERS, PIES — CONT.														
Cakes[1], cont.														
Boston cream pie	1 pce	120	302	3	52	2	10	3	5.3	1.2	44	28	.46	173
Coffee:														
Piece, ⅙ of cake	1 pce	72	229	4	38	1	7	1.3	2.8	2.3	35	98	1.04	303
Devil's food:														
Piece, 1/16 of cake	1 pce	69	253	3	38	2	11	3.2	6.2	1.3	32	30	1.52	230
Cupcake, 2½″ diam	1 ea	42	154	2	23	1	7	1.9	3.8	.8	19	18	.93	140
Gingerbread:														
Piece, ⅑ of cake	1 pce	63	195	3	32	2	6	1.6	3.5	.8	22	43	2.09	289
Yellow:														
Piece, 1/16 of cake	1 pce	69	262	3	38	1	12	3.3	6.7	1.4	38	25	1.44	233
Carrot cake, cream cheese frosting:[2]														
Piece, 1/16 of cake, 2¼ × 3¼″ slice	1 pce	112	488	5	53	1	30	5.5	7.3	15.2	60	28	1.41	276
Pound cake:														
Piece, 1/17 of loaf, ½″ slice	1 pce	28	109	2	14	<1	6	3	1.5	.31	0	5	.1	88
Cheesecake:														
Piece, 1/12 of cake	1 pce	92	295	5	23	2	21	10.6	7.1	1.3	51	47	.58	190
Strawberry shortcake, fresh	1 ea	254	327	5	40	4	17	10.1	4.9	1	53	209	2.33	510
White, white frosting 2 layer:														
Piece, 1/16 of cake	1 pce	71	266	2	45	1	10	2.8	4.2	2.5	6	34	.57	166
Cookies made with enriched flour:														
Brownies with nuts:														
Commercial w/frosting, 1½ × 1¾ × ⅞″	1 ea	25	101	1	16	1	4	1.1	2.1	.6	4	7	.56	78
Home recipe, 1¾ × 1¾ × ⅞″[3]	1 ea	20	93	1	10	<1	6	1.5	2.2	1.9	15	11	.37	69
Chocolate chip:														
Commercial, 2¼″ diam	4 ea	42	192	1	25	1	10	3.1	5.5	1.1	0	6	1.02	137
Home recipe, 2¼″ diam	4 ea	40	195	2	23	1	11	3.2	4.2	3.4	13	16	.99	144
From refrigerated dough, 2¼″ diam	4 ea	48	213	2	29	1	10	3.3	4.8	1	11	12	1.08	100
Fudge, fat free, Snackwell	1 ea	16	53	1	12	<1	<1	.1	.1	<.1	0	3	.29	71
Granola cookie, fat free	3 ea	28	85	2	19	2	0	0	0	0	0	—	.72	80
Oatmeal raisin, 2⅝″ diam	4 ea	52	226	3	36	2	8	1.7	3.6	2.6	17	52	1.38	280
Peanut Butter, home recipe, 2⅝″ diam[3]	4 ea	48	228	4	28	1	11	2.1	5.2	3.5	15	19	1.08	249
Shortbread, commercial, small	4 ea	32	161	2	21	1	8	2	4.3	1	6	11	.88	146
Sugar, from refrigerated dough, 2″ diam	4 ea	48	232	2	31	<1	11	2.8	6.2	1.4	15	43	.89	225
Vanilla wafers	10 ea	40	176	2	29	8	6	1.4	2.4	1.5	23	19	.96	125
Corn chips	1 oz	28	151	2	16	1	9	1.3	2.7	4.7	0	36	.37	179
Crackers:[4]														
Cheese	10 ea	10	50	1	6	<1	3	.9	.9	.5	1	15	.48	99
Rice cakes, unsalted	2 ea	18	69	1	14	<1	1	.2	.2	.2	0	2	.37	5
Saltine®[5] 4 ea	12	52	1	9	<1	1	.3	.8	.2	0	14	.65	156
Saltine®, unsalted tops	2 ea	6	25	1	4	0	1	0	0	0	0	—	.36	50
Snack-type, round like Ritz	3 ea	9	45	1	5	<1	2	.4	1	.8	0	11	.32	76
Wheat, thin	4 ea	8	38	1	5	1	2	.7	.8	.2	2	3	.25	69
Whole-wheat wafers	2 ea	8	35	1	5	1	1	.2	.8	.2	0	4	.25	53

[1]Excepting angel food cake, cakes were made from mixes containing vegetable shortening, and frostings were made with margarine. All mixes use enriched flour.
[2]Made with vegetable oil.
[3]Made with vegetable shortening.
[4]Crackers made with enriched white (wheat) flour except for rye wafers and whole-wheat wafers.
[5]Made with lard.
(For purposes of calculations, use "0" for t, <1, <.1, <.01, etc.)

Food Composition

FOOD DESCRIPTION	MEASURE	WT (G)	ENER (CAL)	PROT (G)	CARB (G)	DIETARY FIBER (G)	FAT (G)	FAT BREAKDOWN (G)			CHOL (MG)	CALC (MG)	IRON (MG)	SODI (MG)
								SAT	MONO	POLY				
BAKED GOODS: BREADS, CAKES, COOKIES, CRACKERS, PIES — CONT.														
Croissants, 4½ × 4 × 1¾″	1 ea	57	231	5	26	1	12	6.7	3.2	.7	43	21	1.16	424
Croutons, seasoned	½ c	15	70	2	10	<1	3	.8	1.4	.4	<1	14	.42	186
Doughnuts:														
Cake type, plain, 3¼″ diam	1 ea	50	211	3	25	1	11	1.9	4.8	4.1	18	22	.98	273
Yeast-leavened, glazed	1 ea	60	242	4	27	1	14	3.5	7.7	1.7	4	26	1.23	205
English muffins:														
Plain, enriched	1 ea	57	134	4	26	2	1	.1	.2	.5	0	99	1.43	264
Toasted	1 ea	50	128	4	25	2	1	.1	.2	5	0	94	1.37	252
Whole wheat	1 ea	50	102	4	20	5	1	.2	.3	.4	0	133	1.23	319
Fruit & fitness bar, fat free	1 ea	38	110	2	27	1	0	0	0	0	0	—	1.08	35
Granola bar, soft	1 ea	42	188	3	29	2	7	3.1	1.6	2.3	<1	45	1.09	118
Granola bar, hard	1 ea	28	132	3	18	2	6	.7	1.2	3.4	0	17	.84	83
Granola bar, fat free:														
Chocolate chip	1 ea	43	140	3	33	3	0	0	0	0	0	20	3.6	10
Muffins 2½″ diam, 1½″ high:														
From commercial mix:														
Blueberry	1 ea	45	135	2	22	1	4	.7	1.6	1.4	21	11	.51	197
Bran, wheat	1 ea	45	124	3	21	4	4	1.1	2.1	.6	31	14	1.14	210
Cornmeal	1 ea	45	144	3	22	2	5	1.3	2.4	.6	28	34	.88	358
Nabisco Newtons fat free:														
Fig	1 ea	23	68	1	16	—	0	0	0	0	—	—	—	76
Pancakes, 4″ diam:														
Buckwheat, from mix w/egg and milk	1 ea	27	56	2	8	1	2	.5	.5	.8	18	69	.51	144
Plain, from home recipe	1 ea	27	61	2	8	<1	3	.6	.7	1.2	16	59	.49	119
Plain, from mix; egg, milk, oil added	1 ea	27	52	1	10	<1	1	.1	.2	.2	3	34	.42	170
Pies, 9″ diam; crust made with vegetable shortening, enriched flour:														
Apple:[1]														
Piece, ⅙ of pie	1 pce	158	374	3	54	3	17	3.3	9.4	3.3	0	17	.71	420
Banana cream:														
Piece, ⅙ of pie	1 pce	198	533	9	65	—	27	7.4	11.3	6.5	101	149	2.08	475
Blueberry:[1]														
Piece, ⅙ of pie	1 pce	158	387	4	53	2	19	4.6	8.1	4.9	0	11	1.96	292
Cherry:[1]														
Piece, ⅙ of pie	1 pce	158	427	4	61	2	19	4.7	8.4	5.1	0	16	2.94	302
Chocolate cream:[2]														
Piece, ⅙ of pie	1 pce	199	561	10	62	1	32	10	13	6.7	105	161	2.04	487
Custard:[1]														
Piece, ⅙ of pie	1 pce	152	319	8	32	2	18	4.2	8.8	2.9	50	122	.88	365
Lemon meringue:[1]														
Piece, ⅙ of pie	1 pce	140	375	2	66	2	12	2.2	5.1	4	63	78	.85	204
Peach:														
Piece, ⅙ of pie	1 pce	158	435	4	63	2	18	4.4	8.2	5.3	3	13	57	445
Pecan:[1]														
Piece, ⅙ of pie	1 pce	138	552	6	79	5	25	5.2	14.9	4.1	44	23	1.45	585
Pumpkin:[1]														
Piece, ⅙ of pie	1 pce	206	433	8	56	6	20	4.2	10.3	3.3	41	124	1.63	581
Pretzels, made with enriched flour:														
Thin sticks, 2¼″ long	10 ea	3	11	<1	2	<1	<1	t	t	t	0	1	.13	51
Dutch twists, 2¾ × 2⅝″	1 ea	16	61	1	13	<1	1	.1	.2	.2	0	6	.69	274

[1]Values from latest USDA data for Baked Goods.
[2]Values based on recipe: pie crust, cooked chocolate pudding, whipped cream topping.
(For purposes of calculations, use "0" for t, <1, <.1, <.01, etc.)

Food Composition

FOOD DESCRIPTION	MEASURE	WT (G)	ENER (CAL)	PROT (G)	CARB (G)	DIETARY FIBER (G)	FAT (G)	FAT BREAKDOWN (G) SAT	MONO	POLY	CHOL (MG)	CALC (MG)	IRON (MG)	SODI (MG)
BAKED GOODS: BREADS, CAKES, COOKIES, CRACKERS, PIES — CONT.														
Pretzels, cont.														
Thin twists, 3¼ × 2¼ × ¼"	10 ea	60	229	5	47	2	2	.4	.8	.7	0	22	2.59	1029
Rolls & buns:														
Hot dog buns	1 ea	40	114	3	20	1	2	.5	1	.4	0	56	1.27	224
Hamburger buns	1 ea	45	129	4	23	1	2	.5	1.1	.4	0	63	1.43	252
Hard roll, white, 3¾" diam, 2" high	1 ea	50	147	5	26	1	2	.3	.6	.9	0	47	1.65	272
Dinner rolls, 2½" diam, 2" high	1 ea	35	112	3	19	1	3	.7	1.1	.7	13	21	1.04	145
Sports/fitness bar:														
Power bar	1 ea	65	225	10	40	3	1	—	—	—	—	300	5.4	20
Tiger sports bar	1 ea	65	230	11	40	4	2	—	—	—	—	350	4.5	100
Toaster pastries, fortified (Poptarts)	1 ea	54	212	3	38	1	6	.8	2.2	2.1	0	14	1.89	226
Tortilla chips:														
Plain	1 oz	28	140	2	18	2	6	2	4.4	1	0	0	0	135
Nacho flavor	1 oz	28	139	2	18	1	7	1.4	4.3	1	1	42	.4	198
Taco flavor	1 oz	28	134	2	18	2	7	1.3	4	1	1	44	.57	221
Tortillas:														
Corn, enriched, 6" diam	1 ea	30	67	2	14	2	1	.1	.2	.3	0	52	.42	48
Flour, 8" diam	1 ea	35	115	3	20	1	2	.4	1	1	0	44	1.17	169
Flour, 10" diam	1 ea	57	185	5	32	1	4	.6	1.6	1.6	0	71	1.88	272
Taco shells	1 ea	14	66	1	9	1	3	.4	1.5	.6	0	22	.35	51
Waffles, 7" diam:														
From home recipe	1 ea	75	218	6	25	1	11	2.1	2.6	5.1	52	191	1.74	383
From mix, egg/milk added	1 ea	75	218	5	26	1	10	1.7	2.7	5.2	52	91	1.23	383
GRAIN PRODUCTS: CEREAL, FLOUR, GRAIN, PASTA AND NOODLES, POPCORN														
Breakfast cereals, hot, cooked:														
Cream of wheat:														
Regular, quick, instant	1 c	244	131	4	27	1	<1	.1	.1	.2	0	51[1]	10.5[1]	141[2]
Oatmeal or rolled oats:														
Regular, quick	1 c	234	145	6	25	4	2	.4	.7	.9	0	19	1.59	2[3]
Instant, fortified:														
Plain, from packet	¾ c	177	104	4	18	3	2	.3	.6	.7	0	162[1]	6.3[1]	283[1]
Flavored, from packet	¾ c	164	167	4	33	2	2	.3	.6	.7	0	172[1]	7[1]	235[1]
Breakfast cereals, ready to eat:														
Cheerios	1 c	23	90	3	16	2	1	.3	.5	.6	0	39	3.66[1]	249
Corn Chex	1 c	28	110	2	25	<1	1	.1	.2	.6	0	3	1.8	268
Corn Flakes, Kellogg's	1¼ c	28	109	2	24	1	<1	t	t	t	0	1	1.8[1]	286
Fortified Oat Flakes	1 c	48	177	9	35	1	1	.1	.3	.3	0	68	13.7	429
40% Bran Flakes, Kellogg's	1 c	39	127	5	31	6	1	.1	.1	.4	0	19	24.8[1]	302
Froot Loops	1 c	28	111	2	25	1	1	.2	.1	.1	0	3	4.52[1]	144
Frosted Flakes	1 c	35	133	2	32	1	<1	t	t	t	0	1	2.21[1]	283
Frosted Rice Krispies	1 c	28	108	1	26	<1	<1	t	t	t	0	1	1.79	237
Granola, low fat, commercial	½ c	47	179	4	36	3	3	0	—	—	0	19	7	47
Grape Nuts	½ c	57	203	7	47	6	<1	t	t	.2	0	5	2.47[1]	396
Honey Nut Cheerios	1 c	33	126	4	27	1	1	.1	.3	.3	0	23	5.3[1]	299
Life	1 c	43	158	8	31	3	1	.1	.2	.4	0	150	11.3	224
Granola, low-fat	⅓ c	31	119	3	25	2	2	0	—	—	0	—	1.8	60
Raisin Bran, Kellogg's	1 c	49	152	5	37	5	1	.2	.1	.4	0	17	22.2[1]	271
Rice Chex	¾ c	19	75	1	17	<1	1	.2	.2	.3	0	3	1.2	158

[1]Nutrient added (values sometimes based on label declaration).
[2]Values for quick cereal.
[3]Cooked without salt. If added according to label recommendation, sodium content is 390 mg for Cream of Wheat; 324 mg for Malt-O-Meal; 374 mg for oatmeal; 385 mg for Farina.
(For purposes of calculations, use "0" for t, <1, <.1, <.01, etc.)

Food Composition

FOOD DESCRIPTION	MEASURE	WT (G)	ENER (CAL)	PROT (G)	CARB (G)	DIETARY FIBER (G)	FAT (G)	FAT BREAKDOWN (G) SAT	MONO	POLY	CHOL (MG)	CALC (MG)	IRON (MG)	SODI (MG)
GRAIN PRODUCTS: CEREAL, FLOUR, GRAIN, PASTA AND NOODLES, POPCORN — CONT.														
Breakfast cereals, ready to eat, cont.														
Rice Krispies, Kellogg's	1 c	29	114	2	25	<1	<1	t	t	.1	0	5	1.83[1]	213
Rice, puffed	1 c	14	56	1	13	<1	<1	t	t	t	0	1	.15[1]	<1
Shredded Wheat	1 c	43	155	5	34	4	1	.2	.2	.5	0	16	1.8	4
Special K	1 c	21	83	4	16	1	<1	t	t	t	<1	6	3.39[1]	196
Total, wheat, with added calcium	1 c	33	116	3	26	4	1	.1	.1	.3	0	282	21[1]	326
Wheaties	1 c	29	101	3	23	3	<1	.1	t	.2	0	44	4.61[1]	276
Macaroni, cooked:														
Enriched	1 c	140	197	7	40	2	1	.1	.1	.4	0	10	1.96	1
Pasta, cooked:														
Fresh	2 oz	57	74	3	14	1	1	.1	.1	.2	19	3	.65	3
Popcorn:														
Air popped, plain	1 c	8	31	1	6	1	<1	<.1	.1	.2	0	1	.21	<1
Microwaved, low fat, low sodium	1 c	6	24	1	4	1	1	.1	.2	.3	0	1	.13	28
Popped in vegetable oil/salted	1 c	11	55	1	6	1	3	.5	.9	1.5	0	1	.31	97
Sugar-syrup coated	1 c	35	151	1	28	2	4	1.3	1	1.6	2	15	.61	72
Rice:														
Brown rice, cooked	1 c	195	216	5	45	4	2	.4	.6	.6	0	19	.82	10
White, enriched, all types:														
Instant, prepared without salt	1 c	165	161	3	35	1	<1	.1	.1	.1	0	13	1.04	5[2]
Spaghetti pasta:														
With salt, enriched	1 c	140	197	7	40	2	1	.1	.1	.4	0	10	1.96	140
MEATS: FISH AND SHELLFISH														
Cod:														
Baked with butter	4 oz	113	150	26	0	0	4	.4	.3	.6	68	23	.56	254
Batter fried	4 oz	113	196	20	8	<1	9	2.2	3.6	2.6	64	43	.9	124
Crab, meat only:														
Dungeness crab, cooked	4 oz	113	124	25	1	0	1	.2	.2	.5	86	67	.49	427
Crab, imitation, from surimi	4 oz	113	115	14	12	0	1	.3	.2	.8	23	15	.44	951
Fish sticks, breaded pollock	2 ea	57	155	9	14	<1	7	1.8	2.9	1.8	64	11	.42	331
Haddock, breaded, fried[3]	4 oz	113	264	22	14	1	13	3.2	5.4	3.3	96	63	1.93	524
Haddock, smoked	4 oz	113	131	29	0	0	1	.2	.2	.4	87	56	1.59	862
Halibut, baked or broiled	4 oz	113	158	30	0	0	3	.5	1.1	1.1	47	68	1.21	78
Lobster meat, cooked w/moist heat	1 c	145	142	30	2	0	1	.2	.2	.1	104	88	.57	551
Oysters:														
Raw	1 c	248	169	18	10	0	6	1.9	.8	2.4	131	112	16.5	523
Salmon:														
Canned pink, solids and liquid	4 oz	113	157	22	0	0	7	1.7	2.1	2.3	62	242[4]	.95	626
Boiled or baked	4 oz	113	244	31	0	0	13	2.2	6	2.7	99	8	.62	75
Atlantic sardines, canned	4 oz	113	235	28	0	0	13	1.7	4.4	5.8	160	433[4]	3.31	572
Scallops, steamed/boiled	½ c	60	64	10	1	0	2	.3	.7	.6	19	15	.15	246
Shrimp:														
Cooked, boiled, 2 large = 11 g	16 ea	86	85	18	0	0	1	.2	.2	.4	167	33	2.65	192
Fried, 2 large = 15 g[3]	12 ea	90	218	19	10	<1	11	1.9	3.6	4.6	159	60	1.13	309
Trout, baked or broiled	4 oz	113	170	26	0	0	7	1.8	2	2.1	78	97	.43	63
Tuna, light, canned:														
Oil pack	3 oz	85	168	25	0	0	7	1.3	2.5	2.4	15	11	1.18	301
Water pack	3 oz	85	98	22	0	0	1	.2	.1	.3	25	9	1.3	287

[1]Nutrient added (values sometimes based on label declaration).
[2]If prepared with salt according to label recommendation, sodium would be 608 mg.
[3]Dipped in egg, bread crumbs, and flour; fried in vegetable shortening.
[4]If bones are discarded, calcium value is greatly reduced.
(For purposes of calculations, use "0" for t, <1, <.1, <.01, etc.)

Food Composition

FOOD DESCRIPTION	MEASURE	WT (G)	ENER (CAL)	PROT (G)	CARB (G)	DIETARY FIBER (G)	FAT (G)	FAT BREAKDOWN (G)			CHOL (MG)	CALC (MG)	IRON (MG)	SODI (MG)
								SAT	MONO	POLY				
MEATS: BEEF, LAMB, PORK, AND OTHERS														
Beef, cooked:[1]														
Braised, simmered, pot roasted:														
Relatively fat, choice chuck blade:														
Lean and fat,														
piece 2½ × 2½ × ¾"	4oz	113	393	30	0	0	29	11.6	12.6	1.1	112	11	3.46	67
Lean only	4 oz	113	297	35	0	0	16	6.3	7	.5	120	15	4.17	81
Relatively lean, like choice round:														
Lean and fat,														
pce 4⅛ × 2½ × ¾"	4 oz	113	311	32	0	0	19	7.2	8.3	.7	109	7	3.54	57
Lean only	4 oz	113	249	36	0	0	11	3.6	4.7	.4	109	6	3.92	58
Ground beef, broiled, patty 3 × ⅝":														
Extra lean, about 16% fat	4 oz	113	299	32	0	0	18	7	7.8	.7	112	10	3.14	93
Lean, 21% fat	4 oz	113	316	32	0	0	20	7.9	8.7	.7	114	14	2.78	101
Roasts, oven cooked, no added liquid:														
Relatively fat, prime rib:														
Lean and fat,														
pce 4⅛ × 2¼ × ½"	4 oz	113	425	25	0	0	35	14.3	15.2	1.3	96	12	2.62	71
Lean only	4 oz	113	274	31	0	0	16	6.6	6.8	.5	90	11	2.96	81
Steak, broiled, relatively lean, choice sirloin:														
Lean and fat,														
pce 2½ × 2½ × ¾"	4 oz	113	320	31	0	0	21	8.7	9.3	.8	102	12	3.4	70
Steak, broiled, relatively fat, choice T-bone:														
Lean and fat	4 oz	113	337	28	0	0	24	9.7	10.1	.9	94	9	3.01	69
Beef, canned, corned	4 oz	113	282	31	0	0	17	7	6.8	.7	97	14	2.36	1136
Beef, dried, cured	1 oz	28	46	8	<1	0	1	.5	.5	.1	12	2	1.28	972
Lamb:														
Chop, arm, braised														
Lean and fat	1 ea	70	242	21	0	0	17	6.9	7.1	1.2	84	18	1.68	50
Lean only	1 ea	55	153	20	0	0	8	2.8	3.4	.5	67	14	1.49	42
Cutlet, avg of lean cuts, cooked	4 oz	113	330	28	0	0	23	9.9	9.9	1.7	110	12	2.27	77
Pork, cured:														
Bacon, medium slices	3 pce	19	109	6	<1	0	9	3.3	4.5	1.1	16	2	.31	303
Breakfast strips, cooked	2 pce	23	106	7	<1	0	8	2.9	3.7	1.3	24	3	.45	483
Canadian-style bacon	2 pce	47	87	11	1	0	4	1.3	1.9	.4	27	5	.38	726
Ham, roasted:														
Lean and fat	4 oz	113	275	24	0	0	19	6.8	8.9	2.1	70	8	1	1341
Lean only	4 oz	113	177	24	0	0	6	2	3	.7	62	8	1	1500
Pork, fresh, cooked:														
Chop, loin														
Braised, lean and fat	1 ea	71	170	19	0	0	10	3.6	4.3	1	57	15	.77	34
Braised, lean only	1 ea	55	112	16	0	0	5	1.9	2.3	1	43	15	.77	34
Veal, cooked:														
Cutlet, braised or broiled	4 oz	113	322	34	0	0	19	7.6	7.6	1.3	134	32	1.24	91
MEATS: POULTRY AND POULTRY PRODUCTS														
Chicken, cooked:														
Fried, batter dipped:[2]														
Breast (5.6 oz with bones)	1 ea	140	364	35	13	<1	18	4.9	7.6	4.3	119	28	1.75	385
Drumstick (3.4 oz with bones)	1 ea	72	192	16	6	<1	11	3	4.6	2.7	62	12	.97	193
Thigh	1 ea	86	238	19	8	<1	14	3.8	5.8	3.3	80	15	1.25	247
Wing	1 ea	49	158	10	5	<1	11	2.9	4.4	2.5	39	10	.63	156

[1]Outer layer of fat removed to about ½" of the lean. Deposits of fat within the cut remain.
[2]Fried in vegetable shortening.
(For purposes of calculations, use "0" for t, <1, <.1, <.01, etc.)

Food Composition

FOOD DESCRIPTION	MEASURE	WT (G)	ENER (CAL)	PROT (G)	CARB (G)	DIETARY FIBER (G)	FAT (G)	FAT BREAKDOWN (G) SAT	MONO	POLY	CHOL (MG)	CALC (MG)	IRON (MG)	SODI (MG)
MEATS: POULTRY AND POULTRY PRODUCTS — CONT.														
Chicken, cooked, cont.														
Roasted:														
All types of meat	1 c	140	266	40	0	0	10	2.9	3.7	2.4	124	21	1.69	120
Dark meat	1 c	140	287	38	0	0	14	3.7	5	3.2	130	21	1.86	130
Light meat	1 c	140	242	43	0	0	6	1.8	2.2	1.4	119	21	1.48	107
Breast, without skin	1 ea	86	141	27	0	0	3	.9	1.1	.7	73	13	.89	64
Drumstick	1 ea	44	95	12	0	0	5	1.4	2	1	41	5	.57	40
Leg, without skin	1 ea	95	163	26	0	0	5	1.4	2	1	88	11	1.26	90
Turkey:														
Roasted, meat only:														
Dark meat	4 oz	113	250	31	0	0	13	4	4	3.5	101	37	2.64	86
Light meat	4 oz	113	223	32	0	0	9	2.7	3.8	2.3	86	24	1.53	71
MEATS: SAUSAGES AND LUNCHMEATS														
Bologna:														
Beef	1 pce	23	72	3	<1	0	7	2.8	3.2	.3	13	3	.38	226
Coldcuts, fat free, deli thin	1 pce	13	10	2	1	0	0	0	0	0	4	0	.18	153
Frankfurters:														
Beef, large link, 8/package	1 ea	57	180	7	1	0	16	6.9	7.7	.8	35	11	.81	585
Beef and pork, large link, 8/package	1 ea	57	182	6	1	0	17	6.2	7.8	1.6	28	6	.66	638
Chicken frankfurter, 10/package	1 ea	45	115	6	3	0	9	2.5	3.8	1.8	45	43	.9	616
Turkey frankfurter, 10/package	1 ea	45	101	6	1	0	8	2.7	2.5	2.2	39	48	.83	641
Ham:														
Chopped ham, packaged	2 pce	42	76	7	1	0	5	1.4	2.1	.5	21	3	.35	576
Ham lunchmeat, regular	2 pce	57	103	10	2	0	6	1.9	2.8	.7	32	4	.56	746
Sandwich spreads:														
Ham salad spread	1 c	240	518	21	26	0	37	12.2	17.3	6.5	89	19	1.42	2188
Pork and beef	2 tbs	30	70	2	4	<1	5	1.8	2.3	.8	11	4	.24	304
Chicken/turkey	2 tbs	26	52	3	2	0	4	.9	.8	1.6	8	3	.16	98
Smoked link sausage, beef and pork	1 ea	68	228	9	1	0	21	7.2	9.7	2.2	48	7	.99	642
Smoked link sausage, pork	1 ea	68	265	15	1	0	22	7.7	9.9	2.6	46	20	.79	1020
MIXED DISHES AND FAST FOODS														
Baked beans, fat free, honey	½ oz	120	110	7	24	7	0	0	0	0	0	40	2.7	135
Beef stew w/vegetables, canned	1 c	245	194	14	17	2	8	2.4	3.1	.3	34	29	2.21	1006
Beef, macaroni, tomato sauce casserole	1 c	226	284	21	25	3	11	4.2	4.7	.6	57	28	3.11	841
Cheeseburger deluxe	1 ea	219	563	28	38	—	33	15	12.6	2	88	206	4.69	1108
Chicken & noodles, homemade	1 c	240	367	22	26	2	18	5.9	7.1	3.5	96	26	2.16	600
Chicken chow mein, canned	1 c	250	95	6	18	2	1	0	.1	.8	8	45	1.25	725
Chicken fajitas	1 ea	223	405	22	50	4	13	2.5	6	3.5	41	83	3.7	439
Chicken pot pie, homemade (⅓)	1 pce	232	545	23	42	3	33	10.9	15.5	6.6	72	70	3.02	594
Chili con carne	½ c	127	128	12	11	2	4	1.7	1.7	.3	67	34	2.62	506
Chop suey with beef & pork	1 c	250	483	26	35	4	25	5.7	9.8	3.9	52	44	4.45	930
Coleslaw[1]	1 c	120	178	2	15	2	13	2	2.9	7.7	6[2]	41	.88	324
Egg roll, meatless	1 ea	64	101	3	10	1	6	1.2	2.5	1.6	30	12	.74	307
Egg roll, with meat	1 ea	64	114	5	9	1	6	1.6	2.9	1.6	38	12	.77	305
Egg salad	1 c	183	586	17	3	0	56	10.6	17.5	24.2	574	74	1.8	666
French toast w/wheat bread, homemade[3]	1 pce	65	151	5	16	<1	7	2	3	1.7	76	64	1.09	311
Hamburger deluxe	1 ea	110	279	13	27	—	14	4.1	5.3	2.6	26	63	2.64	504

[1]Recipe: 41% cabbage; 12% table cream; 12% sugar; 7% green pepper; 6% lemon juice; 4% onion; 3% pimento; 3% vinegar; 2% each for salt, dry mustard, and white pepper.

[2]From dairy cream in recipe.

[3]Recipe: 35% whole milk, 32% white bread, 29% egg, and cooked in 4% margarine.

(For purposes of calculations, use "0" for t, <1, <.1, <.01, etc.)

Food Composition

FOOD DESCRIPTION	MEASURE	WT (G)	ENER (CAL)	PROT (G)	CARB (G)	DIETARY FIBER (G)	FAT (G)	FAT BREAKDOWN (G) SAT	MONO	POLY	CHOL (MG)	CALC (MG)	IRON (MG)	SODI (MG)
MIXED DISHES AND FAST FOODS — CONT.														
Lasagna:														
With meat, homemade	1 pce	245	382	22	39	3	15	7.7	5	.8	56	258	3.43	745
Without meat, homemade	1 pce	218	298	15	39	3	9	5.4	2.4	.6	31	252	2.5	714
Macaroni & cheese, canned[1]	1 c	240	228	9	26	1	10	4.2	3.1	1.4	24	199	.96	730
Macaroni & cheese, homemade[2]	1 c	200	430	17	40	1	22	8.9	8.8	3.6	42	362	1.8	1086
Potato salad with mayonnaise and eggs[3]	½ c	125	179	3	14	2	10	1.8	3.1	4.7	85	24	.81	661
Pizza, combination, 1/12 of 12" round	1 pce	53	123	9	14	—	4	1	1.7	.6	14	68	1.03	255
Pizza, pepperoni, 1/12 of 12" round	1 pce	47	121	7	13	—	5	1.5	2.1	.8	10	43	.63	178
Ramen noodles, cooked	1 c	227	156	5	29	3	2	.4	.4	.4	38	20	1.78	1349
Ravioli, meat	½ c	125	194	11	18	1	9	3	3.6	1	84	33	1.99	619
Fried rice (meatless)	1 c	166	264	5	34	1	11	1.7	2.9	6.2	42	30	1.84	286
Spaghetti (enriched) in tomato sauce:														
With cheese:														
Canned	1 c	250	190	5	38	2	1	0	.4	.5	8	40	2.75	955
Homemade	1 c	250	260	9	37	2	9	2	5.4	1.2	8	80	2.25	955
With meatballs:														
Canned	1 c	250	258	12	28	6	10	2.1	3.9	3.9	22	52	3.25	1220
Homemade	1 c	248	332	19	39	8	12	3.3	6.3	2.2	74	124	3.72	1009
Sweet and sour pork	1 c	226	231	14	25	1	8	2.8	3.8	2.9	38	28	1.49	1220
Sweet & sour chicken breast	1 ea	131	117	8	15	1	3	.6	.8	1.5	23	16	.8	732
Tuna salad[4]	1 c	205	383	33	19	1	19	3.2	5.9	8.4	27	35	2.05	824
FAST FOODS AND SANDWICHES														
Burrito[5], beef & bean	1 ea	175	385	17	50	4	14	6.3	5.3	.9	37	80	3.71	1011
Burrito, bean	1 ea	174	358	11	57	7	11	5.5	3.8	1	3	90	3.62	790
Cheeseburger with bun, regular	1 ea	112	261	13	20	—	14	6.7	5.2	1.1	38	132	1.93	710
Cheeseburger with bun, 4-oz patty	1 ea	194	487	25	41	—	25	10.2	9.1	3.1	70	200	4	1228
Enchilada	1 ea	230	451	14	40	—	27	15	8.9	1.1	62	458	1.86	1106
Fish sandwich:														
Regular, with cheese	1 ea	140	400	16	36	<1	22	6.2	6.8	7.2	52	141	2.67	718
Hamburger with bun, regular	1 ea	98	252	12	30	1	9	3.2	3.4	1.6	39	47	2.25	516
Hamburger with bun, 4-oz patty	1 ea	174	466	26	31	—	26	9.7	11.4	2.2	84	75	4.49	600
Hot dog/frankfurter with bun	1 ea	85	210	9	16	—	13	4.4	5.9	1.5	38	20	2.01	581
Lunchables:														
Bologna & American cheese	1 ea	128	450	18	19	0	34	15	—	—	85	300	2.7	1620
Pizza, cheese, 1/8 of 15" round[6]	1 pce	120	268	15	39	2	6	2.9	1.9	.9	18	222	1.1	640
Sandwiches:														
Bacon, lettuce & tomato:														
On white bread, soft	1 ea	135	401	12	34	2	24	6	9	8	28	60	2.33	731
On whole wheat	1 ea	149	421	14	37	6	26	6	9.6	8	26	62	3.18	818
Cheese, grilled:														
On white bread, soft	1 ea	117	393	17	29	1	23	12.2	7.6	2.1	55	393	1.79	1129
Chicken salad:														
On white bread, soft	1 ea	105	371	10	28	1	24	4	7.3	12	32	56	1.98	447
On whole wheat	1 ea	118	389	12	32	5	25	4	7.6	12	31	58	2.58	526
Corned beef & swiss on rye	1 ea	147	457	28	25	3	28	9.8	9	6.4	79	307	2.75	1064

[1]Made with corn oil.
[2]Made with margarine.
[3]Recipe: 62% potatoes; 12% eggs; 8% mayonnaise; 7% celery; 6% sweet pickle relish; 2% onion; 1% each for green pepper, pimento, salt, and dry mustard.
[4]Made with drained chunk light tuna, celery, onion, pickle relish, and mayonnaise-type dressing.
[5]Made with a 10½"-diameter flour tortilla.
[6]Crust made with vegetable shortening and enriched flour.
(For purposes of calculations, use "0" for t, <1, <.1, <.01, etc.)

Food Composition

FOOD DESCRIPTION	MEASURE	WT (G)	ENER (CAL)	PROT (G)	CARB (G)	DIETARY FIBER (G)	FAT (G)	FAT BREAKDOWN (G)			CHOL (MG)	CALC (MG)	IRON (MG)	SODI (MG)
								SAT	MONO	POLY				
FAST FOODS AND SANDWICHES — CONT.														
Sandwiches, cont.														
Egg salad:														
On white bread, soft	1 ea	111	380	9	29	1	26	4.5	8	11.8	147	65	2.21	507
On whole wheat	1 ea	125	403	11	33	5	27	4.7	8	12	147	69	2.81	592
Ham:														
On rye bread	1 ea	116	241	16	20	3	10	2.2	3.8	3.6	35	38	1.72	1289
On white bread, soft	1 ea	122	260	17	23	1	11	2.3	4.1	3.6	36	47	1.86	1263
Ham & cheese:														
On white bread, soft	1 ea	151	388	21	29	1	20	7.8	6.8	4.6	59	224	2.2	1564
On whole wheat	1 ea	165	411	24	33	5	22	8	7.1	4.9	57	228	2.93	1655
Ham and swiss on rye	1 ea	145	368	23	25	3	19	7.2	6.2	4.6	56	309	1.99	1289
Peanut butter & jelly:														
On white bread, soft	1 ea	100	345	10	47	3	14	2.7	6.6	3.9	2	61	2.23	290
On whole wheat	1 ea	114	368	13	51	7	15	2.9	6.9	4.2	0	64	2.97	375
Roast beef:														
On a bun	1 ea	150	374	23	36	—	15	3.9	7.3	1.8	55	58	4.56	855
On white bread, soft	1 ea	122	315	23	27	1	13	2.7	4.3	4.9	34	47	3.21	1243
Tuna salad:														
On white bread, soft	1 ea	116	331	13	32	2	17	3	5	8	16	56	2	543
Turkey:														
On white bread, soft	1 ea	122	270	19	22	1	11	2	3.5	5	34	44	1.57	1238
On whole wheat	1 ea	136	294	21	26	4	12	2.2	3.8	5.3	35	47	2.19	1339
Taco	1 ea	78	168	9	12	—	9	5.2	3	.4	26	101	1.1	366
Tostada:														
With refried beans	1 ea	157	243	10	29	8	11	5.9	3.3	.8	33	229	2.06	592
Vege-burger	½ c	108	110	22	4	1	1	.1	.1	.4	0	32	2.7	190
NUTS, SEEDS, AND PRODUCTS														
Almonds:														
Dry roasted, salted	1 c	138	810	22	33	14	71	6.7	46.2	14.9	0	389	5.24	1076
Cashew nuts, salted:														
Dry roasted:	1 c	137	786	21	45	4	64	12.5	37.4	10.7	0	62	8.22	877[1]
Coconut, dried, shredded/grated:														
Unsweetened	1 c	78	514	5	19	13	50	44.6	2.1	.6	0	20	2.59	29
Sweetened	1 c	93	465	3	44	4	33	29.3	1.4	.4	0	14	1.79	243
Filberts/hazelnuts, chopped:	1 c	115	726	15	18	9	72	5.3	56.4	6.9	0	216	3.76	3
Mixed nuts:														
Dry roasted, salted	1 c	137	814	24	35	12	71	9.4	43	14.7	0	96	5.07	917[2]
Peanuts:														
Oil roasted, salted:	1 c	144	837	38	27	10	71	9.8	35.3	22.5	0	126	2.64	624[3]
Oil roasted, unsalted	1 c	144	837	38	27	9	71	9.8	35.3	22.5	0	126	2.64	9
Peanut butter:	½ c	129	759	32	27	8	64	12.3	30.4	18.6	0	44	2.15	617[4]
Tablespoon	2 tbs	32	188	8	7	2	16	3.1	7.6	4.6	0	11	.54	153[4]
Pistachios, dried, shelled	1 oz	28	162	6	7	3	14	1.7	9.3	2.1	0	38	1.92	2[5]
Pistachios, dry roasted, salted, shelled	1 c	128	776	19	35	14	68	8.6	45.6	10.2	0	90	4.06	998

[1]Dry-roasted cashews without salt contain 21 mg sodium per cup, or 4 mg per ounce.
[2]Mixed nuts without salt contain about 15 mg sodium per cup.
[3]Peanuts without salt contain 22 mg sodium per cup, or 4 mg per ounce.
[4]Peanut butter without added salt contains 3 mg sodium per tablespoon.
[5]Salted pistachios contain approx 221 mg sodium per ounce.
(For purposes of calculations, use "0" for t, <1, <.1, <.01, etc.)

Food Composition

FOOD DESCRIPTION	MEASURE	WT (G)	ENER (CAL)	PROT (G)	CARB (G)	DIETARY FIBER (G)	FAT (G)	FAT BREAKDOWN (G) SAT	MONO	POLY	CHOL (MG)	CALC (MG)	IRON (MG)	SODI (MG)
NUTS, SEEDS, AND PRODUCTS — CONT.														
Sunflower seed kernels:														
Dry	¼ c	36	205	8	7	2	18	1.9	3.4	11.8	0	42	2.44	11[1]
Oil roasted	¼ c	34	209	7	5	2	19	2	3.7	12.9	0	19	2.28	11[1]
Trail Mix w/chocolate chips	1 c	146	707	21	66	—	47	8.9	19.8	16.5	5.84	159	4.96	177
Black walnuts, chopped:	1 c	125	758	30	15	6	71	4.5	15.9	46.9	0	73	3.85	1
English walnuts, chopped:	1 c	120	770	17	22	5	74	6.7	17	47	0	113	2.93	12
Ounce	1 oz	28	180	4	5	1	17	1.6	4	11.1	0	27	.69	3
SWEETENERS AND SWEETS														
Jams or preserves:														
Jellies:	1 tbs	18	49	<1	13	<1	<1	t	t	t	0	1	.04	6
Packet	1 ea	14	38	<1	10	<1	<1	t	t	t	0	1	.03	5
Popsicle/ice pops	1 ea	95	68	0	18	0	0	0	0	0	0	0	0	11
Sugars:														
Brown sugar	1 c	220	827	0	214	0	0	0	0	0	0	187	4.2	86
White sugar, granulated:	1 c	200	774	0	200	0	0	0	0	0	0	2	.13	2
Tablespoon	1 tbs	12	46	0	12	0	0	0	0	0	0	<1	.01	<1
Packet	1 ea	6	23	0	6	0	0	0	0	0	0	<1	<.01	<1
White sugar, powdered, sifted	1 c	100	389	0	100	0	<1	0	0	0	0	1	.06	1
Sweeteners:														
Equal, packet	1 ea	1	4	1	0	0	0	0	0	0	0	<1	.02	<1
Sweet 'N Low, packet	1 ea	1	4	0	1	0	0	0	0	0	0	<1	—	1
Syrups:														
Chocolate:														
Hot fudge type	2 tbs	38	131	2	22	<1	5	2.2	1.4	1.2	5	38	.46	49
Thin type	2 tbs	38	83	1	22	1	<1	.2	.1	<.1	0	5	.81	36
Pancake table syrup (corn and maple)	¼ c	79	227	0	60	0	0	0	0	0	0	1	.07	66
VEGETABLES AND LEGUMES														
Alfalfa sprouts	1 c	33	10	1	1	1	<1	t	t	.1	0	11	.32	2
Artichokes, cooked globe	1 ea	120	60	4	13	6	<1	t	t	.1	0	54	1.55	114
Asparagus, green, cooked:														
From fresh:														
Spears, ½" diam at base	6 ea	90	22	2	4	2	<1	.1	t	.1	0	18	.66	10
Lima beans:														
Thick seeded (Fordhooks),														
cooked from frozen	½ c	85	85	5	16	6	<1	.1	t	.1	0	19	1.16	45
Thin seeded (Baby), cooked from frozen	½ c	90	95	6	18	6	<1	.1	t	.1	0	25	1.76	26
Bean sprouts (mung):														
Raw	1 c	104	31	3	6	2	<1	.1	t	.1	0	14	.95	6
Cooked, stir-fried	1 c	124	62	5	13	4	<1	.1	.1	.1	0	16	2.36	11
Beets, cooked from fresh:														
Sliced or diced	½ c	85	37	1	8	1	<1	t	t	.1	0	14	.67	65
Broccoli, raw:														
Chopped	1 c	88	25	3	5	3	<1	.1	t	.2	0	42	.77	24
Spears	1 ea	151	42	4	8	5	1	.1	t	.3	0	72	1.33	41
Broccoli, cooked from fresh:														
Spears	1 ea	180	50	5	9	5	1	.1	t	.3	0	83	1.51	47
Chopped	1 c	156	44	5	8	5	1	.1	t	.3	0	72	1.31	41
Brussels sprouts, cooked from fresh	½ c	78	30	2	7	4	<1	.1	t	.2	0	28	.94	16

[1]Unsalted sunflower seeds contain 1 mg sodium per ¼ cup.
(For purposes of calculations, use "0" for t, <1, <.1, <.01, etc.)

Food Composition

FOOD DESCRIPTION	MEASURE	WT (G)	ENER (CAL)	PROT (G)	CARB (G)	DIETARY FIBER (G)	FAT (G)	FAT BREAKDOWN (G)			CHOL (MG)	CALC (MG)	IRON (MG)	SODI (MG)
								SAT	MONO	POLY				
VEGETABLES AND LEGUMES — CONT.														
Cabbage, savoy, coarsely chopped raw	1 c	70	19	1	4	2	<1	t	t	t	0	24	.28	20
Cabbage, savoy, cooked	1 c	145	35	3	8	4	0	<.1	<.1	.1	0	44	.55	35
Carrots, raw:														
Whole, 7½ × 1⅛″	1 ea	72	31	1	7	2	<1	t	t	.1	0	19	.36	25
Grated	½ c	55	24	1	6	2	<1	t	t	t	0	15	.27	19
Carrots, cooked, sliced, drained:														
From fresh	½ c	78	35	1	8	2	<1	t	t	.1	0	24	.48	51
From frozen	½ c	73	26	1	6	3	<1	t	t	t	0	20	.34	43
Cauliflower, flowerets:														
Raw	½ c	50	12	1	3	1	<1	t	t	.1	0	11	.22	15
Cooked from fresh, drained	½ c	62	14	1	3	1	<1	.1	t	.1	0	10	.2	9
Celery, pascal type, raw:														
Large outer stalk, 8 × 1½″	1 ea	40	6	<1	1	1	<1	t	t	t	0	16	.16	35
Celeriac/celery root, cooked	3½ oz	99	25	1	6	4	<1	<.1	<.1	.1	0	26	.43	61
Corn, cooked, drained:														
From fresh, on cob, 5″ long	1 ea	77	83	3	19	2	1	.2	.3	.5	0	2	.47	13
From frozen on cob, 3½″ long	1 ea	63	59	2	14	2	<1	.1	.1	.2	0	2	.38	3
Kernels, cooked from frozen	½ c	82	66	2	17	2	<1	t	t	t	0	2	.25	4
Corn, canned:														
Cream style	½ c	128	92	2	23	2	1	.1	.2	.3	0	4	.49	364[1]
Whole kernel, vacuum pack	½ c	105	83	3	20	6	1	.1	.2	.3	0	5	.44	286[2]
Cucumber slices with peel	7 pce	28	4	<1	1	<1	<1	t	t	t	0	4	.07	1
Eggplant, cooked	1 c	160	45	1	11	4	<1	.1	t	.2	0	10	.56	5
Kidney beans, canned	1 c	256	217	13	40	16	1	.1	.1	.5	0	61	3.23	873
Leeks, raw, chopped	1 c	104	63	2	15	3	<1	t	t	.2	0	61	2.18	21
Lentils, cooked from dry	½ c	99	115	9	20	5	<1	.1	.1	.2	0	19	3.3	2
Lettuce:														
Butterhead/Boston types:														
Head, 5″ diameter	¼ ea	41	5	1	1	1	<1	t	t	.1	0	13	.12	2
Leaves, inner or outer	4 ea	30	4	<1	1	<1	<1	t	t	t	0	10	.09	2
Iceberg/crisphead:														
Wedge, ¼ head	1 ea	135	18	1	3	1	<1	t	t	.1	0	25	.67	12
Looseleaf, chopped	½ c	28	5	<1	1	<1	<1	t	t	t	0	19	.39	3
Romaine, chopped	½ c	28	4	<1	1	<1	<1	t	t	t	0	10	.31	2
Romaine, inner leaf	3 ea	30	5	<1	1	<1	<1	t	t	t	0	11	.33	2
Mushrooms:														
Raw, sliced	½ c	35	9	1	2	<1	<1	t	t	.1	0	2	.43	1
Cooked from fresh, pieces	½ c	78	21	2	4	2	<1	t	t	.1	0	5	1.36	2
Navy beans, cooked from dry	1 c	182	258	16	48	16	1	.3	.1	.4	0	127	4.51	2
Onions:														
Raw, chopped	1 c	160	61	2	14	3	<1	t	t	.1	0	32	.35	5
Onion rings, breaded, heated f/frozen	2 ea	20	81	1	8	<1	5	1.7	2.2	1	0	6	.34	75
Parsley:														
Raw, sprigs	5 ea	5	2	<1	<1	<1	<1	t	t	t	0	6	.31	3
Peas:														
Black-eyed, cooked:														
From frozen, drained	½ c	85	112	7	20	7	1	.2	.1	.2	0	20	1.8	4
Green, canned, drained	½ c	85	59	4	11	3	<1	.1	t	.1	0	17	.81	186[2]
Green, cooked from frozen	½ c	80	62	4	11	4	<1	t	t	.1	0	19	1.26	70
Split, green cooked from dry	½ c	98	116	8	21	3	<1	.1	.1	.2	0	14	1.26	2

[1]Low sodium pack contains 4 mg sodium per ½ cup.
[2]Low sodium pack contains 6 mg sodium per cup.
(For purposes of calculations, use "0" for t, <1, <.1, <.01, etc.)

Food Composition

FOOD DESCRIPTION	MEASURE	WT (G)	ENER (CAL)	PROT (G)	CARB (G)	DIETARY FIBER (G)	FAT (G)	FAT BREAKDOWN (G) SAT	MONO	POLY	CHOL (MG)	CALC (MG)	IRON (MG)	SODI (MG)
VEGETABLES AND LEGUMES — CONT.														
Peas & carrots, cooked from frozen	½ c	80	38	2	8	3	<1	.1	t	.2	0	18	.75	54
Peppers, sweet, green:														
Whole pod (90 g with refuse) raw	1 ea	74	20	1	5	1	<1	t	t	.1	0	7	.34	1
Cooked, chopped														
(1 pod cooked = 73 g)	½ c	68	19	1	5	1	<1	t	t	.1	0	6	.31	1
Peppers, sweet, red:														
Raw, chopped	1 c	100	27	1	6	2	<1	t	t	.1	0	9	.46	2
Pinto beans, cooked from dry	½ c	85	116	7	22	7	<1	t	.1	.2	0	41	2.23	2
Potatoes:[1]														
Baked in oven, 4¾ × 2⅓″ diam:														
With skin	1 ea	202	220	5	51	5	<1	.1	1	.1	0	20	2.75	16
Baked in microwave, 4¾ × 2⅓″ diam:														
With skin	1 ea	202	212	5	49	5	<1	.1	t	.1	0	22	2.5	16
Flesh only	1 ea	156	156	3	36	2	<1	t	t	.1	0	8	.64	11
Skin only	1 ea	58	77	3	17	2	<1	t	t	t	0	27	3.45	9
Boiled, about 2½″ diam:														
Peeled after boiling	1 ea	136	118	3	27	2	<1	t	t	.1	0	7	.42	5
Peeled before boiling	1 ea	135	116	2	27	2	<1	t	t	.1	0	11	.42	7
French fried, strips 2–3½″ long:														
Oven heated	10 pce	50	163	2	19	1	9	3.8	4.2	.9	0	6	.83	306
Fried in vegetable oil	10 ea	50	155	2	19	2	8	2.5	4	1.2	0	8	.68	82
Hashed browns from frozen	1 c	156	340	5	44	3	18	7	8	2.1	0	23	2.36	53
Mashed:														
Home recipe with whole milk[2]	½ c	105	81	2	18	2	1	.3	.2	.1	2	27	.28	318
Prepared from flakes; water,														
milk, margarine, salt added	½ c	110	124	2	17	1	6	1.6	2.5	1.7	4[3]	54	.24	365
Potato products, prepared:														
Au gratin:														
From dry mix	½ c	122	114	3	16	2	5	3.2	1.4	.2	6	102	.39	536
Scalloped:														
From dry mix	½ c	122	114	3	16	1	5	3.2	1.5	.2	13	44	.47	416
Soybean products:														
Miso	½ c	138	284	16	39	7	8	1.2	1.8	4.7	0	92	3.76	5033
Tofu (soybean curd, regular)	½ c	124	94	10	2	1	6	.9	1.3	3.3	0	130	6.65	9
Spinich:														
Raw, chopped	1 c	56	12	2	2	2	<1	t	t	.1	0	55	1.52	44
Cooked, from fresh, drained	½ c	90	21	3	3	2	<1	t	t	.1	0	122	3.21	63
Squash, summer varieties, cooked:														
Varieties averaged	½ c	90	18	1	4	1	<1	.1	t	.1	0	24	.32	1
Zucchini	½ c	90	14	1	4	1	<1	t	t	t	0	12	.31	3
Squash, winter varieties, cooked:														
Average of all varieties, baked:														
Mashed	1 c	245	96	2	21	7	2	.3	.1	.7	0	34	.81	2
Cubes	1 c	205	80	2	18	6	1	.3	.1	.5	0	29	.68	2
Sweet potatoes:														
Baked in skin, peeled, 5 × 2″ diam	1 ea	114	140	3	28	4	<1	t	t	.1	0	32	2	11
Boiled without skin, 5 × 2″ diam	1 ea	151	159	3	37	3	<1	.1	t	.2	0	32	.85	20

[1]Vitamin C varies with length of storage. After 3 months of storage approximately two-thirds of the ascorbic acid remains; after 6 to 7 months, about one-third remains.

[2]Recipe: 84% potatoes, 15% whole milk, 1% salt.

[3]Data is for margarine; if butter is used, cholesterol = 25 mg for 29 total mg.

(For purposes of calculations, use "0" for t, <1, <.1, <.01, etc.)

Food Composition

FOOD DESCRIPTION	MEASURE	WT (G)	ENER (CAL)	PROT (G)	CARB (G)	DIETARY FIBER (G)	FAT (G)	FAT BREAKDOWN (G) SAT	MONO	POLY	CHOL (MG)	CALC (MG)	IRON (MG)	SODI (MG)
VEGETABLES AND LEGUMES — CONT.														
Tomatoes:														
Raw, whole, 2⅗″ diam	1 ea	123	26	1	6	1	<1	.1	.1	.2	0	6	.55	11
Raw, chopped	1 c	180	38	2	8	2	1	.1	.1	.2	0	9	.81	16
Cooked from raw	1 c	240	65	3	14	2	1	.1	.2	.4	0	14	1.34	26
Canned, solids and liquid	1 c	240	48	2	10	2	1	.1	.1	.2	0	62[1]	1.46	391[2]
Tomatoes, sundried:	1 c	54	139	8	30	7	2	.2	.3	.6	0	59	4.91	1131
Pieces	10 pce	20	52	3	11	2	1	.1	.1	.2	0	22	1.82	419
Tomato, raw	1 ea	123	26	1	6	1	<1	.1	.1	.2	0	6	.55	11
Tomato juice, canned	1 c	244	41	2	10	1	<1	t	t	.1	0	22	1.42	881[3]
Tomato products, canned:														
Paste	1 c	262	220	10	49	11	2	.3	.4	.9	0	92	7.83	2070[4]
Puree	1 c	250	102	4	25	6	<1	t	t	.1	0	37	2.33	998[5]
Sauce	1 c	245	73	3	18	3	<1	.1	.1	.2	0	34	1.89	1482[6]
MISCELLANEOUS														
Catsup:	¼ c	61	64	1	17	1	<1	t	t	.1	0	12	.43	723
Tablespoon	1 tbs	15	16	<1	4	<1	<1	t	t	t	0	3	.1	178
Mustard, country dijon	1 tsp	5	5	0	0	0	0	0	0	0	0	—	—	120
Mustard, prepared (1 packet = 1 tsp)	1 tsp	5	4	<1	<1	<1	<1	t	.2	t	0	4	.1	63
Pickles:														
Dill, medium, 3¾ × 1¼″ diam	1 ea	65	12	<1	3	1	<1	t	t	.1	0	6	.34	833
Fresh pack, slices, 1½ diam × ¼″	2 pce	15	3	<1	3	<1	<1	t	t	t	0	5	.08	192
Sweet medium	1 ea	35	41	<1	11	<1	<1	t	t	t	0	1	.21	328
Pickle relish, sweet	2 tbs	30	41	<1	10	1	<1	.1	t	.1	0	6	.24	214
Potato chips	14 ea	28	150	2	15	1	10	3.1	2.8	3.5	0	7	.46	166[7]
SOUPS, SAUCES, AND GRAVIES														
Cream of celery	1 c	251	181	3	18	2	11	2.8	2.6	5	28	80	1.26	1900
Clam chowder, New England	1 c	248	164	9	17	1	7	2.9	2.3	1.1	22	186	1.49	992
Tomato	1 c	248	161	6	22	1	6	2.9	1.6	1.1	17	159	1.81	932
Chicken noodle	1 c	241	75	4	9	1	2	.7	1.1	.6	7	17	.77	1106
Chicken rice	1 c	241	60	4	7	1	2	.5	.9	.4	7	17	.75	815
Minestrone	1 c	241	82	4	11	1	3	.6	.7	1.1	2	34	.92	911
Vegetable beef	1 c	244	78	6	10	<1	2	.9	.8	.1	5	17	1.12	956
BURGER KING														
Whopper sandwiches:														
Whopper	1 ea	265	618	27	44	3	38	10.8	10.8	12.8	88	59	4.4	834
Whopper with cheese	1 ea	289	708	32	44	3	45	15.7	12.8	12.8	113	246	4.4	1248
Hamburger	1 ea	109	275	15	30	1	11	4	5	1	32	42	1.9	529
Cheeseburger	1 ea	120	313	18	29	1	15	6.3	6.3	1	47	104	1.88	741
Chicken sandwich	1 ea	230	703	26	54	2	43	8	11	20.1	60	100	3.62	1406
BK broiler chicken sandwich	1 ea	248	540	30	41	2	29	6	—	—	80	40	5.4	480
French fries (salted)	1 svg	74	255	3	27	2	13	3	6	1	0	6	.69	153
Milk shake, chocolate	1 ea	273	298	9	52	3	7	3.9	3.9	0	19	192	1.73	221
Milk shake, vanilla	1 ea	273	298	9	51	1	7	3.9	2.9	0	19	288	—	221

[1]Calcium is added as a firming agent.
[2]Dietary pack contains 31 mg sodium.
[3]If no salt is added, sodium content is 24 mg.
[4]If salt is added, sodium content is 2070 mg.
[5]If salt is added, sodium content is 998 mg.
[6]With salt added.
[7]If no salt added, sodium = 2 mg.
(For purposes of calculations, use "0" for t, <1, <.1, <.01, etc.)

Food Composition

FOOD DESCRIPTION	MEASURE	WT (G)	ENER (CAL)	PROT (G)	CARB (G)	DIETARY FIBER (G)	FAT (G)	FAT BREAKDOWN (G) SAT	MONO	POLY	CHOL (MG)	CALC (MG)	IRON (MG)	SODI (MG)
DAIRY QUEEN														
Ice cream cones:														
Small vanilla	1 ea	85	140	4	22	0	4	3	1	—	15	100	.4	60
Regular vanilla	1 ea	142	230	6	36	0	7	5	1	1	20	150	.7	95
Large vanilla	1 ea	213	340	9	53	0	10	7	1	1	30	200	1.4	140
Chocolate dipped	1 ea	156	330	6	40	<1	16	8	4	3	20	300	.7	100
Chocolate sundae	1 ea	177	300	6	54	<1	7	5	1	1	20	150	1.1	140
Banana split	1 ea	383	529	9	97	2	11	8.3	3.1	.4	31	311	3.74	259
Peanut Buster Parfait	1 ea	305	710	16	94	1	32	10	10	9	30	350	3.6	410
Milk shake, regular	1 ea	418	548	13	93	<1	15	8.4	2.1	2.1	47	421	1.52	242
Misty slush, small	1 ea	454	220	0	56	0	0	0	0	0	0	0	0	20
KENTUCKY FRIED CHICKEN														
Original recipe:														
Center breast	1 ea	95	240	23	8	<1	13	3.5	7.2	1.8	85	28	.83	562
Side breast	1 ea	69	204	14	7	<1	12	3.5	7.3	1.7	65	57	.92	502
Dinners:														
2-pce dinner, white	1 ea	322	702	32	56	2	39	9.5	18.4	7.9	119	215	3.71	1854
2-pce dinner, dark	1 ea	346	721	33	57	1	40	10.1	17.9	8.5	164	197	3.84	1738
2-pce dinner, combo	1 ea	341	741	32	58	1	42	10.7	19.3	8.8	160	217	3.88	1801
Extra crispy recipe:														
Center breast	1 ea	104	291	25	9	<1	17	4	9.5	1.9	66	29	.62	652
Side breast	1 ea	84	290	17	11	<1	20	4.2	9.3	1.7	54	14	.61	514
Drumstick	1 ea	58	170	11	5	<1	11	3	6.8	1.5	58	12	.59	277
Thigh	1 ea	107	373	18	13	<1	29	7.6	15.7	4	88	48	1.08	510
Wing	1 ea	53	216	10	8	<1	15	4	9.6	2	58	18	.05	287
McDONALD'S														
Big Mac	1 ea	215	508	25	46	3	26	9	7.4	4.1	76	201	4.3	928
McChicken	1 ea	187	486	17	41	2	28	5	8.4	10	52	127	2.5	789
Quarter-pounder	1 ea	166	403	22	34	2	20	8	7	1	68	123	4	672
Quarter-pounder with cheese	1 ea	194	507	27	34	2	28	12	1	2	94	139	4	1132
Filet-O-Fish	1 ea	142	357	13	40	2	16	3.6	4	5	36	121	1.81	735
Hamburger	1 ea	102	251	12	33	2	8	3	2.7	.9	27	119	2.7	490
Cheeseburger	1 ea	116	302	14	34	2	12	5	3.6	1	40	127	2.7	725
French fries, small serving	1 ea	68	207	3	26	2	10	1.7	3.1	2.5	0	9	.53	110
Chicken McNuggets	6 ea	112	303	19	16	0	18	3.8	5.7	3.7	65	15	1.08	580
Sauces (packet):														
Hot mustard	1 ea	30	63	5	8	<1	4	.47	1.1	2	3	7	.8	85
Barbecue	1 ea	32	53	<1	12	<1	<1	.1	.1	.2	0	4	0	277
Sweet & sour	1 ea	32	55	<1	14	<1	<1	.1	.1	.3	0	2	.17	158
Breakfast items:														
Egg McMuffin	1 ea	138	292	18	29	1	13	6.1	1	4.1	235	152	2.76	726
Hashbrown potatoes	1 ea	53	130	1	15	1	8	1.4	7.3	2	0	7	.27	330
Sausage McMuffin	1 ea	117	377	13	28	2	24	8.6	8.5	3	49	138	2.34	667
PIZZA HUT														
Pan pizza:														
Cheese	2 pce	205	492	30	57	5	18	8.6	5.5	2.7	34	630	5.4	940
Pepperoni	2 pce	211	540	29	62	5	22	9.2	9.3	3.4	42	520	6.3	1127
Supreme	2 pce	255	589	32	53	7	30	13.8	11.9	4.3	48	500	5	1363
Super supreme	2 pce	257	563	33	53	6	26	12	—	—	55	540	6.7	1447

(For purposes of calculations, use "0" for t, <1, <.1, <.01, etc.)

Food Composition

FOOD DESCRIPTION	MEASURE	WT (G)	ENER (CAL)	PROT (G)	CARB (G)	DIETARY FIBER (G)	FAT (G)	FAT BREAKDOWN (G)			CHOL (MG)	CALC (MG)	IRON (MG)	SODI (MG)
								SAT	MONO	POLY				
PIZZA HUT — CONT.														
Personal pan pizza:														
Pepperoni	1 ea	256	675	37	76	8	29	12.5	12.1	4.5	53	730	5.8	1335
Supreme	1 ea	264	647	33	76	9	28	11.2	12.4	4.4	49	520	6.7	1313
TACO BELL														
Burritos:														
Bean with red sauce	1 ea	191	414	14	58	11	13	6.4	4.4	1.1	9	136	3.22	1064
Beef with red sauce	1 ea	191	457	23	44	4	19	9.7	6.9	.8	53	106	3.46	1215
Burritos, cont.														
Big beef supreme	1 ea	298	525	25	51	—	25	11	—	—	72	200	4.5	1418
Chicken burrito	1 ea	171	345	17	41	—	13	5	—	—	57	140	2.52	854
Tacos:														
Taco	1 ea	78	183	10	11	1	11	4.6	4.5	.8	32	84	1.07	276
Soft taco	1 ea	92	225	12	18	1	12	5.4	4.3	1.2	32	116	2.27	554
Soft taco supreme	1 ea	124	262	13	20	2	15	7.3	—	—	44	78	1.74	533
Soft taco, chicken	1 ea	128	223	14	20	—	10	4	—	—	58	60	1.44	553
Soft taco, steak	1 ea	100	217	12	21	—	9	4	—	—	31	50	1.08	569
WENDY'S														
Hamburgers:														
Single on white bun, no toppings	1 ea	119	350	21	29	<1	16	—	—	—	65	100	4.5	420
Big classic	1 ea	241	470	26	36	—	25	—	—	—	80	40	4.5	900
Cheeseburgers:														
Bacon cheeseburger	1 ea	147	460	29	23	<1	28	13	13	2	65	136	3.6	860
Double with lettuce & tomato	1 ea	215	548	30	32	2	33	12.9	11.8	5.4	84	177	4	864
Baked potatoes:														
Plain	1 ea	250	250	6	52	4	<1	t	t	.1	0	40	2.7	60
With bacon & cheese	1 ea	350	570	19	57	4	30	11.8	11.4	5.6	22	200	3.7	180
With cheese	1 ea	350	590	16	55	4	34	12.5	12.7	7.1	22	350	3.6	450
French fries	1 ea	106	306	4	38	1	15	7	5	2	15	13	1.02	105
Frosty dairy dessert	1 c	216	354	7	53	0	13	5	3	2	44	257	.86	194

(For purposes of calculations, use "0" for t, <1, <.1, <.01, etc.)

Appendix B
Wellness Directory

In this directory, you will find a list of organizations and clearinghouses that can provide you with answers to your questions and help you make more informed lifestyle choices.

General Information Resources

National Health Information Center
P.O. Box 1133
Washington, DC 20013
800-336-4797
http://nhic-nt.health.org/

Office of Minority Health Resource Center
P.O. Box 37337
Washington, DC 20013
800-444-6472
http://www.omhrc.gov/

American Self-Help Clearinghouse
Northwest Covenant Medical Center
25 Pocono Road
Denville, NJ 07834
201-625-7101
http://www.cmhc.com/selfhelp

Alcohol and Drug Abuse

Al-Anon and Alateen
1372 Broadway
New York, NY 10018
800-356-9996
http://www.al-anon.alateen.org

Alcoholics Anonymous World Services (AA)
P.O. Box 459 Grand Central Station
New York, NY 10163
212-870-3400
http://www.alcoholics-anonymous.org

Mothers Against Drunk Driving (MADD)
511 E. John Carpenter Freeway
Suite 700
Irving, TX 75062-8187
http://www.madd.org
800-438-MADD

Narcotics Anonymous
19737 Nordhoff Place
Chatsworth, CA 91311
818-773-9999
http://www.wsoinc.com

National Clearinghouse for Alcohol and Drug Information
P.O. Box 2345
Rockville, MD 20847
800-729-6686
http://www.health.org/

National Institute on Drug Abuse Helpline
800-662-4357
http://www.nida.hih.gov/

Cocaine Anonymous World Services
http://www.ca.org/

CDC Office on Smoking and Health
4770 Buford Highway, NE, MS-K 50
Atlanta, GA 30341
800-CDC-1311; 770-488-5701
http://www.cdc.gov/nccdphp/osh

Chronic Diseases

American Cancer Society
1599 Clifton Road, NE
Atlanta, GA 30329
800-227-2345
http://www.cancer.org

American Diabetes Association, Inc.
1660 Duke Street
Alexandria, VA 22314
800-342-2383
http://www.diabetes.org

American Heart Association
7272 Greenville Avenue
Dallas, TX 75231
214-373-6300; 800-242-8721
http://www.americanheart.org

Cancer Information Service
National Cancer Institute
9000 Rockville Pike
Building 31, Room 10A16
Bethesda, MD 20892-0001
800-4-CANCER
http://www.nci.nih.gov/

Centers for Disease Control and Prevention (CDC)
1600 Clifton Road, NE
Atlanta, GA 30333
404-639-3534
http://www.cdc.gov

Leukemia Society of America, Inc.
600 Third Avenue
New York, NY 10016
800-955-4LSA
http://www.leukemia.org/

National Heart, Lung, and Blood Institute
4733 Bethesda Avenue
Suite 530
Bethesda, MD 20814
301-951-3260
http://www.nhlbi.nih.gov/nhlbi/nhlbi.htm

Consumer Information

Bureau of Consumer Protection
Federal Trade Commission
Division of Advertising Practices
6th St. and Pennsylvania Ave., NW
Washington, DC 20580
800-876-7060
http://www.ftc.gov/ftc/consumer.htm

Consumer Information Center (CIC)
General Services Administration
18th & F Street, NW
Room 6-142
Washington, DC 20405
888-8PUEBLO
http://www.pueblo.gsa.gov

Fraud Division
Chief Postal Inspector
U.S. Postal Service
475 L'Enfant Plaza
Washington, DC 20260
800-372-8347

Environmental Health

National Center for Environmental Health
Centers for Disease Control
1600 Clifton Road, NE
Atlanta, GA 30333
404-639-3534
http://www.cdc.gov/nceh/ncehhome.htm

Environmental Protection Agency (EPA)
Public Information Center
PM 211-B
401 M Street, SW
Washington, DC 20460
202-260-2080
http://www.epa.gov/

Greenpeace, USA
1436 U Street, NW
Washington, DC 20009
202-462-1177
http://www.greenpeace.org

Sierra Club
730 Polk Street
San Francisco, CA 94109
415-776-2211
http://www.sierraclub.org/

World Wildlife Fund
90 Eglinton Avenue, East
Suite 504
Toronto, Ontario M4P 2Z7
416-489-8800
http://www.worldwildlife.org/

Fitness

American Council on Exercise
5820 Oberlin Drive, Suite 102
San Diego, CA 92121
800-529-8227
http://www.acefitness.org

American College of Sports Medicine
P.O. Box 1440
Indianapolis, IN 46206
317-637-9200
http://www.acsm.org/sportsmed

Psychological Health

**American Anorexia/Bulimia Association, Inc.
(AABA)**
165 West 46th Street #1108
New York, NY 10036
212-575-6200
http://members.aol.com/amanbu/index.htm

American Psychiatric Association
1400 K Street, NW
Washington, DC 20005
202-682-6000
http://www.psych.org

American Psychological Association
1200 17th Street, NW
Washington, DC 20036
202-955-7600
http://www.apa.org

**Anorexia Nervosa and Related Eating Disorders,
Inc.**
P.O. Box 5102
Eugene, OR 97405
503-344-1144

**National Depressive and Manic-Depressive
Association (NDMDA)**
730 N. Franklin Street
Suite 501
Chicago, IL 60610
800-82-NDMDA
http://www.ndmda.org

Anxiety Disorders Association of America
11900 Parklawn Drive
Rockville, MD 20852
301-231-9350
http://www.adaa.org

**National Clearinghouse for Mental Health
Information**
Public Inquiries Section
5600 Fishers Lane, Room 11A-21
Rockville, MD 20857
301-443-4356; 800-421-4211
http://www.nimh.gov/home.htm

Nutrition

American Institute of Nutrition
9650 Rockville Pike
Bethesda, MD 20814
301-530-7050

American Dietetic Association
216 West Jackson Blvd., Suite 800
Chicago, IL 60606
800-877-1600; 800-366-1655
http://www.eatright.org

Food and Drug Administration (FDA)
Office of Consumer Affairs
Public Inquiries
5600 Fishers Lane (HFE-88)
Rockville, MD 20857
301-443-3170
http://vm.cfsan.fda.gov/list.html

Food and Nutrition Board
National Academy of Science
Institute of Medicine
2101 Constitution Avenue, NW
Washington, DC 20418
202-334-2238
http://www2.nas.edu/iom/

Rape

National Clearinghouse on Marital and Date Rape
2325 Oak Street
Berkeley, CA 94708
510-524-1582
http://members.aol.com/ncmdr/index.html

National Coalition Against Sexual Assault
P.O. Box 21378
Washington, DC 20009
202-483-7165
http://www.cs.utk.edu/~bartley/ncasa/ncasa.html

Sex Education

American Association of Sex Educators, Counselors, and Therapists
435 North Michigan
Suite 1717
Chicago, IL 60611
312-644-0828

Planned Parenthood Federation of America
810 Seventh Avenue
New York, NY 10019
212-541-7800
http://www.ppfa.org/ppfa

Sexuality Information and Education Council of the United States (SIECUS)
130 W. 42nd St., Suite 2500
New York, NY 10036
212-819-9770
http://www.siecus.org/

STDs and AIDS

National STD Hotline
800-227-8922

National AIDS Hotline
800-342-AIDS
800-344-SIDA (Spanish)
800-AIDS-TTY (hearing impaired)

American Social Health Association
P.O. Box 13827
RTP, NC 27709
919-361-8400
http://sunsite.unc.edu/ASHA

National AIDS Information Clearinghouse
P.O. Box 6003
Rockville, MD 20850
800-458-5231
http://www.cdcnac.org/

Shanti Project
525 Howard Street
San Francisco, CA 94105

Index

Credits

This page constitutes an extension of the copyright page. We have made every effort to trace the ownership of all copyrighted material and to secure permission from copyright holders. In the event of any question arising as to the use of any material, we will be pleased to make the necessary corrections in future printings. Thanks are due to the following authors, publishers, and agents for permission to use the material indicated.

Chapter 1: 18: Box 1.7 From *Wellness Interactive Network* web site, used by permission.

Chapter 2: 45: Table 2.2; **46:** Table 2.3 From W. L. Kenney, et al, *Guidelines for Exercise Testing and Prescription, 5th Ed.* Copyright © 1995 American College of Sports Medicine. Published by Williams & Wilkins. Reprinted by permission. **51:** Box 2.4 From *Fitness Partner Connection Jumpsite* web site, used by permission of Vicki Pierson. **54:** Box 2.1 Reprinted from the 1994 revised version of the Physical Activity Readiness Questionnaire (PAR-Q and YOU). The PAR-Q and YOU is a copyrighted, pre-exercise screen owned by the Canadian Society for Exercise Physiology. Reprinted by permission.

Chapter 3: 58: Figure 3.1; **59:** Figure 3.2 Adapted from W. D. McArdle, F. I. Katch, and V. I. Katch, *Exercise Physiology: Energy, Nutrition, and Human Performance, 3rd Ed.* Copyright © 1991 by Lea & Febiger. Reprinted by permission. **59:** Figure 3.3 From E. Larson, *Fitness, Health, and Work Capacity, 5E.* All rights reserved. Reprinted/adapted by permission of Allyn & Bacon. **60:** Figure 3.4 From Elaine Marieb, *Human Anatomy and Physiology, 2E.* Redwood City, CA: Benjamin/Cummings, 1992. Copyright © 1992 Benjamin/Cummings Publishing Company. Reprinted by permission. **61:** Figure 3.5 From Diane Hales, *An Invitation to Health, 6th Ed.,* Redwood City, CA: Benjamin/Cummings. Copyright © 1994 Benjamin/Cummings Publishing Company. Reprinted by permission. **62:** Figure 3.6 From S. Alters and W. Schiff, *Concepts for Healthy Living.* Copyright © 1998 Brooks/Cole Publishing Company. All rights reserved. Reprinted by permission. **64:** Table 3.1 Adapted from B. J. Sharkey, *New Dimensions in Aerobic Fitness.* Champaign, IL: Human Kinetics Press, 1991. **71:** Figure 3.7 From Gary A. Klug and Janice Lettunich, *Wellness: Exercise and Physical Fitness.* Copyright © 1992 The Dushkin Publishing Group, Inc., Guilford, CT. All rights reserved. Reprinted by permission. **73:** Box 3.4 From *Dis-*

abled Sports USA web site. Copyright © 1995–1998, Disabled Sports USA. Used by permission. **81:** Exercise 3.9 Adapted from B. Getchell, *Physical Fitness: A Way of Life, 4th Ed.* Copyright © 1992. All rights reserved. Reprinted/adapted by permission of Allyn & Bacon.

Chapter 4: 89: Figure 4.1 From Gary A. Klug and Janice Lettunich, *Wellness: Exercise and Physical Fitness.* Copyright © 1992 The Dushkin Publishing Group, Inc., Guilford, CT. All rights reserved. Reprinted by permission. **90:** Figure 4.2 From Elaine Marieb, *Human Anatomy and Physiology, 2E,* Redwood City, CA: Benjamin/Cummings, 1992. Copyright © 1992 Benjamin/Cummings Publishing Company. Reprinted by permission. **112:** Box 4.6 From *Strength Training* website. Used by permission of Georgia State University, Department of Kinesiology. **120:** Exercise 4.9 Reprinted by permission from Heyward, V., 1991, *Advanced Fitness and Exercise Prescription, 2nd ed.* (Champaign, IL: Human Kinetics), 109.

Chapter 5: 125: Figure 5.1 From Elaine Marieb, *Human Anatomy and Physiology, 2E,* Redwood City, CA: Benjamin/Cummings, 1992. Copyright © 1992 Benjamin/Cummings Publishing Company. Reprinted by permission. **152:** Box 5.6 From web site: *Yogaaahhh* used by permission of Mindy Maxwell. **156:** Table 5.2 Reprinted from L. Golding, C. Meyers and W. Sinning, *Y's Way to Physical Fitness,* 1983, with permission of the YMCA of the USA, 101 N. Wacker, Chicago, IL 60606. Table 5.3 Data from B. L. Johnson, J. K. Nelson, *Practical Measurements for Evaluation in Physical Education, 4th Ed.,* 1986. Macmillan Pub. Co. **157:** Table 5.4 Reprinted by permission from E. T. Howley and B. D. Franks, 1997, *Health Fitness Instructor's Handbook, 3rd ed.* (Champaign, IL: Human Kinetics), 253. **158:** Exercise 5.2 *The New York Physical Fitness Test: A Manual for Teachers of Physical Education,* New York State Education Department, HPER, 1958.

Chapter 6: 162: Table 6.1 Adapted from T. D. Fahey, *Athletic Training: Principles and Practice,* 1986, Mayfield Publishing Company, Mountain View, CA. Reprinted by permission. **166:** Table 6.2 Adapted from Roy and Irwin, *Sports Medicine.* Copyright © 1983. All rights reserved. Reprinted/adapted by permission of Allyn & Bacon. **168:** Figure 6.3 From J. M. Booher, G. A.Thibodeau, *Athletic Injury Assessment, 3rd Ed.,* St. Louis, MO: C. V. Mosby, 1994. Reprinted by permission. **170:**

Figure 6.5 From Letha Y. Hunter-Griffin, *Athletic Training and Sports Medicine, 2nd Edition*, American Academy of Orthopedic Surgeons 1991. Reprinted by permission. **173:** Figure 6.9 From Elaine Marieb, *Human Anatomy and Physiology, 2E*, Redwood City, CA: Benjamin/Cummings, 1992. Copyright © 1992 Benjamin/Cummings Publishing Company. Reprinted by permission. **178:** Table 6.5 Adapted from Roy and Irwin, *Sports Medicine*, Copyright © 1983. All rights reserved. Reprinted/adapted by permission of Allyn & Bacon. **181:** Box 6.7 From Emory University web site: *MedWeb—Sports Medicine* used by permission.

Chapter 7: 188: Figure 7.1 From Diane Hales, *An Invitation to Health, 6th Ed.*, Redwood City, CA: Benjamin/Cummings. Copyright © 1994 Benjamin/Cummings Publishing Company. **191:** Figure 7.3; **192:** Figure 7.4 From Janet Christian and Janet Greger, *Nutrition for Living, 4th Ed.*, Redwood City, CA; Benjamin/Cummings, 1994. Copyright © 1994 Benjamin/Cummings Publishing Co. Reprinted by permission. **197:** Table 7.4 Data: RDA Subcommittee, 1989; H. E. Shils and V. R.Young 1988, *Modern Nutrition in Health & Disease,* Philadelphia: Lea & Feiber, 1988. **202:** Table 7.6 From Janet Christian and Janet Greger, *Nutrition for Living, 4th Ed.,* Redwood City, CA; Benjamin/Cummings, 1994. Copyright © 1994 Benjamin/Cummings Publishing Co. Reprinted by permission. **209:** Figure 7.6 Wheat Thins®, Courtesy of Nabisco, Inc. **213:** Box 7.6 From *CyberDiet* web site. Reprinted by permission.

Chapter 8: 227: Figure 8.2 From Janet Christian and Janet Greger, *Nutrition for Living, 4th Ed.*, Redwood City, CA; Benjamin/Cummings, 1994. Copyright © 1994 Benjamin/Cummings Publishing Co. Reprinted by permission. **229:** Table 8.1 From W. D. McArdle, F. I. Katch, and V. I. Katch, *Exercise Physiology: Energy, Nutrition, and Human Performance, 3rd ed.,* Philadelphia: Lea & Febiger, 1991. Reprinted by permission. **232:** Table 8.2 From Metropolitan Life Insurance Co., 1959. **233:** Table 8.3 From Metropolitan Life Insurance Co., 1983. **240:** Figure 8.9 From Janet Christian and Janet Greger, *Nutrition for Living, 4th Ed.*, Redwood City, CA; Benjamin/Cummings, 1994. Copyright © 1994 Benjamin/Cummings Publishing Co. Reprinted by permission. **250:** Box 8.11 From *Something Fishy Website on Eating Disorders.* Used by permission. Copyright 1996-1998 Something Fishy Music & Publishing. **259:** Exercise 8.1 From M. L. Pollock, and J. H. Wilmore, Philadelphia, Saunders 1990, *Exercise in Health and Disease.*

Chapter 9: 285: Box 9.8 From CMCH Systems web site: *Mental Health Net* used by permission.

Chapter 10: 296: Figure 10.12 From Donatelle and Davis, *Access to Health, 5e.* Reprinted by permission of Allyn & Bacon, Inc. **300:** Exhibit 1 Adaptation from Brigid Schulte, "Relaxing and Managing Stress Are Important to Reducing Heart Disease" as appeared in Knight-Ridder Newspapers, October 19, 1997. Reprinted by permission of the author. **302:** Table 10.2 From T. H. Holmes and R. H. Rahe, "The Social Readjustment Rating Scale" reprinted from the *Journal of Psychosomatic Research,* Vol.11, 1967 with permission from Elsevier Science. **318:** Box 10.8 From

Duquesne University web site, *The Digital Duke.* Used by permission of The Duquesne Duke & The Digital Duke Newspapers. **325:** Exercise 10.1 From T. H. Holmes and R. H. Rahe, "The Social Readjustment Rating Scale" reprinted from the *Journal of Psychosomatic Research*, Vol.11, 1967 with permission from Elsevier Science.

Chapter 11: 334: Table 11.2 From "Binge Drinking on American College Campuses: A New Look at An Old Problem" from Harvard School of Public Health, August 1995. Reprinted by permission. **336:** Table 11.3 From Glen Evans and Robert O'Brien, *The Encyclopedia of Alcoholism.* Copyright © 1991 by Facts on File and Greenspring Inc. Reprinted with permission of Facts On File Inc., New York. **351:** Table 11.4 Copyright © Sacred Heart General Hospital, 1988. **355:** Box 11.14 From NACoA web site: *National Association for Children of Alcoholics* used by permission. **356:** Table 11.5 From G. A. Marlatt. & J. R. Gordon, eds., Relapse Prevention, Guilford Press, 1985. Reprinted by permission. **360:** Box 11.1 Reprinted from the brochure "Alcohol: Decisions on Tap," with permission from the American College of Health Association, P.O. Box 28937, Baltimore, MD 21240-8937. **361:** Exercise 11.2 Adapted by permission, from Richard Benyo, 1990, *The Exercise Fix*, (Champaign, IL: Human Kinetics), 5-6. **362:** Exercise 11.3 From Gamblers Anonymous, Inc., Los Angeles, CA. Reprinted with permission.

Chapter 12: 392: Box 12.14 From Christopher Filkins web site *The Safer Sex Page* used by permission.

Chapter 13: 398: Figure 13.1 From L. Brannon and J. Feist, *Health Psychology: An Introduction to Behavior and Health*, p. 213. Copyright © 1997 Brooks/Cole Publishing Company. All rights reserved. **399:** Figure 13.2 From Elaine Marieb, *Human Anatomy and Physiology, 2E,* Redwood City, CA: Benjamin/Cummings, 1992. Copyright © 1992 Benjamin/Cummings Publishing Company. Reprinted by permission. **401:** Figure 13.3 From G. S. Berenson, et al. "Risk factors in early life as predictors of adult heart disease: The Bogalusa Heart Study," *American Journal of the Medical Sciences,* 298, 1989. Reprinted by permission of Lippincott-Raven Publishers. **407:** Figure From "Cancer Facts and Figures- 1997." Reprinted by permission of the American Cancer Society, Inc. **408:** Figure 13.8 Reprinted by permission of the American Cancer Society, Inc. **410:** Figure 13.9 Reprinted by permission of the American Cancer Society, Inc. **415:** Warning Signs of Cancer, American Cancer Society. **416:** Figure 13.10 Adapted from "Caring for Your Breasts," pp. 10, 12-13. Customized Communications. 1-800-476-2253. Reprinted by permission. **421:** Table 13.3 American Diabetes Association, Inc., 1992. Diabetes '92, Winter, p. 2. Reprinted by permission. **427:** Box 13.8 From *American Cancer Society* web site, used by permission. **432:** Exercise 13.1 Reproduced with permission. RISKO, A Heart Health Appraisal, 1994. Copyright American Heart Association.

Appendix: From F. Sizer and E. Whitney, Nutrition: *Concepts and Controversies, 7th Edition*, pp. A-1–A-113. Copyright © 1997 Wadsworth Publishing Company. Reprinted by permission.

Photo Credits

Chapter 1: 1, Kevin Fleming / Corbis-Bettmann; **5**, PhotoDisc, Inc.; **8**, PhotoDisc, Inc.; **13**, Karl Weathers / Corbis-Bettmann; **19**, (top background) Bob Krist / Corbis-Bettmann, (lower foreground) © Mary Kate Denny / PhotoEdit.

Chapter 2: 31, PhotoDisc, Inc.; **37**, (top) Corbis-Bettmann, (bottom) Paul A. Souders / Corbis-Bettmann.

Chapter 3: 57, PhotoDisc, Inc.; **60**, Sean Aidan, Eye Ubiquitous / Corbis-Bettmann; **70**, PhotoDisc, Inc.; **89**, (top) © Michael Newman / PhotoEdit, (middle) © Michael Newman / PhotoEdit, (bottom) © Michael Newman / PhotoEdit.

Chapter 4: 93, PhotoDisc, Inc.; **104**, PhotoDisc, Inc.; **105**, © David Young-Wolff / PhotoEdit; **106**, (top) PhotoDisc, Inc., (bottom) Karl Weatherly / Corbis-Bettmann.

Chapter 5: 133, Joseph Sohm, Chromosohm Inc. / Corbis-Bettmann; **136**, PhotoDisc, Inc.; **154**, Joseph Sohm, Chromosohm Inc. / Corbis-Bettmann.

Chapter 6: 177, Karl Weatherly / Corbis-Bettmann; **182**, Karl Weatherly / Corbis-Bettmann; **183**, Karl Weatherly / Corbis-Bettmann; **184**, Karl Weatherly / Corbis-Bettmann; **196**, PhotoDisc, Inc.; **177**, © Jeff Greenberg / PhotoEdit.

Chapter 7: 205, PhotoDisc, Inc.; **232**, PhotoDisc, Inc.; **233**, Corbis-Bettmann.

Chapter 8: 245, PhotoDisc, Inc.; **248**, PhotoDisc, Inc.; **250**, Corbis-Bettmann; **253**, Corbis-Bettmann; **254**, (left) Corbis-Bettmann, (right) © Bonnie Kamin / PhotoEdit; **258**, © D. Young-Wolff / PhotoEdit; **261**, © D. Young-Wolff / PhotoEdit.

Chapter 9: 287, © Bonnie Kamin / PhotoEdit; **290**, PhotoDisc, Inc.; **291**, (left) PhotoDisc, Inc.; **291**, (right) PhotoDisc, Inc.

Chapter 10: 321, © Gary Conner / PhotoEdit; **327**, (left) © Bonnie Kamin / PhotoEdit, (right) PhotoDisc, Inc.; **333**, © Ulrike Welsch / PhotoEdit; **343**, PhotoDisc, Inc.; **345**, © Tony Freeman / PhotoEdit.

Chapter 11: 359, courtesy of the American Cancer Society; **370**, (top) © Rudi Von Briel / PhotoEdit, (bottom) PhotoDisc, Inc.; **371**, PhotoDisc, Inc.; **373**, AP Wide/World; **376**, Corbis-Bettmann; **381**, © Mark Richards / PhotoEdit.

Chapter 12: 395, PhotoDisc, Inc.; **398**, PhotoDisc, Inc.; **400**, Corbis-Bettmann; **406**, Corbis-Bettmann; **410**, (top) © Biophoto Associates / Photo Researchers, Inc., (bottom) © NIH / Science Source / Photo Researchers, Inc.; **412**, Medichrome; **417**, AP Wide/World; **421**, AP Wide/World; **421**, AP Wide/World; **423**, PhotoDisc, Inc.

Chapter 13: 418, Corbis-Bettmann; **431**, AP Wide/World; **433**, Corbis-Bettmann; **448**, © Spencer Grant / PhotoEdit; **461**, Corbis-Bettmann.